Breast Cancer Screening

An Examination of Scientific Evidence

Edited by

Nehmat Houssami
Professor of Public Health, and National Breast Cancer Foundation (NBCF Australia) Breast Cancer Research Leader Fellow, School of Public Health, Sydney Medical School, University of Sydney, Australia

Diana Miglioretti
Dean's Professor in Biostatistics, UC Davis School of Medicine, Department of Public Health Sciences, University of California, Davis, CA, United States and
Senior Investigator, Group Health Research Institute, Group Health Cooperative, Seattle, WA, United States

ELSEVIER

AMSTERDAM • BOSTON • HEIDELBERG • LONDON
NEW YORK • OXFORD • PARIS • SAN DIEGO
SAN FRANCISCO • SINGAPORE • SYDNEY • TOKYO

Academic Press is an imprint of Elsevier

Academic Press is an imprint of Elsevier
125 London Wall, London EC2Y 5AS, UK
525 B Street, Suite 1800, San Diego, CA 92101-4495, USA
50 Hampshire Street, 5th Floor, Cambridge, MA 02139, USA
The Boulevard, Langford Lane, Kidlington, Oxford OX5 1GB, UK

Library of Congress Cataloging-in-Publication Data
A catalog record for this book is available from the Library of Congress

British Library Cataloguing-in-Publication Data
A catalogue record for this book is available from the British Library

ISBN: 978-0-12-802209-2

For information on all Academic Press publications
visit our website at http://elsevier.com/

Typeset by MPS Limited, Chennai, India

Contents

List of Contributors

Susan Astley
Genesis Breast Cancer Prevention Centre and Nightingale Breast Screening Centre, University Hospital of South Manchester, Manchester, United Kingdom; Manchester Academic Health Science Centre, University Hospital of South Manchester, The University of Manchester, Manchester, United Kingdom; Centre for Imaging Sciences, Institute for Population Health, University of Manchester, Manchester, United Kingdom

Alexandra L. Barratt
School of Public Health, University of Sydney, NSW, Australia

Mireille J. M. Broeders
Radboud Institute for Health Sciences, Radboud University Medical Center, Nijmegen, The Netherlands; Dutch Reference Centre for Screening, Nijmegen, The Netherlands

David Cameron
Edinburgh Cancer Research Centre, Western General Hospital, Edinburgh, United Kingdom

Stacy M. Carter
Centre for Values, Ethics and the Law in Medicine (VELiM), The University of Sydney, Sydney, NSW, Australia

Anna M. Chiarelli
Prevention and Cancer Control, Cancer Care Ontario, Toronto, ON, Canada; Dalla Lana School of Public Health, University of Toronto, Toronto, ON, Canada

Geertruida H. de Bock
Department of Epidemiology, University Medical Center Groningen, University of Groningen, Groningen, The Netherlands

J. Michael Dixon
Edinburgh Breast Unit, Western General Hospital, Edinburgh, United Kingdom

Joann G. Elmore
Professor of Medicine School of Medicine and Adjunct Professor of Epidemiology School of Public Health, Harborview Medical Center, Seattle, WA, United States

D. Gareth Evans
Genesis Breast Cancer Prevention Centre and Nightingale Breast Screening Centre, University Hospital of South Manchester, Manchester, United Kingdom; Genomic Medicine, Manchester Academic Health Sciences Centre, University of Manchester and Central Manchester Foundation Trust, Manchester, United Kingdom; Manchester Academic Health Science Centre, University Hospital of South Manchester, The University of Manchester, Manchester, United Kingdom; Consultant Clinical Geneticist, Genomic Medicine, MAHSC, St. Mary's Hospital, Manchester, United Kingdom

Rongwei Fu
Pacific Northwest Evidence-Based Practice Center and Departments of Public Health and Preventive Medicine, Medical Informatics and Clinical Epidemiology and Emergency Medicine, Oregon Health & Science University, Portland, OR, United States

Russell P. Harris
School of Medicine, the Cecil G. Sheps Center for Health Services Research, UNC; School of Public Health, University of North Carolina at Chapel Hill, Chapel Hill, NC, United States

Jolyn Hersch
Screening and Test Evaluation Program (STEP) and Centre for Medical Psychology and Evidence-based Decision-making (CeMPED), Sydney School of Public Health, The University of Sydney, Sydney, NSW, Australia

Nehmat Houssami
School of Public Health, Sydney Medical School, University of Sydney, Sydney, NSW, Australia

Anthony Howell
Genesis Breast Cancer Prevention Centre and Nightingale Breast Screening Centre, University Hospital of South Manchester, Manchester, United Kingdom; Manchester Academic Health Science Centre, University Hospital of South Manchester, The University of Manchester, Manchester, United Kingdom; The Christie NHS Foundation Trust, Manchester, United Kingdom

Rebecca A. Hubbard
Department of Biostatistics and Epidemiology, Perelman School of Medicine, University of Pennsylvania, Philadelphia, PA, Unites States

Linda L. Humphrey
Pacific Northwest Evidence-Based Practice Center and Departments of Medical Informatics and Clinical Epidemiology and Medicine, Oregon Health & Science University, Portland, OR, United States; Veterans Affairs Portland Health Care System, Portland, OR, Unites States

Gemma L. Jacklyn
School of Public Health, University of Sydney, Sydney, NSW, Australia

Jesse Jansen
Screening and Test Evaluation Program (STEP) and Centre for Medical Psychology and Evidence-based Decision-making (CeMPED), Sydney School of Public Health, The University of Sydney, Sydney, NSW, Australia

Karla Kerlikowske
General Internal Medicine Section, Department of Veteran Affairs, San Francisco, CA, and Departments of Medicine and Epidemiology and Biostatistics, University of California, San Francisco, CA, Unites States

Janie M. Lee
Department of Radiology, University of Washington, Seattle, WA, United States

Anthony J. Maxwell
Genesis Breast Cancer Prevention Centre and Nightingale Breast Screening Centre, University Hospital of South Manchester, Manchester, United Kingdom; Manchester Academic Health Science Centre, University Hospital of South Manchester, The University of Manchester, Manchester, United Kingdom; Centre for Imaging Sciences, Institute for Population Health, University of Manchester, Manchester, United Kingdom

Kirsten McCaffery
Screening and Test Evaluation Program (STEP) and Centre for Medical Psychology and Evidence-based Decision-making (CeMPED), Sydney School of Public Health, The University of Sydney, Sydney, NSW, Australia

Diana L. Miglioretti
Department of Public Health Sciences, University of California, Davis, CA, United States; Group Health Research Institute, Seattle, WA, United States

Heidi D. Nelson
Pacific Northwest Evidence-Based Practice Center and Departments of Medical Informatics and Clinical Epidemiology and Medicine, Oregon Health & Science University, Portland, OR, United States; Providence Cancer Center, Providence Health & Services, Portland, OR, United States

Lisa M. Parker
Centre for Values, Ethics and the Law in Medicine (VELiM), The University of Sydney, Sydney, NSW, Australia

Xuan-Anh Phi
Department of Epidemiology, University Medical Center Groningen, University of Groningen, Groningen, The Netherlands

Theodora M. Ripping
Radboud Institute for Health Sciences, Radboud University Medical Center, Nijmegen, The Netherlands

Clyde B. Schechter
Department of Family & Social Medicine, Albert Einstein College of Medicine, Bronx, NY, United States

Mara A. Schonberg
Division of General Medicine and Primary Care, Beth Israel Deaconess Medical Center, Harvard Medical School, Boston, MA, United States

Jeffrey A. Tice
Division of General Internal Medicine, Department of Medicine, University of California, San Francisco, CA, Unites States

Nicolien T. van Ravesteyn
Department of Public Health, Erasmus Medical Center, Rotterdam, The Netherlands

Sophia Zackrisson
Department of Translational Medicine, Diagnostic Radiology, Lund University, Skåne University Hospital, Malmö, Skåne, Sweden

Foreword

A large body of evidence on population breast cancer screening with mammography has accumulated over five decades, including evidence from randomized controlled trials demonstrating efficacy.[1,2] Despite this, little in population health practice has received more attention, critique, praise, reinterpretation, and forensic-like scrutiny than mammography screening. The debate around breast cancer screening is unlikely to diminish as we move into a future of precision medicine, potentially competing screening technologies, and increasingly effective cancer treatments that require, more than ever before, working collaboratively to answer important questions about breast screening, based on the best available evidence. These questions include the optimal ages to start and stop routine screening, how often to screen, which modalities to use given a woman's personal characteristics and risk factors, and how to ensure women are adequately informed about the benefits and harms of breast screening.

It is well-established that mammography screening has the potential to confer benefit for many women by reducing breast cancer deaths through early-detection and treatment of the disease. Relative to younger or older counterparts, women aged 60–69 years are likely to benefit the most from mammography screening, given breast cancer is more common in this age-group than in younger women, and competing risk of death from other causes is still relatively low compared to older women.[3] Although there is heterogeneity in estimates of the relative reduction in breast cancer mortality attributed to screening, reflecting differences in the design of studies and whether there was adjustment for screening participation, all estimates indicate the potential for benefit.[1–3] Given this evidence of benefit, *why is breast cancer screening still so controversial?* The very same package through which this highly valued health benefit from mammography screening is achieved also causes harms. Harms include those associated with the technique itself comprising the relatively small risk associated with radiation exposure from mammography, and the inconvenience of an examination that briefly transitions the woman to a "patient" receiving an intervention. Because mammography is not a perfect test, somewhat more serious harms are false-positive interpretations, which result in additional imaging and biopsies of women without breast cancer.

Perhaps the most serious harms of screening are overdiagnosis and overtreatment,[3–6] outcomes of the biologic process inherent in early-detection of asymptomatic disease. Overdiagnosis is not unique to breast cancer screening, and is known to occur in the context of screening for other conditions. Just as calibration of an instrument determines the extent of true-positive versus false-positive results, the biologic mechanism underlying early-detection leading to prevention of breast cancer death also yields diagnosis of "disease" that would have never become clinically apparent, or caused harm, in the individual's lifetime (hence an overdiagnosed cancer). However, our present level of scientific knowledge is not ready, nor able, to "calibrate" the biologic mechanisms of early-detection that lead to screening-related benefit and conversely to overdiagnosis. Because it is not possible to determine which cancers are overdiagnosed and which will progress and potentially cause death, women with screen-detected breast cancer receive treatments with potentially serious side-effects, leading to overtreatment.

Whereas harms from false-positive screening can be accurately measured, and strategies can be put in place to limit or to at least monitor the frequency with which they occur, the harm of overdiagnosis is much more challenging at many levels: overdiagnosis is complex in terms of defining, quantifying, monitoring, and mitigating. Consequently, there is both heterogeneity and substantial uncertainty around estimates of overdiagnosis from breast screening.[3] Hence, the *balance* of benefit and harms from population breast cancer screening (which varies between settings and age-groups) is not only a challenge to quantify, but is built around uncertain estimates and inherently requires value judgement, societal, or individual.

In this increasingly complex and political environment for population breast cancer screening, it is disheartening that the divergent interpretations and views on the outcomes or impact of breast screening are so polarized that efforts are frequently channeled into relentless debate. This may be obscuring a way forward to achieve some level of consensus as we move into the future, and may be diverting effort away from finding solutions toward enhancing the balance between benefit and harms of screening and supporting evidence-based screening policy decisions. To contribute toward more balanced scientific discussion, and to define priorities for breast screening research and practice as we move into the future, we present this book on the scientific evidence on breast screening.

The contributions assembled in this book cover three *themes* and gather leading experts from around the world to address key topics within each breast cancer screening theme. The book's introductory chapter eloquently discusses the factors that have shaped the history of breast cancer screening, and provides insights into how breast screening practice has been driven by a delicate balance between scientific evidence and culture, politics, and media. It also underscores the importance of the book's chosen themes in terms of understanding the past and steering the future of breast cancer screening practice. The book's first theme focuses on the efficacy and the outcomes of population breast cancer screening, the benefit and the harms, and the trade-off between these outcomes, and considers methodological aspects of screening evaluations. The risk-based screening theme highlights the evidence surrounding screening "younger" and "older" women, and reviews the evidence in relation to risk defined by breast density, cancer gene mutations or a strong family history, and a personal history of breast cancer. It also outlines the challenges surrounding implementation of risk-based screening.

Issues that are increasingly relevant to the future of breast cancer screening are addressed in the third theme, including the evolution of mammography technologies for breast cancer screening, overtreatment of screen-detected breast cancer, and ethical and societal considerations in population screening. It also discusses how to potentially support individuals to make informed decisions about breast cancer screening, an issue that has received little attention until recently and one that emphasizes the emerging need for shared decision-making in breast cancer screening and more broadly in healthcare.

We sincerely thank all contributing authors who have provided their time, insights, and expertise to developing this book. We hope that our readers find this work a timely and balanced overview of the evidence on breast cancer screening.

Nehmat Houssami[1] and Diana L. Miglioretti[2,3]

[1]Sydney School of Public Health, Sydney Medical School, The University of Sydney, Sydney, Australia, [2]Department of Public Health Sciences, University of California, Davis, CA, United States, [3]Group Health Research Institute, Seattle, WA, United States

REFERENCES

1. Independent UK Panel on Breast Cancer Screening The benefits and harms of breast cancer screening: an independent review. *Lancet* 2012;**380**(9855):1778–86.
2. Lauby-Secretan B, Scoccianti C, Loomis D, Benbrahim-Tallaa L, Bouvard V, Bianchini F, et al. Breast-cancer screening—viewpoint of the IARC working group. *N Engl J Med* 2015;**372**(24):2353–8.

3. Myers ER, Moorman P, Gierisch JM, Havrilesky LJ, Grimm LJ, Ghate S, et al. Benefits and harms of breast cancer screening: a systematic review. *JAMA* 2015;**314**(15):1615–34.
4. Keating NL, Pace LE. New guidelines for breast cancer screening in US women. *JAMA* 2015;**314**(15):1569–71.
5. Barratt A. Overdiagnosis in mammography screening: a 45 year journey from shadowy idea to acknowledged reality. *BMJ* 2015;**350**:h867.
6. Biesheuvel C, Barratt A, Howard K, Houssami N, Irwig L. Effects of study methods and biases on estimates of invasive breast cancer overdetection with mammography screening: a systematic review. *Lancet Oncol* 2007;**8**(12):1129–38.

CHAPTER

BREAST CANCER SCREENING: BALANCING EVIDENCE WITH CULTURE, POLITICS, MONEY, AND MEDIA

1

Joann G. Elmore

Professor of Medicine School of Medicine and Adjunct Professor of Epidemiology School of Public Health, University of Washington, Harborview Medical Center, Seattle, WA, United States

CHAPTER OUTLINE

Breast Cancer Screening. DOI: http://dx.doi.org/10.1016/B978-0-12-802209-2.00001-2

PLAIN LANGUAGE SUMMARY

Culture, politics, money, and media intersect to influence the interpretation of scientific evidence, directly affecting the lives of women. Before venturing into detailed chapters reviewing the scientific evidence on breast cancer screening, we begin this textbook with an overview of the history of the breast, of breast cancer screening, and of the perfect storm of politics and science surrounding this topic. We examine the complex forces that shape the way many well-intentioned individuals view the same scientific evidence, yet arrive at vastly different interpretations.

This chapter provides a brief overview on the history of the breast, breast cancer screening, scientific evidence for and against different screening strategies, and important influences on the development of screening strategies.

HISTORY

HISTORY OF THE BREAST

Over the years, well-intentioned individuals have reviewed the scientific evidence on breast cancer screening, yet come to surprisingly different conclusions. While many chapters in this textbook describe the scientific evidence surrounding breast cancer screening dating back decades, the interpretation of this evidence is influenced by complex factors. Individual interpretation of scientific medical information is colored by a heightened fear of breast cancer, mass media campaigns promoting screening, political involvement, and financial incentives all colliding with the complicated culture that surrounds women's health in general, and breast health in particular. While a financial conflict of interest might be concrete and obvious, an emotional conflict of interest is subtle and can be deeply rooted. Just as a Rorschach ink blot might be interpreted quite differently by individuals, the interpretation of scientific evidence remains challenging in the area of breast cancer screening with multiple and variable interpretations.

To understand the complex nature of breast cancer screening scientific data, a reflection on the history of the breast is a helpful starting point. While thousands of pages have been written on this topic,[1–5] a summary of key themes is briefly covered here.

The breast was depicted in ancient art as a symbol of motherhood, comfort, and nourishment. For example, this ancient Greek sculpture (Fig. 1.1) depicts a mother feeding her twins, with the mother's right hand gently playing with the foot of one of the infants. The mother seems relaxed in this nurturing context. Sculptor Jean-Jacques Caffieri's marble statue titled *Hope Nourishes Love* shows a young woman who represents Hope nursing a winged Cupid, personifying love (Fig. 1.2). Fig. 1.3 depicts Artemis, goddess of the hunt and wild animals, in her temple at Ephesus (in present-day Turkey) with striking rows of pendant objects on her torso. Most scholars have identified these pendant objects as breasts. The nourishing breast is tied to power and strength in this hunter-goddess's statue. Just as scientists variably interpret medical data, the interpretation of art has varied over the years. While most assume that the repeated paired objects on this statue are breasts, a scientist in 1978 claimed that, as no nipples were depicted, the round objects represent bulls' testicles,[6] adding an example of variability in interpretation of visual data based on the viewer's perspective.

While historic depictions have also sexualized the breast, over the centuries, artistic depictions of the breast became increasingly sensual. Representations of the breast moved from scenes of nourishment between Madonna and Child to increasingly sexualized images. In the last century, the slender

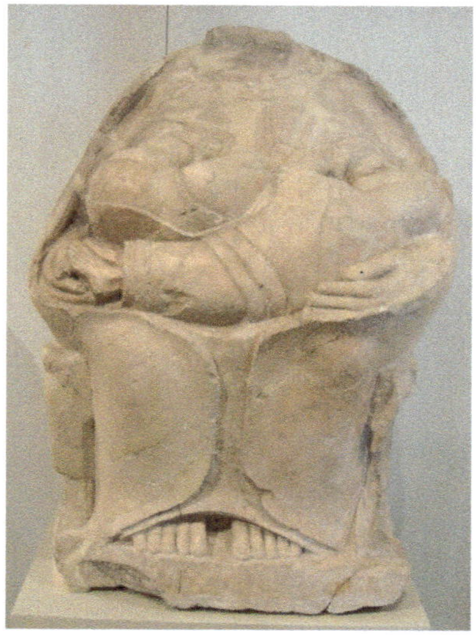

FIGURE 1.1

Kourotrophos statue from Paolo Orsi Museum (Siracusa, Sicily).

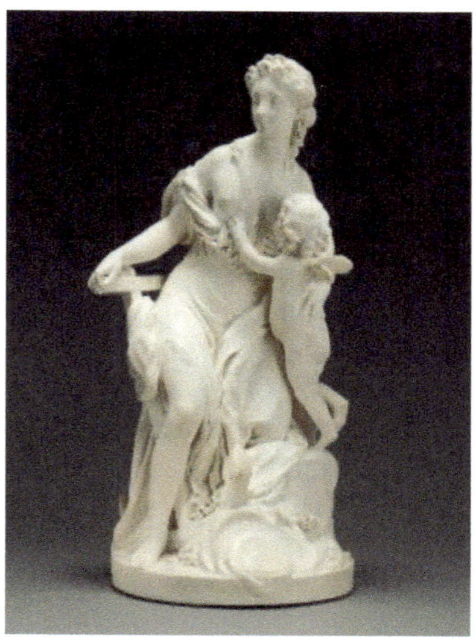

FIGURE 1.2

Hope Nourishes Love sculpture by Jean-Jacques Caffieri (1769).

Digital image courtesy of the Getty's Open Content Program.

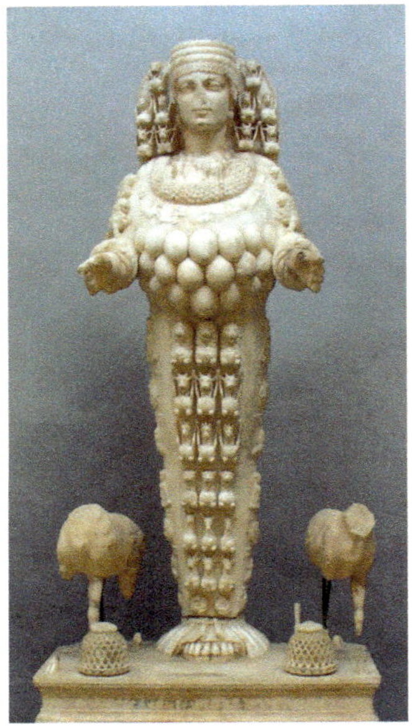

FIGURE 1.3

Artemis at Ephesos (Turkey, 2nd century).

Artemis of Ephesus *by QuartierLatin1968/Wikimedia Commons/CC BY-SA 2.0.*

flapper image of a woman was replaced with full-bodied women and the breast came to represent a key feature of a woman's sexuality. Push-up bras and breast augmentation became commonplace and were openly discussed in conversations.

Breast cancer is one of the most feared afflictions in modern society because of its potential devastation of both the woman and her family, given the nurturing, comforting, and sexual attributes of breasts, in addition to the risk of death from the disease. Descriptions of breast cancer treatments date back thousands of years and include the cauterization of breast tumors and ulcers as described in Egyptian textbooks. In describing breast cancer, authors of the past bluntly stated: "There is no treatment."[7] Thankfully, this is no longer the case. However, early treatments included extensive surgical resections. As the surgical treatments for breast cancer were developed, images of mastectomy scars came to represent mutilation of the body and death. This new symbolism was evident in artist and former fashion model Matuschka's stunning self-portrait, featured on the cover of *The New York Times Magazine* in 1993, in which she boldly exposed the remnants of her postmastectomy breast. The juxtaposition of the model's lithe body and the taboo scar forced readers to confront breast cancer and its raw physical impact.

HISTORY OF MEDICAL SCREENING

Given the historical value society has placed on women and the breast, it is no surprise that breast cancer screening remains in the forefront of societal focus. With the development of successful treatment for early-stage breast cancer, early detection screening programs became a possible approach to consider.

Table 1.1 Key Requirements When Evaluating the Evidence of a Medical Screening Test

Disease requirements
• Disease is serious • Effective treatment exists • Natural history of disease is understood • Disease occurs frequently • Other diseases or conditions may be detected
Screening test requirements
• Test is quick to perform • Test is easy to administer • Test is inexpensive • Test is safe • Test is acceptable to participants • Sensitivity, specificity, and other operating characteristics are acceptable
Health care system requirements
• Method meets the requirements for screening in a community setting • Method meets the requirement for case finding in a medical care setting
Adapted from Katz DL, Elmore JG, Wild DMG, Lucan SC. Jekel's epidemiology, biostatistics, preventive medicine and public health, Fourth Edition. 2014. Copyright Elsevier (2014).

Effective medical screening includes consideration of whether earlier treatment of disease improves prognosis and whether screening tests are accurate and able to detect disease at an early stage.[8,9] Over time, the criteria for evaluating the usefulness and appropriateness of medical screening tests expanded to take into consideration characteristics of the specific disease, such as its severity and frequency in the target population, and characteristics of the screening test, such as cost and acceptability. Additionally, the impact of implementing screening exams in the target health care system became a requirement for consideration as well (Table 1.1).

The success of mass screening programs, such as cervical cancer screening on reducing morbidity and mortality, has been impressive. These successes have increased enthusiasm for the general concept of screening to allow early-stage detection of disease while it is easier to treat. Screening for many diseases has now become a vital part of public health efforts to improve health and health outcomes.

HISTORY OF SCREENING WITH BREAST SELF-EXAM AND CLINICAL BREAST EXAM

As improved treatment options became available to women with early-stage breast cancers and following the hypothesis that earlier detection saves lives, scientists and health care practitioners set out to identify the best strategies for finding breast cancer early via screening. Initially, a three-pronged approach was formulated involving screening mammography, clinical breast exam, and breast self-exam. The idea behind this comprehensive tactic was that: (1) breast self-exams would keep breast screening at the forefront of a woman's health care practice and remind her to screen; (2) clinician breast exam would provide a good opportunity for the physician and woman to discuss breast health and screening; and (3) all three tactics would provide a thorough screening that improved the woman's chance of finding a cancerous lesion early.

From the 1960s through 2000s, clinicians were encouraged to perform screening breast exams on their patients in the clinic, and clinicians instructed their patients in how to perform monthly breast self-examinations. As scientific evidence was collected,[10] however, it became apparent that breast self-examination is not associated with a reduction in breast cancer mortality, though it does increase the risk of having a biopsy with benign results.[11,12]

Studies of screening clinical breast examination performed by clinicians have been limited. The Canadian National Breast Screening Study found the 25-year cumulative mortality from breast cancer to be similar between women screened with mammography and clinical breast examinations and women screened with clinical breast examinations alone.[13] However, the quality of these exams may have exceeded that of the standard community practice: the clinicians providing clinical breast examinations in the study were well-trained, spent 5–10 minutes examining each breast, and were periodically evaluated for examination quality.[14] In general, clinical breast exams performed in the community setting were noted to have lower sensitivity compared with mammography.[15] A US study found examination sensitivity to be only 21.6% in asymptomatic women who received a clinical breast examination within 1 year of breast cancer diagnosis but died of breast cancer within 15 years of diagnosis.[15]

While the evidence on screening for breast cancer by breast self-examination and clinician breast examination is not covered in this textbook, and less research has been done on these topics, in general they are no longer recommended as part of most breast cancer screening programs in developed countries.

HISTORY OF MAMMOGRAPHY SCREENING

For many diseases, detection is best achieved through visualization. Initial advances in breast imaging occurred in the early 1900s when Dr Albert Salomon, a German surgeon, began using X-rays to image the breasts of symptomatic women.[16] Mammography exams were initially evaluated as a diagnostic tool and not considered as a screening tool. With technological advances, the first dedicated mammography systems were in place the mid-1960s. As with any new, unproven device these mammography units were initially met with cautious regard by many practicing physicians, including breast surgeons, until their worth as a diagnostic aid was demonstrated.

The use of mammography as a screening tool took shape in the later part of the 1900s. In 1969, R.L. Egan published an article in *Cancer* describing screening mammography as having a "certain magic appeal" and saying that the patient "feels something special is being done for her."[17] The availability of a tool to identify early-stage breast cancer in order to improve treatment and survival helped to establish breast cancer screening as a common practice. Women wanted to do anything possible to reduce their risk of dying of breast cancer, and breast cancer screening with mammography was seen as promising.

In the 1960s, breast imaging became a radiology subspecialty in medical schools in the United States, and the Health Improvement Program (HIP) in New York—the first randomized controlled trial (RCT) of screening mammography—began in 1963.[18] In 1972, the results of this HIP trial were published with much fanfare. This study reported a statistically significant reduction in breast cancer mortality among women randomized to the screening mammography arm of the study. This promising result was followed by additional studies including more RCTs (see chapter: Estimates of Screening

Benefit: The Randomized Trials of Breast Cancer Screening), observational studies (see chapter: The Importance of Observational Evidence to Estimate and Monitor Mortality Reduction From Current Breast Cancer Screening), statistical modeling (see chapter: The Role of Microsimulation Modeling in Evaluating the Outcomes and Effect of Screening), and even studies designed to identify best ways to promote mammography in different communities.[19] Research on mammography and breast cancer screening in community settings became a primary focus in the early 1990s as the National Cancer Institute (NCI) initiated funding for the Breast Cancer Surveillance Consortium (BCSC). The consortium is a collaborative network of multiple, nationwide mammography registries with linkage to cancer registries for the sole purpose of research on breast cancer detection and identification.[20] The BCSC has been in operation since 1994 and has been the source of more than 550 research articles about breast cancer.[21]

HISTORY OF THE MEDIA AND MARKETING RELATED TO BREAST CANCER SCREENING

Alongside the rapidly growing and extensive body of scientific evidence on breast cancer screening, media messages geared toward women and their families have promoted breast cancer screening. Throughout the past century, a "war on cancer"[1] has been waged. This war initially began as a push to get women to seek evaluation as soon as they noted a breast abnormality. Women's activism and war rhetoric against breast cancer has been traced back to the Women's Field Army which was formed in the 1930s to educate the public about breast cancer and encourage women to seek medical attention as soon as they noted a breast abnormality.[22] This war rhetoric soon moved from encouraging diagnostic evaluation to encouraging screening for earlier cancer detection.

Increased interest in diagnostic evaluation and screening has had fiscal ramifications, as breast cancer charities have gained popularity and become a strong political force. Additionally, the massive funding stream into breast cancer research began to flow in the mid-1990s and continues to be a tremendous resource today.[22]

While media attention has helped to inspire charitable contributions toward research and clinical programs, there have been negative results as well. In the media, breast cancer is often characterized as imminently life threatening—the anxiety-fueling "one in eight" statistic—and screening mammography is considered to be the only way to combat the resulting sense of vulnerability. Many misconstrue that one in eight women will die of breast cancer or that one in eight women will be diagnosed with breast cancer in the immediate year ahead. Rather, this is a statistic that one in eight women will be diagnosed with (but not die of) breast cancer in her lifetime. Most of these women will live long lives after their diagnosis with many remaining in remission indefinitely.

In addition to feeding anxiety, media marketing of breast cancer screening has been unbalanced, often covering only the benefits of mammography without discussing the harms and placing blame on and causing guilt in women. Ad campaigns have stated that women who died from breast cancer "could have been saved" had they been screened. Slogans include: "Mammography saves lives, and one of them might be yours,"[23] and "If you haven't had a mammogram, you need more than your breasts examined."[24]

The supply of information guiding individual screening decisions extends beyond research and big business; the actions of famous individuals inform and sway the public as well. Awareness of breast cancer being diagnosed in prominent women fueled the breast screening movement through the media. In 1974, Margaretta (Happy) Rockefeller, the wife of former American Vice President Nelson Rockefeller, underwent a double mastectomy 2 weeks after Betty Ford, then First Lady of the United States, underwent the same procedure. It is suspected that the media attention surrounding prominent women such as these led to increased attendance at breast cancer screening programs and the subsequent increase in the incidence of breast cancer cases in the United States.[25]

Prime examples of other prominent women in the media include Amy Robach, an anchor on a US national morning news show, who had a screening mammogram on live television and revealed months later that the mammogram had found breast cancer. Robach's message to her audience: "If I got the mammogram on air and it saved one life, then it's all worth it. It never occurred to me that the life would be mine."[26] There is also former First Lady of the United States Nancy Reagan, who publicly chose mastectomy as her form of breast cancer treatment, which resulted in a subsequent increase in women choosing mastectomy.[27,28] Finally, in 2013 actress Angelina Jolie Pitt announced her *BRCA1* gene mutation status and her decision to undergo prophylactic mastectomy and bilateral salpingo-oophorectomy.[29] Jolie Pitt encouraged women to make informed decisions, keeping their own health histories in mind and knowing the best decision for them, not basing their decision on what other people do. Referral to genetics services increased in the months following Jolie Pitt's news story.[28]

Balanced information is not always included in marketing media. Mammography is now an estimated $8 billion annual business in the United States,[30,31] with active marketing by hospitals and facilities to entice women to their centers. Such facilities advertise that they are using the most recent technologies, operating under the assumption that new technology is superior to "old" technology.

At what point does marketing overshadow medical reason and evidence? One US hospital promotes monthly "Mingle and Mammograms" parties with pampering to calm the nerves of women before they receive a screening exam.[32] These parties include appetizers, chocolate, foot massages, pink carnations, and bags emblazoned with the phrase "Fight Like a Girl." In addition to appetizers, women would benefit from digestible information that will aid them in making informed medical decisions about their own participation in screening. *Women need balanced information on potential harms and benefits of screening.*

HISTORY OF SCIENCE ON BREAST CANCER SCREENING

A primary area of focus in this book is a comprehensive review of the evidence demonstrating the potential benefits and harms of breast cancer screening. Chapters "Estimates of Screening Benefit: The Randomized Trials of Breast Cancer Screening" through "Challenges in Understanding and Quantifying Over-Diagnosis and Over-Treatment" provide an in-depth examination of the scientific evidence produced to date showing the benefits and harms of different screening strategies. Below is a brief summary providing the historical background for the chapters that follow in this text.

THE ACCUMULATION OF EVIDENCE ON THE BENEFITS

The gold standard study design to evaluate cancer screening is the RCT. The first RCT about mammography, the HIP trial, was initiated in New York in 1963. The study reported positive results in women 50–69 years of age suggesting that mammography screening is effective in reducing breast cancer mortality.[33,34] These promising results encouraged many physicians and health plans to begin offering mammography screening to the general public. The HIP trial also encouraged scientists to conduct other RCTs to verify the findings. The early reports of these other RCTs were generally positive—screening women with mammography was associated with a statistically significant reduction in subsequent breast cancer mortality.[35,36] Chapter "Estimates of Screening Benefit: The Randomized Trials of Breast Cancer Screening" provides a comprehensive review of breast screening RCTs.

These large, expensive RCTs collectively followed hundreds of thousands of women over many years of screening with additional follow-up over the ensuing decades to collect mortality data. It was challenging to get all of the women to comply with the screening intervention, with compliance rates of about 80%.[37–39] Additionally, as the news spread that breast cancer screening was possibly beneficial, it was also increasingly challenging to conduct a trial in which women randomized to the control arm did not seek out and receive mammography. Some RCTs reported that approximately 20–30% of women in the control arm received screening mammography.[40] The screening programs varied among these RCTs in numerous other ways, such as the number of screening images per breast, the time interval between screens, and the age of women entering into the screening program.

As more RCTs were completed, some RCTs did not reach statistical significance, especially in subgroup analyses.[41] As the quality of these trials was extensively reviewed, heated arguments ensued, helping to push the development of systematic reviews and meta-analysis. Scientists were able to employ techniques of meta-analysis to merge together the data to assess overall impact on a larger scale. One great challenge of studying breast cancer screening is the fact that breast cancer is not as common as many think, and a large number of women are required to participate in these trials to adequately assess an impact. This challenge is particularly pertinent when evaluating subgroups, such as examining the impact of screening on women in certain risk or age groups. As the overall number of meta-analyses performed has grown, even these meta-analyses have produced conflicting results (see chapters: Estimates of Screening Benefit: The Randomized Trials of Breast Cancer Screening and Weighing the Benefits and Harms: Screening Mammography in the Balance). Different methods have been used over time, including the underlying inclusion and exclusion of trials in the analyses, which obviously has a major impact on the overall findings.

Given the cost and time required for RCTs, and as breast cancer screening became a standard of care in clinical practice in many countries, RCTs became unfeasible. Scientists then turned to other study designs. Case-control studies evaluated mortality differences between screened and unscreened women, but these studies were tricky methodologically, with many potential sources of bias. The selection of cases, controls, and definitions of "screening" varied among these case-control studies, as did their results.

Scientists have increasingly evaluated the accuracy of mammography using secondary outcomes rather than its impact on mortality. As large populations underwent screening, observational and ecological data became available. In the United States, the BCSC provided a wealth of standardized data. Other countries evaluated the impact of screening on their entire population of women who participated in standardized programs (see chapter: The Importance of Observational Evidence to Estimate and Monitor Mortality Reduction From Current Breast Cancer Screening).

With this proliferation of big data, methods of statistical modeling were developed (see chapter: The Role of Microsimulation Modeling in Evaluating the Outcomes and Effect of Screening). Unfortunately, these statistical models rely on many underlying assumptions that remain uncertain, such as the amount of time it takes lesions to progress from atypia to ductal carcinoma in situ (DCIS) to invasive breast

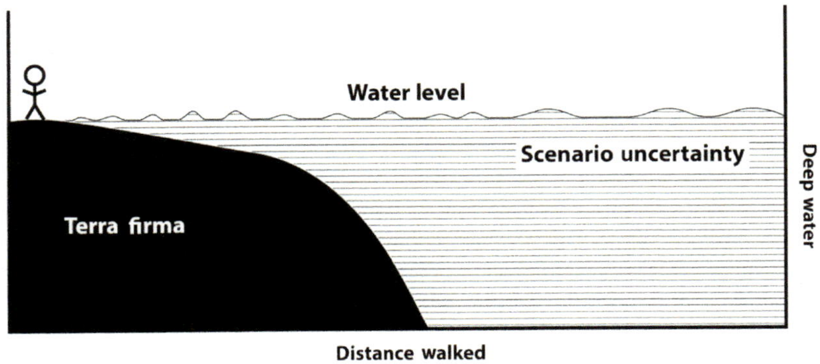

FIGURE 1.4

Depiction of statistical model uncertainty as we move from firm ground to modeling with uncertain parameters and inputs.

Reprinted with permission from Barnett S. Kramer and Joann G. Elmore. J Natl Cancer Inst 2015;107(7):djv145.

cancer. As we wade into the scientific literature using statistical modeling to evaluate whether screening has a positive impact on mortality, it is unclear if the bottom of this pool of data lies within inches or miles of our feet (Fig. 1.4). In an effort to combat this issue, scientific consortiums such as the Cancer Intervention and Surveillance Modeling Network (CISNET) were formed so that scientific groups could work together, though they each used different inputs and statistical methods. These groups share the same goal of modeling the impact of breast cancer screening on mortality reduction.[42]

With the vast number of scientific publications on mammography, the interpretations of the extent of the benefits vary. For some women, participating in breast cancer screening is important as it allows them to be engaged in an effort that is important to their health and, when they have normal screening exams, to be reassured until the next screening exam. While the absolute mortality benefit of screening mammography is less than we had hoped for,[43] if you are the woman whose life was "saved" that benefit is important.

THE ACCUMULATION OF SCIENTIFIC EVIDENCE ON POTENTIAL HARMS

While initial publications on breast cancer screening were aimed at determining whether breast cancer screening is beneficial and might save lives, over time, the possible harms of screening have become an increasingly important consideration. The potential risks are particularly relevant because breast cancer screening imposes a medical screening test on otherwise healthy women with the goal of saving lives through the early diagnosis of cancer.

Most RCTs only evaluated women undergoing a few rounds of screening. Yet, as breast cancer screening programs are implemented into clinical practice, women are increasingly screened annually over many decades. With this longer perspective, the accumulation of potential harms has become an increasingly important consideration. Questions were raised about the safety of imaging, given the repeated radiation exposure. Scientifically, there is no easy way to answer this question, but the amount of radiation per exam was lowered over time in response to these concerns.

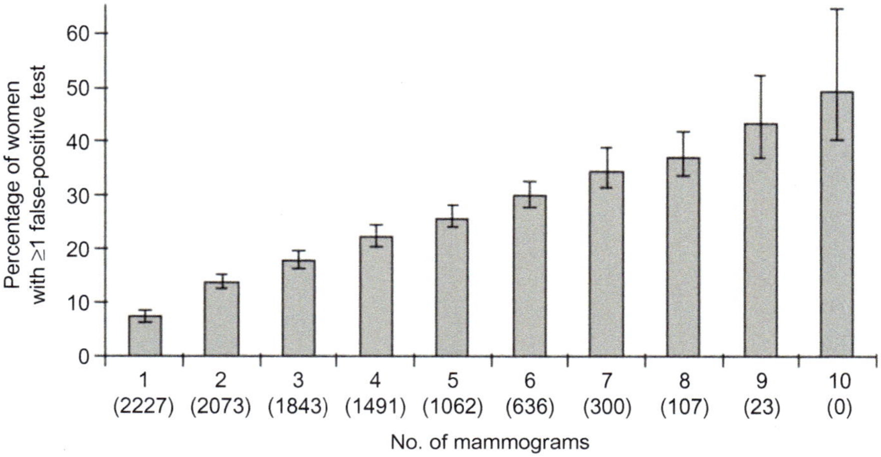

FIGURE 1.5

A woman's estimated risk of having at least one false-positive screening mammogram according to the total number of screening mammograms performed. The numbers in parentheses are the numbers of women with at least that many mammograms. The I bars indicate 95% confidence intervals.

Reprinted with permission from Joann G. Elmore et al. NEJM 1998;338:1089–1096.

After the early introduction of screening mammography into clinical practice, scientists began questioning the methods for studying cancer screening. Prominent among these individuals was Dr Bailar, a statistician from the US NCI of the National Institutes of Health (NIH), who described such concerning topics as lead time and length biases in an *Annals of Internal Medicine* article in 1976.[44]

Women also began reporting extreme anxiety as a result of being called back for additional testing after their screening mammogram. Many women did not like receiving letters or telephone calls stating, "An abnormality has been noted on your screening mammogram and additional testing is recommended." The majority of women called back for additional testing after screening mammograms have false-positive exams. One early study of women in the United States noted that after a decade of annual screening (1983–1993), about half of the women had experienced at least one false-positive mammography exam and about 20% had experienced a false-positive breast biopsy (Fig. 1.5).[45]

As breast cancer screening programs diffused into clinical practice, variable measures of sensitivity and specificity were also noted to be influenced by characteristics of the patients and the experience of the radiologists. Indeed, variability was even noted in the same radiologist who interpreted cases on two separate occasions.[46]

Interestingly, the false-positive rate after screening mammography varies between countries. Most women recalled for additional testing after a screening mammogram will not have cancer (and are thus a false-positive), as illustrated by the recall rate noted in publications from North America compared with other countries (Fig. 1.6). It is apparent that the recall rate in North America is generally much higher.[47] There are many potential reasons for the higher rate, including differences in the underlying

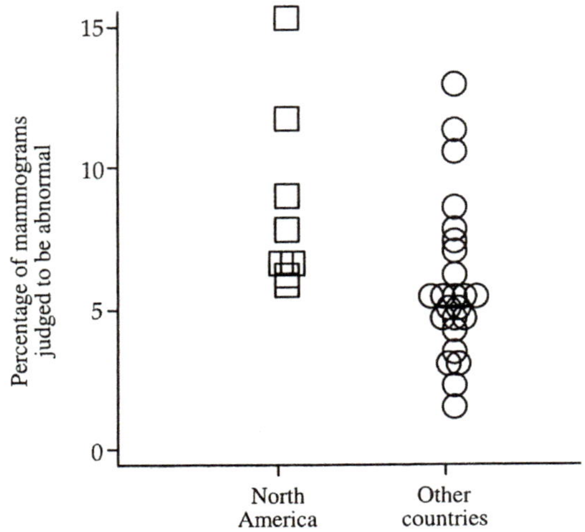

FIGURE 1.6

Percentage of mammograms judged to be abnormal from published studies by screening program location. North American screening programs ($n = 8$) are shown as *open squares*, and programs from other countries ($n = 24$) are shown as *open circles*. The weighted mean percentage of mammograms judged to be abnormal was statistically significantly higher in North American programs than it was in programs from other countries (8.4% vs 5.6%; difference in weighted mean percentage = 2.8%, 95% confidence interval = 0.5–5.1%; $p = 0.018$).

Reprinted with permission from Joann G. Elmore et al. J Natl Cancer Inst. 2003;95:1384–1393.

patient population, age of women being screened, the threshold used by radiologists for calling women back after a screening mammogram, financial incentives, and the fear of medical malpractice litigation if cancer is missed. Table 1.2 lists some of the potential reasons for these striking differences between countries.

In the last decade, the topic of overdiagnosis has joined the list of the harms of cancer screening. Overdiagnosis was not considered, or even mentioned, in many early reviews and guidelines on breast cancer screening, but now most scientists acknowledge that overdiagnosis is occurring. We have seen very little reduction in advanced-stage breast cancer in the face of huge increases in early-stage breast cancer and DCIS, and it has been difficult to determine if these increased rates of early-stage breast cancer and DCIS detection are helping women. During the two decades from 1982 to 2002, a total of 16 publications concerned overdiagnosis related to breast cancer screening in medical journals; this number jumped to 103 publications in the next decade. Published reports on this topic provide a frustratingly wide range of results, with estimates of overdiagnosis ranging from less than 10% to over 50%.[48–52] The actual extent of overdiagnosis remains unclear, and we are unable to identify which women are actually "overdiagnosed." The scientific challenges in studying this phenomenon are deserving of an entire chapter within this text (see chapter: Challenges in Understanding and Quantifying Over-Diagnosis and Over-Treatment).

Table 1.2 Possible Explanations for the Variability Noted Among Published Studies of Screening Mammography

Characteristics of the population screened
• Age (eg, percentage of women <50 years of age) • Initial vs subsequent screening examination • Presence of risk factors for breast cancer • Presence of breast symptoms • Self-referral versus physician referral • Cultural differences
Features of the mammography examination
• Equipment type and year • One or two views of each breast • Single or double readings • Technician training
Features of physicians interpreting the mammogram
• Experience of the physician • Level of personal comfort with ambiguity • Individual thresholds to label film as abnormal
Features of the health care system
• Malpractice concerns • Financial incentives • Private vs academic/public programs • Different stated goals for the percentage of mammograms judged abnormal and positive predictive value • Quality control and auditing procedures • Variability of definitions used to calculate outcome
Reprinted from Elmore JG, CY Nakano, TD Koepsell, LM Desnick, CJ D'Orsi, and DF Ransohoff. International variation in screening mammography interpretations in community-based programs. Journal of the National Cancer Institute. 95.18 (2003): 1384–93.

HISTORY OF VARIABILITY IN GUIDELINE RECOMMENDATIONS AND QUALITY

As the scientific data on the benefits and harms of breast cancer screening expanded, task forces and review groups were created around the world to evaluate the evidence and to make recommendations for screening of specific groups of women. Over the years, there has been variability in the guidelines and they have changed as the evidence accumulated. Chapter "Weighing the Benefits and Harms: Screening Mammography in the Balance" provides a detailed review of today's prominent guidelines. Below is a brief historical summary.

In 1976, 5 years after the first published results of the New York HIP trial, the Canadian Task Force on Preventive Health Care was established. Interestingly, this Canadian Task Force made recommendations to, not from, the government. The Task Force based its recommendations on evidence in the medical literature by considering the basic requirements for evaluating the effectiveness of screening tools, a method that is still used today (Table 1.1). Using their evaluations of the data, the Canadian Task Force incorporated an evidence-based grading system into their recommendations, giving more weight to well-designed randomized trials than to cohort, or other, study designs. The Canadian Task Force also assigned an overall grade to their screening test recommendations.[53]

In 1984 the US Preventive Services Task Force (USPSTF), an independent panel of experts in primary care, prevention, and research methods was formed. This group is charged by US law to review scientific evidence and to make recommendations for clinical preventive services to clinicians and the public. The USPSTF has updated its approach over the years, incorporating systematic reviews, meta-analyses, and modeling into its review methods and considering how to estimate uncertainty, how to standardize the breast screening process, and how to be more transparent in reporting study findings and the process used to develop the guidelines. By law, the USPSTF cannot consider the cost–effectiveness of the screening program.

The late 1990s were a period of increasing attention to quality of mammography and heated debates. In 1997, responding to growing concerns about the variable quality of mammography, the Mammography Quality Standards Act (MQSA)[54] law was passed in the United States in an effort to improve mammography quality and to promote standardization. Mammography is now one of the most highly regulated medical tests in the United States. Because of MQSA regulation, mammograms use lower doses of radiation per exam, and health care facilities use standardized reporting and auditing that facilitates the study of large populations.[55]

In 1997, an NIH Consensus Conference was held to review the extent of the accumulated evidence at that time. The NIH Consensus Conference was led by a panel of individuals with no known conflicts of interest. The panel's conclusion was as follows: "The data currently available do not warrant a universal recommendation for mammography for all women in their 40s. Each woman should decide for herself whether to undergo mammography."[56] The public and scientific reaction to this NIH consensus conference was rapid and, in many ways, harsh. The director of the NCI at NIH said that he was "shocked" by the results, and the head of NIH, Bernadine Healy, was "very disturbed that a group of so-called experts challenged the notion of early detection."[57] The US senate voted 98-to-0 in favor of screening women in their 40s.[58]

Over the next decade heated discussions in the United States centered on whether to invite women in their 40s to screening, with definite differences among guideline groups in their recommendations. Conflicts of interest may sway committee recommendations and have been a source of concern. A study of 12 mammography screening guideline committees (of which the majority cited the same eight main RCTs) found that recommendations reflect the committee member's specialty and intellectual interests.[59] Guidelines developed by radiologists were more likely to recommend routine screening for women aged 40–49 years, while guidelines that did not recommend routine screening in this age group did not have a radiologist on the review committee. Guideline groups are increasingly attempting to be more transparent in sharing their evaluation processes with the public.[60]

In 2002 after more data were published on the topic, the USPSTF reviewed the updated evidence and recommended routine screening mammography in women 40 years or older every two years.[61]

The benefits of screening in younger women were noted, however, to be less than anticipated, especially when considered from an absolute risk reduction perspective. In 2009, the USPSTF again reviewed updated evidence and published their recommendations on November 9, 2009 as follows: "The USPSTF recommends against routine screening mammography in women aged 40–49 years. The decision to start regular, biennial screening mammography before the age of 50 years should be an individual one and take into account patient context, including the patient's values regarding specific benefits and harms…." This 2009 Task Force recommendation touched off a powerful media firestorm as many became upset by the vacillating recommendations. Interestingly, on December 4, 2009, the USPSTF dropped the first sentence of their November 9, 2009 recommendation statement, putting them in line with current guidelines—a recommendation to leave the decision up to women and to help women make an informed decision that takes into account their own values regarding potential benefits and harms.

In an effort to reduce harms, more scientific groups in the United States now recommend screening every 2 years instead of every year. These updated guidelines more closely align US recommendations with other countries, the majority of which do not offer screening to women in their 40s and recommend 2- or 3-year screening intervals.

There is extensive variation among and within countries regarding recommendations for and support of breast cancer screening.[62] Some countries recommend starting at age 50, while many guideline groups in the United States recommend starting at age 40 or 45. Some guideline groups recommend annual mammograms, while others recommend every two or more years. The United States has been distinct in having so many groups actively encouraging annual screening starting at age 40. In fact, most other countries start later (eg, age 50) and recommend screening less frequently (eg, every 2–3 years).

Mammography screening programs require large outlays of financial support. Guidelines can have dramatic financial impact. This is clearly stated in a 2014 editorial entitled "The cost of breast cancer screening in the United States: A picture is worth… a billion dollars?"[31] The costs of implementing three different screening strategies in the United States—biennial screening, following the USPSTF guidelines, or annual screening—can lead to estimated differences between these strategies as large as $8 billion.[30] This value is approximately twice the amount of the annual budget for the NCI, the major funding agency in the United States for research on all types of cancers. This estimate does not include inflation or costs of treating overdiagnosed cases.

Varying guidelines may lead to confusion about when and how to screen for both clinicians and women. With mixed information, clinicians may not know how to inform their patients about screening, which in turn affects womens' trust and confidence in the screening process. Despite the variability in guidelines regarding starting age and screening interval, one growing area of agreement is that women should be helped to make informed medical decisions based on their own values and understanding of the benefits-harms balance.

HISTORY OF INFORMED MEDICAL DECISION MAKING

In the midst of all of the scientific evidence, every day, women are trying to both make the decision about whether to screen and how to deal with the outcome. Most guidelines now include statements about the importance of informed medical decision-making (see chapter: Informed and Shared

Decision-making in Breast Screening). Many guidelines now recommend that women discuss screening with their health care provider. However, conveying nuance and uncertainty is not the strong suit of many health care providers, especially when patients seek black and white answers.

Unfortunately, most women report receiving very little helpful information before undergoing screening mammography exams. Health care providers are more likely to discuss the benefits of screening than the harms, and they do not routinely elicit patient preferences. In one survey, 96.3% of women in the United States reported discussing the pros of breast cancer screening with their health care providers, while only 19.5% said there was a discussion of the cons. Less than half were asked about their screening preference.[63]

Concerns about the inadequacy of information received by women in the United Kingdom screening program actually led to action, including public consultations and a specially convened "citizens' jury" made up of screening-eligible women.[64] The jurors met to hear evidence from experts and make recommendations on the best way to present information on the pros and cons of mammography. After this experience, one participant remarked: "I can't believe how much I didn't know."[65]

Physicians in clinical practice are often faced with inadequate time for fully informed discussions and might be quick to recommend screening mammography, hoping that it will save lives. Physicians may also fear medical malpractice lawsuits and poor quality performance ratings if they do not encourage screening. However, patient and physician fears are not conducive to truly informed, shared decision-making about a complex choice.

One avenue to support informed medical decision-making is via decision aids. Providing decision aids to women has been associated with improved decision quality and fewer women reporting that they will undergo screening. A large, well-conducted randomized clinical trial in Australia studied decision aids related to mammography and found that overall, women understood the concept of overdiagnosis and wanted to receive this information during health care visits.[66]

Providers seek to individualize care for their patients; while it is challenging to apply individual-level risk models, doctors can work with their patients to shape screening to individual preferences. Women want and need information on the benefits and harms of breast cancer screening. Understanding the scientific evidence, as described in this book, is an important first step.

HISTORY OF PATIENT ACTIVISM, POLITICS, AND LAW IN SCREENING

As described above, there are many influential elements involved in the breast screening decision-making process. Perhaps one of the most important influential elements is the patient herself. Women and their loved ones have been trying to find their way in this complex cultural setting. One method of coping has involved turning fear and anxiety into activism. Support and engagement has spread on a large scale as evidenced by events such as Breast Cancer Awareness Month, when the world seems to turn pink in October each year.

In the United States, patient activism, politics, and legislation have begun to influence screening recommendations. This is apparent in the management of women who are identified as having dense breast tissue. This story begins with a single patient, Nancy Cappello, PhD. On February 3, 2004, Nancy Cappello was diagnosed with stage 3c breast cancer. She had a decade-long history of "normal" annual screening mammograms, including a normal exam six weeks before her diagnosis. When she questioned why her breast cancer had not been detected on the most recent screening mammogram, the oversight was attributed to her dense breast tissue.

She soon learned that high breast density is a risk factor for breast cancer and it is associated with less accurate mammography. Frustrated that she had not known this information, she set out to educate other women through organizing advocacy groups to educate women about breast density. This movement was instrumental in establishing state laws in the United States that require medical providers to inform women about their breast density and the risks associated with higher breast density on their mammography reports. A few state laws also require insurance coverage for additional screening options such as ultrasound, magnetic resonance imaging (MRI), or both.

Dr. Cappello's story is a prime example of how personal experience and influential people can drive policy and medical standards despite a lack of strong scientific evidence to support the position. The advocacy groups were motivated by caring and well-intentioned individuals working under assumptions that additional testing is better for women.

Research has found that women with dense breasts have double the relative risk of developing breast cancer, but the absolute five-year risk of a diagnosis (not death) appears to only increase from 0.7% to 1.3%. Additionally, when women in the highest two categories of breast density (heterogeneously or extremely dense breasts) are compared to women with scattered fibroglandular densities, they have 1.43 and 1.85 times greater lifetime risks of developing breast cancer, respectively.[67] Despite these findings of increased risk of a diagnosis, dense breast tissue is not associated with increased breast cancer mortality.[68]

While research indicates that coupling ultrasound, or even MRI, with mammography increases the detection of early-stage cancers in women with dense breast tissue, there is no evidence that incorporating ultrasound into mass screening saves lives. No RCTs have been conducted to provide guidance on how women with dense breast tissue should be screened using mortality as an endpoint.

Density ratings are subjective, and studies report concerning low rates of intrarater agreement. Moreover, most published ultrasound screening studies report outcomes of ultrasounds interpreted by experienced physicians. Yet, expanding ultrasound to mass screening would likely require the involvement of less experienced technologists and clinicians, potentially leading to lower quality exams, in turn exposing patients to diagnostic errors and physicians to malpractice lawsuits. The cost-effectiveness ratio of adding ultrasound screening is also high, estimated at $325,000 per quality-adjusted life year (QALY) gained.[69] While there is disagreement about the appropriate cost-effective threshold, adding ultrasound screening is definitely above what most would accept. Few decision makers will conclude that interventions that cost more than $175,000 per QALY are justifiable.

Women should be informed of their breast density, the limitations of mammography in finding cancer in dense breast tissue, and risks associated with dense breast tissue. Thus, informing women of their breast density seems ethical and necessary. We should be educating women regardless of the law. However, we do not know how to best give this information or whether giving women this information helps in any way or just increases anxiety. Perhaps we need research on the effects of giving women this information.

Much of the drive for legislation stems from an historic lack of communication between the medical and scientific community and its patients with regard to the limitations of mammography. We may have oversold medical technology and our breast cancer screening tools. As clinicians and scientists, *we need to welcome patient advocacy groups and to work together to encourage evidence-based advocacy.*

METHODS TO IDENTIFY HIGH-RISK WOMEN FOR SCREENING

The evidence surrounding risk-based screening is a primary topic of this book with multiple aspects covered in chapters "Challenges and Opportunities in the Implementation of Risk-Based Screening for Breast Cancer" through "Imaging Surveillance of Women With a Personal History of Breast Cancer." Current recommendations and standards that apply to different populations are discussed at length, including screening in older women (see chapter: Breast Cancer Screening in the Older Woman), addressing the issue in younger women (see chapter: Screening Women in Their 40s), screening women with dense breast tissue (see chapter: Screening for Breast Cancer in Women With Dense Breasts), and women with a personal history of breast cancer (see chapter: Imaging Surveillance of Women with a Personal History of Breast Cancer).

As research advances, other sciences, including genetics, have helped develop screening algorithms for breast cancer. Most notable was the discovery of the *BRCA1* gene on chromosome 17 in 1990,[70] followed a few years later by the discovery of *BRCA2*.[71] The chapter "Screening Women with Known or Suspected Cancer Gene Mutations" describes in detail how genetic mutations contribute toward the development of breast cancer and how they are being factored into breast cancer screening.

Given the growing concerns about potential harms from screening, we are increasingly considering how to individualize screening to target women at high risk for breast cancer and how to identify women who will receive the most benefit of screening (eg, by age, breast density, genetic mutations, personal history of cancer). Increased attention has been paid to developing prediction models to identify high-risk women and to minimize the harm to those least likely to benefit from screening.

Intuitively, risk stratification seems like a good idea. For example, from an individual woman's perspective, low-risk women may be reassured by their lessened risk and may require less screening or be able to start screening at a later age. High-risk women are informed about their likelihood of developing cancer, giving them the opportunity to consider screening at an earlier age or with a different (or supplemental) imaging technology. From society's perspective, knowing which women are most likely to be diagnosed with breast cancer would allow concentrated screening and diagnostic efforts on women most likely to benefit from the test.

While risk stratification may be helpful to identify subgroups of populations at high versus low risk, it unfortunately falls short at the level of the individual woman. An individual woman either does or does not develop breast cancer, so her risk is either 0% or 100%. It is only in *groups*, or populations of women that one sees a range of risk from 0% to 100%.

A risk stratification tool for individual women should discriminate among individual women, such that the estimates from the risk model are consistently higher for women who develop breast cancer compared to those who do not develop cancer. Fig. 1.7a shows an example of a fictitious risk stratification tool that clearly and perfectly differentiates women at low risk who do not get cancer compared to women at high risk who are ultimately diagnosed with cancer. Unfortunately, our current ability to risk stratify is far from perfect. For example, the five-year risk estimates for all of the women from the Nurses' Health Study according to the Gail model is shown in Fig. 1.7b. The two lines in the figure represent the groups of women who ultimately developed breast cancer compared to women who did not over a five-year period. Effective risk stratification should separate these two groups of women so that the curves are not overlapping consistently higher estimated risks. The Gail model did not separate the two groups.

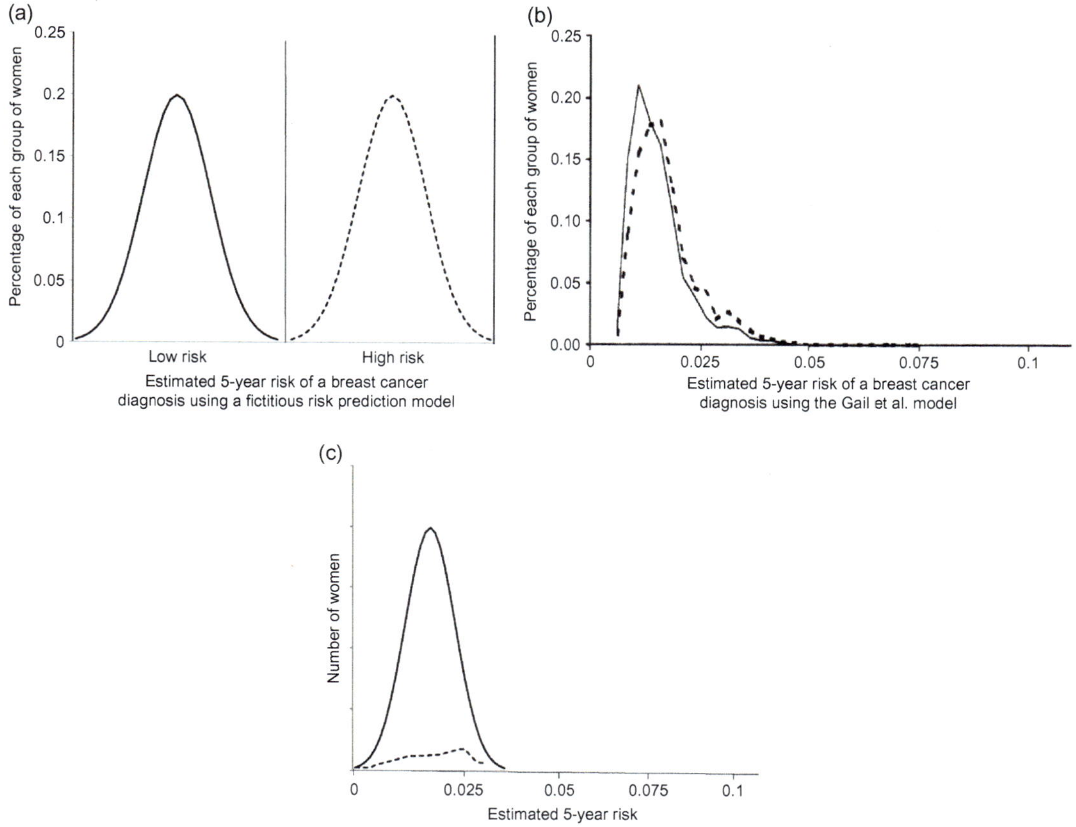

FIGURE 1.7

(a) Ability of a fictitious cancer risk prediction model to discriminate between women who will be diagnosed with breast cancer and women who will not. Concordance statistic = 1.0. *Solid line*, women with no diagnosis of breast cancer; *dashed line*, women with a breast cancer diagnosis. (b) Ability of the Gail risk cancer risk prediction model to discriminate between women who will be diagnosed with breast cancer and women who will not. *Solid line* indicates women with no diagnosis of breast cancer; *dashed line* indicates women with a breast cancer diagnosis. (c) Example showing how (b) might look by number of women on the *y*-axis, not percent of each group of women. Not based on actual numbers.

(a) Adapted from Joann G. Elmore and Suzanne W. Fletcher. J Natl Cancer Inst. 2006;98:1673–1675. (b) Reprinted with permission from Rockhill Levine B and from Joann G. Elmore and Suzanne W. Fletcher. J Natl Caner Inst. 2006;98:1673–1675.

It is important to remember that Fig. 1.7b shows proportions of women on the *y*-axis, not absolute numbers. Almost 80,000 women in the Nurses' Health Study did not develop breast cancer in this 5-year period, whereas 1354 women developed breast cancer. Fig. 1.7c is an example of what the absolute numbers might look like. It is estimated that for every woman classified as "high-risk" who is subsequently diagnosed with breast cancer, another 46 women are classified as "high-risk" but do not have breast cancer.[72]

Except for age, no factors with very large relative risks were included in the original Gail model. In an attempt to improve risk stratification, other risk prediction models have been developed. It has been suggested that for a risk factor (or combination of risk factors) to detect about half the individuals with a disease, with a 5% false-positive rate, a relative risk of about 200 is required.[73] Relative risks of this magnitude are rare. While the relative risk is high for women with genetic mutations, most other variables are not associated with very high relative risks.

Another condition that has been considered a risk factor for breast cancer is atypical ductal hyperplasia (atypia). Some experts suggest annual MRI screening for women with atypia diagnosed by biopsy.[74] However, diagnostic interpretation of atypia by pathologists on breast biopsies varies. A study of 115 US pathologists' interpretation of breast biopsies indicated only 48% agreement on diagnoses of atypia compared with a reference consensus standard.[75] An example slide defined by the reference consensus standard as atypia as can be seen in Fig. 1.8, with diagnoses of practicing pathologists who independently interpreted this same slide ranging from benign without atypia to DCIS. Thus, a risk assessment based on a previous atypia diagnosis might lead to unnecessary screening of women who, in reality, do not even have this risk factor.

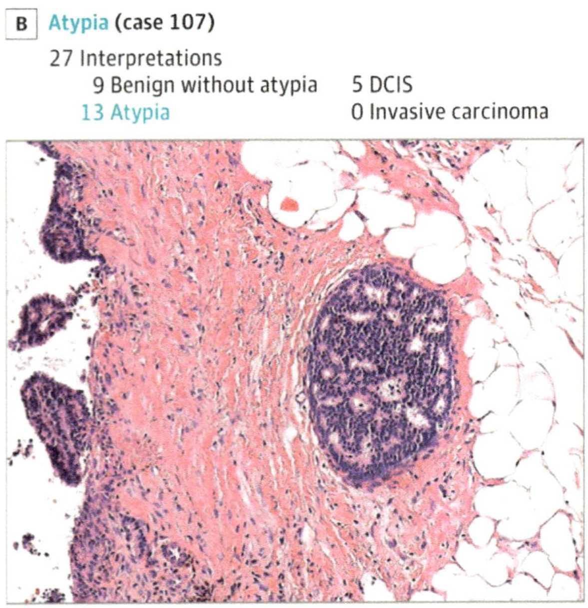

FIGURE 1.8

Example slide of atypia (atypical ductal hyperplasia) from a study of pathologists' interpretations of breast biopsies. *Blue* indicates interpretations concordant with the reference diagnosis of atypia (13 of the 27 pathologists who interpreted this slide gave a diagnosis of atypia) Slide is hematoxylin-eosin stain (original magnification × 100).

Adapted from Elmore JG, Longton G, Carney PA, et al. Diagnostic concordance among pathologists interpreting breast biopsy specimens. JAMA. 2015;313(11):1122–1132.

In summary, risk stratification may be helpful when developing breast cancer screening programs at a population level. Risk models help to make screening programs more efficient and to reduce harms. However, *risk prediction is difficult at the level of individual women* because most known risks for breast cancer are small and spread out over the entire population. The risk factor data from genetic mutations may be an exception. Future developments in breast cancer research may improve our ability to identify other small groups of women with large risks. However, until that happens, risk prediction models should be evaluated not only for their calibration, that is, how well they work for the whole group, but also for their discrimination: how well they can separate individual women who are, and are not, going to develop disease.

STUDYING RAPIDLY EVOLVING NEW TECHNOLOGIES AND OUR GENERAL TECHNOPHILIA

From the beginning of time, humans have survived and thrived based on our ability to adapt, understand, and evolve. Naturally, we are constantly in search of better methods, strategies, and technologies. With regard to breast cancer screening, we seem to trust technology and feel that if scientific studies show that mammography is not the perfect screening tool, we should move on to newer, fancier medical technology. I refer to this as "technophilia"—our love of technology.

Scientists are faced with the daunting task of adapting scientific methods to keep pace with ongoing and rapid technological advancements in medicine. Over time, newer mammography, such as digital breast tomosynthesis (also called 3D mammography), and other imaging technologies, such as ultrasound, computed tomography, and MRI, have been considered as possible diagnostic and screening tools, but these newer technologies have not been studied in large-scale RCTs for screening the general population.

All of the original RCTs on the impact of screening mammography on breast cancer mortality were done using film-screening mammography, which is now a largely outdated technology. Digital mammography has almost completely replaced film-screen mammography in developed countries. It is logistically easier to immediately obtain digital images and to view and store them rather than to view film screen exams, which require light boxes. Publication of one large clinical trial comparing the accuracy of digital mammography to film screen mammography, the Digital Mammography Imaging Screening trial,[76] was received with much fanfare. However, an improvement in accuracy using the digital exams was only noted among women in their 40s and those with dense breast tissue. It is impractical to have facilities maintain both digital and film mammography machines and to schedule women based on these criteria. Digital mammography has therefore rapidly expanded into clinical practices for many reasons beyond the scientific evidence, including the ease of obtaining, storing, and sharing images.

One example of "technophilia" is the technology added to digital mammography machines called computer-aided detection (CAD) programs. CAD programs add marks to alert radiologists to potentially suspicious areas on an image. Some CAD systems mark up to four areas on each exam. While the addition of CAD programs at face-value seemed to be a good idea—letting computers aid the human interpreter so that cancers are not missed—it remains unclear if this technology is actually helping. CAD does not improve sensitivity and may raise the false-positive rate.[77] Despite early scientific evidence published in the *New England Journal of Medicine* in 2007 that CAD may not be helping,[77] these systems rapidly diffused into clinical practice. From January 1, 2001 through December 31, 2009, annual CAD prevalence among Medicare screening mammograms in the United States increased from 3.5% to 79.7%.[78,79] A large 2015 study using digital mammography pointed out, again, that CAD use is not improving accuracy.[80] Given the accumulation of scientific evidence on CAD, the authors of the primary scientific article and the accompanying editorial in 2015[81] questioned why CAD continues to be used and paid for if it is not improving accuracy. These are good questions!

In general, as new technologies for breast cancer screening are developed, they require careful evaluation and consideration (see chapter: Evolution of Mammography Screening: From Film Screen to Digital Breast Tomosynthesis). However, these technologies are often introduced into clinical practice for diagnostic imaging, for evaluating patients with symptoms or clinical concerns, rather than mass screening of asymptomatic women. Thus, less attention has been paid to their potential impact than if they were unleashed on the much larger screening population of healthy, asymptomatic women. Once in clinical practice, however, these *new technologies seem to move into screening practices, often without adequate consideration or evidence.* [82]

THOUGHTS ON THE FUTURE

Breast cancer screening is the most studied cancer screening technique, yet interpretation of the overall benefits and harms remains variable. From a scientific standpoint, we are limited by the fact that it takes hundreds of thousands of women followed over many years to complete a RCT, and by the time a trial is done technologies are likely to have improved.

New technologies have been developed and recommended for breast cancer screening, yet large-scale RCTs of these newer screening tools will likely never be done. Screening mammography has rapidly moved from film to digital mammography and now from digital to 3D tomosynthesis mammography (see chapter: Evolution of Mammography Screening: From Film Screen to Digital Breast Tomosynthesis). Scientific methods to study the efficacy of breast cancer screening need to be developed to keep pace with rapidly developing technology.

After reviewing the evidence on breast cancer screening and realizing both how challenging it is to study and how small the absolute benefit is and how real the potential harms are, some may want to develop different approaches altogether. Two possibilities include optimizing breast cancer treatment or conversely, optimizing primary prevention. First, as our treatments for breast cancer have improved over time, we are able to cure a substantial proportion of women with breast cancer regardless of stage at diagnosis. If the cure rate from treatments, especially if they could be less morbid treatments, could be increased to 100%, then screening would not be necessary to save lives. The second approach is primary prevention; if we could prevent breast cancer, there would no longer be a need for screening.

We have a long way to go before prevention and/or treatment leads us to no longer need to consider screening for breast cancer. Until then, we should be cautious in our scientific methods of studying cancer screening and careful in our interpretation of existing data.

CONCLUSION

Amid the extensive scientific evidence on breast cancer screening, women, their physicians, and public policy administrators are trying to understand the relative benefits and harms. Interpreting the extensive and complicated evidence is challenging. I encourage readers of this book to review the scientific evidence and interpret the facts while considering all of the potential external influences that affect our decision making. As Marie Curie remarked, "Nothing in life is to be feared, it is only to be understood. Now is the time to understand more, so that we may fear less."[83]

GLOSSARY

BRCA1*/*BRCA2 human genes expressed in the cells of the breast and other tissues specific for repairing damaged DNA. Risk of breast cancer is found to increase when either of these genes is damaged by mutation.

Breast self-exam manual examination of the breasts performed by the patient.

Canadian Task Force on Preventive Health Care establishes evidence-based preventive health care guidelines for primary care providers. Breast cancer guidelines address the use of imaging and screening modalities by risk and age group.

Cancer Intervention and Surveillance Modeling Network (CISNET) a US National Cancer Institute-funded consortium of investigators that collaborates to conduct research on statistical modeling and its implications for cancer interventions, from screening to treatment.

Case-control studies studies comparing participants with the disease of interest to participants who do not have the disease.

Clinical breast exam manual examination of the breasts performed by a health care provider.

Computer-aided detection a supplemental, automated technology designed to aid radiologists in the detection of radiological abnormalities.

Digital breast tomosynthesis a method of mammographic imaging that composes multiple X-rays into a three-dimensional representation of the breast.

False-positive exam an exam in which an abnormality is detected when no disease is actually present.

Fibroglandular tissue areas of fibrous and glandular tissue present in the breast; also a breast density classification.

Gail model a breast cancer risk assessment tool that combines information about a woman's personal characteristics (age, race, etc.) to determine her likelihood of being diagnosed with breast cancer.

Lead time bias a discrepancy in the measurement of survival time between preclinical cancers detected via mammography and clinically symptomatic cancers. Survival time for cancers detected during screening includes a presymptomatic period that is not included for cancers detected after the development of symptoms.

Length bias occurs because conditions with longer preclinical phases present more opportunities for detection and are generally associated with better outcomes, regardless of screening.

Mammography X-ray image of the breast using specialized equipment.

Mammography Quality Standards Act enacted by the US Congress on October 27, 1992 to ensure access to mammography and promote early detection of breast cancer through the accreditation, certification, and inspection of mammography facilities.

Meta-analysis statistical approach used to consider results from multiple studies.

Modeling study scientific process in which data are accumulated and used to develop algorithms designed to best simulate a population of interest with and without an intervention.

Observational study studies in which participants are observed and data are collected to determine differences. There is no direct intervention.

Overdiagnosis diagnosis of disease that, if left untreated, would never progress to clinical significance over the course of an individual's lifetime.

Prophylactic mastectomy preventive removal of one or both breasts to reduce the risk of developing breast cancer.

Quality-adjusted life year a quantification of disease burden that accounts for duration and quality of life (one quality-adjusted life year represents one year of perfect health). Most frequently used in cost-value evaluations of medical interventions.

Technophilia a love of technology.

LIST OF ACRONYMS AND ABBREVIATIONS

BCSC Breast Cancer Surveillance Consortium
CAD Computer-aided detection
CISNET Cancer Intervention and Surveillance Modeling Network
DCIS Ductal carcinoma in situ
HIP Health Improvement Program
MQSA Mammography Quality Standards Act
NIH National Institutes of Health
NCI National Cancer Institute
RCT Randomized controlled trial
US United States
USPSTF US Preventive Services Task Force

REFERENCES

1. Lerner BH. *The breast cancer wars: hope, fear, and the pursuit of a cure in twentieth-century America*. New York: Oxford University Press; 2001.
2. Love SM, Lindsey K. *Dr. Susan Love's breast book*. Cambridge, MA: Da Capo Press; 2010.
3. Williams F. *Breasts: a natural and unnatural history*. New York: WW Norton & Company; 2012.
4. Yalom M. *A history of the breast*. A History of the Breast (Hardcover), Published June 7th 1999 by Knopf, Hardcover; 1999:331. ISBN: 0679434593 (ISBN13: 780679434597).
5. Olson JS. *Bathsheba's breast: women, cancer, and history*. Baltimore, MD: JHU Press; 2002.
6. Seiterle G. Artemis-Die Grosse Gottin von Ephesos. Eine neue Deutung der Vielbrüstigkeit eroffnet einen Zugang zum bisher unbekannten Kult der Gottin. (Artémis, la Grande Déesse d'Ephèse. Une nouvelle interprétation des seins multiples ouvre un accès au culte de la déesse jusque-là inconnu). *Antike Welt Zürich* 1979;**10**(3):3–16.
7. Breasted JH. *The Edwin Smith surgical papyrus: hieroglyphic transliteration, translation and commentary*. Whitefish, MT: Kessinger Publishing; 2006.
8. Rose G, Barker DJ. Epidemiology for the uninitiated. Screening. *Br Med J* 1978;**2**(6149):1417–8.
9. Morabia A, Zhang FF. History of medical screening: from concepts to action. *Postgrad Med J* 2004;**80**(946):463–9.
10. Elmore JG, Armstrong K, Lehman CD, Fletcher SW. Screening for breast cancer. *JAMA* 2005;**293**(10):1245–56.
11. Kosters JP, Gotzsche PC. Regular self-examination or clinical examination for early detection of breast cancer. *Cochrane Database Systemat Rev* 2003(2):CD003373.
12. Thomas DB, Gao DL, Ray RM, Wang WW, Allison CJ, Chen FL, et al. Randomized trial of breast self-examination in Shanghai: final results. *J Natl Cancer Inst* 2002;**94**(19):1445–57.
13. Miller AB, Wall C, Baines CJ, Sun P, To T, Narod SA. Twenty five year follow-up for breast cancer incidence and mortality of the Canadian National Breast Screening Study: randomised screening trial. *BMJ* 2014;**348**:g366.
14. Baines CJ, Miller AB, Bassett AA. Physical examination. Its role as a single screening modality in the Canadian National Breast Screening Study. *Cancer* 1989;**63**(9):1816–22.
15. Fenton J, Barton M, Geiger A, Herrington LJ, Rolnick SJ, Harris EL, et al. Screening clinical breast examination: how often does it miss lethal breast cancer? *JNCI Monogr* 2005;**35**:67–71.
16. Gold RH, Bassett LW, Widoff BE. Highlights from the history of mammography. *Radiographics* 1990;**10**(6):1111–31.

17. Egan RL. Roles of mammography in the early detection of breast cancer. *Cancer* 1969;**24**(6):1197–200.
18. Lerner BH. "To see today with the eyes of tomorrow": a history of screening mammography. *Can Bullet Med Hist* 2003;**20**(2):299–321.
19. Urban N, Taplin SH, Taylor VM, Peacock S, Anderson G, Conrad D, et al. Community organization to promote breast cancer screening among women ages 50–75. *Prevent Med* 1995;**24**(5):477–84.
20. Ballard-Barbash R, Taplin SH, Yankaskas BC, Ernster VL, Rosenberg RD, Carney PA, et al. Breast Cancer Surveillance Consortium: a national mammography screening and outcomes database. *Am J Roentgenol* 1997;**169**(4):1001–8.
21. National Cancer Institute. *Breast Cancer Surveillance Consortium.* [Web]. <http://breastscreening.cancer.gov/>; 2015 [accessed 11.03.15].
22. Lerner BH. Breast cancer activism: past lessons, future directions. *Nat Rev Cancer* 2002;**2**(3):225–30.
23. Radiology ACo. *Mammography saves lives.* [Website]. <http://mammographysaveslives.org>; 2014 [accessed 02.07.14].
24. Woloshin S, Schwartz LM, Black WC, Kramer BS. Cancer screening campaigns—getting past uninformative persuasion. *New Engl J Med* 2012;**367**(18):1677–9.
25. Braun S. The history of breast cancer advocacy. *Breast J* 2003;**9**(s2):S101–3.
26. Kim EK. 'Brave' Amy Robach reveals breast cancer detected by on-air mammogram. *Today News.* <http://www.today.com/news/brave-amy-robach-reveals-breast-cancer-detected-air-mammogram-2D11577476>; 2013 [accessed 11.02.15].
27. Nattinger AB, Hoffmann RG, Howell-Pelz A, Goodwin JS. Effect of Nancy Reagan's mastectomy on choice of surgery for breast cancer by US women. *JAMA* 1998;**279**(10):762–6.
28. Evans DG, Barwell J, Eccles DM, Collins A, Izatt L, Jacobs C, et al. The Angelina Jolie effect: how high celebrity profile can have a major impact on provision of cancer related services. *Breast Cancer Res* 2014;**16**(5):442.
29. Jolie A. My medical choice. The New York Times. May 14, 2013: A25.
30. O'Donoghue C, Eklund M, Ozanne EM, Esserman LJ. Aggregate cost of mammography screening in the United States: comparison of current practice and advocated guidelines. *Ann Internal Med* 2014;**160**(3):145–53.
31. Elmore JG, Gross CP. The cost of breast cancer screening in the United States: a picture is worth... a billion dollars? *Ann Internal Med* 2014;**160**(3):203.
32. Ferraro N. Hastings hospital's mammogram parties offer women a dose of pampering to calm the nerves. *St. Paul Pioneer Press.* January 20, 2011.
33. Shapiro S, Venet W, Strax P, Venet L. *Periodic screening for breast cancer: the health insurance plan project and its sequelae, 1963–1986.* Baltimore, MD: The Johns Hopkins University Press; 1988.
34. Shapiro S, Venet W, Strax P, Venet L, Roeser R. Ten- to fourteen-year effect of screening on breast cancer mortality. *J Natl Cancer Inst* 1982;**69**(2):349–55.
35. Nystrom L, Andersson I, Bjurstam N, Frisell J, Nordenskjold B, Rutqvist LE. Long-term effects of mammography screening: updated overview of the Swedish randomised trials. *Lancet* 2002;**359**(9310):909–19.
36. Tabar L, Fagerberg G, Duffy SW, Day NE. The Swedish two county trial of mammographic screening for breast cancer: recent results and calculation of benefit. *J Epidemiol Commun Health* 1989;**43**(2):107–14.
37. Miller AB, To T, Baines CJ, Wall C. The Canadian National Breast Screening Study-1: breast cancer mortality after 11 to 16 years of follow-up. A randomized screening trial of mammography in women age 40 to 49 years. *Ann Internal Med* 2002;**137**(5 Part 1):305–12.
38. Miller AB, Baines CJ, To T, Wall C. Canadian national breast screening study: 2. Breast cancer detection and death rates among women aged 50 to 59 years. *CMAJ* 1992;**147**(10):1477–88.
39. Frisell J, Eklund G, Hellstrom L, Lidbrink E, Rutqvist LE, Somell A. Randomized study of mammography screening—preliminary report on mortality in the Stockholm trial. *Breast Cancer Res Treatment* 1991;**18**(1):49–56.

40. Andersson I, Aspegren K, Janzon L, Landberg T, Lindholm K, Linell F, et al. Mammographic screening and mortality from breast cancer: the Malmo mammographic screening trial. *BMJ* 1988;**297**(6654):943–8.
41. Moss SM, Cuckle H, Evans AL, Johns L, Waller M, Bobrow L, et al. Effect of mammographic screening from age 40 years on breast cancer mortality at 10 years' follow-up: a randomised controlled trial. *Lancet* 2006;**368**(9552):2053–60.
42. Mandelblatt JS, Cronin KA, Bailey S, Berry DA, de Koning HJ, Draisma G, et al. Effects of mammography screening under different screening schedules: model estimates of potential benefits and harms. *Ann Internal Med* 2009;**151**(10):738–47.
43. Pace LE, Keating NL. A systematic assessment of benefits and risks to guide breast cancer screening decisions. *JAMA* 2014;**311**(13):1327–35.
44. Bailar III JC. Mammography: a contrary view. *Ann Internal Med* 1976;**84**(1):77–84.
45. Elmore JG, Barton MB, Moceri VM, Polk S, Arena PJ, Fletcher SW. Ten-year risk of false positive screening mammograms and clinical breast examinations. *New Engl J Med* 1998;**338**(16):1089–96.
46. Elmore JG, Wells CK, Lee CH, Howard DH, Feinstein AR. Variability in radiologists' interpretations of mammograms. *New Engl J Med* 1994;**331**(22):1493–9.
47. Elmore JG, Nakano CY, Koepsell TD, Desnick LM, D'Orsi CJ, Ransohoff DF. International variation in screening mammography interpretations in community-based programs. *J Natl Cancer Inst* 2003;**95**(18):1384–93.
48. Gotzsche PC, Jorgensen KJ, Maehlen J, Zahl PH. Estimation of lead time and overdiagnosis in breast cancer screening. *Br J Cancer* 2009;**100**(1):219. author reply 220.
49. Duffy SW, Lynge E, Jonsson H, Ayyaz S, Olsen AH. Complexities in the estimation of overdiagnosis in breast cancer screening. *Br J Cancer* 2008;**99**(7):1176–8.
50. Gotzsche PC, Jorgensen KJ. Screening for breast cancer with mammography. *Cochrane Database Systemat Rev (Online)* 2013;**6**:CD001877.
51. Zackrisson S, Andersson I, Janzon L, Manjer J, Garne JP. Rate of over-diagnosis of breast cancer 15 years after end of Malmo mammographic screening trial: follow-up study. *BMJ* 2006;**332**(7543):689–92.
52. Bleyer A, Welch HG. Effect of three decades of screening mammography on breast-cancer incidence. *New Engl J Med* 2012;**367**(21):1998–2005.
53. Tonelli M, Connor Gorber S, Joffres M, Dickinson J, Singh H, Lewin G, et al. Recommendations on screening for breast cancer in average-risk women aged 40–74 years. *CMAJ* 2011;**183**(17):1991–2001.
54. U.S. Food and Drug Administration. Consumer information (MQSA). *Radiation-emitting products.* <http://www.fda.gov/Radiation-EmittingProducts/MammographyQualityStandardsActandProgram/ConsumerInformation/default.htm>; 2014 [accessed 01.05.15].
55. U.S. Government Accountability Office. *Mammography services: impact of federal legislation on quality, access, and health outcomes.* Washington, DC: US General Accounting Office; 1997.
56. NIH Consensus Development Panel. National Institutes of Health Consensus Development conference statement: breast cancer screening for women ages 40–49, January 21–23, 1997. *J Natl Cancer Inst* 1997;**89**(14):1015–26.
57. Kolata G. Stand on mammograms greeted by outrage. *New York Times C* 1997;**1**:C8.
58. A resolution expressing the sense of the Senate concerning the need for accurate guidelines for breast cancer screening for women between the ages of 40 and 49. Snowe OJ, *trans. S.Res.47.* 105th Congress ed1997.
59. Norris SL, Burda BU, Holmer HK, Ogden LA, Fu R, Bero L, et al. Author's specialty and conflicts of interest contribute to conflicting guidelines for screening mammography. *J Clin Epidemiol* 2012;**65**(7):725–33.
60. Brawley O, Byers T, Chen A, Pignone M, Ransohoff D, Schenk M, et al. New American Cancer Society process for creating trustworthy cancer screening guidelines. *JAMA* 2011;**306**(22):2495–9.
61. U.S. Preventive Services Task Force. Screening for breast cancer: recommendations and rationale. *Ann Internal Med* 2002;**137**(5 Part 1):344–6.
62. International Cancer Screening Network. Breast Cancer Screening Programs in 26 ICSN Countries, 2012: Organization, Policies, and Program Reach. 2013; <http://appliedresearch.cancer.gov/icsn/breast/screening.html>; 2014 [accessed 04.09.14].

63. Hoffman RM, Lewis CL, Pignone MP, et al. Decision-making processes for breast, colorectal, and prostate cancer screening: the DECISIONS survey. *Med Decision Making* 2010;**30**(5 Suppl.):53S–64S.
64. Hawkes N. "Citizens' jury" disagrees over whether screening leaflet should put reassurance before accuracy. *BMJ* 2012;**345**:e8047.
65. Coulter A. UK citizen's jury advises on communication about the benefits and harms of breast screening. Healthnewsreview.org: Gary Schwitzer; 2013:Guest blog post.
66. Hersch J, Barratt A, Jansen J, Irwig L, McGeechan K, Jacklyn G, et al. Use of a decision aid including information on overdetection to support informed choice about breast cancer screening: a randomised controlled trial. *Lancet* 2015;**385**:1642–52.
67. Barlow WE, White E, Ballard-Barbash R, Vacek PM, Titus-Ernstoff L, Carney PA, et al. Prospective breast cancer risk prediction model for women undergoing screening mammography. *J Natl Cancer Inst* 2006;**98**(17):1204–14.
68. Gierach GL, Ichikawa L, Kerlikowske K, Brinton LA, Farhat GN, Vacek PM, et al. Relationship between mammographic density and breast cancer death in the Breast Cancer Surveillance Consortium. *J Natl Cancer Inst* 2012;**104**(16):1218–27.
69. Sprague BL, Stout NK, Schechter C, van Ravesteyn NT, Cevik M, Alagoz O, et al. Benefits, harms, and cost-effectiveness of supplemental ultrasonography screening for women with dense breasts. *Ann Internal Med* 2015;**162**(3):157–66.
70. Hall JM, Lee MK, Newman B, Morrow JE, Anderson LA, Huey B, et al. Linkage of early-onset familial breast cancer to chromosome 17q21. *Science* 1990;**250**(4988):1684–9.
71. Wooster R, Neuhausen SL, Mangion J, Quirk Y, Ford D, Collins N, et al. Localization of a breast cancer susceptibility gene, BRCA2, to chromosome 13q12-13. *Science* 1994;**265**(5181):2088–90.
72. Rockhill B, Spiegelman D, Byrne C, Hunter DJ, Colditz GA. Validation of the Gail et al. model of breast cancer risk prediction and implications for chemoprevention. *J Natl Cancer Inst* 2001;**93**(5):358–66.
73. Wald NJ, Hackshaw AK, Frost CD. When can a risk factor be used as a worthwhile screening test? *BMJ* 1999;**319**(7224):1562–5.
74. Hartmann LC, Degnim AC, Santen RJ, Dupont WD, Ghosh K. Atypical hyperplasia of the breast—risk assessment and management options. *New Engl J Med* 2015;**372**(1):78–89.
75. Elmore JG, Longton G, Carney PA, Geller BM, Onega T, Tosteson AN, et al. Diagnostic concordance among pathologists interpreting breast biopsy specimens. *JAMA* 2015;**313**(11):1122–32.
76. Pisano ED, Gatsonis C, Hendrick E, Yaffe M, Baum JK, Acharyya S, et al. Diagnostic performance of digital versus film mammography for breast-cancer screening. *New Engl J Med* 2005;**353**(17):1773–83.
77. Fenton JJ, Taplin SH, Carney PA, Abraham L, Sickles EA, D'Orsi C, et al. Influence of computer-aided detection on performance of screening mammography. *New Engl J Med* 2007;**356**(14):1399–409.
78. Rao VM, Levin DC, Parker L, Cavanaugh B, Frangos AJ, Sunshine JH. How widely is computer-aided detection used in screening and diagnostic mammography? *J Am College Radiol* 2010;**7**(10):802–5.
79. Fenton JJ, Lee CI, Xing G, Baldwin LM, Elmore JG. Computer-aided detection in mammography: downstream effect on diagnostic testing, ductal carcinoma in situ treatment, and costs. *JAMA Internal Med* 2014;**174**(12):2032–4.
80. Lehman CD, Wellman RD, Buist DS, Kerlikowske K, Tosteson AN, Miglioretti DL. Diagnostic accuracy of digital screening mammography with and without computer-aided detection. *JAMA Internal Med* 2015:1–10.
81. Fenton JJ. Is it time to stop paying for computer-aided mammography? *JAMA Internal Med* 2015:1–2.
82. Nass SJ, Henderson IC, Lashof JC. *Mammography and beyond: developing technologies for the early detection of breast cancer*. Washington, DC: National Academy Press; 2001.
83. Chang L. *Wisdom for the soul: five millennia of prescriptions for spiritual healing*. Washington, DC: Gnosophia Publishers; 2006.

CHAPTER

ESTIMATES OF SCREENING BENEFIT: THE RANDOMIZED TRIALS OF BREAST CANCER SCREENING

2

Heidi D. Nelson[1,2], Linda L. Humphrey[1,3] and Rongwei Fu[4]

[1]Pacific Northwest Evidence-Based Practice Center and Departments of Medical Informatics and Clinical Epidemiology and Medicine, Oregon Health & Science University, Portland, OR, United States, [2]Providence Cancer Center, Providence Health & Services, Portland, OR, United States, [3]Veterans Affairs Portland Health Care System, Portland, OR, United States, [4]Pacific Northwest Evidence-Based Practice Center and Departments of Public Health and Preventive Medicine, Medical Informatics and Clinical Epidemiology and Emergency Medicine, Oregon Health & Science University, Portland, OR, United States

CHAPTER OUTLINE

Breast Cancer Screening. DOI: http://dx.doi.org/10.1016/B978-0-12-802209-2.00002-4

PLAIN LANGUAGE SUMMARY

The benefits of mammography screening have been studied in nine randomized controlled trials comparing women screened with those not screened. Randomized controlled trials are regarded as the strongest type of study to determine whether screening is effective because they provide the most reliable results about the differences in outcomes between screening and nonscreening groups. It is important to appreciate the differences between the trials and their limitations in order to understand the results.

The trials began between 1965 and 1991, and involved over 600,000 women in the United States, Canada, United Kingdom, and Sweden. The trials varied in their recruitment of women, the numbers of women enrolled, and methods of assigning screening. Some trials enrolled only women in their 40s or 50s, while others included various broader age groups ranging from 39 to 74. In some trials, women were screened every 12 months, while others screened every 33 months. The lengths of screening varied from 4 to 10 years, and follow-up ranged from 11 to 25 years. The trials also differed in the ways they counted breast cancer cases and analyzed their results.

Several limitations of the trials have been recognized. An important concern has been whether the screening and control groups are truly similar at the start of the trials, as well as throughout their duration. Also, the relevance of the screening trials to current populations and practice is likely to have diminished over time. All of the trials were conducted in the past when imaging technologies and breast cancer therapies were markedly different than today. Whether results from trials using these outdated practices would be the same if they were conducted today is questionable. In addition, as with all research studies, the effects of screening for women in trials may be different than for women in the general population. Research has found that women who enrolled in some of the breast cancer screening trials were more educated and had higher risks of breast cancer compared with the general population.

When the results of the trials were combined using statistical methods, summary estimates indicated that death from breast cancer was lower for women undergoing screening compared to those who were not screened, but results varied by age. Results for women in their 40s and 50s were of borderline statistical significance and varied by how cases were counted in the trials. Trials did not enroll enough women age 70 and older to provide reliable results for older women. Assuming that differences actually exist, the estimates can be expressed as the number of breast cancer deaths prevented for 10,000 women screened for 10 years as: 3 deaths for women age 40–49; 5–8 deaths for age 50–59; and 12–21 deaths for age 60–69. The trials also reported that age-specific deaths from all causes, not just death from breast cancer, were not reduced with screening. Cases of advanced breast cancer were reduced for women age 50 and older, but not younger women.

Although the screening trials provide the strongest type of research to determine whether mammography screening is beneficial, the trials are outdated and may not represent current practices. Results indicate only small reductions in breast cancer deaths among women who were screened, but vary by age, with the largest effects (the most benefit) among women age 60–69.

INTRODUCTION

The benefits of mammography screening have been studied in nine main randomized controlled trials (RCT) beginning between 1965 and 1991, and involving over 600,000 women in the United States, Canada, United Kingdom, and Sweden. Trials provide estimates of the effectiveness of routine mammography screening by comparing breast-cancer specific mortality between women randomized to screening versus no screening. Additional outcomes related to benefit include reduced all-cause mortality and incidence of advanced breast cancer.

Age is an important factor in the design, analysis, and interpretation of the screening trials because the risk for breast cancer,[1] types of breast cancer,[2] and performance of screening technologies[3] differ by age. Accordingly, guideline development groups depend on age-specific evidence to provide screening recommendations. To address these issues, this chapter presents results of the trials according to the age of participants when available.

RCTs are regarded as the strongest study design to determine effectiveness, because a well-designed RCT is less susceptible to bias than other study designs.[4] Bias refers to any effect of the design or conduct of a study that systematically favors one comparison group over others. Studies with greater risks of bias are more likely to yield incorrect results. RCTs provide direct comparisons between screened and unscreened groups, while studies of women who are screened but not compared with unscreened women are unable to account for other factors that may explain outcomes.

Randomization is an important aspect of a RCT's design and refers to how participants are allocated to screening and control groups. A truly randomized method of allocation means that the assignment of screening or control groups is not predictable by the participant, researchers, and others. Randomization largely eliminates the problem of selection bias and associated confounding. With successful randomization and a large enough sample size, important confounders are equally distributed among comparison groups, including confounders that are unrecognized or not measured. Ideally, in this way, the comparison groups are similar except for whether they are screened or not, and differences in outcomes can be correctly attributed to screening.

In general, the strength of evidence is determined by judging how well individual studies were designed and executed to reduce bias, as well as their place on a study design-based evidence hierarchy (Fig. 2.1).[4] Results of appropriately performed RCTs are generally more reliable than results of nonrandomized or observational studies, and they are placed at the highest level of the evidence hierarchy. However, the evidence hierarchy assumes that RCTs are well conducted. A poor-quality RCT could yield results that are as or more misleading than those from studies lower in the evidence hierarchy. That is why it is important to critically evaluate and understand the quality of each trial and its contribution to the overall strength of evidence in order to determine the effectiveness of breast cancer screening.

BREAST CANCER SCREENING TRIALS

The nine main RCTs of breast cancer screening include the Health Insurance Plan of Greater New York (HIP) trial,[5] Edinburgh trial,[6] Canadian National Breast Screening Study 1 (CNBSS-1),[7,8] Canadian National Breast Screening Study 2 (CNBSS-2),[9,10] United Kingdom Age trial,[11] Stockholm trial,[12] Malmö Mammographic Screening Trial (referred to separately as MMST I and MMST II),[13] Gothenburg trial,[14] and Swedish Two-County Study (referred to separately as Östergötland and Kopparberg).[15] For some trials, results are sometimes combined (eg, Canadian) or provided separately (eg, CNBSS-1, CNBSS-2) leading to different ways of counting the number of trials. The descriptions of trials and metaanalyses in this chapter are based on a systematic review of the most recent trial results.[16,17] In these analyses, the number of trials was counted as the number of discrete data sources contributing to each summary estimate.

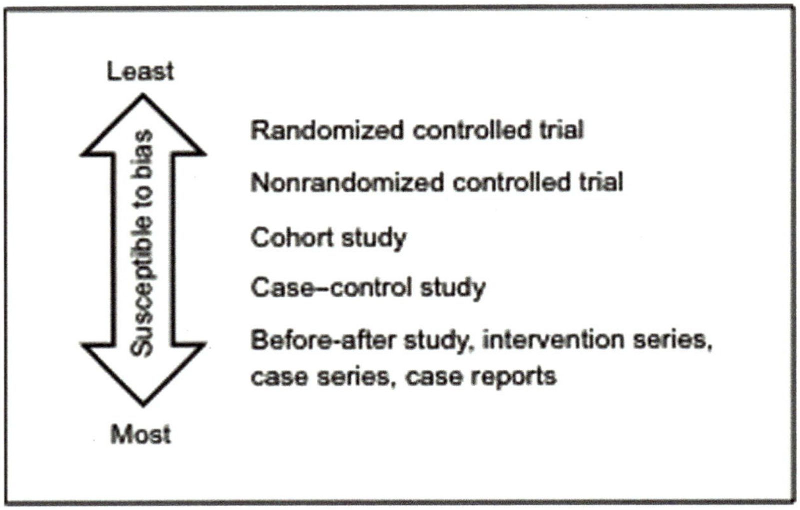

FIGURE 2.1

Hierarchy of evidence. The evidence hierarchy reflects the inherent strengths and limitations of different study designs and their susceptibility to bias. Results of studies least susceptible to bias, such as randomized trials, are generally more reliable than results of studies more susceptible, such as case series.

DESIGN AND METHODS

All trials were designed as RCTs, although they varied in their recruitment of participants and controls, sizes, methods of randomization, and screening protocols (Tables 2.1 and 2.2). Some trials enrolled only women in their 40s (CNBSS-1 and Age)[7,11] or 50s (CNBSS-2),[9] while others included various broader age ranges.[5,6,12–15] The two Canadian trials recruited volunteers, the Age trial identified women from general practice lists, and the HIP trial recruited women enrolled in a health insurance plan. The other trials enrolled participants based on their residence in communities.

The Gothenburg trial used individual (82%) and cluster (18%) randomization methods, and the Swedish Two-County and Edinburgh trials used cluster randomization by community. The other five trials randomized participants at the individual level with some stratifying randomization by age (HIP, CNBSS-1, CNBSS-2, Malmö), clinical center (CNBSS-1, CNBSS-2, Age), or other factors (HIP, Stockholm, Swedish Two County). Seven trials established control groups that received usual care. At the time of the trials, screening mammography was not usually provided as usual care, or only offered at specific age thresholds. Participants in the Canadian trials received baseline clinical breast examinations and instructions in breast self-examination before randomization to either screening or control groups.

None of the trials used digital or three-dimensional digital mammography (digital breast tomosynthesis) for screening. The HIP trial used direct-exposure film mammography and the other trials used screen-film mammography. The Age trial and four Swedish trials provided mammography alone, and the other trials provided mammography combined with clinical breast examination. Protocols varied,

Table 2.1 Breast Cancer Screening Trials

Trial	Age, *y*	Year Trial Began	Screening, *n*; Control, *n*[a]	Population	Comparison Groups	Method of Randomization
Health Insurance Plan of New York (HIP)	40–64	1965	30,239; 30,765	New York health plan members	Mammography + clinical breast examination vs usual care	Individual based on stratification by age and family size and drawn from a list
Canadian National Breast Screening Studies (CNBSS-1 & CNBSS-2)	CNBSS-1: 40–49; CNBSS-2: 50–59	1980	CNBSS-1: 25,214; 25,216; CNBSS-2: 19,711; 19,694	Self-selected from 15 centers in Canada	Mammography + clinical breast examination vs usual care[b]	Block stratified by center and 5-year age group
Edinburgh	45–64	1978	28,628; 26,015	All women from 87 general practices in Edinburgh, Scotland	Mammography + clinical breast examination vs usual care	Cluster based on general practitioner practices
Malmö Mammographic Screening Trial (MMST I & II)	43–69	1976–78	MMST I: 21,088; 21,195; MMST II: 9581; 8212	All women born between 1908 and 1945 living in Malmö, Sweden	Mammography vs usual care	Individual within birth year
Stockholm	40–64	1981	40,318; 19,943	Residents of Stockholm, Sweden	Mammography vs usual care	Individual by day of month
Swedish Two-County	40–70	1977	77,080; 55,985	Women from Östergötland and Kopparberg counties in Sweden	Mammography vs usual care	Cluster based on demographically homogeneous geographic units
Gothenburg	39–59	1982	21,650; 29,961	All women born between 1923 and 1944 living in Gothenburg, Sweden	Mammography vs usual care	Cluster based on day of birth for women born 1923–35 (18%); individual for women born 1936–44 (82%)
Age	39–41	1991	53,884; 106,956	Women from 23 National Health Service breast screening units in England, Scotland, and Wales	Mammography vs usual care	Individual stratified by general practitioner group[c]

Adapted from Ref. 16.
[a]*Numbers of participants in screening and control groups vary by publication.*
[b]*All women were prescreened with clinical breast examinations and instructed in breast self-examination. For women 50–59, usual care involved annual clinical breast examinations.*
[c]*Used random number generation between 1991 and 1992, then Health Authority computer system.*

Table 2.2 Protocols for Breast Cancer Screening Trials

Trial	Screening Interval, months	Rounds, *n*	Views, *n*	Adherence, %	Screening Duration, *y*	Controls Screened	Longest Follow-Up, *y*
Health Insurance Plan of New York (HIP)	12	4	2	46	4	After trial completed	18
Canadian National Breast Screening Studies (CNBSS-1 & CNBSS-2)	12	4–5	2	85	4.5	At age ≥50 after trials completed	25
Edinburgh	24	2–4 varied by cohort	1–2	61	2–8 varied by cohort	After 6–10 years, varied by cohort	10–14 varied by cohort
Malmö Mammographic Screening Trial (MMST I & II)	18–24	9	1–2	70	10+	After 14 years	11–13; 15.5
Stockholm	24–28	2	1	81	4.8	After 5 years	11.4
Swedish Two-County	24–33	3	1	84	7	After 7 years	20; 15.5
Gothenburg	18	5	1–2	75	9	After 5 years	12
Age	12	4–6, varied by center	2	57	9	At ages 50–52	17

Adapted from Ref. 16.

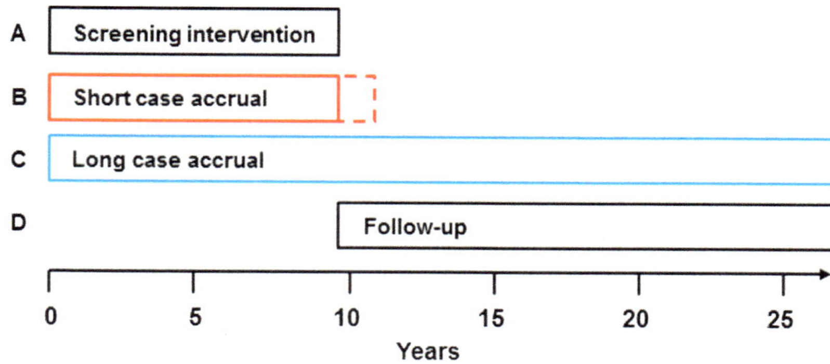

FIGURE 2.2

Methods of case accrual in trials. Short case accrual includes deaths occurring among cases diagnosed during the screening intervention period (A), and in some trials, within an additional defined case accrual period. Long case accrual includes deaths occurring among cases diagnosed during the screening intervention period plus the follow-up period (A + D).

Adapted from Ref. 16.

with screening intervals ranging from 12 to 33 months; rounds from 2 to 9; and durations from 4 to over 10 years. Follow-up ranged from 11 to 25 years.

Breast cancer mortality was the main outcome measure in all of the screening trials. Most trials also reported all-cause mortality and breast cancer incidence. Ductal carcinoma in situ (DCIS) was included in breast cancer case reporting for most trials (Gothenburg, Stockholm, Malmö, Swedish Two-County, Age, Edinburgh, HIP), while the Canadian trials included only invasive breast cancer in their latest update. All of the trials provided information on the stage, size, or lymph node involvement of cases. However, these outcomes were reported differently across the trials using various descriptions and levels of severity. All trials compared differences between screening and control groups using intention-to-screen analysis.

Two methods of accrual of breast cancer cases and deaths were used in determining outcomes in the trials (Fig. 2.2).[16,17] These methods affect the analysis of outcomes and are important to recognize when interpreting trial results. The long case accrual method counts all of the breast cancer cases contributing to breast cancer deaths diagnosed during the screening intervention period plus the follow-up period. This method has been referred to as the "follow-up" method of analysis by some investigators. While this method includes the most cases, it has the potential to dilute a true benefit because participants from the control group may have been screened after the study intervention period ended.

The short case accrual method includes only deaths occurring among cases of breast cancer diagnosed during the screening intervention period, and in some trials, within an additional defined case accrual period. This has been referred to as the "evaluation method" of analysis by some investigators. This method always involves the evaluation of fewer breast cancer cases for mortality outcomes because the duration of case accrual is shorter than for the long accrual method.

LIMITATIONS

Methodological limitations of the trials have been widely described. A major concern has been comparability of screening and control groups at the time of randomization, as well as maintenance of comparability during the trial and follow-up periods. For example, differences between baseline characteristics of participants in the Edinburgh trial have been considered important enough to invalidate its randomization.[6] For this reason, the results of the Edinburgh trial are usually not included in quantitative metaanalysis of the screening trials. However, few baseline characteristics were collected in most trials, and data are lacking to determine whether differences in important variables, such as family history of breast cancer, may actually exist.

Also, the clinical relevance (applicability) of the screening trials to current populations and practice is likely to have diminished over time. All of the trials were conducted in the past when imaging technologies and breast cancer therapies were markedly different than today. Whether the results of screening with film mammography, particularly with only one view as used in some trials, are similar to screening with two views using current technology is questionable. Also, advances in breast cancer treatment, particularly more widespread use of adjuvant therapies and new types of therapies, have improved mortality even for women diagnosed at later stages. As a result, the use of more effective treatments may have diminished the impact of screening.[18]

As with all clinical trials, the effects of screening in trial participants may not represent effects in general populations. Women who enroll in trials and attend screening interventions frequently differ from those who do not, underscoring the importance of intention-to-screen analysis to evaluate outcomes. Adherence rates varied widely across the trials, from 46% in the HIP trial to 85% in the Canadian trials. These differences provide additional insights when interpreting the results of the trials and considering their applicability to clinical populations.

Two trials that enrolled participants based on their membership in an insurance plan (HIP) or residence in a specific city (Stockholm) evaluated differences between women randomized to the intervention group who attended the screenings compared with those who did not attend. In these trials, attendees had higher risks of breast cancer and lower risks of all-cause mortality than nonattendees.[19,20] In the Canadian trials, volunteers were recruited from several communities. Compared with the general population, trial participants were more educated, had fewer pregnancies, and had overall higher risks for breast cancer.[7,9] These findings suggest that women who were more knowledgeable about breast cancer, recognized their individual risks, and were interested in improving their health were more likely to participate in mammography screening. These are important differences that could introduce bias and influence results.

INDIVIDUAL TRIALS

HIP of Greater New York

The HIP trial began in 1963, and was the first RCT of mammography screening.[5,20–24] Nonpregnant women age 40–64 without prior breast cancer with 1 year of membership in the insurance plan were eligible. Age and family size-stratified pairs of women were drawn from a list and individually randomized to either intervention or usual care control groups.

The intervention consisted of two-view film mammography, a clinical breast examination performed by a physician (usually a surgeon), and an interview to obtain relevant demographic information and health history. Adherence with the initial exam was 67% and only adherent women were offered subsequent screening with three annual exams. Independence between screening mammography, clinical breast examination, and interview results was strictly maintained. Few women in the control group had mammography screening during the trial. Cases of breast cancer were ascertained using insurance plan records, claims files, death records, cancer registry, and the National Death Index. All causes of death were determined by blind record review.

The two randomized groups were similar in terms of age, religion, marital status, prior pregnancies, and all-cause mortality. Although prior breast cancer was a prespecified exclusion criterion for entry, prior mastectomy status was more completely ascertained for the screening than control group, resulting in differences in the groups' sizes (30,239 vs 30,756) and potential noncomparability. However, when breast cancer deaths were evaluated, only deaths occurring among breast cancer cases diagnosed within the study period or in a defined period of observation were considered, depending on the analysis.

Information important for critical appraisal of the trial varied across over 40 publications. Limitations of the HIP trial include inadequate description of blinding, low adherence, inconsistent reporting of the numbers of participants in publications, and inadequate reporting of outcomes in screening and control groups.

CNBSS-1 and CNBSS-2

The CNBSS-1 evaluated the effectiveness of mammography, annual clinical breast examination by physicians or nurses, and breast self-examination instruction compared with usual care in reducing breast cancer mortality among women age 40–49.[7,8] The trial was conducted in 15 centers in Canada from 1980 to 1985. Volunteers without prior breast cancer or mammography in the prior 12 months were recruited using mass media advertising. After a clinical breast examination and instruction on breast self-examination, 25,214 women were randomized to receive two-view mammography plus clinical breast examination for 4–5 annual screens, and 25,216 women were randomized to usual care. Usual care was based on general care in the community that did not include routine mammography screening, and breast self-examination was reinforced for those returning to the clinical centers. Abnormalities detected during the study were evaluated through referral to the CNBSS review clinic, where the study surgeon reviewed the case and mammogram with the study radiologist and made recommendations to the participant's physician for evaluation and follow-up.

The CNBSS-2 was designed to determine the incremental benefit of adding mammography to annual clinical breast examination by physicians or nurses and breast self-examination instruction in reducing breast cancer mortality among women age 50–59.[9,10] Study participants were recruited through mass media advertising and randomized after clinical breast examinations to either annual clinical breast examination alone (19,694 participants) or annual clinical breast examination plus two-view mammography (19,711 participants) for 5 annual screens. In addition, breast self-examination instruction was provided at the first visit and reinforced at each screening visit for participants in both screening and control groups.

The Canadian trials differed from the other screening trials because they obtained medical histories and clinical breast examinations on all participants before randomization, and the trials enrolled volunteers with different breast cancer risk profiles and health habits than the general population, as detailed above in Limitations. Adherence for both trials was 85%. At the initial screen, more women age 40–49 had breast cancer with 4 or more positive nodes in the screening compared with the control group

(17 vs 5),[7] suggesting that groups may not have been entirely comparable. However, this could also be the result of mammography detection of advanced as well as early breast cancer and was observed in other trials as well.

Edinburgh trial

Edinburgh was one of the screening centers enrolled in the nonrandomized UK Trial of the Early Detection of Breast Cancer.[6,25] The investigators added a randomization component in 1978. The only exclusion criterion was prior breast cancer; however, this was generally ascertained after randomization. Women age 45–64 were identified from 84 general practices, stratified by practice, and cluster randomized to screening and control groups. Different cohorts were enrolled over time and the initial cohort experienced up to 4 rounds of screening, while the latest cohort had 2 rounds. A total of 23,226 women were randomized to baseline clinical breast examination and two-view mammography followed by annual clinical breast examination and biennial one-view mammography. The control group of 21,904 continued to receive usual care. Adherence with the initial screen was 61%, but lower with follow-up screening. Importantly, women in the control group had lower socioeconomic status and higher all-cause mortality than women in the screening group, suggesting inadequate randomization. The noncomparability of screening and control groups invalidates estimates of screening effectiveness from the trial.

MMST I and MMST II

The MMST I began in 1976 and included a 50% random sample of women age 44–69 identified in the Malmö population registry. These women were individually randomized by birth cohort to screening or usual care groups.[13,26,27] A total of 21,088 women were invited to screening with two-view mammography every 18–24 months for 2 rounds followed by either one- or two-view mammography thereafter (6–8 rounds), and 21,195 received usual care. In 1978, women age 43–49 were randomized in a similar fashion for the MMST II. This trial enrolled 9582 women to screening (1–7 rounds) and 8212 to control groups. Fourteen years after the trial began, screening was offered to women in the control group. Women previously treated for breast cancer were followed for breast cancer death and included only if a new breast cancer was diagnosed. A blinded endpoint committee determined causes of death by reviewing records and postmortem reports.

During the trial, mammography was available outside the screening program. A sample of 500 women in the control group indicated that 25% had mammography during the trial, but most had only one exam. However, these rates ranged from 13% among women age 60–69 to 35% among women age 45–49. Other limitations include inadequate descriptions of the randomization process and less than 75% adherence with screening. Also, additional details of MMST II are often inadequately described.

Stockholm trial

The Stockholm Trial began in 1981 and included women age 40–64 from the community.[12,28] Individual randomization was conducted by birth date. A total of 40,318 participants were invited to screening using one-view mammography for two screens separated by 24–28 months, and 19,943 received usual care. After the second screen in 1985, the control design of the study was broken and participants in the control group were invited for screening mammography in 1986. Adherence in the intervention group was approximately 81% for both screens, while 77% of the control group was screened after the second intervention screening.

The initial analysis of results evaluated mortality outcomes based on whether breast cancer was present at death, rather than as the cause of death. However, subsequent evaluations of causes of death by an independent and blinded committee indicated similar outcomes.[29]

Swedish Two-County Study

The Swedish Two-County Study began in 1977 and involved cluster randomization of women age 40–74 from Östergötland and Kopparberg counties.[15,30,31] The screening group included 77,080 participants, and the usual care group 55,985. Screening consisted of one-view mammography every 24 months for women age 40–49, and every 33 months for age 50–74. Overall adherence was 89% with the first invitation to screening and 83% for the second screening. After the second round of screening, invitations to women ages 70–74 were discontinued because of poor response rates. The control group was invited for screening approximately 7–8 years after randomization in 1985. In addition, 13% of women in the control group had mammography during the trial.

Causes of deaths were classified after full review of clinical and pathologic records. Although the review was originally not blinded, a blinded review was subsequently conducted.[29,32,33] Mortality rates were determined for all breast cancer cases diagnosed in both groups up to and including the first screen of the control group and a final screen of the screening group. The trial was limited by inadequate descriptions of blinding and lack of information to assess comparability of groups.

Gothenburg trial

The Gothenburg Trial began in 1982 to evaluate mammography screening among the entire female population of Gothenburg, Sweden born between 1923 and 1944 (age 39–59) without prior breast cancer.[14,34,35] Randomization was individual for 82% of participants and cluster for 18%. A total of 21,650 women were randomized to screening approximately every 18 months that included initial two-view mammography followed by one-view incident mammography unless two views were more appropriate based on the initial screen. Attendance at the first screening round was above 80% and varied by age. A control group of 29,961 women received usual care.

All breast cancer cases diagnosed up to and including the fifth screen of the screening group, and the first screen of the control group at approximately year 7, were followed for breast cancer mortality. After the trial was closed, women in both groups were invited to regular screening. Breast cancer cases were ascertained through treatment centers, pathology laboratories, and the national cancer registration system, and follow-up was conducted through 1996. Mortality from breast cancer was determined by the Swedish Cause of Death Register and two blinded independent endpoint committees.

Age trial

The Age trial was designed to evaluate the effectiveness of mammography screening for women in their 40s.[11] The trial enrolled 160,921 women age 39–41 stratified by group practice in the United Kingdom from 1991 to 1997. Women were randomized to screening with 7 rounds of annual mammography until age 48 or usual care. The baseline screen used two-view mammography and subsequent screens were one view. Follow-up was conducted through the National Health Service central register, and the analysis included deaths from breast cancer during the trial and during follow-up. Sixty eight percent attended the prevalent screen, and overall, 81% of women attended at least one screen. The mean number of screens in the trial was 4.5. Limitations include lack of reporting of the use of mammography in the control group and low adherence (<70%).

Trial	Relative risk (95% CI)
Malmö II	0.64 (0.39–1.06)
Kopparberg	0.73 (0.37–1.41)
Östergötland	1.02 (0.52–1.99)
Age	0.93 (0.80–1.09)
Gothenburg	0.69 (0.45–1.05)
HIP	0.75 (0.53–1.05)
Stockholm	1.52 (0.80–2.88)
Malmö I	0.74 (0.42–1.29)
CNBSS-1	1.04 (0.87–1.24)
Overall (I^2 = 24.0%, p = 0.230)	**0.92 (0.75–1.02)**

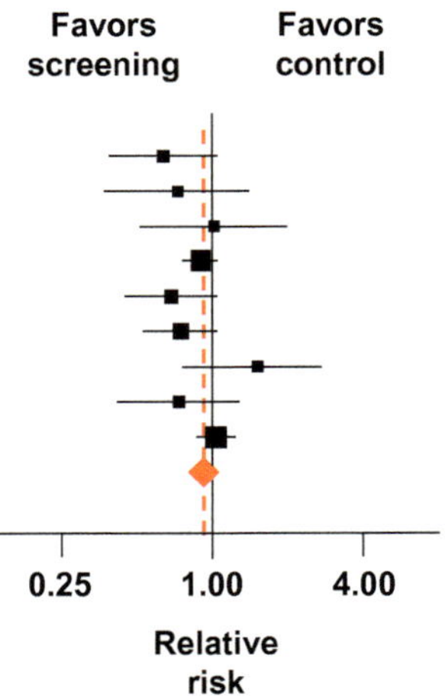

FIGURE 2.3

Effects of screening on breast cancer mortality age 40–49 years. Results of a metaanalysis of nine trials with estimates based on the longest case accrual methods available.

Adapted from Ref. 16.

BREAST CANCER MORTALITY OUTCOMES

RELATIVE RISK REDUCTION

Six trials reported breast cancer mortality outcomes by age using the long case accrual method (ie, breast cancer cases contributing to breast cancer deaths diagnosed during the screening and follow-up periods) (Swedish Two-County (Kopparberg and Östergötland),[15] Age,[11] Gothenburg,[14] and CNBSS-1 and CNBSS-2[36]). The HIP,[24] Malmö I,[37] Malmö II,[37] and Stockholm[37] trials used only short case accrual methods. Using the longest case accrual available across all trials, mean durations of screening were 3.5–18.8 years, case accrual 7.0–21.9 years, and follow-up 11.2–21.9 years.

Age-specific summary estimates of breast cancer mortality reduction were derived from metaanalyses that combined results from these trials.[16,17] For women age 40–49, neither the individual trials nor the combined estimate indicated statistically significant differences between screening and control groups (relative risk (RR), 0.92; 95% confidence interval (CI), 0.75–1.02; 9 trials)[14–17,24,36–38] (Fig. 2.3). Results for ages 50–59 (RR, 0.86; 95% CI, 0.68–0.97; 7 trials)[14,15,24,36,37] and 60–69 years (RR, 0.67; 95% CI, 0.54–0.83; 5 trials)[15,24,37] were consistent with statistically significantly lower risks of breast cancer death in the screening groups[15–17,24,37] (Fig. 2.4).

The numbers of women and events in the three trials providing results for women age 70–74 were much lower than for other age groups.[15,37] Neither the individual trials nor the combined estimate indicated statistically significant differences between screening and control groups (RR, 0.80; 95% CI, 0.51–1.28; 3 trials).[16,17]

The metaanalyses were repeated using estimates from trials with short case accrual methods to examine differences related to how outcomes were captured. Point estimates differed only slightly

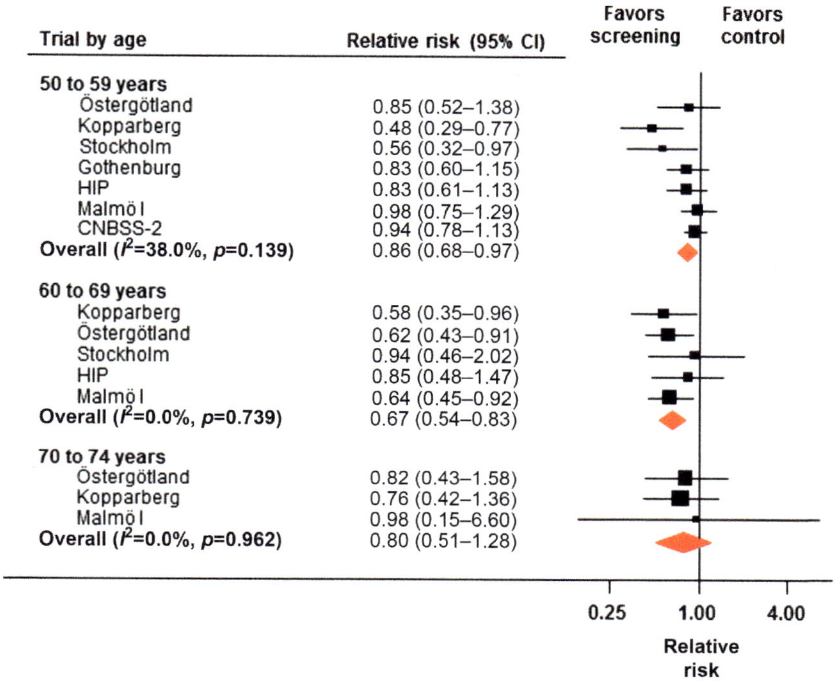

FIGURE 2.4

Effects of screening on breast cancer mortality age ≥50 years. Results of metaanalyses of trials with estimates based on the longest case accrual methods available.

Adapted from Ref. 16.

from those with long case accrual, although differences between screening and control groups for ages 40–49, 50–59, and 70–74 included or crossed 1.0[16,17] using this approach.

ABSOLUTE RISK REDUCTION

Absolute rates of breast cancer mortality reduction were derived from results of metaanalyses of RCTs (Fig. 2.5). Using estimates from the long case accrual metaanalyses, the numbers of deaths reduced (prevented) per 10,000 women screened for 10 years were 2.9 (95% CI, −0.6 to 8.9) for age 40–49; 7.7 (95% CI, 1.6 to 17.2) for age 50–59; 21.3 (95% CI, 10.7 to 31.7) for age 60–69; and 12.5 (95% CI, −17.2 to 32.1) for age 70–74.[16,17] Results for analyses of trials using short case accrual methods indicated lower absolute rates of risk reduction because fewer cancer cases were included in the calculation.

ALL-CAUSE MORTALITY

All-cause mortality outcomes were reported by all of the trials, although not all trials reported them according to age groups, and the CNBSS-1 and CNBSS-2 trials reported combined results (40–49 and 50–59). Individual trials indicated no statistically significant differences in all-cause mortality. Combining

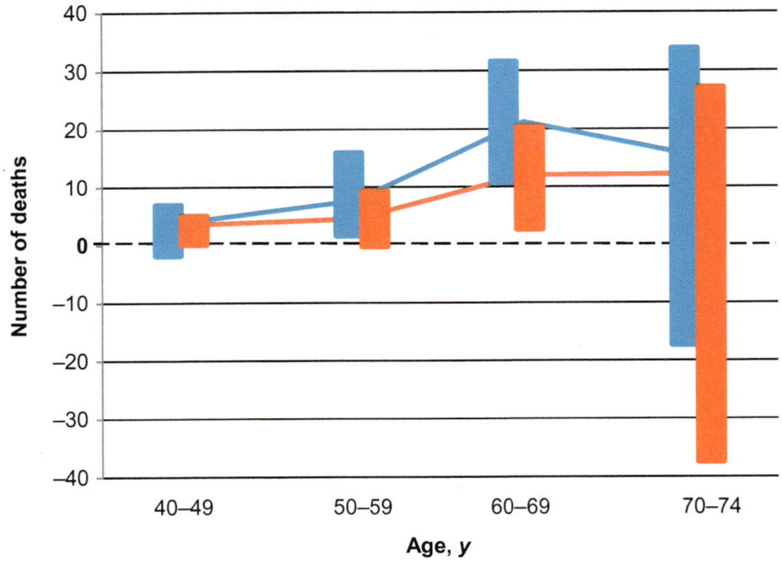

Number of deaths prevented for 10,000 women over 10 years (95% CI)

Case accrual	Age, *y* 40–49	50–59	60–69	70–74
Long (blue)	2.9 (−0.6 to 8.9)	7.7 (1.6 to 17.2)	21.3 (10.7 to 31.7)	12.5 (−17.2 to 32.1)
Short (red)	2.9 (0.1 to 6.5)	4.5 (−0.2 to 9.8)	12.1 (3.4 to 20.7)	12.2 (−37.7 to 26.9)

FIGURE 2.5

Age-specific rates of breast cancer mortality reductions with screening. Number of deaths prevented when 10,000 women are screened over 10 years based on results of trials included in the metaanalyses. Estimates using both the long (*blue line*) and short (*red line*) case accrual methods are included. Most estimates have confidence intervals that include 0 deaths except for women age 60–69.

all age groups, a metaanalysis of trials using the longest case accrual methods available indicated no differences between screening and control groups (RR, 0.99; 95% CI, 0.97–1.002; 9 trials)[11,16,17,22,36,37] (Fig. 2.6). Results were similar for each age group and when using short case accrual methods.[16,17]

EFFECTS OF SCREENING INTERVALS ON MORTALITY

No trials directly compared the effect of different screening intervals. The HIP, Age, and Canadian trials used mammography screening intervals of 12 months, while the Swedish Two-County trial had screening intervals ranging from 24 to 36 months that varied by age group. However, these trials differed by

Trial	Age, *y*	Relative risk (95% CI)
HIP	40–64	0.99 (0.93–1.05)
Gothenburg	39–59	0.94 (0.88–1.00)
Östergötland	40–74	0.98 (0.95–1.01)
Stockholm	40–64	0.99 (0.95–1.03)
Malmö II	43–49	1.03 (0.89–1.20)
Malmö I	45–70	0.99 (0.97–1.01)
Age	39–49	0.98 (0.93–1.03)
CNBSS-1 & 2	40–59	1.02 (0.98–1.06)
Overall (I^2 = 0.0%, *p* = 0.591)		0.99 (0.97–1.002)

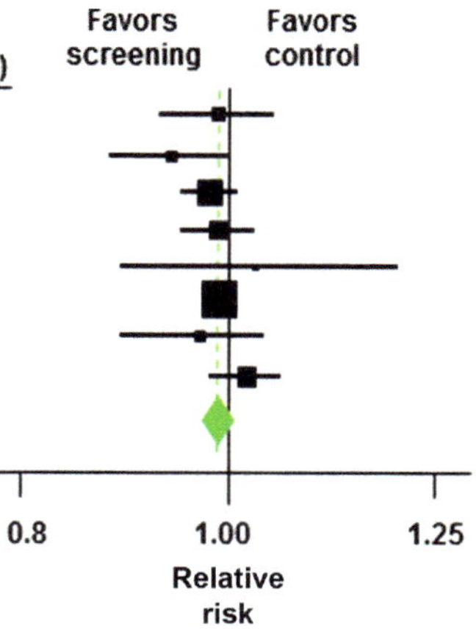

FIGURE 2.6

Effects of screening on all-cause mortality. Results of a metaanalysis of eight trials with estimates based on the longest case accrual methods available.

Adapted from Ref. 16.

many other factors, such as population, randomization, and adherence; and they did not provide enough information to determine the specific effects of screening intervals.

EFFECTS OF IMAGING MODALITY ON MORTALITY

No trials of screening using digital mammography, tomosynthesis, ultrasound, or MRI provide mortality outcomes. The HIP and Canadian trials combined mammography and clinical breast examination in the screening groups,[20,24,36] and women in the control group of the CNBSS-2 trial received clinical breast examinations. However, neither study was designed to determine the effectiveness of the combined versus single screening approach.

INCIDENCE OF ADVANCED BREAST CANCER

The incidence of advanced breast cancer is another clinically important outcome in determining the effectiveness of screening. The RCTs provided several measures including clinical stage (Stage 0–IV),[12,13,23,39] number of involved lymph nodes (0, 1–3, 4+),[7,9,14,15,40] and tumor size (mm),[8,10,15] although these measures varied across trials. However, most comparisons between screening and control groups using these categories provided differences between groups in relatively early stages of disease, rather than advanced stages.

A published analysis of trials defined advanced breast cancer as Stage II disease or higher, size 20 mm or greater, or having one or more positive lymph nodes.[41] These outcomes are all consistent with

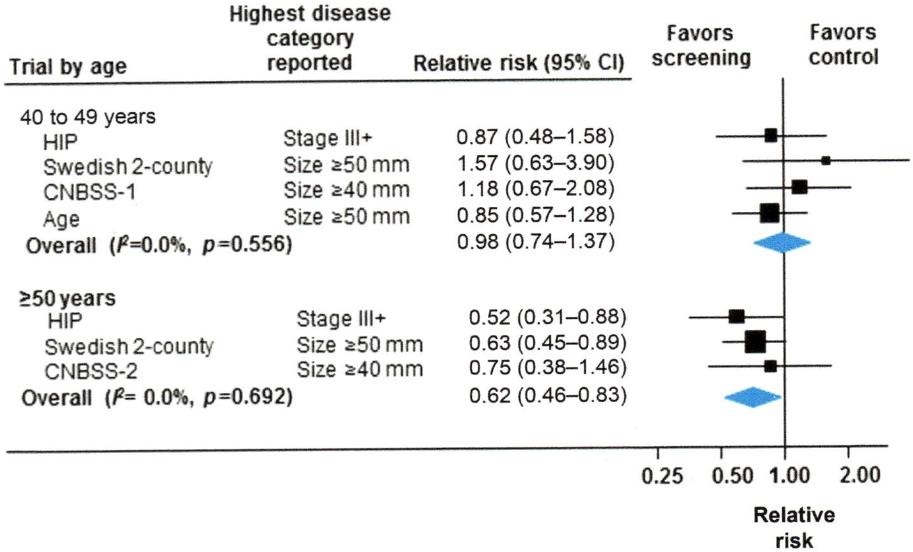

FIGURE 2.7

Effects of screening on advanced cancer outcomes. Results of metaanalyses of trials using the highest breast cancer disease category reported for each trial.

Adapted from Ref. 16.

Stage IIA disease (ie, localized) or higher according to the AJCC TNM system.[42] Using these definitions, the eight trials indicated statistically significantly reduced risks of node positive disease with screening for women age 39–49 in the Gothenburg trial[14]; and Stage II+ disease and large size tumors for women age 40–74 in the Swedish Two-County Study.[15] Other differences between screening and control groups were not statistically significant. Combining estimates based on these definitions of advanced cancer in a metaanalysis indicated no statistically significant overall differences between the screening and control groups.[16,17]

A separate analysis used higher levels of disease to define advanced breast cancer based on the most severe disease categories available in the trials.[16,17] These included Stage III and IV disease (ie, regional and metastatic), size 50 mm or greater, or having four or more positive lymph nodes. Combining estimates based on these definitions of advanced cancer in a metaanalysis indicated no difference with screening for women age 40–49 years (RR, 0.98; 95% CI, 0.74–1.37; 4 trials)[8,15,23,40]; but reduced risk of advanced cancer with screening for age 50 and older (RR, 0.62; 95% CI, 0.46–0.83; 3 trials)[10,15–17,23] (Fig. 2.7).

TREATMENT RELATED MORBIDITY

Outcomes related to breast cancer treatment provide another measure of benefit. Although these were reported by some of the screening trials, they may not be applicable to current practice because treatment has changed over time, practice standards vary, and patient preferences increasingly influence decisions. In a Cochrane review, treatments between randomized groups in five screening trials were compared, including the CNBSS-1, CNBSS-2, Malmö, Kopparberg, and Stockholm trials.[43] Results indicated that women randomized to screening were significantly more likely to have surgical therapy and radiation therapy, and less likely to have hormone therapy, while use of chemotherapy was similar between groups.

CONCLUSIONS

RCTs of mammography screening involving over 600,000 women provide the strongest evidence of the effectiveness of routine mammography screening by comparing breast cancer specific mortality between women randomized to screening versus no screening. Additional trial outcomes related to effectiveness include all-cause mortality and incidence of advanced breast cancer. However, the trials are limited by questions of the comparability of screening and control groups and how well participants in the trials represent women in the general population. Also, the clinical relevance of the trials to current cohorts of women, technologies, and treatments has likely diminished over time. In addition, each trial has inherent methodological limitations.

Regardless of these shortcomings, the trials provide an important foundation of the evidence base for mammography screening. Metaanalyses of the screening trials indicated reduced breast cancer mortality with screening that was dependent on age. Results for ages 40–49 and 50–59 years were of borderline statistical significance and varied depending on how cases were accrued in trials. Assuming that differences actually exist, the absolute breast cancer mortality reduction per 10,000 women screened for 10 years ranged from 3 for age 39–49 years; 5–8 for age 50–59 years; and 12–21 for age 60–69 years. Estimates for age 70–74 years were limited by low numbers of events in trials that had smaller numbers of women in this age group.

All-cause mortality did not differ between randomized groups in metaanalyses of trials, regardless of whether trials were analyzed in combined or separate age groups. Screening reduced advanced breast cancer outcomes (Stage III+IV disease, size $\geq$50 mm) for women age 50 years and older, but not for women in their 40s. This reduction in advanced cancer outcomes reinforces results indicating reductions in breast cancer mortality with screening for older women.

Several important questions have not been adequately addressed by the screening trials. Trials were not designed to evaluate the effectiveness of different screening intervals or imaging modalities, and none evaluated outcomes on the basis of risk factors besides age. Comparisons of different types of therapies in use at the time of the trials are not relevant to current practice because they are outdated. Additional research needs to focus on these gaps. New imaging technologies, such as tomosynthesis, are becoming more widely used without definitive studies of their effects on screening outcomes (further details in chapter: Evolution of Mammography Screening: From Film Screen to Digital Breast Tomosynthesis). Efforts to individualize screening decisions are limited by the lack of trial evidence to support effective approaches. Data for specific groups of women, based on risk factors, racial and ethnic background, access to screening, or existence of comorbidities, for example, could inform screening practices. Although trials indicated only slight benefit, if any, for screening women age 40–49, it would be important to determine whether benefits exist for specific women within this age group. Studies of older women are essential in order to determine appropriate screening regimens for them including when to discontinue screening (further details in chapter: Breast Cancer Screening in the Older Woman). Focusing on these areas could expand research beyond the landmark investigations of the initial screening trials and, ideally, lead to optimal screening practices.

ACKNOWLEDGMENTS

Miranda Pappas and Monica Daegas assisted with preparation of this chapter.

GLOSSARY

Absolute risk expresses risk for disease in terms of numbers in a population over a specified time period (eg, 2 per 1000 women over 1 year).

Adherence rate the proportion of participants in a trial who actually participate in the activities of the trial (eg, complete screening examinations and follow-up).

All-cause mortality mortality due to any cause of death.

Bias refers to any effect of the design or conduct of a study that systematically favors one comparison group over others. Studies with greater risks of bias are more likely to yield incorrect results.

Birth cohort all of the individuals born within a specified time period.

Blinding methods used to keep participants, health care providers, and other study personnel unaware of treatment assignments.

Breast-cancer mortality deaths due to breast cancer.

Clinical relevance (applicability) refers to how well the research findings from a study translate to other patient populations, settings, and circumstances.

Cluster randomization participants in a study are randomized according to the clinic they attend, area in which they live, or other similar factor.

Cochrane review a systematic review conducted by the Cochrane international collaborative using standardized methods.

Evidence hierarchy ranking of study designs based on their potential risk of bias and reliability of results. Well-conducted randomized controlled trials are considered the least biased study design.

Individual randomization participants in a study are randomized at the individual level.

Intention-to-screen analysis analyzing the results of the study according to the groups that participants were assigned, regardless of whether or not they were actually screened. This approach is critical because it preserves the benefits of randomization in minimizing selection bias.

Long case accrual method counts all of the breast cancer cases contributing to breast cancer deaths diagnosed during the screening intervention period plus the follow-up period. This method has been referred to as the "follow-up" method of analysis by some investigators.

Metaanalysis statistical methods to combine results from two or more studies to provide summary estimates.

Randomization the assignment of screening or control groups is not predictable by the participant, researchers, and others and important confounders are equally distributed among comparison groups, including confounders that are unrecognized or not measured.

Randomized controlled trial (RCT) provides direct comparisons between screened and control groups; is regarded as the strongest study design to determine effectiveness, because a well-designed RCT is less susceptible to bias than other study designs.

Relative risk (RR) expresses risk for disease in terms of one group of individuals compared to another (eg, women randomized to the screening group versus control group).

Short case accrual method includes only deaths occurring among cases of breast cancer diagnosed during the screening intervention period, and in some trials, within an additional defined case accrual period. This has been referred to as the "evaluation method" of analysis by some investigators.

Strength of evidence determined by judging how well individual studies are designed and executed to reduce bias, as well as their place on a study design-based evidence hierarchy.

LIST OF ACRONYMS AND ABBREVIATIONS

AJCC TNM	American Joint Committee on Cancer system based on tumor size (T), lymph node involvement (N), and presence of metastasis (M)
CI	Confidence interval
CNBSS-1	Canadian National Breast Screening Study 1
CNBSS-2	Canadian National Breast Screening Study 2
DCIS	Ductal carcinoma in situ
HIP	Health Insurance Plan of Greater New York
MMST	Malmö Mammographic Screening Trial
RCT	Randomized controlled trial
RR	Relative risk

REFERENCES

1. Altekruse S, Kosary C, Krapcho M, Neyman N, Aminou R, Waldron W, et al. *SEER Cancer Statistics Review, 1975–2007*. Bethesda, MD: National Cancer Institute. http://seer.cancer.gov/csr/1975_2007/, based on November 2009 SEER data submission, posted to the SEER web site; 2010.
2. Li CI, Uribe DJ, Daling JR. Clinical characteristics of different histologic types of breast cancer. *Br J Cancer* 2005;**93**:1046–52.
3. Kerlikowske K, Zhu W, Hubbard RA, Geller B, Dittus K, Braithwaite D, et al. Outcomes of screening mammography by frequency, breast density, and postmenopausal hormone therapy. *JAMA Intern Med* 2013;**173**:807–16.
4. Nelson HD. *Systematic reviews to answer health care questions*. Philadelphia, PA: Lippincott Williams & Wilkins, a Wolters Kluwer Business; 2014.
5. Shapiro S, Venet W, Strax P, Venet L, Roeser R. Ten- to fourteen-year effect of screening on breast cancer mortality. *J Natl Cancer Inst* 1982;**69**:349–55.
6. Alexander FE, Anderson TJ, Brown HK, Forrest AP, Hepburn W, Kirkpatrick AE, et al. 14 years of follow-up from the Edinburgh randomised trial of breast-cancer screening. *Lancet* 1999;**353**:1903–8.
7. Miller AB, Baines CJ, To T, Wall C. Canadian National Breast Screening Study: 1. Breast cancer detection and death rates among women aged 40 to 49 years. *CMAJ* 1992;**147**:1459–76.
8. Miller AB, To T, Baines CJ, Wall C. The Canadian National Breast Screening Study-1: breast cancer mortality after 11 to 16 years of follow-up. A randomized screening trial of mammography in women age 40 to 49 years. *Ann Intern Med* 2002;**137**:305–12.
9. Miller AB, Baines CJ, To T, Wall C. Canadian National Breast Screening Study: 2. Breast cancer detection and death rates among women aged 50 to 59 years. *CMAJ* 1992;**147**:1477–88.
10. Miller AB, To T, Baines CJ, Wall C. Canadian National Breast Screening Study-2: 13-year results of a randomized trial in women aged 50–59 years. *J Natl Cancer Inst* 2000;**92**:1490–9.
11. Moss SM, Cuckle H, Evans A, Johns L, Waller M, Bobrow L, et al. Effect of mammographic screening from age 40 years on breast cancer mortality at 10 years' follow-up: a randomised controlled trial. *Lancet* 2006;**368**:2053–60.
12. Frisell J, Lidbrink E, Hellstrom L, Rutgvist LE. Followup after 11 years—update of mortality results in the Stockholm mammographic screening trial. *Breast Cancer Res Treat* 1997;**45**:263–70.
13. Andersson I, Aspegren K, Janzon L, Landberg T, Lindholm K, Linell F, et al. Mammographic screening and mortality from breast cancer: the Malmö mammographic screening trial. *BMJ* 1988;**297**:943–8.

14. Bjurstam N, Bjorneld L, Warwick J, Sala E, Duffy SW, Nystrom L, et al. The Gothenburg Breast Screening Trial. *Cancer* 2003;**97**:2387–96.
15. Tabár L, Fagerberg G, Chen HH, Duffy SW, Smart CR, Gad A, et al. Efficacy of breast cancer screening by age. New results from the Swedish Two-County Trial. *Cancer* 1995;**75**:2507–17.
16. Nelson HD, Cantor A, Humphrey L, Fu R, Pappas M, Daeges M, Griffin J. *Screening for breast cancer: a systematic review to update the 2009 U.S. Preventive Services Task Force Recommendation*. Evidence Synthesis No. 124. AHRQ Publication No. 14-05201-EF-1. Rockville, MD: Agency for Healthcare Research & Quality; 2016.
17. Nelson HD, Fu R, Cantor A, et al. Effectiveness of breast cancer screening: systematic review and meta-analysis to update the 2009 U.S. Preventive Services Task Force Recommendation. *Ann Intern Med*, published online Jan 12, 2016.
18. Kalager M, Zelen M, Langmark F, Adami HO. Effect of screening mammography on breast-cancer mortality in Norway. *N Engl J Med* 2010;**363**:1203–10.
19. Lidbrink E, Frisell J, Brandberg Y, Rosendahl I, Rutgvist LE. Nonattendance in the Stockholm mammography screening trial: relative mortality and reasons for nonattendance. *Breast Cancer Res Treat* 1995;**35**:267–75.
20. Shapiro S, Venet W, Strax P, Venet L, Roeser R. Current results of the breast cancer screening randomized trial: the Health Insurance Plan (HIP) of greater New York Study. *Screening for Breast Cancer*. Toronto: Hans Huber; 1988.3.15.
21. Shapiro S. Periodic screening for breast cancer: the HIP Randomized Controlled Trial. *J Natl Cancer Inst Monogr* 1997;**22**:27–30.
22. Aron JL, Prorok PC. An analysis of the mortality effect in a breast cancer screening study. *Int J Epidemiol* 1986;**15**:36–43.
23. Chu KC, Smart CR, Tarone RE. Analysis of breast cancer mortality and stage distribution by age for the Health Insurance Plan clinical trial. *J Natl Cancer Inst* 1988;**80**:1125–32.
24. Habbema JD, van Oortmarssen GJ, van Putten DJ, Lubbe JT, van der Maas PJ. Age-specific reduction in breast cancer mortality by screening: an analysis of the results of the Health Insurance Plan of Greater New York study. *J Natl Cancer Inst* 1986;**77**:317–20.
25. Roberts MM, Alexander FE, Anderson TJ, Chetty U, Donnan PT, Forrest P, et al. Edinburgh trial of screening for breast cancer: mortality at seven years. *Lancet* 1990;**335**:241–6.
26. Andersson I, Janzon L. Reduced breast cancer mortality in women under age 50: updated results from the Malmö Mammographic Screening Program. *J Natl Cancer Inst Monogr* 1997;**22**:63–7.
27. Andersson I, Janzon L, Sigfusson BF. Mammographic breast cancer screening—a randomized trial in Malmö, Sweden. *Maturitas* 1985;**7**:21–9.
28. Frisell J, Eklund G, Hellström L, Lidbrink E, Rutgvist LE, Somell A, et al. Randomized study of mammography screening—preliminary report on mortality in the Stockholm trial. *Breast Cancer Res Treat* 1991;**18**:49–56.
29. Nyström L, Rutqvist LE, Wall S, Lindgren A, Lindgvist M, Ryden S, et al. Breast cancer screening with mammography: overview of Swedish randomised trials. *Lancet* 1993;**341**:973–8.
30. Tabár L, Chen HH, Fagerberg G, Duffy SW, Smith TC. Recent results from the Swedish Two-County Trial: the effects of age, histologic type, and mode of detection on the efficacy of breast cancer screening. *J Natl Cancer Inst Monogr* 1997;**22**:43–7.
31. Tabár L, Vitak B, Chen HH, Duffy SW, Yen MF, Chian CF, et al. The Swedish Two-County Trial twenty years later. Updated mortality results and new insights from long-term follow-up. *Radiol Clin North Am* 2000;**38**:625–51.
32. Rohan TE, Jain M, Howe GR, Miller AB. A cohort study of dietary carotenoids and lung cancer risk in women (Canada). *Cancer Causes Control* 2002;**13**:231–7.
33. Tabár L, Fagerberg G, Duffy SW, Day NE. The Swedish two county trial of mammographic screening for breast cancer: recent results and calculation of benefit. *J Epidemiol Community Health* 1989;**43**:107–14.

34. Bjurstam N, Bjorneld L, Duffy SW, Smith TC, Cahlin E, Erikson O, et al. The Gothenburg Breast Cancer Screening Trial: preliminary results on breast cancer mortality for women aged 39-49. *J Natl Cancer Inst Monogr* 1997;**22**:53–5.
35. Bjurstam N, Bjorneld L, Duffy SW, Smith TC, Cahlin E, Eriksson O, et al. The Gothenburg breast screening trial: first results on mortality, incidence, and mode of detection for women ages 39–49 years at randomization. *Cancer* 1997;**80**:2091–9.
36. Miller AB, Wall C, Baines CJ, Sun P, To T, Narod SA. Twenty five year follow-up for breast cancer incidence and mortality of the Canadian National Breast Screening Study: randomised screening trial. *BMJ* 2014;**348**:g366.
37. Nyström L, Andersson I, Bjurstam N, Frisell J, Nordenskjold B, Rutgvist LE, et al. Long-term effects of mammography screening: updated overview of the Swedish randomised trials. *Lancet* 2002;**359**:909–19.
38. Moss S, Wale C, Smith R, Evans A, Cuckle H, Duffy SW. Effect of mammographic screening from age 40 years on breast cancer mortality in the UK Age trial at 17 years' follow-up: a randomised controlled trial. *Lancet Oncol* 2015;**16**:1123–32.
39. Duffy SW, Tabár L, Vitak B, Yen MF, Warwick J, Smith RA, et al. The Swedish Two-County Trial of mammographic screening: cluster randomisation and end point evaluation. *Ann Oncol* 2003;**14**:1196–8.
40. Moss S, Thomas I, Evans A, Thomas B, Johns L, Trial Management Group. Randomised controlled trial of mammographic screening in women from age 40: results of screening in the first 10 years. *Br J Cancer* 2005;**92**:949–54.
41. Autier P, Hery C, Haukka J, Boniol M, Byrnes G. Advanced breast cancer and breast cancer mortality in randomized controlled trials on mammography screening. *J Clin Oncol* 2009;**27**:5919–23.
42. Edge S, Byrd DR, Compton C, Fritz AG, Greene FL, Trotti A. *AJCC cancer staging manual*, 7th ed. New York, NY: Springer; 2010.
43. Gotzsche PC, Jorgensen KJ. Screening for breast cancer with mammography. *Cochrane Database Syst Rev* 2013;**6**:CD001877.

CHAPTER

3

WEIGHING THE BENEFITS AND HARMS: SCREENING MAMMOGRAPHY IN THE BALANCE

Mireille J. M. Broeders[1,2], Theodora M. Ripping[1] and Rebecca A. Hubbard[3]

[1]Radboud Institute for Health Sciences, Radboud University Medical Center, Nijmegen, The Netherlands, [2]Dutch Reference Centre for Screening, Nijmegen, The Netherlands, [3]Department of Biostatistics and Epidemiology, Perelman School of Medicine, University of Pennsylvania, Philadelphia, PA, United States

CHAPTER OUTLINE

Breast Cancer Screening. DOI: http://dx.doi.org/10.1016/B978-0-12-802209-2.00003-6

PLAIN LANGUAGE SUMMARY

Breast cancer affects millions of women worldwide. Screening mammography has the potential to detect breast cancer early, leading to more effective treatment, reduced chance of metastasis, and better survival and quality of life for the patient. Large trials performed in the 1970s and 1980s showed that breast cancer mortality was lower in women who were invited for mammography screening. This led to widespread implementation of breast cancer screening, predominantly in Western Europe and North America. However, the implementation of screening introduced harms in addition to benefits. The major harm of breast cancer screening is overdiagnosis, the detection of a breast cancer that would never have become symptomatic during a woman's lifetime in the absence of screening. False-positive test results, a positive screening mammography result in a woman who does not have breast cancer, are the most common harm. Over recent decades, a debate has been ongoing as to whether the benefits of breast cancer screening outweigh the harms. In an effort to guide decision-making, a number of organizations have summarized the available evidence in reviews, balance sheets, and screening recommendations, aiming to help women and their physicians make an informed choice about screening. Despite the fact that all reviews are based on evidence from similar sets of trials and observational studies, some have concluded that screening should be stopped, while others recommend continuation of screening activities. In this chapter, we show that the differences between these reviews are at least partly related to choices about which studies to include, which screening strategies to consider, and how screening harms and benefits are defined. One of the challenges is that estimates of breast cancer mortality reduction due to screening are generally based on "old trials" and do not consider more recent observational studies that have evaluated mortality reductions using data from modern screening programs. Harms, on the other hand, are almost exclusively assessed based on today's screening practice. Another factor that complicates the comparability of the reviews is that the benefits and harms are not expressed in the same way, using different measures and populations. Finally, there are differences across countries in the organization of health care, cultural factors, and medicolegal considerations that shift the relative balance of harms and benefits. This is best illustrated in the large difference in the risk of a false-positive screening result, which is much higher in the United States compared to Europe. Future evaluations of the benefits and harms of breast cancer screening should base estimates of breast cancer mortality, overdiagnosis, and false-positives on the same screening setting, including time period, age, screening test, screening frequency, and organization of screening. If the aim is to compare the balance of harms and benefits between countries, it is important to ensure that the balances are indeed comparable. Finally, those creating or applying balance sheets should be aware that additional challenges lie ahead with the implementation of new screening tests and more personalized screening strategies. All of these are likely to affect the current balance of benefits and harms.

INTRODUCTION

The primary aim of breast cancer screening is to reduce mortality from the disease, but it is well-understood that screening does harm as well as good. Mammography is the preferred screening test for early detection of breast cancer and has been studied in more than 600,000 women in 11 randomized trials over the past 50 years. Over the past several decades, mammographic breast cancer screening has been the subject of controversy, with some questioning whether the benefit in terms of mortality reduction is large enough to justify the recognized harms of screening, in particular overdiagnosis.[1] Others reviewing essentially the same accumulated evidence have concluded that the pros outweigh the cons.[2]

In light of this debate, this chapter focuses on reviews that evaluate the balance of screening mammography benefits and harms that have been used to guide decision-making or provide recommendations for breast cancer screening. We have selected the reviews to represent evidence from different settings where screening practices vary, but acknowledge that many more reviews could potentially have been included. In this sense, the selected reviews serve as examples to illustrate how researchers and decision-makers reach conclusions on the balance of benefits and harms. This provides the background for a discussion of the methodologies used to determine this information and present results and conclusions.

The balance of the benefits and harms of a breast screening program can be communicated in a number of ways and to a variety of audiences. The format depends on the purpose of the balance and the intended audience. In this chapter, the focus is on benefit/harm balance sheets as presented in the scientific literature rather than communication to individual women or decision-makers. However, these scientific balance sheets should serve as the primary source of information for estimates communicated to women in the target population, health professionals and policy-makers. Outcome measures may be chosen according to the purpose of communication, but by necessity should be based on the same evidence. However, recommendations based on the same evidence may still differ, depending on the relative weight that is placed on different outcomes.

BENEFITS

BREAST CANCER MORTALITY REDUCTION

Screening mammography aims to reduce breast cancer mortality through detection and treatment of tumors at an early stage, leading to better survival than symptomatically detected tumors. As such, there is agreement across all reviews presenting a harm/benefit balance sheet on relative or absolute reductions in breast cancer mortality as the main benefit of screening. Nevertheless, some authors have suggested adopting all-cancer or all-cause mortality as the main outcome measure in order to avoid overestimation of the benefit due to bias in cause-of-death classification.[3] Several studies have explicitly assessed the quality of cause-of-death determination in relation to mammographic screening and have found no significant evidence of bias.[4–6] Further, the randomized trials of screening mammography were not designed to estimate overall or all-cancer mortality and were thus not powered to adequately estimate these outcome measures. Absence of evidence for an effect on these outcomes can thus not be taken to indicate evidence for absence of an effect. Estimates of screening benefit from randomized trials and observational studies are further detailed in chapters "Estimates of Screening Benefit: The Randomized Trials of Breast Cancer Screening" and "The Importance of Observational Evidence to Estimate and Monitor Mortality Reduction From Current Breast Cancer Screening," respectively.

Effects of screening on breast cancer mortality can be quantified as lives saved or life-years saved. Evidence reviews typically translate decreases in breast cancer mortality risk into absolute effects in terms of lives saved. However, since absolute risk is higher among older women, most of the benefit accrues at older ages in which the total number of life-years saved may be relatively small.[7] Life-years saved attributable to breast cancer screening have been reported by some cost-effectiveness analyses,[8] but are not generally included in evidence reviews.

OTHER BENEFITS

Early detection of breast cancer only confers benefit if it is followed by appropriate treatment, resulting in a more favorable outcome than would have been achieved had the treatment been given later in the course of disease or not at all. Early detection and treatment are also expected to improve quality of life for the women diagnosed, since less invasive procedures are more likely to be an option when the tumor is detected at a more favorable stage, for example, breast conserving surgery as opposed to mastectomy. Thus the majority of women participating in screening do not experience a benefit, and even those with a screen-detected cancer benefit only if earlier treatment leads to reduced morbidity and mortality. Although improved quality of life is expected to result from screening for some women, this benefit is not typically considered in balance sheets.

Since the ultimate impact of service screening on breast cancer mortality is inevitably long term, there are several indicators that can assess the performance of a screening program in its early phases and that can also be used to predict whether an effect on breast cancer mortality is likely. These early benefits are mostly related to the stage shift that is introduced with screening and is expected to result in a higher rate of small cancers and a lower rate of advanced cancers.[9] Although these measures are intuitive, there are many methodological challenges associated with their definition and interpretation.[10,11] Moreover, assumptions need to be made in order to estimate their consequent effect on breast cancer mortality.[2] The latter may explain why these outcomes are not usually considered in the evidence reviews.

HARMS

OVERDIAGNOSIS AND OVERTREATMENT

Overdiagnosis, and resulting overtreatment, is regarded as the major harm of breast cancer screening. In cancer screening, overdiagnosis is defined as the detection of cancers that would not present symptomatically during one's lifetime in the absence of screening. Although there is ongoing research focusing on identification of overdiagnosed tumors,[12] at present the extent of overdiagnosis can only be estimated on the population level by comparing breast cancer incidence in the presence and absence of screening or by using simulation models.

Overdiagnosis is harmful in two major ways. The first harm is simply due to the unnecessary detection of a breast cancer. This diagnosis transforms women into cancer patients, a transformation that would not have taken place in the absence of screening. The second and major harm of overdiagnosis is overtreatment. Although some tumors will not become life-threatening during the life span of the woman, it is currently not possible to distinguish dangerous from nonlife-threatening cancers. As a consequence, women with an overdiagnosed cancer receive unnecessary treatment, referred to as overtreatment. To prevent unnecessary treatment, a few trials have begun to compare usual care with active surveillance, a "wait-and-see"-procedure, for cancers that have a high risk of being overdiagnosed, that is, low-grade ductal carcinoma in situ (DCIS). In a "wait-and-see"-procedure cancers are only treated if and when they progress.[13,14]

The extent of overdiagnosis in breast cancer screening remains highly uncertain, with estimates ranging from 0% to 54%.[15,16] A major reason for this disagreement is the difficulty in estimating overdiagnosis. Overdiagnosis in cancer screening can be estimated with a variety of study designs, including randomized trials, pathological or imaging studies, modeling studies, and observational studies.[15,17]

In breast cancer screening, the most common designs are randomized trials,[2,3] observational studies,[16] and modeling studies.[17,18] However, each design has limitations. In randomized trials and observational studies, overdiagnosis is estimated by comparing breast cancer incidence in the presence and absence of screening. Breast cancer screening works by identifying cancers at an earlier, more treatable stage. As a result, after the initiation of screening there will be a transient increase in breast cancer incidence. In the absence of overdiagnosis, this increased incidence will be compensated for by a subsequent decrease in cancer diagnoses.[15] To determine if the cancers diagnosed during screening were attributable to early detection or overdiagnosis, women should be followed after leaving screening to account for this effect. Ideally, this follow-up after leaving screening should be until death.[2] In randomized trials, there may be incomplete adjustment for early detection, although women were followed for 15 years after leaving screening in the Canadian trials[19] and in the Malmö trial.[20] This leads to overestimation of the extent of overdiagnosis. In observational studies, longer follow-up periods are possible, but there is no comparable population that is not offered screening. As a result, breast cancer incidence in the absence of screening is estimated using extrapolation of prescreening trends,[21] control regions,[22] nonattenders,[23,24] or adjustment for the effect of screening.[25] Because unscreened populations may differ from screened populations in characteristics that are also related to breast cancer incidence, all observational studies of overdiagnosis have the potential for bias. The primary limitation of using modeling studies to estimate overdiagnosis is the heavy dependence of overdiagnosis estimates from these studies on modeling assumptions such as lead time.[15]

FALSE-POSITIVES

False-positive test results are the most common harm of screening mammography. Conceptually, a false-positive is defined as a positive screening mammography result in a woman who is cancer free. In the United States and other settings where screening mammography interpretation is performed according to the American College of Radiology Breast Imaging Reporting And Data Systems (BI-RADS) Atlas,[26] a positive examination has been operationalized as a screening mammography initial assessment of 0:Needs Additional Evaluation, 3:Probably Benign, 4:Suspicious, or 5:Highly Suggestive of Malignancy. In organized screening programs such as those in Europe and Australia, a positive screening result is defined by recall for further evaluation. Typically, recalled women who are determined to be cancer free at the end of diagnostic evaluation and for 1 year after the recall are considered to have experienced a false-positive. False-positive results can be subdivided into those receiving further evaluation with imaging only and those that undergo invasive procedures including biopsy or fine needle aspiration.

False-positive test results have a number of negative consequences. The greater the false-positive risk, the lower the efficiency of the screening program and the more unnecessary imaging is performed. This adds to the overall resource use and cost of screening. False-positives also have negative psychological consequences for the affected women. Studies have found that women receiving false-positive test results experience increased anxiety and psychological distress.[27] This anxiety and distress is greater in women who undergo invasive procedures rather than additional imaging only.[28] However, a recent study found that the associated anxiety resolved quickly once the women were determined to be cancer free.[29] The experience of receiving false-positive test results can also be a deterrent to participation in future screening. This has been found to be the case in several of the organized screening programs in Europe and Canada.[30] Conversely, in the United States women receiving false-positive test results have been found to be more likely to return for future screening.[31] Finally, false-positive results lead to additional radiation exposure through subsequent mammography and mammography-guided biopsy. Although radiation exposure due to mammography is small,[32–35] the aggregate burden among women experiencing repeated false-positives could become large and should be minimized to avoid the increased risk of radiation-induced cancer.

False-positive screening mammography results are common, occurring in approximately 10% of exams in the United States[36] and 1–7% of mammograms in European service screening programs.[37] False-positives are generally more common in younger women and those with dense breasts.[36] Because false-positive mammography results are common, the proportion of women participating in regular screening who receive a false-positive result over the course of their screening participation is large. Most evaluations of the balance of harms and benefits have quantified this harm in terms of the cumulative false-positive risk of screening mammography, defined as the probability that a woman will receive at least one false-positive mammography result over the course of a fixed number of screening mammograms, typically either 10 or the total number recommended by the screening program.

OTHER HARMS

There are a variety of screening mammography harms that are not typically explicitly included when evaluating the balance of benefits and harms. When considering the harms of screening, it is important to consider not only direct harms but harms that result indirectly from downstream effects of the screening process, such as unnecessary treatment resulting from incidental findings.[38] However, evidence reviews have not typically included indirect harms.

Additional direct harms not typically considered by evidence reviews, can be divided into harms that are serious but very rare and those that are common but have a generally minor impact. A false-negative screening mammography result is one harm that is very serious but relatively rare. A false-negative occurs when a woman is diagnosed with cancer following a negative screening mammography assessment (in the BI-RADS lexicon, an assessment of 1:Negative or 2:Benign). A negative mammography result could give a woman false reassurance that she is cancer free and may lead to delays in seeking care for new symptoms.[39] Some evaluations of screening mammography include measures of the diagnostic accuracy of screening mammography interpretation, which typically provide an assessment of false-negatives at a single screening round.[36,40–42] However, these are not commonly included in evaluations of the balance of harms and benefits. Radiation-induced cancer is another harm that is very serious but considered extremely rare.[34,43] Radiation-induced cancer may be more of a concern in women with very large breasts or breast augmentation who require extra views at each exam for full coverage of breast tissue.[35] Additional minor harms of screening mammography include the pain of the examination itself. A systematic review found that 28–77% of women report experiencing pain associated with mammography.[32] Pain due to mammography has been found to be associated with discontinuation of screening.[44]

REVIEWING THE BALANCE OF HARMS AND BENEFITS

We have selected a number of influential reviews from North America and Europe to serve as examples for the comparison of reviews of benefits and harms of breast cancer screening. In this section, we will describe the context of these reviews, the general approach adopted by the authors, the sources of data used and the main outcomes of the reviews, both in relative and absolute measures. Tables 3.1–3.3 summarize the data from these reviews for breast cancer mortality, overdiagnosis, and the cumulative risk of false-positives.

NORTH AMERICA

In North America, the landscape of guidelines for screening mammography is characterized by recommendations from numerous groups. A variety of independent panels, professional societies, and advocacy groups issue screening recommendations. Several of these conduct an evaluation of the balance of harms and benefits in order to support their recommendations, while others rely on existing evaluations. Canadian provinces offer a defined screening mammography program to women age 50–69 but practices for younger and older women vary across provinces. No defined screening program exists in the United States, where it is left to individual providers and patients to make decisions that are informed by recommendations. Guidelines issued by the US Preventive Services Task Force (USPSTF) are particularly influential because they inform Medicare coverage decisions and many private insurers follow the same coverage practices as the Center for Medicare and Medicaid Services. Below we summarize the evidence review conducted by the USPSTF[45] as well as that of the Canadian Task Force on Preventive Health Care (Canadian Task Force),[46,47] a similar independent panel for Canada. Finally, we discuss the American Cancer Society (ACS) guideline statement[48] as an example of an influential North American organization issuing recommendations related to screening mammography.

US Preventive Services Task Force

The USPSTF is an independent panel authorized by the US Congress and supported by the Agency for Healthcare Research and Quality (AHRQ) to make evidence-based recommendations about clinical preventive services. The USPSTF commissioned a review of the evidence on benefits and harms of screening mammography in preparation for an update to their recommendations on screening mammography issued in 2015. The review included evidence on harms and benefits of mammography for all women age 40 years and older. Evidence on harms and benefits of other screening modalities including breast MRI and digital breast tomosynthesis was also reviewed. The USPSTF in conjunction with AHRQ developed the key questions used to structure the review. The review itself was then conducted by an independent contractor sponsored by AHRQ, the Pacific Northwest Evidence-based Practice Center.

The primary benefit of screening mammography as defined by the draft USPSTF evidence review was reduction in breast cancer mortality.[45] Other benefits considered included reductions in all-cause mortality, advanced breast cancer cases, and treatment-related morbidity. Harms were radiation exposure, pain during procedures, patient anxiety and other psychological responses, false-positive and false-negative test results, overdiagnosis, and overtreatment. Evidence on breast cancer mortality was obtained from randomized controlled trials of screening mammography in women age 40 and over. The evidence review identified eight eligible studies by searching the Cochrane Register of Controlled Trials, Cochrane Database of Systematic Reviews, and MEDLINE, as well as by manually reviewing references. Observational studies and systematic reviews were also included, although quantitative evaluation of breast cancer benefits was based on RCTs. A variety of evidence sources were used for evaluating harms. Systematic reviews and metaanalyses were included as well as recently published primary studies. Primary analysis of observational data on screening mammography from the Breast Cancer Surveillance Consortium (BCSC) was conducted to provide information on performance

Table 3.1 Breast Cancer Mortality in Evidence Reviews

	Study Designs Selected; Included Studies	Intervention (Study Period; Age Groups; Screening Test; Screening Interval)	Relative Effect	Absolute Effect
Cochrane	Randomized trials • 4/11 eligible trials included as adequately randomized: Malmo I, Canada I and II, UK age trial • 6/11 eligible trials included as suboptimally randomized: HIP, Malmo II, Kopperberg, Östergötland, Stockholm, Göteborg • Edinburgh trial excluded	• Adequately randomized trials: trials conducted between1976–1997; 293,135 women in age range 39–69; mammography with/without physical examination and/or self-examination; interval 12–24 months • Subadequately randomized trials: trials starting between 1963 and 1981; 355,796 women in age range 38–75; mammography and physical examination; interval 12–33 months	Four trials with adequate randomization did not show a statistically significant reduction in breast cancer mortality at 13 years (relative risk (RR) 0.90, 95% confidence interval (CI) 0.79–1.02); five trials with suboptimal randomization showed a significant reduction in breast cancer mortality with an RR of 0.75 (95% CI 0.67–0.83). The RR for all nine trials combined was 0.81 (95% CI 0.74–0.87) after 13 years. Malmo II trial excluded from 13-year follow-up analysis	Assuming a 15% mortality reduction: For every 2000 women invited for screening throughout 10 years, one will avoid dying of breast cancer
Independent UK Panel	Randomized trials. 10/11 eligible trials included. Edinburgh trial excluded	Trials conducted between 1963 and 1997; 648,931 women in the age range 38–74 years; mammography with/without physical examination and/or self-examination; interval 12–33 months	Metaanalysis of these trials with 13 years of follow-up estimated a 20% reduction in breast cancer mortality in women invited for screening (RR = 0.80, 95% CI 0.73–0.89)	• Assuming a 20% mortality reduction: For 10,000 UK women invited to screening from age 50 for 20 years, 43 deaths from breast cancer will be prevented • For every 10,000 women attending screening from age 50–70 years, about 56 deaths from breast cancer would be prevented

USPSTF	Randomized trials. Selection depends on age: • 39–49 years, 9/11 eligible trials included: HIP, Malmo I and II, Kopperberg, Östergötland, Canada I, Stockholm, Göteborg, and UK age trial • 50–59 years, 7/11 eligible trials included: Malmo I and II, Kopperberg, Östergötland, Canada II, Stockholm, and Göteborg • 60–69 years, 5/11 eligible trials included: Malmö I and II, Östergötland • 70–74 years, 3/11 eligible trials included: Östergötland, Kopparberg, Malmo I	• 39–49 years: Trials conducted between 1963 and 1997; 609,472 women in the age range 38–75 years; mammography with/without physical examination and/or self-examination; interval 12–33 months • 50–59 years: Trials starting between 1976 and 1981; 386,551 women in the age range 38–75; mammography with/without physical examination and/or self-examination; interval 12–33 months • 60–69 years: trials starting between 1976–1978; 112,298 women in the age range 43–75; mammography with/without self-examination; interval 18–33 months • 70–74 years: trial starting in 1978; 92,934 women in the age range 38–75; mammography with/without self-examination; interval 24–33 months	In metaanalysis, RR for breast cancer mortality in women age 39–49 based on nine trials was 0.88 (95% CI 0.73–1.003), for women 50–59 based on seven trials was 0.86 (95% CI 0.68–0.97), based on five trials for women 60–69 was 0.67 (95% CI 0.54–0.83), and for women 70–74 based on three trials was 0.80 (95% CI 0.51–1.28)	• Assuming a 12% mortality reduction: For every 10,000 women screened aged 40–49 for 10 years, four deaths from breast cancer will be prevented • Assuming a 14% mortality reduction: For every 10,000 women screened aged 50–59 for 10 years, eight deaths from breast cancer will be prevented • Assuming a 33% mortality reduction: For every 10,000 women screened aged 60–69 for 10 years, 21 deaths from breast cancer will be prevented • Assuming a 20% mortality reduction: For every 10,000 women screened aged 70–74 for 10 years, 13 deaths from breast cancer will be prevented

(Continued)

Table 3.1 Breast Cancer Mortality in Evidence Reviews (Continued)

	Study Designs Selected; Included Studies	Intervention (Study Period; Age Groups; Screening Test; Screening Interval)	Relative Effect	Absolute Effect
American Cancer Society	Metaanalysis of 9 randomized trials (13-year follow-up).[3] Metaanalysis of 14 observational studies: seven incidence-based mortality studies and seven case–control studies.[58] One modeling study providing seven estimates[71]	• Metaanalysis of RCTs: Trials published 1963–1991; 599,090 women age 39–74; screening mammography; interval not reported but available from the original study • Metaanalysis of population-based observational studies: Studies published 1997–2012; >2 million women age >40; screening mammography; interval not reported but available from the original study • Model-based estimates from seven models	• See Cochrane review: The RR for all nine trials combined was 0.81 (95% CI 0.74–0.87) after 13 years • See EUROSCREEN: Pooled estimates of breast cancer mortality reduction among invited women were 0.75 (95% CI 0.69–0.81) in incidence-based mortality studies and 0.69 (95% CI 0.57–0.83) in case–control studies. Estimates for women actually screened were 0.62 (95% CI 0.56–0.69) in incidence-based mortality studies and 0.52 (95% CI 0.42–0.65) in case–control studies, corrected for self-selection. Interval not reported but available from the original study • Model-based estimates: median reduction of 15% (range 7–23%)	• Assuming a 20% mortality reduction: 1770 women age 40–49, 1087 women age 50–59, and 835 women age 60–69 would need to be screened biennially for 15 years to prevent one breast cancer death • Assuming a 40% mortality reduction: 753 women age 40–49, 462 women age 50–59, and 355 women age 60–69 would need to be screened biennially for 15 years to prevent one breast cancer death
Canadian Taskforce	Randomized trials. 10/11 eligible trials included. Selection depends on age: • 39–49 years, 9/11 eligible trials included: HIP, Malmo I and II, Kopperberg, Östergötland, Canada I, Stockholm, Göteborg and UK age trial • 50–69 years, 8/11 eligible trials included: HIP, Malmo I and II, Kopperberg, Östergötland, Canada II, Stockholm, Göteborg • 70–74 years, 1/11 eligible trials included: Kopperberg, Östergötland	• 39–49 years: Trials conducted between 1963 and 1997; 211,270 women in the age range 39–74 years; mammography with/without physical examination and/or self-examination; interval 12–33 months • 50–69 years: Trials starting between 1976 and 1981; 250,274 women in the age range 50–69; mammography with/without physical examination and/or self-examination; interval 12–33 months • 70–74 years: trial starting in 1978; 17,646 women above 70; mammography with/without self-examination; interval 24–33 months	Pooled estimate of breast cancer reduction from eight trials in women 40–49 of 0.85 (95% CI 0.75–0.96), seven trials of women 50–69 of 0.79 (95% CI 0.68–0.90), and two trials of women 70–74 of 0.68 (95% CI 0.45–1.01). Results are reported after a median follow-up of 11.4 years	• Assuming a 15% mortality reduction: 2108 women aged 40–49 need to be screened to prevent one breast cancer death • Assuming a 21% mortality reduction: 721 women aged 50–69 need to be screened to prevent one breast cancer death • Assuming a 32% morality reduction: 451 women aged 70–74 need to be screened to prevent one breast cancer death

EUROSCREEN	Systematic search of PubMed up to February 2011; European observational studies, ie, trend studies ($n = 17$), incidence-based mortality (IBM) studies ($n = 20$) and case–control studies ($n = 8$)	Studies reporting on programs implemented between 1970 and 2007; including at least some of the age groups between 50–69; mammography; interval 2–3 years; population-based screening programs (study has at least a three years' overlap with the current regional or national program)	Pooled estimates of breast cancer mortality reduction among invited women were 0.75 (95% CI 0.69–0.81) in incidence-based mortality studies and 0.69 (95% CI 0.57–0.83) in case–control studies. Estimates for women actually screened were 0.62 (95% CI 0.56–0.69) in incidence-based mortality studies and 0.52 (95% CI 0.42–0.65) in case–control studies, corrected for self-selection	Assuming a 25–38% mortality reduction: For every 1000 women screened from age 50 to 69, seven to nine breast cancer deaths are prevented

Table 3.2 Overdiagnosis in Evidence Reviews

	Study Designs Selected; Included Studies	Intervention (Study Period; Age Groups; Screening Test; Screening Interval; Screening Organization)	Relative Effect	Absolute Effect
Cochrane	Randomized trials that did not invited the control group at the end of the screening phase (3/11: Malmö I, Canada I and II) and recent observational studies mentioned in discussion	Trials started screening between 1976 and 1980; 132,214 women in age range 40–69; mammography with/without physical examination and/or self-examination; interval 12–24 months	There were 30% more cancers in the screened groups than in the control groups. Large observational studies support these findings	Assuming 30% overdiagnosis: For every 2000 women invited for screening throughout 10 years, 10 healthy women who would not have had a breast cancer diagnosis if there had not been screening will be diagnosed as cancer patients, and will be treated unnecessarily
Independent UK Panel	Randomized trials that did not invited the control group at the end of the screening phase (3/11: Malmö I, Canada I and II)	Trials started screening between 1976 and 1980; 132,214 women in age range 40–69; mammography with/without physical examination and/or self-examination; interval 12–24 months	The frequency of overdiagnosis was of the order of 11% from a population perspective, and about 19% from the perspective of a woman invited to screening	Assuming 19% overdiagnosis from an individual women perspective: For every 10,000 UK women invited to screening from age 50 for 20 years, 129 cancers will be overdiagnosed
USPSTF	A review of eight trials,[72] a metaanalysis of three trials,[2,50] a systematic review of 13 individual studies,[16] and 25 primary studies estimating overdiagnosis[20,73–79]	Details on intervention factors can be found in the metaanalysis,[2,50] systematic review of randomized trials[72] and observational studies[16] and the 25 primary studies[19–22,24,61,73–91]	The relative overdiagnosis estimate was based on the metaanalysis of three trials. The rate of overdiagnosis was estimated at 19%	No absolute estimate provided
American Cancer Society	Review of observational studies, modeling studies, and trials that did not invite the control group at the end of screening	Details on intervention factors are not reported in the review	The review notes that overdiagnosis estimates range from <5% to >50% with estimates based on modeling studies generally lower than those based on empirical studies	No absolute numbers provided. They conclude that there is good evidence that overdiagnosis does occur but no high-quality evidence on the magnitude of overdiagnosis

Canadian Taskforce	The USPSTF review, a systematic review and four primary studies estimating overdiagnosis	Details on intervention factors can be found in the included systematic review[21] and the four primary studies[86,87,92,93]	The frequency of overdiagnosis ranges from 0.4% to 52% s in the included studies.[46] In the main report of the review, the frequency of overdiagnosis ranges from 30% to 52%[47]	For every 1000 women aged 39 years and older who are screened using mammography, five will have an unnecessary lumpectomy or mastectomy as a result of overdiagnosis
EUROSCREEN	Literature review of observational studies that provided estimates of breast cancer overdiagnosis in European population-based mammographic screening programs	Studies reporting on programs implemented between 1970 and 2007; there were 13 primary studies reporting 16 estimates of overdiagnosis in seven European countries (the Netherlands, Italy, Norway, Sweden, Denmark, United Kingdom, and Spain)	Unadjusted estimates ranged from 0% to 54%. Reported estimates adjusted for breast cancer risk and lead time were 2.8% in the Netherlands, 4.6% and 1.0% in Italy, 7.0% in Denmark and 10% and 3.3% in England and Wales. The average estimate of the individual estimates was 6.5% of the incidence in the absence of screening	Assuming 6.5% overdiagnosis: For every 1000 women screened biennially from ages 50 to 51 years until ages 68–69 years and followed up until age 79 years, four cases are overdiagnosed

Table 3.3 Cumulative Risk of False-Positives in Evidence Reviews

	Study Designs Selected; Included Studies	Intervention (Study Period; Age Groups; Screening Test; Screening Interval; Screening Organization)	Relative Effect	Absolute Effect
Cochrane	Observational studies mentioned in the discussion[94–101]	Details on the intervention are not reported in the review and can be found in the included studies[94–101]	The cumulative risk of a false-positive result after 10 mammograms ranges from about 20% to 60%	For every 2000 women invited for screening throughout 10 years, it is likely that more than 200 women will experience important psychological distress for many months because of false-positive findings
Independent UK Panel	*No quantitative assessment of false-positive risk*			
USPSTF	Observational studies from the United States[97,99,102] and unpublished data from the BCSC	• 1983–1995, 40–69 years old, annual vs biennial screening, United States[97] • 1994–2006, 169,456 women aged 40–59, annual vs biennial screening, United States[99] • 1994–2008, 11,474 women with and 9,222,624 women without breast cancer aged 40–74, annual vs biennial vs triennial screening, United States[102] BCSC data was used from women undergoing screening from 2003 to 2011; 405,191 women aged 40–89 years; mammography; one mammogram in the previous 2 years	The observational studies reported a 10-year cumulative risk for false-positive mammography results of 61% for annual and 41% for biennial screening[97,99,102]	The BCSC provided the absolute number of false-positives per 1000 women screened per age category: • 40–49 years: 121.2 • 50–59 years: 93.2 • 60–69 years: 80.8 • 70–79 years: 69.6 • 80–89 years: 65.2

American Cancer Society	Observational studies from the United States[97,99,102]	Details on intervention factors are not reported in the review and can be found in the included studies[97,99,102]	The observational studies reported a 10-year cumulative risk for false-positive mammography results of 61% for annual and 41% for biennial screening and for false-positive results leading to a biopsy recommendation of 7% for annual and 5% for biennial screening[97,99,102]	No absolute numbers provided
Canadian Taskforce	The USPSTF review and one additional primary study[60]	Details on intervention factors are not reported in the review and can be found in the included studies[59,60,97,98]	Data from the BCSC, as reported in the USPSTF review, gave a cumulative false-positive risk of 49%-77% after 10 screening rounds The observational studies on 49.1% and 20.8%[97,98]	The absolute number of false-positive results per 1000 women screened for a median of 11 years was reported per age group: • 40–49 years: 327 • 50–69 years: 282 • 70–74 years: 212
EUROSCREEN	Systematic review of studies of the cumulative risk of a false-positive result in European screening program. Four studies were included[95,98,101,103]	Studies published between 1955–2001 were incorporated; 390,000 women starting at ages 50–51 and continuing to ages 68–69; mammography; interval of 2 years; population-based screening program in a European country	Pooled estimates were derived from studies that estimated the risk over 10 years (364,991 women). The estimated cumulative risk of a false-positive screening result in women aged 50–69 undergoing 10 biennial screening tests varied from 8% to 21% in the three studies examined (pooled weighted estimate 19.7%). The cumulative risk of an invasive procedure with benign outcome ranged from 1.8% to 6.3% (pooled weighted estimate 2.9%)	Assuming a 20% false-positive recall and 3% false-positive recall with invasive work-up: For every 1000 women screened biennially from ages 50 to 51 years until ages 68–69 years and followed up until age 79 years, 170 women have at least one recall followed by noninvasive assessment with a negative result, and 30 women have at least one recall followed by invasive procedures yielding a negative result

characteristics of screening mammography. Simulation modeling from the Cancer Intervention Surveillance Network (CISNET) as well as a new simulation model for radiation exposure were also incorporated.

A metaanalysis of the 8 trials included in the draft USPSTF evidence review estimated a relative risk (RR) of breast cancer mortality of 0.88 (95% CI: 0.73–1.00) for women age 39–49 years. Similar estimates were obtained for women 50–59 and 60–69. For women over age 70 three trials met inclusion criteria, but results of the metaanalysis in this age group had broad confidence intervals indicating substantial uncertainty in the benefit (RR = 0.80, 95% CI: 0.51–1.28). The evidence review summarized the absolute benefit corresponding to these RRs in terms of breast cancer deaths prevented by screening for 10 years per 10,000 women screened. The number of breast cancer deaths prevented was estimated at 4.1 (95% CI: –0.1–9.3) for women aged 39–49, 7.7 (95% CI: 1.6–7.2) for women aged 50–59, 21.3 (95% CI: 10.7–31.7), and 12.5 (95% CI: –17.2–32.1) for women aged 70–74. The number needed to invite (NNI) the number of women who must be invited to participate in screening mammography for 10 years in order to prevent one breast cancer death. For women age 40–49 and 50–59 the NNI was estimated at approximately 2000 women. The draft USPSTF evidence review also included a summary of breast cancer mortality reduction based on observational studies using the results of the EUROSCREEN review (see section: Europe). However, estimates based on observational studies were not incorporated into numerical summaries of breast cancer mortality reduction due to the risk of bias inherent in observational studies.

The evidence review for overdiagnosis found that estimates varied substantially across studies and methodologies. Included studies consisted of a metaanalysis of five trials, a systematic review of observational studies, and 17 individual studies. A metaanalysis of three trials considered to be least biased, estimated overdiagnosis to be 19% (95% CI: 15–23). In observational and modeling studies using varied methodologies, overdiagnosis estimates ranged from <1% to 54%. The risk of false-positive mammography at a single screening round was estimated using data from the BCSC. Estimates ranged from 65 to 121 per 1000 examinations across age groups. Two observational studies of cumulative false-positive risk from the United States were identified that met inclusion criteria. Overall, cumulative false-positive risk after 10 years of annual mammography was estimated at 61%. Risk was higher among women 40–49 with heterogeneously dense breasts (69%) or extremely dense breasts (66%).

Overall, the evidence review found a significant benefit of screening mammography coupled with relatively frequent harms, with more modest benefits and more common harms in women under 50 years of age. On the basis of this review, the USPSTF issued new draft guidelines in 2015 supporting biennial mammography for women age 50–74 years. Routine screening for women younger than 50 was not recommended.

Canadian Task Force on preventive health care

The Canadian Task Force is an independent panel that makes recommendations on preventive clinical services, similar to the USPSTF in the United States. They commissioned the Evidence Review and Synthesis Centre to undertake a review of screening mammography to support updated recommendations in 2011. Because the USPSTF had conducted an evidence review using similar methodology in support of their 2009 breast cancer screening guidelines, the Canadian Task Force used the USPSTF evidence review and updated this review with studies published in the intervening period. The USPSTF review was used for evidence up to 2008 and updated with additional data through October 2011. The

Canadian Task Force review identified breast cancer mortality as the benefit of screening mammography and expressed their results in terms of the number needed to screen (NNS) defined as the number of women who would need to be screened once every 2 years over about 11 years to prevent one breast cancer death. Results from nine trials were included in estimates of the benefit of screening mammography. The estimated NNS for women 40–49 was 2108, while for women 50–69 it was only 721. On the basis of a review of four primary studies and one prior systematic review, the Canadian Task Force estimated the overdiagnosis rate at 5 per 1000 women screened. Unlike the USPSTF review, evidence reviewed on false-positive risk did not incorporate primary data and was expressed only in terms of the number of false-positives associated with one breast cancer death prevented, not as a cumulative false-positive risk. The false-positive risk was found to be highest in the youngest age group at 690 false-positives per breast cancer death averted compared to only 204 in the 50–69 year age group.

The conclusions of the Canadian Task Force echo those of the USPSTF. The benefit of screening mammography was found to be smaller in younger women and harms were found to be more common. Screening every 2–3 years for women aged 50–74 was recommended. Routine screening was not recommended for women under 50 years of age.

American Cancer Society

In 2015, the ACS updated their breast cancer screening guidelines based on an independent systematic review conducted by the Duke University Evidence Synthesis Group, new analyses of observational data conducted by the BCSC, and data on burden of disease provided by the ACS Surveillance and Health Services Research Program. The benefit of screening mammography for the ACS review was defined as reduction in breast cancer mortality and increase in life expectancy and quality-adjusted life expectancy. Evidence on breast cancer mortality from RCTs, recent observational studies including at least 1000 women, and simulation modeling studies were included. New metaanalyses were not conducted, but pooled estimates of the RR of breast cancer mortality from metaanalyses conducted by the Canadian Task Force, UK Independent Panel, and Cochrane review were considered (see section: Europe). Absolute mortality benefit was expressed as the NNS biennially for 15 years to prevent one breast cancer death. Assuming a 20 or 40% mortality reduction, the NNS was 1770 or 753 for women 40–49, 1087 or 462 for women 50–59, and 835 or 355 for women 60–69. The ACS guideline group concluded that there was evidence that screening mammography leads to increases in life expectancy and quality-adjusted life expectancy but concluded that uncertainty about key parameters related to life expectancy precluded quantification of this benefit.

Harms included in the ACS evidence review were false-positive results, overdiagnosis, and overtreatment. Evidence on false-positive results was derived from two observational studies using data from the BCSC. Both observational and modeling studies of overdiagnosis were reviewed, but the ACS concluded that all existing studies relied upon unverifiable assumptions or were subject to potential biases. They therefore concluded that the risk of overdiagnosis could not be quantified using the available evidence.

On the basis of this evidence, the ACS recommended annual mammography for women aged 45–54 years and biennial mammography for women 55 years and older, as long as they are healthy and have a life expectancy of at least 10 years. Because the absolute risk of breast cancer is similar among women 45–49 and those aged 50–54, the ACS concluded that benefits outweigh harms beginning at age 45 years. Among women under 45, the harms were judged to likely outweigh the benefits.

EUROPE

Early evidence on the efficacy of mammography screening became available with the first publications of the randomized controlled trials in the early 1980s. Thus, when the Europe Against Cancer (EAC) program was initiated in 1986 in an effort to control cancer in Europe, its Committee of Cancer Experts decided that secondary prevention should be included.[49] Breast, cervical, and colorectal cancers were considered. For breast cancer, a European Network was created in 1989, cofunded by the European Community, to implement mammography screening pilot programs in a number of member states. The target population in the pilots was women aged 50–64, but variation was allowed in the starting and stopping ages. It was expected that these pilots would provide a practical basis for the implementation of nationwide breast cancer screening programs. At the time of implementation of the pilots, population-based screening programs were already established in a limited number of countries, including the United Kingdom, the Netherlands, Finland, and Sweden.

The positive results of the EAC program prompted the European Council to publish a recommendation on cancer screening in 2003. In this recommendation, member states were invited to take common action to implement national cancer screening programs with a population-based approach, according to European quality assurance guidelines where they existed. Following this recommendation, numerous additional programs were established in Western Europe in the 1990s and, more recently, also in Eastern Europe. The first report on cancer screening in the European Union noted that in 2007 breast cancer screening programs were running or being established in at least 26 of the 27 member states. The majority of the programs have a 2-year screening interval and invite at least women in the age group 50–69, as specified in the Council Recommendation. However, despite this broad consensus, the way screening programs are implemented still varies across the EU.

The debate on breast cancer screening in Europe, and elsewhere, was not new but reignited with the publication of the first Cochrane Review in 2001. Below we summarize the outcomes of the Cochrane Review,[3] based on its last update in 2013. We further summarize the reviews performed by the UK Independent Panel[2,50] and the EUROSCREEN group[51,52] that were initiated in response to the continuing debate and were published in 2012.

Nordic Cochrane review

The Cochrane Collaboration is an international, independent, not-for-profit organization, funded by a variety of sources including governments, universities, hospital trusts, charities, and personal donations. The first Cochrane review on screening for breast cancer with mammography was performed following a request of the Danish National Board of Health in 1999 and published in 2001. Updates were published in 2006, 2009, 2011, and 2013. The last review in 2013 was declared stable as no new randomized controlled trials on mammography screening had been identified. No further updates are expected.

The authors of the Cochrane review aimed to study the effect of screening for breast cancer with mammography on mortality and morbidity. A broad search strategy was used in Pubmed to identify both randomized trials and observational studies, as the latter were considered to provide important new knowledge, for example, in relation to evidence on overdiagnosis and other harms of screening. References were manually searched and letters, abstracts, gray literature, and unpublished data retrieved where possible. The outcome measures of the review included mortality from breast cancer, mortality from cancer, all-cause mortality, use of surgical interventions, use of adjuvant therapy, and harms of mammography.

The Cochrane review identified eight eligible randomized clinical trials, but excluded one because it was not adequately randomized. Intention to treat analyses were performed for breast cancer mortality, even though the authors judged breast cancer mortality to be an unreliable outcome, biased in favor of screening, and recommended overall mortality as primary outcome measure. Trials using less reliable randomization methods were evaluated separately. The pooled RR for the three trials with adequate randomization was 0.90 (95% CI: 0.79–1.02) and did not show a significant effect of screening on breast cancer mortality. The four trials classified as having suboptimal randomization had a pooled RR of 0.75 (95% CI: 0.67–0.83) indicating a 25% reduction in breast cancer mortality. The overall estimate for all seven trials combined was 0.81 (95% CI: 0.74–0.87), consistent with a 19% reduction after 13 years. The authors further assessed the impact of screening on all-cause mortality as well as deaths ascribed to any cancer and found no reductions. To express the results in absolute numbers, the authors assumed a 15% reduction in breast cancer mortality after 13 years of follow-up which means that for every 2000 women invited for screening throughout 10 years, one will avoid dying of breast cancer. Data from the randomized trials were further assessed for surgical interventions and radiotherapy, with significantly more operations performed in the study groups and more women receiving radiotherapy. Little information was found on other adjuvant therapy and no comparative data was reported on psychological morbidity.

In contrast to outcomes relating to benefit, the harms of screening were summarized only in the discussion section. The review does not state explicitly how the randomized trials and/or observational studies referred to in this section were selected. The outcomes discussed include overdiagnosis and overtreatment, in particular the increase in mastectomies, false-positives, psychological distress and pain. Based on the references selected, the authors conclude that the level of overdiagnosis and overtreatment was about 30% in the trials that did not introduce early screening in the control group and somewhat larger in the trials with suboptimal randomization. These findings were supported in a number of observational studies with overdiagnosis estimates ranging from 18% to 60%. In terms of absolute numbers, the authors estimated that for every 2000 women invited for screening throughout 10 years, 10 women would be overdiagnosed and overtreated, under the assumption that the level of overdiagnosis is 30%. For false-positive results, the cumulative risk after 10 mammograms was found to range from about 20% to 60%, with the highest risk reported for the United States. No mention is made of the estimate used to calculate the absolute numbers, but the authors stated that it is likely that more than 200 women will experience false-positive findings and psychological distress for every 2000 women invited for screening throughout 10 years.

The authors of the Cochrane review concluded that the evidence reported in the review cast doubts on the effectiveness of breast cancer screening and that "the time has come to re-assess whether universal mammography screening should be recommended for any age group." In their view, women should be made more aware of the harms associated with attending screening, since the benefits are small at best.

United Kingdom

The Independent UK Panel on Breast Cancer Screening (referred to below as the independent UK panel) issued a report in 2012 that was jointly commissioned by Cancer Research UK and the Department of Health (England). The group was convened to review the evidence for the benefits and harms of breast screening in the United Kingdom. Members of the independent UK panel had relevant expertise but had not previously published on breast screening in order to ensure an objective and independent assessment of the evidence. A patient advocate was an integral member of the independent UK panel.

The evidence considered included randomized controlled trials of breast screening as well as observational studies, including prospective follow-up and case–control studies. The independent UK panel reviewed the literature, but did not perform a formal systematic review, and heard testimony from experts in the field, from both sides of the debate. The key outputs of the review were an estimate of the effect of breast screening on breast cancer mortality, as the main benefit, and an estimate of the risk of overdiagnosis, as the main harm. Besides these, the independent UK panel considered other relevant issues, including additional harms through invitation, screening, diagnosis, and treatment, as well as women's perceptions and cost-effectiveness. Although the independent UK panel did not make a systematic appraisal of evidence in all these areas, it did provide comments on each of these issues.

The independent UK panel's estimate of the quantitative effect of breast screening on breast cancer mortality is based on randomized trials of screening, while acknowledging that these trials are not perfect. The analysis focused on 10 of the 11 randomized trials (excluding Edinburgh) and the metaanalysis conducted in the Cochrane review, using 13 years of follow-up (published in 2011). A RR reduction in breast cancer mortality of 20% (95% CI: 11–27) was estimated for groups invited to screening. The absolute risk reduction was expressed as the number of women needed to be screened for 20 years to prevent one death from breast cancer and was estimated at 180 women. The independent UK panel estimated that for 10,000 women attending screening from age 50 for 20 years, 43 deaths would be prevented. The independent UK panel looked at observational studies as a possible guide to more contemporary estimates of the benefit of breast cancer screening. They noted that in general these studies showed beneficial effects in the same direction as those seen in the trials, but expressed concern about inadequate control for the potential noncomparability of screened and unscreened women (self-selection bias).

The independent UK panel based its estimate of the risk of overdiagnosis on three randomized trials that did not systematically screen the control group at the end of the screening period. Estimates were on the order of 11% (95% CI: 9–12) from a population perspective, and about 19% (95% CI: 15–23) from the perspective of a woman invited to screening. In absolute terms, the independent UK panel estimated that for every 10,000 UK women invited to screening from age 50 for 20 years, about 681 cancers will be found of which 129 will represent overdiagnosis. Information from observational studies was also considered, but the independent UK panel concluded that these studies could not give reliable estimates of the extent of overdiagnosis. For the specific case of diagnosing DCIS via a screening program, it was noted that diagnoses of DCIS do not solely represent overdiagnosis, but that these diagnoses undoubtedly contribute to the cases of overdiagnosis. The independent UK panel did not mention the cumulative risk of false-positive results among the other harms of breast screening, but noted that a false-positive result can cause psychological distress.

The independent UK panel concluded that breast screening reduces breast cancer mortality, but that some overdiagnosis occurs. Based on the estimates for the United Kingdom, one breast cancer death is prevented for every three overdiagnosed cases identified and treated. Evidence from a focus group further showed that many women feel that accepting the offer of breast screening is worthwhile.

EUROSCREEN

The effort of the EUROSCREEN group to summarize the accumulated evidence on the impact of population-based breast cancer screening in Europe was launched in the context of the European Screening Network in 2010. EUROSCREEN is a self-initiated cooperative group that includes scientists and professionals experienced in planning and evaluating most of the population-based screening programs running in Europe. In contrast to the other reviews presented in this chapter, EUROSCREEN focused on observational studies to systematically assess the impact of established service screening programs in Europe. The aim was to develop the best current estimate of the impact of service screening on breast cancer mortality, as well as screening harms, in particular the risk of overdiagnosis and false-positive screening results. Outcomes of EUROSCREEN were published in eight peer-reviewed papers, including a summary of main findings in the form of a balance sheet. The series of literature reviews further addressed the methodological standards of evaluation and the importance of using appropriate statistical methodology to design and analyze observational studies of mammography.

EUROSCREEN defined the reduction in breast cancer mortality for women invited versus not invited and/or women screened versus not screened as the primary benefit, and overdiagnosis of breast cancer and false-positive screening tests as the most important harms. A systematic search of Pubmed identified observational studies reporting on breast cancer mortality in relation to service screening programs in Europe implemented between 1970 and 2007. In line with European policy recommendations, eligible studies had to include at least part of the age group between 50 and 69. Since the aim of the review was to report on estimates from ongoing population-based screening programs, the studies had to have at least a three years' overlap with the current regional or national screening program. Based on these criteria, 83 studies were selected and grouped according to study design, that is, trend studies, incidence-based mortality studies, and case–control studies. The trend studies that aimed to quantify the impact on breast cancer mortality were too different to produce a pooled estimate of the effect of screening. Pooled estimates of breast cancer mortality reduction based on incidence-based mortality studies and case–control studies were on the order of 25–31% for women invited and 38–48% for women actually screened. The search strategy for overdiagnosis identified 13 studies that provided 16 explicit estimates from European population-based screening programs. Unadjusted estimates varied widely with estimates in the range of 0–54%. Studies were further classified according to the adjustment for breast cancer risk and lead time bias. Adequately adjusted studies report estimates of overdiagnosis in the range of 1–10%. Literature review and manual search of references for studies of the cumulative risk of a false-positive result in European service programs identified three unique studies. The pooled estimate from these studies indicated a cumulative risk of 20% for women aged 50–69 undergoing 10 biennial screening tests. The cumulative risk of a false-positive result in women undergoing needle biopsy was reported in two studies with a pooled estimate of 3%.

The evidence from the literature reviews was further summarized in the form of a balance sheet. For every 1000 women screened biennially from ages 50 to 51 years until ages 68–69 years and followed up until age 79 years, an estimated seven to nine breast cancer deaths are avoided, four cases are overdiagnosed, 170 women have at least one recall followed by noninvasive assessment with negative results, and 30 women have at least one recall followed by invasive procedures yielding a negative result. In conclusion, the pooled experience in European countries showed that the chance of saving a woman's life is greater than that of overdiagnosis. EUROSCREEN recommended continuing the population-based screening programs currently ongoing in Europe.

DIFFERENCES BETWEEN EVIDENCE REVIEWS

In the section Reviewing the Balance of Harms and Benefits, we gave an overview of the existing evidence reviews and showed that they differed in both methodology and outcomes (Tables 3.1–3.3). In this section, we provide a detailed explanation of some of the methodological differences between the reviews that partly explain variations in their conclusions. We focus on four methodological issues: study design, screening setting, outcome measure and reference population.

STUDY DESIGN

There are a number of epidemiological study designs used to quantify breast cancer mortality reduction, overdiagnosis and cumulative risk of a false-positive result attributable to screening mammography. The well-known hierarchy of research evidence puts systematic reviews and metaanalyses at the top. Single studies are classified as to their strength of evidence in the following order: randomized controlled trials, cohort studies (ie, incidence-based mortality studies), case–control studies, and ecological studies (ie, trend studies). We will discuss the study designs selected by the reviews separately for breast cancer mortality reduction, overdiagnosis, and false-positives.

Breast cancer mortality reduction

Five reviews estimated breast cancer mortality reduction on the basis of randomized trials, but the number of trials included in each review differed (see Table 3.1). In total, there have been 11 randomized trials of mammography: HIP, Malmö I and II, Swedish Two County (Kopperberg and Östergötland), Canada I and II, Stockholm, Göteborg, Edinburgh, and UK Age trial. All reviews excluded the Edinburgh trial because of methodological limitations. The Nordic Cochrane Review made a distinction between adequately and suboptimally randomized trials. Four trials were included as adequately randomized (Malmö I, Canada I and II, UK Age trial) and the other trials, except for the Edinburgh trial, were included as suboptimally randomized.

EUROSCREEN based their estimate of breast cancer mortality reduction predominantly on incidence-based mortality studies and case–control studies from Europe. They reported separate pooled estimates for incidence-based mortality studies (25%) and case–control studies (31%). Because trend studies have major methodological limitations in evaluating the effect of screening on breast cancer mortality,[53] the outcomes were reported but not pooled.

The USPSTF, ACS, and the independent UK panel also considered observational data on mortality as a guide for more contemporary estimates of screening because the randomized controlled trials, which are older, are limited in their ability to estimate the effect of modern mammographic screening. These reviews concluded that the effect of mammographic screening was larger in incidence-based mortality and case–control studies than in randomized trials. Comparison of the reviews reveals a similar picture: metaanalyses of randomized trials show a smaller breast cancer mortality reduction than metaanalyses of incidence-based mortality and case–control studies. It remains unknown, however, whether this difference is due to limitations in observational studies, such as selection bias, or differences in the details of screening practice, as will be discussed in section "Screening Setting."

Overdiagnosis

Of the six reviews, only the Nordic Cochrane Review and the independent UK panel created a single overdiagnosis estimate, while EUROSCREEN used the average of the most plausible overdiagnosis estimates. The three reviews from North America included overdiagnosis, but did not report a single estimate.

Two out of the three reviews, that is, Nordic Cochrane review and the independent UK panel, based their estimates of overdiagnosis on RCTs. They both included three trials that did not offer screening to women in the control group at the end of the trial; Malmö I, Canada I, and II.

EUROSCREEN estimated overdiagnosis in European population-based mammographic screening programs using observational studies. They included both cohort studies and ecological studies.[16] Case–control studies estimating overdiagnosis in Europe were not published at that time and therefore, could not be included. EUROSCREEN did not classify the studies estimating overdiagnosis according to study design, but on the basis of two methodological limitations relating to overdiagnosis, adjustment for lead time and underlying breast cancer risk.

Both trials and observational studies have limitations when it comes to estimating overdiagnosis. The major limitation of trials is the short follow-up period after the end of screening. This limitation can be overcome in observational study designs. However, these designs lack a comparable nonscreened control group. A nonscreened control group is often created by extrapolating prescreening trends, using control regions, using nonattenders or other approaches. All of these approaches require assumptions, which can have a large impact on the overdiagnosis estimate, and do not necessarily create a comparable nonscreened control group.[50]

False-positives

Five reviews reported the cumulative risk of a false-positive result: the Nordic Cochrane review, EUROSCREEN, USPSTF, the Canadian Task Force, and the ACS. The independent UK panel did not consider the cumulative risk of false-positives, because they felt there was more agreement about the nature and magnitude of false-positives.[2] When reported, the cumulative risk of false-positives was always based on observational study designs.

EUROSCREEN was the only review that systematically searched the literature for studies on the cumulative risk of false-positives. The Nordic Cochrane review provides a range of cumulative risks based on several studies which were not obtained using a systematic search. The USPSTF showed both the cumulative risk of false-positives in percentages and absolute numbers, but based on different studies. In total, two studies were listed for the cumulative risks and unpublished results from the BCSC were used for false-positive estimates at a single screening round. The same two observational studies were used by the ACS to inform estimates of cumulative false-positive risk. The Canadian Task Force also reports the absolute number of false-positives per 1000 women without clearly mentioning the basis for this estimate.

SCREENING SETTING

Although the research hierarchy of epidemiological studies is widely accepted in the medical literature, it is not absolute or fixed. Well-executed studies of lower order might provide more valid evidence than poorly executed studies of higher order. Furthermore, other factors relating to external validity may make studies of lower order more relevant than studies of higher order. In this section, we will discuss factors relating to the external validity of the executed studies. To this end, we will compare current screening practice to the intervention delivered in the trials and observational studies in terms of study period, age groups, screening test, and screening organization.

Breast cancer mortality reduction

The differences between breast cancer mortality estimates in the reviews can largely be explained by the period during which the studies were conducted. One study[54] indicated that the effectiveness of mammographic screening has increased over time. Screening mammography programs have improved over time, and some studies show increased breast cancer detection with newer technologies, such as digital mammography[55] and digital breast tomosynthesis.[56,57] Randomized trials were executed between 1963 and 1991, while most incidence-based mortality and case–control studies were executed more recently.[58] This might explain why EUROSCREEN estimated a higher breast cancer mortality reduction based on observational studies than the other reviews which based their estimated on the randomized trials. Potential factors that have changed over time and may have contributed to this effect are improvements in screening tests and treatments and a growing awareness of breast cancer among women.

Another factor that differs between randomized trials and observational studies is age. The randomized trials included women in the age range 38–74. The mean age of the trial participants is not reported, but will be relatively low given that three trials focused solely on women below age 50. In most European screening programs, as evaluated by EUROSCREEN, the starting age is 40 or 50 and stopping age is 69 or 74. Because most studies in Europe are executed in countries that start screening at age 50, the age range included in trials and studies included in the EUROSCREEN review might differ. This may have affected the estimates, because some studies show a larger effect of screening in older women.[59]

Overdiagnosis

Age and screening test are known to influence overdiagnosis. The risk of overdiagnosis increases substantially at older ages,[7] because of a higher risk of death due to competing events. Screening tests with improved sensitivity, such as digital mammography, also increase the risk of overdiagnosis,[60,61] because more life-threatening as well as nonlife-threatening breast cancers can be detected.

Although overdiagnosis is influenced by the details of screening practice, it is difficult to determine which factors explain the differences in overdiagnosis estimates between the reviews. Currently, there is much discussion about the optimal methodology to estimate overdiagnosis.[15,17] Factors, such as the length of follow-up after the end of screening and the underlying breast cancer incidence rate may have a larger influence on the overdiagnosis estimates than screening policy. As a consequence, the differences in overdiagnosis estimates are likely primarily explained by methodological differences rather than differences in screening practice.

False-positives

Difference in screening organization is the major factor explaining the differences between the cumulative false-positive risks reported in the reviews. This is best illustrated by comparing the cumulative risk reported by the ACS and USPSTF with the risk reported by EUROSCREEN. The US evidence reviews reported cumulative risks of false-positives about double or triple the risks of false-positives estimated in Europe and Australia.[30] This difference may be partially explained by the fact that in the United States typically a single radiologist decides whether to recall or not, while in Europe and Australia two or three radiologists make this decision. As a consequence, recall rates are generally higher in the United States.[62,63] Additionally, the requirements for screening radiologist accreditation differ between the United States and other countries. For example, the United States requires 960 mammograms read in the prior 2 years to maintain accreditation,[64] while the European guidelines for quality assurance in breast cancer screening and diagnosis recommend that each screening radiologist should read a minimum of 5000 screening cases per year in a centralized program.[65]

Other details of screening practice also influence the cumulative risk of a false-positive, including screening test,[60] screening interval,[7] and age.[36,47] In general, cultural factors, organization of health care, and the medicolegal context also affect the threshold used to determine whether to recall, and thus the cumulative risk of false-positive recall in different screening settings.

OUTCOME MEASURE

Here we consider the measures used to quantify breast cancer mortality reduction, overdiagnosis, and cumulative risk of false-positives. For example, overdiagnosis can be expressed as a percentage of cancers in the presence or absence of screening. Even when the absolute number of overdiagnosed cases per 1000 women is the same, this leads to different overdiagnosis estimates. The resultant major drawback is the incomparability of estimates across reviews due to differences in choice of outcome measures. We will discuss several differences in outcome measures that at least partially explain differences between the reviews.

Breast cancer mortality reduction

Across outcome measures, the percentage breast cancer mortality reduction reported by the reviews ranges from 10% to 48%. However, the range is reduced to 10–33% when expressed as the breast cancer mortality reduction in women invited to screening. Trials and incidence-based mortality studies usually estimate the breast cancer mortality reduction in women invited to screening, for example, intention to treat. In case–control studies, the effect of screening on breast cancer mortality is most often expressed in women actually screened. EUROSCREEN calculated the breast cancer mortality reduction in both women invited and women screened, thereby increasing comparability with estimates based on trials.

Another factor that affects the estimated breast cancer mortality reduction is length of follow-up. The independent UK panel and Nordic Cochrane review both used a 13-year follow-up period for the randomized trials. EUROSCREEN defined adequate follow-up as "at least 10 years from the date of full coverage by invitation."[58]

Overdiagnosis

The extent of overdiagnosis depends greatly on the method of estimating overdiagnosis and all reviews used a different method. EUROSCREEN pooled overdiagnosis estimates with different denominators and concluded that overdiagnosis was on average 6.5% in the absence of screening (average of the most plausible overdiagnosis estimates).[52] However, they did not report the age range for breast cancers included in the absence of screening, which has a large influence on the overdiagnosis estimate. Including breast cancers diagnosed in women outside the age range of the screened population provides an estimate reflective of the overdiagnosis risk among the total population of women. However, this estimate will be lower than overdiagnosis estimates including only women of screening age since women outside the screened age range are not at risk of having cancers overdiagnosed. The independent UK panel expressed overdiagnosis as a percentage of breast cancers in women invited to screening. They also proposed two age ranges, that is, breast cancers in all ages and breast cancers in the invited age range. Because of the difference in methods, the percentages of overdiagnosis from the reviews are incomparable.

The extent of overdiagnosis is also dependent on the type of breast cancer studied: overdiagnosis estimates of invasive breast cancer are lower than overdiagnosis estimates of invasive breast cancer plus DCIS. Although the effect of the type of breast cancer studied can be large,[25] it is not directly visible in the reviews because the choice of denominator masks this difference.

False-positives

All reviews use more or less the same definition to calculate the cumulative risk of false-positives. If there are any differences between the reviews in the definition of the cumulative risk of false-positive, these will be minimal, for example, inclusion or exclusion of false-positive recalls due to insufficient technical quality.[30] Therefore, differences in outcome measures will have a minor effect on the difference in the cumulative risk of false-positives between the reviews.

REFERENCE POPULATION

In all reviews, the relative breast cancer mortality reduction was translated to absolute numbers. Overdiagnosis and cumulative false-positive risks were also expressed in absolute terms by all reviews except for ACS. For these purposes, each review uses a so-called "reference population," that is, the breast cancer incidence and mortality of a certain population under a particular screening scenario.[52] The absolute risk estimates for each of the outcome measures depend largely on the underlying breast cancer mortality and incidence in the reference population[50] as we will show here.

Breast cancer mortality reduction

All reviews used a reference population to obtain the absolute numbers of breast cancer deaths prevented by screening. The Cochrane review used the control groups of the trials, which had low breast cancer mortality because of the low mean age.[50] The independent UK panel and EUROSCREEN calculated absolute numbers with a different approach, but both based their estimates on the screened age range in the United Kingdom. The USPSTF and Canadian Taskforce did not clearly describe which reference population was used to obtain the absolute breast cancer mortality reduction estimate. The ACS estimate was based on incidence-based mortality among US women reported by SEER but does not clearly describe the included age range.

The absolute number of breast cancers prevented by breast cancer screening ranges from 0.4 to 9 per 1000 women across the reviews. The USPSTF reports the lowest number of breast cancers prevented in the age group 39–49 (0.4) and EUROSCREEN reports the highest number of breast cancers prevented (7–9). The reviews from North America report absolute breast cancer mortality reductions that are on the lower end, 0.8 for women 50–59 years and 2.1 for 60–69 years reported by the USPSTF and 1.4 by the Canadian Taskforce. The independent UK panel reports that 5.6 breast cancer deaths are prevented per 1000 women screened. Since the reported absolute numbers are based on different reference populations and screening scenarios, they are not comparable.

When applying the UK reference population to the relative mortality reductions estimated by each review, the absolute number of breast cancer deaths prevented ranges from 2 to 11 per 1000 women screened (see Table 3.4). For all reviews, these absolute estimates are higher than those provided in the review, with the exception of the independent UK panel which provided the reference population. The Nordic Cochrane review still reports the lowest number of breast cancers prevented and EUROSCREEN the highest. The change in absolute breast cancer deaths prevented was most notable for the Canadian Taskforce, which reported a RR reduction equal to the independent UK panel and an absolute risk reduction of 4.2 per 1000 less than the independent UK panel before recalculation. After applying the reference population of the independent UK panel, the Canadian Taskforce reported absolute risk reductions equal to the independent UK panel.

Table 3.4 Reported and Recalculated Absolute Breast Cancer Mortality Reduction per 1000 Women for Each Evidence Review

Balance	Absolute Breast Cancer Mortality Reduction per 1000 Women		
	Absolute Reduction as Reported	**Percent Reduction for Invited Women**	**Absolute Reduction Recalculated**[a]
USPSTF	39–49 years: 0.4 50–59 years: 0.8 60–69 years: 2.1 70–74 years: 1.3	39–49 years: 12 50–59 years: 14 60–69 years: 33 70–74 years: 20	39–49 years: 3 50–59 years: 4 60–69 years: 11 70–74 years: 6
ACS	40–49 years: 0.6–1.3 50–59 years: 0.9–2.2 60–69 years: 1.2–2.8	Not provided	
EUROSCREEN	50–69 years: 7–9	25 and 31	7–10
Independent UK panel	50–69 years: 4.3 (invited) 5.6 (screened)	20	6
Nordic Cochrane Institute	0.5[b]	10	2
Canadian Taskforce	40–49 years: 0.5 50–69 years: 1.4 70–74 years: 2.2	40–49 years: 15 50–69 years: 21 70–74 years: 32 All ages: 18	40–49 years: 4 50–69 years: 6 70–74 years:10 All ages: 5

[a]*The recalculated absolute mortality reductions are based on UK mortality rates (2008–2010) and independent UK panel's calculations.*[42] *In 2008–2010, 1.70% of the women aged 50 are expected to die from breast cancer between age 55 and 79. The absolute risk reduction (r) is the breast cancer mortality risk in absence of screening (=1.70/$RR_{invited}$) minus the breast cancer mortality risk in presence of screening (=1.70). The absolute number of breast cancer mortality cases prevented was calculated as the inverse of the risk reduction (1/r) times the coverage rate of the screening program in the United Kingdom (0.77).*

[b]*The Nordic Cochrane review did not explicitly mention the age range of the absolute breast cancer mortality reduction. They based their absolute reduction on the control group (age range 39–69).*

Overdiagnosis

The underlying breast cancer incidence in the reference population is an important determinant of the absolute number of overdiagnosed cases. Unfortunately, we were not able to recalculate the absolute number of overdiagnosed cases, because the absolute number of breast cancers in the denominator was unknown in most reviews. However, it can be expected that the choice of reference population has a similar or even larger effect on overdiagnosis compared to its effect on breast cancer deaths prevented.

False-positives

The influence of the reference population on the absolute number of false-positives is limited, because false-positives are not highly dependent on breast cancer incidence and/or mortality. The risk of a false-positive is likely to increase with a higher risk of breast cancer. For example, some studies indicate that women with a family history of breast cancer, and therefore a higher risk of having breast cancer themselves, also have a higher risk of false-positives. However, this effect is likely too minor to explain the differences between reviews.

CONCLUSION

This chapter provided an overview of reviews of the benefits and harms of mammographic screening and discussed factors that can explain the differences between reviews. In this concluding section, we provide recommendations to those designing and applying harm/benefit balance sheets. We conclude with a discussion of some future challenges, including the introduction of new screening modalities and personalized screening, which are likely to affect the current balance between benefits and harms.

RECOMMENDATIONS

Most reviews quantified breast cancer mortality reduction using estimates from randomized trials. The majority of these randomized trials were executed at least 25 years ago and estimated the effect of mammography using older technology and screening protocols tested in different populations than those for whom recommendations are being made. The continued reliance on these older trials reflects the fact that the validity of breast cancer mortality reduction estimates is valued more highly than their generalizability. As we discussed in this chapter, both study design and screening policy can affect estimates of breast cancer mortality reduction. Given that breast cancer screening continues to improve and new randomized controlled trials investigating the effect of breast cancer screening including an unscreened arm are unlikely to be executed, we recommend putting more weight on the generalizability of breast cancer mortality estimates and thus on estimates from well-executed observational studies. Estimates of cancer incidence and mortality from observational studies are potentially affected by healthy screened bias.[66] Many factors may also differ between screened and unscreened populations or individuals screened more or less frequently, leading to possible confounding. Development of rigorous methodological criteria for the validity of observational studies of cancer screening is therefore needed.

Furthermore, it may be misleading to use breast cancer mortality reduction estimates from randomized controlled trials in combination with overdiagnosis and cumulative false-positive risk estimates based on observational studies of current screening programs, as this may distort the balance of benefits and harms. Breast cancer mortality reduction, overdiagnosis and cumulative risk of false-positives are strongly related to each other via features of the mammography screening program.[67] When breast cancer mortality reduction is greater, overdiagnosis and the cumulative false-positive risk are also likely to be greater. Therefore, the harm/benefit balance should be based on estimates of breast cancer mortality, overdiagnosis, and false-positives from the same screening setting, including period, age, test, interval, and organization of screening.

There is also geographical variation in the harm/benefit balance, especially with regard to the cumulative risk of false-positives. The cumulative risk of false-positives is strongly dependent on a country's screening organization, the organization of health care, cultural factors, and the medicolegal context. The largest differences are observed between the United States compared to Europe and Australia.[30] Therefore, balances should only include cumulative risks of false-positives from countries with similar screening settings.

Those creating and applying balances should further be aware of the effect of the choice of reference population. The absolute numbers of breast cancer deaths prevented and overdiagnosed cases depend on breast cancer incidence and mortality in the reference population. Consequently, the absolute numbers of breast cancer deaths prevented and cases overdiagnosed cannot be compared directly between reviews. For this reason, the relative effects should be preferred above the absolute effects for comparison between reviews. Furthermore, those creating balance sheets should clearly identify the reference population used to calculate absolute estimates, thereby allowing readers to evaluate the generalizability of their estimates.

The reviews differed most in their estimates of overdiagnosis. This is likely because there is still much uncertainty and disagreement about the optimal methodology for estimating overdiagnosis and the outcome measure of overdiagnosis. The reviews were generally less systematic in their choice of which studies on overdiagnosis to include and used different outcome measures for overdiagnosis. These and other challenges regarding understanding and quantifying overdiagnosis are further discussed in chapter "Challenges in understanding and quantifying overdiagnosis and overtreatment." Balance sheets reporting on overdiagnosis should include clear descriptions of the methodology, outcome measures, and reference populations used in order to facilitate comparisons across reviews.[68]

FUTURE CHALLENGES

Overdiagnosis, resulting in overtreatment, is undoubtedly the most serious harm of breast cancer screening. Currently, all breast cancers, including DCIS, are treated as if they are life-threatening. However, this may be changing as current research seeks to identify characteristics of tumors that are not likely to progress and that can therefore safely be left untreated. This research would resolve the ambiguity in distinguishing life-threatening from nonlife-threatening cancers, thereby substantially alleviating the uncertainty about overdiagnosis which fuels much of the current controversy about the relative harms and benefits of screening mammography.

The introduction of new screening modalities is a topic of current research that will pose new challenges to estimates of the balance of benefits and harms. The existing randomized trials of screening mammography all used older technology. Currently screening mammography is conducted almost exclusively using full-field digital mammography while the randomized trials used film-screen technology. Digital mammography has been shown to have increased sensitivity at the cost of somewhat decreased specificity relative to film-screen mammography.[69,70] The balance of benefits and harms is likely to differ for digital mammography compared to film-screen with higher sensitivity increasing the possible mortality benefit as well as overdiagnosis[61] and lower specificity leading to more false-positives.

Other new imaging technologies are rapidly being introduced into clinical practice, such as digital breast tomosynthesis, breast magnetic resonance imaging, and whole breast ultrasound. These technologies are already being used for screening in the United States and may increasingly be used in other screening settings in the future. This evolution is further detailed in chapter "Evolution of Mammography Screening: From Film Screen to Digital Breast Tomosynthesis." Of interest, these technological advances take place too rapidly for clinical trials with mortality endpoints to be feasible. In order for benefit/harm balance sheets to remain relevant it will be critical to incorporate clinical trial results using alternative endpoints, such as stage shift, interval cancer reduction, and results from observational studies.

Another challenge is presented by the shift toward personalized screening, as highlighted by the chapters discussing risk-based screening in this book. Decision-makers increasingly recognize that the balance of harms and benefits may be optimized for low-risk women by providing less intensive screening and for high-risk women by intensifying screening regimens. The evidence for personalized screening recommendations is derived entirely from observational studies and microsimulation models. While personalization has the potential to shift the overall balance of benefits and harms in a favorable direction, obtaining unbiased estimates to support personalized screening decisions is challenging. Given the potential for bias, observational studies of harms and benefits of personalized screening strategies must adhere to rigorous methodological standards.

LIST OF ACRONYMS AND ABBREVIATIONS

ACS	American Cancer Society
AHRQ	Agency for Healthcare Research and Quality
BCSC	Breast Cancer Surveillance Consortium
BI-RADS	Breast Imaging Reporting and Data Systems
CI	confidence interval
CISNET	Cancer Intervention Surveillance Network
DCIS	ductal carcinoma in situ
EAC	Europe Against Cancer
HIP	Health Insurance Plan
IBM	incidence-based mortality
NNS	number needed to screen
RCT	randomized controlled trial
RR	relative risk
SEER	Surveillance Epidemiology and End Results
UK	United Kingdom
US	United States
USPSTF	United States Preventive Services Task Force

REFERENCES

1. Jorgensen KJ, Keen JD, Gotzsche PC. Is mammographic screening justifiable considering its substantial over-diagnosis rate and minor effect on mortality? *Radiology* 2011;**260**(3):621–7.
2. Independent UK panel on Breast Cancer Screening. The benefits and harms of breast cancer screening: an independent review. *Lancet* 2012;**380**(9855):1778–86.
3. Gotzsche PC, Jorgensen KJ. Screening for breast cancer with mammography. *Cochrane Database Syst Rev* 2013;**6**:CD001877.
4. Goldoni CA, Bonora K, Ciatto S, Giovannetti L, Patriarca S, Sapino A, et al. Misclassification of breast cancer as cause of death in a service screening area. *Cancer Causes Control* 2009;**20**(5):533–8.
5. Nystrom L, Larsson LG, Rutqvist LE, Lindgren A, Lindgvist M, Ryden S, et al. Determination of cause of death among breast cancer cases in the Swedish randomized mammography screening trials. A comparison between official statistics and validation by an endpoint committee. *Acta Oncol* 1995;**34**(2):145–52.

6. Tabar L, Duffy SW, Yen MF, Warwick J, Vitak B, Chen HH, et al. All-cause mortality among breast cancer patients in a screening trial: support for breast cancer mortality as an end point. *J Med Screen* 2002;**9**(4):159–62.
7. Mandelblatt JS, Cronin KA, Bailey S, Berry DA, de Koning HJ, Draisma G, et al. Effects of mammography screening under different screening schedules: model estimates of potential benefits and harms. *Ann Intern Med* 2009;**151**(10):738–47.
8. Norum J. Breast cancer screening by mammography in Norway. Is it cost-effective? *Ann Oncol* 1999;**10**(2):197–203.
9. Tabar L, Yen AM, Wu WY, Chen SL, Chiu SY, Fann JC, et al. Insights from the breast cancer screening trials: how screening affects the natural history of breast cancer and implications for evaluating service screening programs. *Breast J* 2015;**21**(1):13–20.
10. Autier P, Boniol M, Middleton R, Dore JF, Hery C, Zheng T, et al. Advanced breast cancer incidence following population-based mammographic screening. *Ann Oncol* 2011;**22**(8):1726–35.
11. Foca F, Mancini S, Bucchi L, Puliti D, Zappa M, Naldoni C, et al. Decreasing incidence of late-stage breast cancer after the introduction of organized mammography screening in Italy. *Cancer* 2013;**119**(11):2022–8.
12. Brouckaert O, Schoneveld A, Truyers C, Kellen E, Van Ongeval C, Vergote I, et al. Breast cancer phenotype, nodal status and palpability may be useful in the detection of overdiagnosed screening-detected breast cancers. *Ann Oncol* 2013;**24**(7):1847–52.
13. Elshof LE, Tryfonidis K, Slaets L, Can Leeuwen-Stok AE, Skinner VP, Dif N, et al. Feasibility of a prospective, randomised, open-label, international multicentre, phase III, non-inferiority trial to assess the safety of active surveillance for low risk ductal carcinoma in situ—The LORD study. *Eur J Cancer* 2015;**51**(12):1497–510.
14. Francis A, Fallowfield L, Rea D. The LORIS trial: Addressing overtreatment of ductal carcinoma in situ. *Clin Oncol* 2015;**27**(1):6–8.
15. Biesheuvel C, Barratt A, Howard K, Houssami N, Irwig L. Effects of study methods and biases on estimates of invasive breast cancer overdetection with mammography screening: a systematic review. *Lancet Oncol* 2007;**8**(12):1129–38.
16. Puliti D, Duffy SW, Miccinesi G, de Koning H, Lynge E, Zappa M, et al. Overdiagnosis in mammographic screening for breast cancer in Europe: a literature review. *J Med Screen* 2012;**19**(Suppl. 1):42–56.
17. Carter JL, Coletti RJ, Harris RP. Quantifying and monitoring overdiagnosis in cancer screening: a systematic review of methods. *BMJ* 2015;**350**:g7773.
18. Mandelblatt JS, Cronin KA, de Koning HJ, Miglioretti DL, Schechter CB, Stout NC. *Collaborative modeling of U.S. breast cancer screening strategies*. Rockville, MD: Agency for Healthcare Research and Quality AHRQ Publication No. 14–05201-EF-4; 2015. [updated 4/2015]. Available from: <http://www.uspreventiveservicestaskforce.org/Page/Document/modeling-report-collaborative-modeling-of-us-breast-cancer-1/breast-cancer-screening1/> [accessed 09.02.15].
19. Miller AB, Wall C, Baines CJ, Sun P, To T, Narod SA. Twenty five year follow-up for breast cancer incidence and mortality of the Canadian National Breast Screening Study: randomised screening trial. *BMJ* 2014;**348**:g366.
20. Zackrisson S, Andersson I, Janzon L, Manjer J, Garne JP. Rate of over-diagnosis of breast cancer 15 years after end of Malmö mammographic screening trial: follow-up study. *BMJ* 2006;**332**(7543):689–92.
21. Jørgensen KJ, Gøtzsche PC. Overdiagnosis in publicly organised mammography screening programmes: Systematic review of incidence trends. *BMJ* 2009;**339**(7714):206–9.
22. Njor SH, Olsen AH, Blichert-Toft M, Schwartz W, Vejborg I, Lynge E. Overdiagnosis in screening mammography in Denmark: population based cohort study. *BMJ* 2013;**346**:f1064.
23. Beckmann KR, Lynch JW, Hiller JE, Farshid G, Houssami N, Duffy SW, et al. A novel case-control design to estimate the extent of over-diagnosis of breast cancer due to organised population-based mammography screening. *Int J Cancer* 2015;**136**(6):1411–21.
24. Falk RS, Hofvind S, Skaane P, Haldorsen T. Overdiagnosis among women attending a population-based mammography screening program. *Int J Cancer* 2013;**133**(3):705–12.

25. Ripping TM, Verbeek AL, Fracheboud J, de Koning HJ, van Ravesteyn NT, Broeders MJ. Overdiagnosis by mammographic screening for breast cancer studied in birth cohorts in The Netherlands. *Int J Cancer* 2015;**137**(4):921–9.
26. D'Orsi CJ SE, Mendelson EB, Morris EA, et al. *ACR BI-RADS® Atlas, breast imaging reporting and data system.* Reston, VA: American College of Radiology; 2013.
27. Salz T, Richman AR, Brewer NT. Meta-analyses of the effect of false-positive mammograms on generic and specific psychosocial outcomes. *Psycho-Oncology* 2010;**19**(10):1026–34.
28. Brett J, Bankhead C, Henderson B, Watson E, Austoker J. The psychological impact of mammographic screening. A systematic review. *Psycho-Oncology* 2005;**14**(11):917–38.
29. Tosteson AN, Fryback DG, Hammond CS, Hanna LG, Grove MR, Brown M, et al. Consequences of false-positive screening mammograms. *JAMA Intern Med* 2014;**174**(6):954–61.
30. Winch CJ, Sherman KA, Boyages J. Toward the breast screening balance sheet: cumulative risk of false positives for annual versus biennial mammograms commencing at age 40 or 50. *Breast Cancer Res Treat* 2015;**149**(1):211–21.
31. Brewer NT, Salz T, Lillie SE. Systematic review: The long-term effects of false-positive mammograms. *Ann Intern Med* 2007;**146**(7):502–10.
32. Armstrong K, Moye E, Williams S, Berlin JA, Reynolds EE. Screening mammography in women 40 to 49 years of age: a systematic review for the American College of Physicians. *Ann Intern Med* 2007;**146**(7):516–26.
33. Hendrick RE. Radiation doses and cancer risks from breast imaging studies. *Radiology* 2010;**257**(1):246–53.
34. Yaffe MJ, Mainprize JG. Risk of radiation-induced breast cancer from mammographic screening. *Radiology* 2011;**258**(1):98–105.
35. Miglioretti DL, Lange J, van Ravesteyn NT, van den Broek JJ, Lee CI, Melnikow J, et al. Radiation-induced breast cancer and breast cancer death from mammography screening. *Ann Intern Med* 2015; in press.
36. Nelson HD, Tyne K, Naik A, Bougatsos C, Chan BK, Humphrey L. Screening for breast cancer: an update for the U.S. preventive services task force. *Ann Intern Med* 2009;**151**(10):727–37.
37. Hofvind S, Ponti A, Patnick J, Ascunce N, Njor S, Broeders M, et al. False-positive results in mammographic screening for breast cancer in Europe: a literature review and survey of service screening programmes. *J Med Screen* 2012;**1**:57–66.
38. Harris RP, Sheridan SL, Lewis CL, Barclay C, Vu MB, Kistler CE, et al. The harms of screening: a proposed taxonomy and application to lung cancer screening. *JAMA Intern Med* 2014;**174**(2):281–5.
39. Renzi C, Whitaker KL, Wardle J. Over-reassurance and undersupport after a 'false alarm': a systematic review of the impact on subsequent cancer symptom attribution and help seeking. *BMJ Open* 2015;**5**(2):e007002.
40. Bennett RL, Sellars SJ, Moss SM. Interval cancers in the NHS breast cancer screening programme in England, Wales and Northern Ireland. *Br J Cancer* 2011;**104**(4):571–7.
41. Hofvind S, Yankaskas BC, Bulliard JL, Klabunde CN, Fracheboud J. Comparing interval breast cancer rates in Norway and North Carolina: results and challenges. *J Med Screen* 2009;**16**(3):131–9.
42. Tornberg S, Kemetli L, Ascunce N, Hofvind S, Anttila A, Seradour B, et al. A pooled analysis of interval cancer rates in six European countries. *Eur J Cancer Prev* 2010;**19**(2):87–93.
43. Hauge IH, Pedersen K, Olerud HM, Hole EO, Hofvind S. The risk of radiation-induced breast cancers due to biennial mammographic screening in women aged 50–69 years is minimal. *Acta Radiol* 2014;**55**(10):1174–9.
44. Whelehan P, Evans A, Wells M, Macgillivray S. The effect of mammography pain on repeat participation in breast cancer screening: a systematic review. *Breast* 2013;**22**(4):389–94.
45. Nelson HD, Cantor A, Humphrey L, Fu R, Pappas M, Daeges M, et al. Screening for breast cancer: a systematic review to Update the 2009 U.S. Preventive Service Task Force Recommendation [draft]; 2015.
46. Canadian Task Force on Preventive Health Care. Breast cancer-systematic [review]; 2011. <http://canadiantaskforce.ca/ctfphc-guidelines/2011-breast-cancer/systematic-review/>.
47. Canadian Task Force on Preventive Health C, Tonelli M, Connor Gorber S, et al. Recommendations on screening for breast cancer in average-risk women aged 40-74 years. *CMAJ* 2011;**183**(17):1991–2001.

48. Oeffinger K.C, Fontham E.T.H, Etzioni R, Herzig A, Michaelson J.S, Shih Y.C.T, et al. Breast cancer screening for women at average risk. guideline update from the American Cancer Society. JAMA 2015;**314**(15): 1599–614.
49. de Waard F, Kirkpatrick A, Perry NM, Tornberg S, Tubiana M, de Wolf C. Breast cancer screening in the framework of the Europe Against Cancer programme. *Eur J Cancer Prev* 1994;**3**(Suppl. 1):3–5.
50. Marmot MG, Altman DG, Cameron DA, Dewar JA, Thompson SG, Wilcox M. The benefits and harms of breast cancer screening: an independent review. *Br J Cancer* 2013;**108**(11):2205–40.
51. Paci E, Broeders M, Hofvind S, Puliti D, Duffy SW, Group EW. European breast cancer service screening outcomes: a first balance sheet of the benefits and harms. *Cancer Epidemiol Biomarkers Prev* 2014;**23**(7): 1159–63.
52. Paci E, Group EW. Summary of the evidence of breast cancer service screening outcomes in Europe and first estimate of the benefit and harm balance sheet. *J Med Screen* 2012;**19**(Suppl. 1):5–13.
53. Moss SM, Nystrom L, Jonsson H, Paci E, Lynge E, Njor S, et al. The impact of mammographic screening on breast cancer mortality in Europe: a review of trend studies. *J Med Screen* 2012;**19**(Suppl. 1):26–32.
54. van Schoor G, Moss SM, Otten JDM, Donders R, Paap E, den Heeten GJ, et al. Increasingly strong reduction in breast cancer mortality due to screening. *Br J Cancer* 2011;**104**(6):910–4.
55. Hofvind S, Skaane P, Elmore JG, Sebuodegard S, Hoff SR, Lee CI. Mammographic performance in a population-based screening program: before, during, and after the transition from screen-film to full-field digital mammography. *Radiology* 2014;**272**(1):52–62.
56. Friedewald SM, Rafferty EA, Rose SL, Durand MA, Plecha DM, Greenberg JS, et al. Breast cancer screening using tomosynthesis in combination with digital mammography. *JAMA* 2014;**311**(24):2499–507.
57. McCarthy AM, Kontos D, Synnestvedt M, Tan KS, Heitjan DF, Schnall M, et al. Screening outcomes following implementation of digital breast tomosynthesis in a general-population screening program. *J Natl Cancer Inst* 2014;**106**:11.
58. Broeders M, Moss S, Nystrom L, Njor S, Jonsson H, Paap E, et al. The impact of mammographic screening on breast cancer mortality in Europe: a review of observational studies. *J Med Screen* 2012;**19**(Suppl. 1):14–25.
59. Nelson HD, Tyne K, Naik A, Bougatsos C, Chan B, Nygren P, et al. Screening for breast cancer: systematic evidence review update for the US Preventive Services Task Force. Rockville, MD; Agency for Healthcare Research and Quality (US) 2009.
60. Bluekens AMJ, Karssemeijer N, Beijerinck D, Deurenberg JJM, van Engen RE, Broeders MJM, et al. Consequences of digital mammography in population-based breast cancer screening: initial changes and long-term impact on referral rates. *Eur Radiol* 2010;**20**(9):2067–73.
61. De Gelder R, Fracheboud J, Heijnsdijk EAM, den Heeten G, Berbeek AL, Broeders MJ, et al. Digital mammography screening: weighing reduced mortality against increased overdiagnosis. *Prev Med* 2011;**53**(3):134–40.
62. Hofvind S, Geller BM, Skelly J, Vacek PM. Sensitivity and specificity of mammographic screening as practised in Vermont and Norway. *Br J Radiol* 2012;**85**(1020):e1226–32.
63. Hofvind S, Vacek PM, Skelly J, Weaver DL, Geller BM. Comparing screening mammography for early breast cancer detection in Vermont and Norway. *J Natl Cancer Inst* 2008;**100**(15):1082–91.
64. Mammography quality standards act regulations. <http://www.fda.gov/Radiation-EmittingProducts/MammographyQualityStandardsActandProgram/Regulations/ucm110906.htm/>; 2002. [accessed 09.03.15].
65. *European guidelines for quality assurance in breast cancer screening and diagnosis*. Luxembourg: Office for Official Publications of the European Communities; 2006.
66. Weiss NS, Rossing MA. Healthy screened bias in epidemiologic studies of cancer incidence. *Epidemiology* 1996;**7**(3):319–22.
67. Roman M, Skaane P, Hofvind S. The cumulative risk of false-positive screening results across screening centres in the Norwegian Breast Cancer Screening Program. *Eur J Radiol* 2014;**83**(9):1639–44.
68. Etzioni R, Gulati R, Mallinger L, Mandelblatt J. Influence of study features and methods on overdiagnosis estimates in breast and prostate cancer screening. *Ann Intern Med* 2013;**158**(11):831–8.

69. Kerlikowske K, Hubbard RA, Miglioretti DL, Geller BM, Yankaskas BC, Lehman CD, et al. Comparative effectiveness of digital versus film-screen mammography in community practice in the United States a cohort study. *Ann Intern Med* 2011;**155**(8):493–502.
70. Pisano ED, Gatsonis C, Hendrick E, Yaffe M, Baum JK, Acharyya S, et al. Diagnostic performance of digital versus film mammography for breast-cancer screening. *N Engl J Med* 2005;**353**(17):1773–83.
71. Berry DA, Cronin KA, Plevritis SK, Fryback DG, Clarke L, Zelen M, et al. Effect of screening and adjuvant therapy on mortality from breast cancer. *N Engl J Med* 2005;**353**(17):1784–92.
72. Moss S. Overdiagnosis and overtreatment of breast cancer: overdiagnosis in randomised controlled trials of breast cancer screening. *Breast Cancer Res* 2005;**7**(5):230–4.
73. de Koning HJ, Draisma G, Fracheboud J, de Bruijn A. Overdiagnosis and overtreatment of breast cancer: microsimulation modelling estimates based on observed screen and clinical data. *Breast Cancer Res* 2006;**8**(1):202.
74. Duffy SW, Agbaje O, Tabar L, Vitak B, Bjurstam N, Bjorneld L, et al. Overdiagnosis and overtreatment of breast cancer: estimates of overdiagnosis from two trials of mammographic screening for breast cancer. *Breast Cancer Res* 2005;**7**(6):258–65.
75. Olsen AH, Agbaje OF, Myles JP, Lynge E, Duffy SW. Overdiagnosis, sojourn time, and sensitivity in the Copenhagen mammography screening program. *Breast J* 2006;**12**(4):338–42.
76. Paci E, Miccinesi G, Puliti D, Baldazzi P, De Lisi V, Falcini F, et al. Estimate of overdiagnosis of breast cancer due to mammography after adjustment for lead time. A service screening study in Italy. *Breast Cancer Res* 2006;**8**(6):R68.
77. Paci E, Warwick J, Falini P, Duffy SW. Overdiagnosis in screening: is the increase in breast cancer incidence rates a cause for concern? *J Med Screen* 2004;**11**(1):23–7.
78. Yen MF, Tabár L, Vitak B, Smith RA, Chen HH, Duffy SW. Quantifying the potential problem of overdiagnosis of ductal carcinoma in situ in breast cancer screening. *Eur J Cancer* 2003;**39**(12):1746–54.
79. Zahl PH, Strand BH, Maehlen J. Incidence of breast cancer in Norway and Sweden during introduction of nationwide screening: prospective cohort study. *BMJ* 2004;**328**(7445):921–4.
80. Bleyer A, Welch HG. Effect of three decades of screening mammography on breast-cancer incidence. *N Engl J Med* 2012;**367**(21):1998–2005.
81. Coldman A, Phillips N. Incidence of breast cancer and estimates of overdiagnosis after the initiation of a population-based mammography screening program. *CMAJ* 2013;**185**(10):E492–8.
82. De Gelder R, Heijnsdijk EAM, Van Ravesteyn NT, Fracheboud J, Draisma G, De Koning HJ. Interpreting overdiagnosis estimates in population-based mammography screening. *Epidemiol Rev* 2011;**33**(1):111–21.
83. Gunsoy NB, Garcia-Closas M, Moss SM. Estimating breast cancer mortality reduction and overdiagnosis due to screening for different strategies in the United Kingdom. *Br J Cancer* 2014;**110**(10):2412–9.
84. Hellquist BN, Duffy SW, Nystrom L, Jonsson H. Overdiagnosis in the population-based service screening programme with mammography for women aged 40 to 49 years in Sweden. *J Med Screen* 2012;**19**(1):14–19.
85. Kalager M, Adami H-O, Bretthauer M, Tamimi RM. Overdiagnosis of invasive breast cancer due to mammography screening: results from the Norwegian screening program. *Ann Intern Med* 2012;**156**(7):491–9.
86. Martinez-Alonso M, Vilaprinyo E, Marcos-Gragera R, Rue M. Breast cancer incidence and overdiagnosis in Catalonia (Spain). *Breast Cancer Res* 2010;**12**(4):R58.
87. Morrell S, Barratt A, Irwig L, Howard K, Biesheuvel C, Armstrong B. Estimates of overdiagnosis of invasive breast cancer associated with screening mammography. *Cancer Causes Control* 2010;**21**(2):275–82.
88. Puliti D, Zappa M, Miccinesi G, Falini P, Crocetti E, Paci E. An estimate of overdiagnosis 15 years after the start of mammographic screening in Florence. *Eur J Cancer* 2009;**45**(18):3166–71.
89. Seigneurin A, Francois O, Labarere J, Oudeville P, Monlong J, Colonna M. Overdiagnosis from non-progressive cancer detected by screening mammography: stochastic simulation study with calibration to population based registry data. *BMJ* 2011;**343**:d7017.

90. Yen AM, Duffy SW, Chen TH, Chen LS, Chiu SY, Fann JC, et al. Long-term incidence of breast cancer by trial arm in one county of the Swedish Two-County Trial of mammographic screening. *Cancer* 2012; **118**(23):5728–32.
91. Zahl PH, Maehlen J. Overdiagnosis of breast cancer after 14 years of mammography screening. *Tidsskr Nor Laegeforen* 2012;**132**(4):414–7.
92. Duffy SWTA, Olsen AH, Vitak B, Allgood PC, Chen THH, Yen AM, et al. Absolute numbers of lives saved and overdiagnosis in breast cancer screening, from a randomized trial and from the Breast Screening Programme in England. *J Med Screen* 2010;**17**(1):25–30.
93. Jorgensen KJ, Zahl PH, Gotzsche PC. Overdiagnosis in organised mammography screening in Denmark. A comparative study. *BMC Women's Health* 2009;**9**:36.
94. Barratt A, Howard K, Irwig L, Salkeld G, Houssami N. Model of outcomes of screening mammography: information to support informed choices. *BMJ* 2005;**330**(7497):936.
95. Castells X, Molins E, Macià F. Cumulative false positive recall rate and association with participant related factors in a population based breast cancer screening programme. *J Epidemiol Community Health* 2006;**60**(4):316–21.
96. Christiansen CL, Wang F, Barton MB, Kreuter W, Elmore JG, Gelfand AE, et al. Predicting the cumulative risk of false-positive mammograms. *J Natl Cancer Inst* 2000;**92**(20):1657–66.
97. Elmore JG, Barton MB, Moceri VM, Polk S, Arena PJ, Fletcher SW. Ten-year risk of false positive screening mammograms and clinical breast examinations. *N Engl J Med* 1998;**338**(16):1089–96.
98. Hofvind S, Thoresen S, Tretli S. The cumulative risk of a false-positive recall in the Norwegian Breast Cancer Screening Program. *Cancer* 2004;**101**(7):1501–7.
99. Hubbard RA, Kerlikowske K, Flowers CI, Yankaskas BC, Zhu W, Miglioretti DL. Cumulative probability of false-positive recall or biopsy recommendation after 10 years of screening mammography: a cohort study. *Ann Intern Med* 2011;**155**(8):481–92.
100. Johns LE, Moss SM, Age Trial Management G. False-positive results in the randomized controlled trial of mammographic screening from age 40 ("Age" trial). *Cancer Epidemiol Biomarkers Prev* 2010;**19**(11):2758–64.
101. Njor SH, Olsen AH, Schwartz W, Vejborg I, Lynge E. Predicting the risk of a false-positive test for women following a mammography screening programme. *J Med Screen* 2007;**14**(2):94–7.
102. Kerlikowske K, Zhu W, Hubbard RA, Geller B, Dittus K, Braithwaite D, et al. Outcomes of screening mammography by frequency, breast density, and postmenopausal hormone therapy. *JAMA Intern Med* 2013;**173**(9):807–16.
103. Salas D, Ibáñez J, Román R, Cuevas D, Sala M, Ascunce N, et al. Effect of start age of breast cancer screening mammography on the risk of false-positive results. *Prev Med* 2011;**53**(1–2):76–81.

CHAPTER

THE IMPORTANCE OF OBSERVATIONAL EVIDENCE TO ESTIMATE AND MONITOR MORTALITY REDUCTION FROM CURRENT BREAST CANCER SCREENING

4

Russell P. Harris[1,2]

[1]*School of Medicine, the Cecil G. Sheps Center for Health Services Research, UNC,* [2]*School of Public Health, University of North Carolina at Chapel Hill, Chapel Hill, NC, United States*

CHAPTER OUTLINE

PLAIN LANGUAGE SUMMARY

The benefits and harms of breast cancer screening have been debated for many years. One reason this debate continues is continuing uncertainty about the magnitude of these benefits and harms. In the past, decision makers have relied on randomized controlled trials (RCTs) to give us the best estimates of the benefit of screening—the breast cancer mortality reduction attributable to screening. However, these RCTs were conducted from 20 to 50 years ago. In that time several important factors have changed: women's breast cancer risk, screening technology, and breast cancer treatment. These factors could change the benefit of screening. Thus, we need current evidence about the reduction in breast cancer mortality from present-day screening. Because of the time required, the cost, and other inherent limitations of RCTs, this study design is not up to the task of providing this necessary information in a timely and ongoing manner.

Breast Cancer Screening. DOI: http://dx.doi.org/10.1016/B978-0-12-802209-2.00004-8

A number of observational studies have recently been conducted to help us better understand the effect of mammography in today's setting on breast cancer mortality. Unfortunately, these studies also have serious methodological limitations. A systematic review of the best of these studies shows much variation in their results. The best estimate from all of these studies is that current mammography is associated with about a 10% relative reduction in breast cancer mortality, which is less than predicted by the older RCTs. But this estimate is also not conclusive, and is likely to change in the future.

There is a need for an international team of experts to develop standards for higher-quality observational studies so that the effect of screening on breast cancer mortality can be better estimated and monitored over time.

INTRODUCTION

To make decisions about whether to start or continue widespread screening programs, and how intensive the screening should be, policy-makers need information about the current benefits and harms of screening. Clinicians need the same information to help their patients make individual decisions about screening. But we live in a constantly changing world, and what we thought we knew before rapidly becomes out of date and less relevant for today's decisions. Screening programs, like all other facets of health care, need to be evaluated at the beginning, and then constantly monitored as key factors change over time. Programs once regarded as high value (ie, providing benefits that clearly justify the harms and costs)[1] may become lower value as the risk of populations, screening technology, and treatment change.

It is important to require a high level of evidence about benefits and harms before implementing a widespread screening program at a particular intensity, and the same level of evidence to determine, periodically, whether the program should be continued at its current intensity. This high level of evidence is needed for at least three reasons: (1) the benefits of screening are often smaller than many would guess, and they may become even smaller over time; (2) the harms of screening are often larger than many would expect, and may grow over time; and (3) the costs of a full screening program are actually larger than many would suspect, and may increase over time. Screening programs that are implemented or continued without adequate supporting evidence may cause more harm than good and drain resources from other important health priorities.[2]

It has been thought that the highest evidence requirement for a screening program is a RCT of screening. But because of several inherent limitations of RCTs of screening, and because of the need for ongoing monitoring, this chapter will suggest that implementation of a new screening program, and determination of whether to continue an existing program at its current intensity, should require *both* an RCT of screening and adequate observational evidence to determine that the benefits of a specific screening strategy clearly outweigh the harms and costs (ie, that it is high value). One, or even several, RCTs of screening without appropriate observational evidence from screening implementation are not enough. Further, prior to implementation or continuation, there should also be a determination of the extent to which the screening program at its proposed intensity would reduce the societal burden of the condition, and whether the cost and effort of the program would be more wisely spent in another way that would have a greater effect on reducing societal burden from the same condition or other health problems. The screening programs that should be implemented or continued are the ones that are both high value (ie, provide—for the people screened—benefits that clearly outweigh the harms and costs) and also relieve a substantial part of society's burden of suffering from the condition.

These suggestions together would lead to a slowing down of implementation of new screening proposals (eg, adjunctive screening for women with dense breasts; changing primary screening from digital mammography to tomosynthesis), and perhaps a rolling back of the intensity of some existing programs. The intent is to increase the certainty that screening as currently practiced or proposed would actually lead to the wise use of resources to improve the health of the public without unduly increasing the harms of intensive health care.

Breast cancer screening has been implemented in many developed countries over the past 50 years, yet questions about the value of intensive screening and the extent to which this screening reduces the societal burden of breast cancer, remain, and may even be growing in importance. At least two of the reasons for this ongoing discussion may be an increasing awareness of the harms of screening, and an increasing concern that changes in population risk, screening technology, and treatment may make the results of the multiple screening RCTs less applicable to today. Although investigators have conducted many observational studies to help estimate current benefits and harms, these studies also have multiple methodologic challenges, and have yet to gain the full confidence of decision makers. The time has arrived when we should reexamine whether to continue breast cancer screening at its current level of intensity.

This review will examine the advantages and disadvantages of the older RCTs of breast cancer screening and the more recent observational evidence in assessing the current balance of benefits and harms of breast cancer screening. It will also make suggestions about how we might improve our evidence base to make better decisions about the appropriate intensity of breast cancer screening programs in the future.

ARE RCTs OF SCREENING THE "GOLD STANDARD"?

This section will briefly review some of the limitations of RCTs of screening. Further details of evidence from RCTs of breast cancer screening are provided in the chapter "Estimates of Screening Benefit: The Randomized Trials of Breast Cancer Screening" of this book. It is important to understand that RCTs of screening are different from RCTs of treatment. Trials of screening start with individuals who do not currently have a past diagnosis, symptoms, or signs of the condition in question; they then randomize participants to invitation to screening invitation or no invitation. Trials of treatment start with people who have the condition and randomize them to treatment "A" or treatment "B." Trials of treatment tell us relatively little about the benefits and harms of a screening program. This is because the issue of screening is whether *earlier* treatment conveys better health outcomes than *later* treatment. That is, the issue is the *timing* of treatment. The only difference between randomized groups in a screening RCT is that the affected individuals in the invited group are, on average, treated earlier than similar affected individuals in the not-invited group. The treatment strategy is the same in both groups—but it is just instituted earlier in the invited versus the not-invited group. The issue examined by RCTs of treatment is different: is treatment A better than treatment B?

But even RCTs of screening have limitations in providing the right evidence to determine the value of a screening program. First, screening RCTs estimate the benefits of a single screening intensity for a limited amount of time. For example, the Health Insurance Plan RCT in the United States, started in 1963, examined the effect on breast cancer mortality of five annual screening rounds of 1960s-type mammography and careful clinical breast examination (CBE) for women of ages 40–64 years. The study found a statistically significant 23–24% reduction in breast cancer mortality at 18 years follow-up.[3] This study provides important and necessary evidence that there is a benefit for some women from screening with annual mammography and careful CBE for 5 years. But the implications for policy-makers are still unclear. For example, is there further benefit from screening the same women for a longer duration? What are the physical and psychological harms of such screening? What is the cost of such screening? Would we gain similar benefit from screening every 2 or even 3 years rather than annually? Would we gain similar benefits from starting even earlier at age 30 and continuing even later to age 80? These questions revolve around the more general issue of intensity and value: how does value (ie, the balance between benefits and harms plus costs) change as we vary screening intensity (ie, the starting and stopping ages that define eligibility for screening and the frequency and sensitivity of the screening test)[1]? An RCT of screening does not vary intensity, nor does it adequately assess the real–life harms and costs of screening in the community.

There are further deficiencies in the evidence provided by RCTs of screening. In many cases, participants in screening RCTs are not representative of the larger potentially-eligible population. In addition, the personnel and technology of screening and treatment in RCTs may be very different from that available in most community settings. Another important limitation of screening RCTs for breast cancer is that the trials were mostly conducted in the 1960s, 1970s, and early 1980s. Since then, the risk of developing breast cancer has changed for the population of screening-eligible women—with the rise and fall of postmenopausal hormone treatment, the increased prevalence of obesity, the increased awareness of women about breast lumps, changes in age at menarche and menopause, change in age at first pregnancy. Also, the technology of screening has changed, increasing its sensitivity and the cancer detection rate. Perhaps most dramatically, the range and effectiveness of treatment has increased. Thus, it is not clear how applicable the results of these older RCTs are to the present day. It may be, in fact, that increased sensitivity of screening tools, which find more lesions that are pathologically "breast cancer," may not have reduced mortality more than older, less sensitive mammography, but may instead have increased overdiagnosis by finding those "breast cancers" that would never progress to clinically important lesions.

In addition, RCTs rarely provide adequate evidence about the potential harms of screening. Without evidence about harms, calculation of the balance between benefits versus harms/costs (ie, the value) of a screening program is impossible.[2] These harms occur throughout the screening process, and can be organized into several categories: physical harms (eg, infection from a breast biopsy), psychological harms (eg, anxiety from a false positive mammogram), financial strain (eg, worry about future anticipated expenses from dealing with a newly detected lesion), opportunity costs (eg, lost opportunities to participate in work or family events due to time needed for testing/treatment or due to distraction from concern over positive screening), or hassles (eg, difficulties in organizing transportation or substitutes for responsibilities).[4] The problem of overdiagnosis, which is a potential problem in nearly every screening program, can have both psychological (eg, labeling) and physical (eg, overtreatment) effects (see also chapter: Challenges in Understanding and Quantifying Overdiagnosis and Overtreatment, for further details on overdiagnosis). For each of these potential harms, decision makers need information about both the frequency and the severity of the harm. RCTs, whether of screening or of treatment, rarely provide adequate information about these harms.

Thus, these inherent limitations of RCTs of screening

- failure to provide comparative evidence about different *intensities* (ie, frequency, starting and stopping ages, test sensitivity) of screening;
- failure to provide evidence about *long-term effects* of screening;

- failure to provide adequate evidence about screening *harms or costs*;
- failure to provide evidence about the benefits and harms of *current-day* screening;
- failure to provide evidence of the effects of screening in usual, *community settings*.

make it unlikely that RCTs of screening alone can provide all the evidence that decision makers need. The "gold standard" of screening RCTs, while necessary to provide evidence that the concept of screening is beneficial, is not sufficient to provide all of the evidence needed to decide about implementing or continuing a screening program.

ADVANTAGES AND PROBLEMS WITH OBSERVATIONAL STUDIES

Well-conducted observational studies of various designs can supplement RCTs to supply the evidence we need to make optimal decisions about screening programs. Prospective cohort and ecologic designs have the greatest potential value, and could be conducted within already existing national databases. Linking national databases that reliably capture information on women's risk characteristics, adherence to a specific screening strategy, types of breast cancers diagnosed, treatment received, and breast cancer deaths, these types of studies can be conducted in an ongoing, monitoring manner, and thus can help us understand changes in mortality as women's risk, screening technology, and treatment change. Thus, if a country expands screening to a younger or older age group, or changes screening technology or frequency, the effects on incidence, mortality, medical procedures (eg, mastectomy), and even false positive screening tests could be assessed. In addition, prospective cohort and ecologic designs can be used to compare trends in breast cancer mortality among countries with different intensities of screening, thus gaining insight into the value of different starting and stopping ages, different frequencies of screening, and different screening strategies with different sensitivities. These study designs are also much less costly than expensive RCTs, and can provide evidence in a more timely fashion.

Prospective cohort designs are most helpful, as they include individual-level data, linking actual screening behavior with incidence and mortality in the same people. These cohorts are most helpful when they are true inception cohorts, such as birth cohorts, and when they are analyzed in a similar way to the way an RCT would be analyzed. This involves minimizing selection bias by including only participants meeting strict eligibility criteria: enrolling only people with similar risk for incidence and mortality, excluding people at the start who do not represent the typical risk profile of the population of interest. Birth cohorts are a particularly good choice as all are exposed similarly to risk-changing external factors over time. Because prospective cohort studies can collect information on various potential confounding factors (ie, factors that are unbalanced between comparison groups, that may explain mortality differences that would otherwise be incorrectly ascribed to screening) over time, they can adjust for these confounders in the analysis, thus minimizing selection bias. Prospective cohort studies also collect data over time on both exposure (ie, particular intensities of screening) and outcome (ie, cancer incidence and mortality) in uniform ways, and thus measurement can be more accurate and reliable, and data can be collected equally between more-intensive and less-intensive screening groups. Prospective cohort studies can also minimize bias and imprecision in assessment of outcomes by using committees blinded to exposure to impose strict criteria for such outcomes as mortality due to breast cancer. Because prospective cohort studies can include large numbers of people and continue over long periods of time, they can examine longer-term effects of screening programs and provide more precise estimates. Finally, prospective cohort studies examine screening as practiced in the community in the current time period, making their results more applicable to the real population and to present-day decision making.

Ecologic studies have many of the same advantages as prospective cohorts, except they do not gather individual-level data, and thus open themselves up the "ecologic fallacy" of drawing conclusions only indirectly on population incidence and mortality from individual screening. They are also more subject to selection bias than prospective cohort studies, as statistical adjustment for potential confounding factors can only be done on a population rather than an individual basis. Finally, measurement bias is also potentially more problematic in ecologic studies than in prospective cohorts because assessment of exposure, potential confounders, and outcome is on a population basis, potentially more prone to systematic and random error than would individual data. Ecologic studies, however, do capture the final result we all care most about—the health of the general public. Whatever the screening or other health program, if it doesn't have an effect on the health of the public on a population level, then it can hardly be said to have succeeded. To the extent that those aspects of health most important to the people involved can and are assessed by ecologic studies, these studies may more rightly be considered the end result of a chain of evidence, the chain being the real "gold standard."

There are important problems, however, with prospective cohort and ecologic studies. Some—related to "internal validity" (risk of bias)—are noted above. Selection bias, measurement bias, and confounding are large challenges that are not easily solved. In general, the risk of bias of these studies is greater than well-conducted RCTs. If well conducted, however, prospective cohort and ecologic studies can still provide more applicable and current information for decision makers. Beyond risk of bias, prospective cohorts and ecologic studies are subject to variation in design features and statistical analysis that make interpretation difficult and result in dueling and conflicting results. Among the design features are studies that do not include information on potentially important confounding variables (eg, use of postmenopausal hormone treatment or change in body mass index) or on accessibility of effective treatment (eg, tamoxifen). Thus, differences in mortality between groups screened at different intensities may reflect factors other than screening.

Among the statistical analysis problems are studies that include adjustment for lead time and for actual (vs invited) screening. These adjustments tend to increase the estimated mortality reduction from more intensive screening, but can be criticized as overadjustment (in the case of lead time) or as addressing a separate question (in the case of actual screening). If a prospective cohort study uses an inception cohort over a lengthy time period, collecting cumulative data on breast cancer incidence and mortality between groups screened more versus less intensively, then adjustment for lead time should not be needed. Likewise, adjustment for actual screening is asking a question for an ideal rather than the real world—what would the mortality reduction be if everyone invited to screening and no one not invited actually underwent screening? Decision makers need an answer to a different question: what would the mortality reduction be in the real world (where some invited people are not screened and some not invited people are) if this screening program at the studied intensity were to be implemented? Adjusting mortality differences to reflect an idealized world answers the wrong question and is unwarranted. Even so, one must realize that screening in the "not-invited" control group in observational studies has the potential to underestimate the effect of instituting a new screening program (or modifying an older program) compared with a totally unscreened area.

One further design problem should be addressed. In considering changes in intensity of screening—including changes in starting or stopping ages, changes in screening frequency, or changes in the sensitivity of screening strategies—observational studies may sometimes focus on intermediate rather than health outcomes. These include changes in interval cancers or in stage of diagnosis rather than breast cancer mortality. The validity of these intermediate outcomes, however, depends entirely on the extent to which they accurately predict health outcomes. Even more difficult is that the change in intermediate outcomes must predict not only the direction but also the *magnitude* of change in the health outcome. It is important to remember that policy-makers must weigh the *magnitude* of benefits (ie, breast cancer mortality reduction) against the *magnitude* of harms and costs in arriving at a fair assessment of the value of a particular screening intensity.[2] Because large observational studies may provide an assessment of only the direction rather than the magnitude of health benefit, and because large observational studies may not adequately assess harms and costs, they must be interpreted with caution. Our current understanding of prognostic factors for breast cancer is incomplete; one should resist the temptation to overinterpret changes in stage at diagnosis or interval cancers as providing adequate evidence for a large magnitude of reduction in breast cancer morbidity or mortality. Overinterpretation of these studies would be an error.

WHAT DO OBSERVATIONAL STUDIES TELL US NOW?

In 2011, we published a systematic review of observational evidence[5] on reduction in breast cancer mortality, with a search strategy ending on Mar. 1, 2011. That review included 17 studies that were large population-based cohort and ecologic studies that estimated the effect of screening on breast cancer mortality (Table 4.1). We excluded studies rated as high risk of bias (including studies that compared "attenders" with "nonattenders") and studies that were extensively based on statistical models. We found methodologic concerns in all 17 studies, with large variation in estimates of mortality reduction. Five studies found either a small or no effect of screening on mortality (ie, from 0% to 12% relative risk reduction (RRR)); four studies found a large effect (ie, over 33% RRR); and eight studies found a moderate effect (ie, between 13% and 32% RRR). All estimates lacked precision, with overlap of confidence intervals at around 20–25% RRR. None of the studies were able to adequately adjust for differences in breast cancer risk, screening technology, or treatment among compared groups. We concluded that methodologic problems prevented a firm estimate, but that, if a previous estimate of about 50% of the observed population mortality reduction is due to screening and 50% due to treatment,[6] then our best estimate would be that the actual RRR was about 50% of 20–25%, or about 10–12.5%. This is lower than has been estimated from the RCTs of screening.

We have recently updated this search, through Sep. 30, 2015. Using the same search strategy and selection criteria, we found an additional five studies that met our inclusion criteria. Two of these studies[7,8] were from Norway, one from Australia,[9] one from Finland,[10] and one from the United States.[11] The two studies from Norway were cohort studies, while the other three were ecologic in design. The US study covered the time period from 2000 to 2010, while the others covered the general time period between the mid-1980s and 2009. One study (the United States) found no association between areas exposed to greater mammography intensity and breast cancer mortality; one study from Norway[5] found a nonstatistically significant relative reduction of 11% in breast cancer mortality for geographic areas after versus before the start of a screening program. The other three studies found RRR for breast cancer mortality between geographic areas invited versus not invited to screening of 21%[9]; 25%, only for women ages 60–74[10]; and 28%.[8] None of these studies was able to adequately adjust for differences in women's risk of breast cancer or treatment of breast cancer over the time periods studied.

Table 4.1 Summary Evidence Table—Observational Study Evidence for Effectiveness of Breast Cancer Screening to Reduce Breast Cancer Mortality

Citation; Study Design[a]; Population(s) Compared (eg, Age, Size, Country)	Study Period; Length of Follow-Up; Frequency of Screening	Type of Control Group(s)	Adjustment for Breast Cancer Treatment as Potential Confounder	a. Overall Relative and Absolute Reduction in Breast Cancer Mortality (Screening, Treatment, and Other) b. Estimated Independent Effect of Screening on Breast Cancer Mortality (If Estimated)	a. Quality Rating[b] b. Interpretability[c] c. Comments
No to Low Effectiveness (0–12% Relative Reduction in Breast Cancer Mortality)					
Törnberg (2006); Ecologic; Ages 50–69; Population size: 40,000 (Helsinki), 190,000 (Stockholm), 52,000 (Copenhagen), 46,000 (Oslo); 4 Scandinavian capitals	Study period varied (1986–96 to 1995–99); 10-year follow-up in 2 sites; Frequency: 24 months	Historical local	No adjustment	a. No reduction in breast cancer mortality (no relative risk reduction (RRR) or absolute risk/rate reduction (ARR) estimates given) b. Not estimated (NE)	a. FAIR b. FAIR c. Low precision, may need longer follow-up
Jørgensen (2010); Ecologic; Compared ages 55–74 vs ages 35–54 and ages 75–84; Population size not given; Copenhagen, Funen, remainder of Denmark	1997–2006; 10-year follow-up; Frequency not stated	Historical and concurrent regional	No adjustment	a. 1% annual RRR (95% confidence interval (CI) 0.96–1.01) in screened group; 2% annual RRR (95% CI 0.97–0.99) in nonscreened group, both in ages 55–74; no ARR estimates given b. NE	a. FAIR b. GOOD c. Good precision, uncertain about potential confounders
Broeders (2001); Ecologic; Ages 50–79; Population size increased by year; Nijmegen, Arnhem, the Netherlands	1969–97; 20+ year follow-up; Frequency not stated	Historical local and concurrent regional	No adjustment	a. RRR ranges from 6% (95% CI 27–31) to 16% (95% CI 17–39), depending on control group; no ARR estimates given b. NE	a. FAIR b. FAIR c. Low precision
Jonsson (2003); Hybrid; Ages 40–64; Population size: 43,749 (1977); Gävleborg, Sweden	1974–98; 22-year follow-up; Frequency not stated	Historical local and 2 concurrent regional	No adjustment	a. Control group 1: 14% RRR (95% CI 5–29) for ages 40–64; Control group 2: 7% RRR (95% CI 11–23) for ages 40–64; no ARR estimates given b. NE	a. FAIR b. FAIR c. Low precision, uncertain treatment effect, uncertain comparability of groups

Jonsson (2001); Hybrid; Ages 50–69; Population size: 260,594 (1987); Sweden	1979–97; 10.6-year mean follow-up; Frequency not stated	Historical local and concurrent regional	No adjustment	a. 12% adjusted RRR for annual underlying cause of death (95% CI 10–26) for ages 50–69; no ARR estimates given b. NE	a. FAIR b. FAIR c. Low precision, uncertain treatment differences, uncertain comparability of groups
Moderate Effectiveness (13–33% Relative Reduction in Breast Cancer Mortality)					
Anttila (2002); Cohort; Ages 50–59; Population size: 144,400 invitations; Helsinki	1986–97; 10-year maximum follow-up; Frequency: every 2 years	Historical local	No adjustment	a. 19% RRR (95% CI 5–38) for ages 50–69; 9.1 deaths per 100,000 woman-years ARR (no CI given) b. NE	a. FAIR b. GOOD c. Low precision, uncertain treatment differences
Otto (2003); Ecologic (population-level data only reviewed); Ages 55–74 (for mortality data); Population size: 27,948; The Netherlands	1980–99; 12-year follow-up; Frequency not stated	Trend	No adjustment	a. 20% RRR (95% CI 14–27) for ages 55–74; no ARR estimates given b. NE	a. FAIR b. GOOD c. Moderate precision, uncertain treatment differences
Jonsson (2007); Cohort; Ages 50–69; Population size: 186,000; 4 counties in Northern Sweden	1988–99; 11-year follow-up; Frequency: every 22–24 months	Historical local and concurrent regional	No adjustment	a. 20% RRR (95% CI 0–36) for ages 50–69; no ARR estimates given b. NE	a. FAIR b. FAIR (multiple adjustments) c. Low precision, historical local control group not clear
Sarkeala (2008); Cohort; Ages 50–69; Population size: 361,848; Areas within Finland	1974–85 and 1992–2003; 9.8-year follow-up; Frequency: every 2 years	Historical local and concurrent regional	No adjustment	a. 22% RRR (95% CI 13–30) for ages 50–69; no ARR estimates given b. NE	a. FAIR b. FAIR c. Moderate precision, uncertain treatment differences, uncertain comparability of groups

(Continued)

Table 4.1 Summary Evidence Table—Observational Study Evidence for Effectiveness of Breast Cancer Screening to Reduce Breast Cancer Mortality (Continued)

Citation; Study Design[a]; Population(s) Compared (eg, Age, Size, Country)	Study Period; Length of Follow-Up; Frequency of Screening	Type of Control Group(s)	Adjustment for Breast Cancer Treatment as Potential Confounder	a. Overall Relative and Absolute Reduction in Breast Cancer Mortality (Screening, Treatment, and Other) b. Estimated Independent Effect of Screening on Breast Cancer Mortality (If Estimated)	a. Quality Rating[b] b. Interpretability[c] c. Comments
Tabar (2003); Ecologic; Ages 20–69; Population size: 210,000; Uppsala and Linköping Sweden	1958–97; 20-year follow-up; Frequency not stated	Historical local	No adjustment	a. 23% RRR (95% CI 15–30) for ages 40–69; no ARR estimates given b. NE	a. FAIR b. FAIR c. Moderate precision, uncertain treatment differences
Olsen (2005); Olsen (2007); Cohort; Ages 50–69; Olsen Population size not stated; Copenhagen, Denmark	1991–2001; 10-year follow-up; Frequency: every 2 years	Historical local, concurrent regional, and historical regional	No adjustment	a. 25% RRR (95% CI 11–37) for ages 50–69; no ARR estimates given b. NE	a. FAIR b. GOOD c. Moderate precision, uncertain treatment differences, uncertain comparability of groups
Swedish Organized Service Screening Evaluation Group (2006); Hybrid; Ages 40–69; Population size: 1,108,610 13 areas within 9 counties in Sweden	1958–2001; 20–44-year follow-up; Frequency not stated	Historical local	No adjustment	a. 27% RRR (95% CI 23–31) for ages 40/50–69; no ARR estimates given b. NE	a. FAIR b. FAIR c. Good precision, uncertain treatment differences, uncertain comparability of groups
Duffy (2010); Ecologic (data from England only considered); Ages 50–69; Population size: not stated; England	1974–2004; 10-year follow-up; Frequency: every 3 years	Historical regional	No adjustment	a. 28% RRR (95% CI 26–30) for ages 50–69; 23.1 deaths per 100,000 woman-years ARR (no CI given) b. NE	a. FAIR b. FAIR c. Good precision, uncertain treatment differences

High Effectiveness (34% or Greater Relative Reduction in Breast Cancer Mortality)					
Parvinen (2006); Hybrid; Ages 55–69; Population size: 1,980,026 total woman-years in study and reference populations); 3 cities in Finland	1976–2001; 15-year follow-up; Frequency: every 2 years	Historical and concurrent local and regional	No adjustment	a. 36% RRR (95% CI 12–53) for ages 55–69; 16.9 deaths per 100,000 woman-years ARR (no CI given) b. NE	a. FAIR b. POOR c. Low precision, uncertain comparability of groups, uncertain treatment differences
Gorini (2004); Ecologic; Ages 55–74; Population size not stated; 2 areas in the province of Florence, Italy	1985–2000; 15-year follow-up; Frequency not stated	Historical local and concurrent regional	Statistical calculation based on changes in control area	a. 42% (95% CI 12–70) for ages 55–64; 65% (95% CI 0–70) for ages 65–74; 16.8 deaths per 100,000 woman-years ARR (no CI given) b. 26% for ages 55–64; 34% for ages 65–74	a. FAIR to POOR b. FAIR c. Low precision; rural vs urban setting and treatment differences are potential confounders
Ascunce (2007); Ecologic; Ages 50–69; Population size not stated; Navarre, Spain	1986/90 compared with 1997/2001; 11-year follow-up; Frequency: every 2 years	Historical local and concurrent regional	No adjustment	a. 42% RRR (95% CI 25–56) for ages 50–69; 21.9 deaths per 100,000 woman-years ARR (no CI given) b. NE	a. FAIR b. POOR c. Low precision, overall country mortality reduced despite minimal screening
Garne (1997); Hybrid; Ages 45–69; Population size: ranged from 118,565 to 136,083; Malmö, Sweden	1964–92; 16-year follow-up; Frequency not stated	Historical and concurrent local and regional	No adjustment	a. 43% RRR (95% CI 26–56) for ages 45–69; 3.1 deaths per 100,000 women over 17 years ARR (no CI given) b. NE	a. FAIR b. GOOD c. Low precision; uncertain comparability of groups; uncertain treatment differences

Description and critical appraisal of 17 observational studies meeting eligibility criteria, assessing the magnitude of the effect of breast cancer screening on mortality from breast cancer.

[a]*Study design: ecologic means both data about exposure to mammography and breast cancer mortality are at the local/regional (not individual) level; hybrid means that data about exposure to mammography are at the local/regional level but data about breast cancer mortality are at the individual level; cohort means that both data about exposure to mammography and breast cancer mortality are at the individual level.*

[b]*Quality rating (good, fair, poor) based on 5 ratings: (1) precision of estimates, (2) validity and reliability of measurements (especially cause of death), (3) comparability of groups, (4) consideration of potential confounders (treatment, patient awareness of breast cancer symptoms, other patient factors), (5) external validity.*

[c]*Interpretability rating (good, fair, poor) based on 2 ratings: (1) clarity and justification of adjustments, (2) relevance to review question (effect on breast cancer mortality of breast cancer screening implementation).*

In all, these studies confirm the prior findings that most cohort or ecologic studies have found that screening programs are associated with a 20–25% reduction in breast cancer mortality. As above, if half of this mortality reduction is attributable to screening (as opposed to treatment or other differences between compared populations), then the *true screening effect may be between 10% and 12.5% reduction in breast cancer mortality*, lower than predicted by several of the RCTs of screening. This likely represents a more realistic estimate of current screening practice.

Despite the general uniformity of findings, there remains much uncertainty about the best interpretation of this evidence. If, for example, differences in factors other than screening between compared groups are larger than statistical adjustments have allowed, then the true screening effect would be less than 10%. If, on the other hand, most of the total reduction in breast cancer mortality over the study periods is in fact attributable to screening, then the true screening effect would be closer to 20%. Note that if the studies had been able to adjust for more potential confounding factors, such as improved treatment, the best interpretation would become clearer. Improved standards for cohort and ecologic studies could help us with future interpretations of these complex data.

Interestingly, other groups, examining many of the same studies, have come to other interpretations. The Independent UK Panel on Breast Cancer Screening[12] determined that the variation in the results of ecologic studies made them not useful in estimating the effects of screening. They also found that cohort studies more often gave estimates of mortality reduction greater than the RCTs. However, the UK Panel was concerned that residual bias could explain these differences, and thus it decided that the older RCTs provide a better estimate of the current effect of screening than the observational evidence.

In the United States, a review for the US Preventive Services Task Force[13] and a review for the American Cancer Society[14] both examined observational evidence primarily through other systematic reviews, principally three reviews by the EUROSCREEN group published in 2012.[15–17] These reviews suffer from several drawbacks:

- inappropriate inclusion of studies that overlapped with other included studies
- inappropriate exclusion of studies that did not adjust for lead time, when this adjustment was itself inappropriate
- inappropriate inclusion of studies that inappropriately adjusted for lead time
- focus on comparing screened versus unscreened populations rather than invited-to-screen versus not invited
- insufficient critical appraisal
- inappropriate pooling of data with substantial heterogeneity
- no appreciation of the failure of the observational studies to adjust for differences among populations in risk, screening technology, and treatment.

For these reasons, the results of these reviews tend to be somewhat inflated compared with our findings. For "trend studies" (ie, studies comparing mortality before and after a screening program is instituted for a single population), they found a range of 28–36% RRR among 12 studies.[16,17] For "incidence-based mortality" studies (ie, cohort or ecologic studies comparing different geographic areas), a pooled analysis found a relative risk of 0.75 (95% CI 0.69–0.81), or a 25% RRR.[15,17] Correctly interpreted, these reviews do not differ markedly from our results.

HOW TO IMPROVE OUR OBSERVATIONAL EVIDENCE?

Although prospective cohort and ecologic studies have the potential to provide useful evidence about the effect of screening on breast cancer mortality under actual conditions today, methodologic problems with many of these studies prevent us from drawing firm conclusions. The potential could be better realized if there were standards for these studies, developed by an independent group of experts, and a consortium of independent investigators who could monitor these data from multiple countries over time. Once established, the evidence base for deciding the appropriate screening intensity for different screening situations could be greatly improved. Clearly, these ongoing studies would need to also monitor such harms as overdiagnosis as well as financial cost as well as mortality. The question to be answered is the value of current screening programs, and whether they should be continued at their present level of intensity. The answer to the value question depends on having good evidence about benefits, harms, and costs, and then about different societies asking whether the magnitude of benefits justifies the associated harms and costs.

Among the methodologic questions that the independent group of experts should clarify are:

- how best to continuously gather data on factors that could modify the effect of screening on mortality (eg, breast cancer risk, exposure to screening at a particular intensity, breast cancer treatment)
- how best to continuously gather data on breast cancer incidence and mortality
- how best to analyze these data in an ongoing manner, dealing with such issues as adjustment for lead time and lack of adherence to screening
- how best to analyze observational data as an RCT
- how best to avoid the ecologic fallacy
- how best to avoid the inappropriate use and interpretation of intermediate outcomes.

What is clearly needed is a uniform set of standards for conducting prospective cohort and ecologic studies, plus validated national databases to collect in an ongoing way the critical variables, and an unbiased international team of investigators to monitor incidence and mortality in multiple countries over time.

CONCLUSIONS

There is no single best way to estimate and monitor the mortality benefit of a program of breast cancer screening. RCTs of screening have helped us understand that the cancer biology, breast cancer risk levels, screening technology, and treatment conditions are in place so that benefit is possible. Unfortunately, these critically important factors are all changing. We struggle now to know whether the benefit is the same as previously, and whether the harms and costs have now overcome any remaining benefit. Observational evidence is necessary to answer these issues. We cannot wait for future RCTs—which may not even occur—and which may well be outdated by the time they publish their results. But neither should we simply assume that breast cancer screening will retain its same benefits, harms, and costs into the indefinite future. Timely, well-conducted observational evidence is necessary to help us answer these questions.

Our review has several important findings:

- the observational literature has many limitations—our certainty in these results is at best moderate;
- it is likely that there continues to be a mortality reduction from breast cancer screening programs—perhaps on the order of a 10% RRR;
- there is no convincing evidence at present that the mortality reduction is declining, although this remains a possibility in the future;
- observational evidence is also needed to examine the harms and costs of screening, to determine whether screening continues to be high enough value that it should be continued.

This final point should be emphasized. Even if there remains a mortality reduction from breast cancer screening, the determination of value—the extent to which the magnitude of benefit is large enough to justify the associated harms and costs—is still to be determined. Only by having good quality evidence about benefits, harms, and costs together can policy-makers, and the public, decide whether screening should continue, and, if so, at what level of intensity.

REFERENCES

1. Harris RP, Wilt TJ, Qaseem A. A value framework for cancer screening: Advice for high-value care from the American College of Physicians. *Ann Int Med* 2015;**162**:712–7.
2. Harris RP, Sawaya GF, Moyer VA, Calonge N. Reconsidering the criteria for evaluating proposed screening programs: Reflections from 4 current and former members of the U.S. Preventive Services Task Force. *Epidemiol Rev* 2011;**33**:20–35.
3. Shapiro S, Venet W, Strax P, Venet L. *Periodic screening for breast cancer*. Baltimore: The Johns Hopkins University Press; 1988.p. 77.
4. Harris RP, Sheridan SL, Lewis CL, Barclay C, Vu MB, Kistler CE, et al. The harms of screening: A proposed taxonomy and application to lung cancer screening. *JAMA Intern Med* 2014;**174**:281–5.
5. Harris R, Yeatts J, Kinsinger L. Breast cancer screening for women ages 50 to 69 years: A systematic review of observational evidence. *Prev Med* 2011;**53**:108–14.
6. Berry DA, Cronin KA, Plevritis SK, Fryback DG, Clarke L, Zelen M, et al. Effect of screening and adjuvant therapy on mortality from breast cancer. *N Engl J Med* 2005;**353**:1784–92.
7. Olsen AH, Lynge E, Njor SH, Kumle M, Waaseth M, Braaten T, et al. Breast cancer mortality in Norway after the introduction of mammography screening. *Int J Cancer* 2013;**132**:208–14.
8. Weedon-Fekjaer H, Pal RR, Vatten LJ. Modern mammography screening and breast cancer mortality: Population study. *BMJ* 2014;**348**:g3701.
9. Morrell S, Taylor R, Roder D, Dobson A. Mammography screening and breast cancer mortality in Australia: An aggregate cohort study. *J Med Screen* 2012;**19**:26–34.
10. Parvinen I, Heinavaara S, Anttila A, Helenius H, Klemi P, Pylkkanen L. Mammography screening in three Finnish residential areas: Comprehensive population-based study of breast cancer incidence and incidence-based mortality 1976–2009. *Br J Cancer* 2015;**112**:918–24.
11. Harding C, Pompei F, Burmistrov D, Welch HG, Abebe R, Wilson R. Breast cancer screening, incidence, and mortality across U.S. Counties. *JAMA Intern Med* 2015;**175**:1483–9.
12. Independent UK Panel on Breast Cancer Screening The benefits and harms of breast cancer screening: An independent review. *Lancet* 2012;**380**:1778–86.

13. Nelson, H.D., Cantor, A., Humphrey, L., Fu, R., Pappas, M., Daeges, M., et al. Screening for breast cancer: A systematic review to update the 2009 U.S. Preventive Services Task Force recommendation. AHRQ publication No. 14-05201-EF-1, 2015 April.
14. Myers ER, Moorman P, Gierisch JM, Havrilesky LJ, Grimm LJ, Ghate S, et al. Benefits and harms of breast cancer screening: A systematic review. *JAMA* 2015;**314**:1615–34.
15. Njor S, Nystrom L, Moss S, Paci E, Broeders M, Segnan N, et al. Breast cancer mortality in mammographic screening in Europe: A review of incidence-based mortality studies. *J Med Screen* 2012;**19**(Suppl. 1):33–41.
16. Broeders M, Moss S, Nystrom L, Njor S, Jonsson H, Paap E, et al. The impact of mammographic screening on breast cancer mortality in Europe: A review of observational studies. *J Med Screen* 2012;**19**(Suppl. 1):14–25.
17. Moss SM, Nystron L, Jonsson H, Paci E, Lynge E, Njor S, et al. The impact of mammographic screening on breast cancer mortality in Europe: A review of trend studies. *J Med Screen* 2012;**19**(Suppl. 1):26–32.

CHAPTER

THE ROLE OF MICROSIMULATION MODELING IN EVALUATING THE OUTCOMES AND EFFECT OF SCREENING

5

Clyde B. Schechter[1] and Nicolien T. van Ravesteyn[2]
[1]*Department of Family & Social Medicine, Albert Einstein College of Medicine, Bronx, NY, United States,*
[2]*Department of Public Health, Erasmus Medical Center, Rotterdam, The Netherlands*

CHAPTER OUTLINE

Breast Cancer Screening. DOI: http://dx.doi.org/10.1016/B978-0-12-802209-2.00005-X

PLAIN LANGUAGE SUMMARY

Microsimulation is a process where complex processes are modeled on computers programmed to combine information about separate components of the process into an overall picture. For breast cancer screening this means combining information about the epidemiology of breast cancer, the use and accuracy of screening to detect tumors earlier, and the response of breast cancer to treatment at different times to draw conclusions about the effect of actual or hypothetical screening programs on the frequency of occurrence of, and death from, breast cancer. In this chapter, we review the use of microsimulation to inform breast cancer screening practices and policy.

This chapter begins with a description of some existing microsimulation models and how they are developed and tested for validity. We then review the use of simulation models to provide deeper understanding of the results of clinical trials of mammography and observational data, highlighting, for example, our enhanced understanding of the relative contributions of mammography and adjuvant hormonal treatment and chemotherapy to the ongoing decline in breast cancer mortality.

A particularly important application of microsimulation is projecting the results of different strategies for using mammography. Numerous conflicting guidelines have been proposed regarding starting age, stopping age, and interval between mammograms. None of these guidelines can be directly supported by evidence because clinical trials have not used precisely those protocols, and have not provided life-long follow-up. Microsimulations fill this gap by implementing the protocols under consideration digitally, applying them to simulated women whose "breast cancer histories" mimic those of real women. In addition to providing insight into screening schedules not studied in clinical trials, microsimulations can shed light on the potential of alternative established or existing imaging techniques to improve breast cancer mortality when used in addition to, or instead of, mammography.

Microsimulations also underlie cost-effectiveness analyses of mammographic screening programs, and several examples are discussed.

This chapter continues with a discussion of the strengths and weaknesses of microsimulation as a source of understanding, and the special advantages associated with the collaborative use of multiple models. And we conclude with an outline of possible future directions.

INTRODUCTION

This book chapter focuses on the role of microsimulation modeling in evaluating the effects of breast cancer screening. We will start by giving a brief description of the history of microsimulation modeling, explaining briefly what microsimulation is, and we will give some examples of existing microsimulation models of breast cancer screening. This introduction is followed by a description of how microsimulation models are developed, including model development and model validation. Then, we describe the role of modeling in evaluating the effects of breast cancer screening by highlighting examples of the role of modeling in interpreting trials and observational studies, monitoring ongoing screening programs, and extrapolating the effects of screening to different settings, technologies, and screening schedules. Then we describe some of the strengths and weaknesses of using microsimulation modeling and note possible future directions.

In this chapter, we mainly discuss studies using models that have been developed specifically for breast cancer, use microsimulation modeling to evaluate the effects of breast cancer screening, use a variety of perspectives (often societal) and lengthy time horizon (often lifetime), report a variety of outcomes (eg, mortality reduction, cost-effectiveness), and compare numerous breast cancer screening scenarios (varying in invited ages, screening intervals, screening modalities) to no screening or current practice, all depending on the problem/research question that is addressed.

A BRIEF HISTORY OF MICROSIMULATION MODELING

Generally, Guy Orcutt, is acknowledged as providing the foundation for the field of microsimulation in 1957, by suggesting that microsimulation models consisting of "various sorts of interacting units which receive inputs and generate outputs" could be used to investigate "what would happen given specified external conditions."[1] However, it took some time before microsimulation modeling was widely used, mainly because of limitations in computing power and the lack of suitable data. With the rise of technology and data collection, these limitations were gradually overcome, and the use of microsimulation increased. Since then, microsimulation models have been used extensively for evaluating social and economic policies, such as income tax, social security, health benefits, or pension policies. Microsimulation of industrial processes to explore ways to improve them is also common. And microsimulation also underlies some newly popular methodologies for data analysis, specifically multiple imputation for dealing with missing data, and Metropolis-Hastings or Gibbs sampling for Bayesian data analysis.

The use of models to answer health policy questions began to evolve in the 1980s with application in a wide range of health care topics, such as hospital scheduling and organization, communicable disease, screening, costs of illness, and economic evaluation.[2] For breast cancer screening, specifically, models were developed to extrapolate the findings of randomized trials.[3–5] For example, when long-term outcomes from breast cancer screening trials were not yet available, models were used to predict the lifetime benefits, risks, and costs.[6] Since the 1980s, the breadth of application, diversity, and complexity of model approaches have rapidly increased.[2,7]

WHAT IS MICROSIMULATION MODELING?

According to Wikipedia, "*microsimulation (from microanalytic simulation) is a category of computerized analytical tools that perform highly detailed analysis of activities such as highway traffic flowing through an intersection, financial transactions, or pathogens spreading disease through a population. Microsimulation is often used to evaluate the effects of proposed interventions before they are implemented in the real world.*"[8]

An important/distinguishable feature of microsimulation models is that individuals (or individual components) are simulated. Typically, with microsimulation modeling, a life history is simulated for each individual using an algorithm that describes the events that make up that life history. Random draws decide if and when specific events occur. For health applications, these events typically include birth and death from other causes, as well as a model part that describes the target disease events, such as diagnosis and death from disease. Because individuals are simulated, microsimulation can produce individual-level artificial data that can be analyzed using standard statistical techniques, while population-level outcomes are obtained by aggregating individual life histories. The impact of changes in influential factors on key outcomes for subgroups as well as aggregates of the population can thus be assessed by testing "what if" scenarios. A disadvantage of microsimulation modeling is that it tends to be computationally intensive. In order to obtain stable estimates of stochastic outcomes, a large number of individuals must be simulated, particularly if small effects need to be estimated with precision.

DESCRIPTION OF SOME AVAILABLE MODELS

To evaluate the effects of breast cancer screening several microsimulation models have been developed. We will describe some of the available microsimulation models below. A comprehensive review of all such models would be impractical, so we have selected those we feel have been most influential.

In 1980, Eddy articulated a mathematical theory of screening that closely resembles the approach used by most modern simulation models.[9] He developed a Markov process-based simulation model, CAN*TROL, which he applied to the evaluation of cancer control policies for several cancer sites. He used his model to advise numerous countries about cancer screening programs. Although the underlying mathematical screening is similar to that used by other models reviewed in this chapter, the CAN*TROL model itself is not a microsimulation model.

One of the first microsimulation models, the "MIcrosimulation SCreening ANalysis" (MISCAN) model, was developed to examine the impact of cancer screening on morbidity and mortality.[10] The MISCAN model was developed to evaluate mass screening for breast cancer,[11] as well as for other types of cancers, such as cervical,[12] prostate,[13] and colorectal cancer.[14] It is a microsimulation model with continuous time and discrete events that simulates a dynamic population. The simulated life histories include date of birth and age at death from other causes than the target disease, a preclinical, screen-detectable disease process, in which breast cancer progresses through states, and survival. The natural course of the disease may be influenced by screening when a preclinical lesion becomes screen-detected. Screen-detection can result in the detection of smaller tumors, which may entail a survival benefit.

Within the Cancer Intervention and Surveillance Modeling Network (CISNET), many models have been developed for different cancer sites. For breast cancer, seven models were developed and extensively discussed and compared.[15] Six of the seven models were classified as microsimulation models[16] and six of the seven models include a natural history component. The natural history of breast cancer is modeled with a time from birth to start of the preclinical screen detectable period (the duration of this period being known as the sojourn time), clinical diagnosis, and a period of survival that ends with either breast cancer death or death from other causes. The time of diagnosis can change if screening takes place during the preclinical screen detectable period, which, in turn, may alter the time and cause of death. In most models, therapy influences survival from time of diagnosis.

Despite the similarities, the models also differ in important ways, for example in their assumptions about sojourn time, the mechanism of screen detection, tumor characteristics at diagnosis, survival following clinical detection and survival following screen detection.[16,17] Most CISNET models include ductal carcinoma in situ (DCIS), but one model includes only invasive breast cancer.[18] Also, assumptions on nonprogression vary: several models specifically assume that some percentage of DCIS are nonprogressive; one model also assumes that some cases of small invasive cancer are nonprogressive. Some groups model breast cancer progression in discrete stages, whereas other models explicitly model continuous tumor growth. The models also differ as to whether treatment affects the hazard of death from breast cancer, results in a cure for some fraction of cases, or both.[17]

Besides these models, many models have been developed over the past years, often to estimate the effects of breast cancer screening for specific countries, and often based on previously developed models. For example, models have been developed to determine the potential costs and effects of a breast cancer screening program for New Zealand[19] as well as Slovenia.[20] For both, it was explicitly stated that the model used was similar to MISCAN. In Spain, a model based on the Lee-Zelen[21] approach (one of the CISNET models) was used to estimate the amount of overdiagnosis from breast cancer screening,[22] as well as to estimate the cost-effectiveness of risk-based screening approaches[23] and the cost implications of switching from film to digital mammography.[24] A similar approach was used to estimate the cost-effectiveness of breast cancer screening in Korea.[25] In addition, specific models have been developed to estimate overdiagnosis in France,[26] Denmark,[27] and the United Kingdom.[28,29]

HOW MODELING IS DONE: THE PROCESS OF MICROSIMULATION MODELING

MODEL DEVELOPMENT: CONCEPTUALIZATION AND PARAMETER ESTIMATION

Most models are developed to answer specific questions and the development of a model is ideally guided by an understanding and conceptualization of the problem that is being represented. The conceptualization of the problem involves addressing factors such as the disease or condition, patient population, analytic perspective, alternative interventions, health and other outcomes, and the time horizon.[30]

With regard to the disease or condition, typically, a single disease (eg, breast cancer) or set of closely related diseases is of interest, but sometimes it is necessary to consider multiple diseases, for example if one is interested in estimating the impact on life expectancy of changes in a factor, such as smoking, that influences risk of multiple diseases. The modeled patient population should reflect the population of interest in terms of features relevant to the decision (eg, geography and patient characteristics, including comorbid conditions, disease prevalence, and stage). Analytic perspectives commonly considered are those of the patient, the health plan or insurer, and society. With regard to the diagnostic or therapeutic actions and interventions, it is crucial to model all practical interventions and their variations,[31] because the choice of comparators has a major impact on estimated effectiveness and efficiency, and the results are only meaningful in relation to the set of interventions considered.[30] In addition, the specific implementations of interventions might differ across countries and often across settings or subpopulations within countries. Thus, despite the same label (eg, "breast cancer screening"), effects may differ, depending on the practice patterns in the target population area. Sources of variation include the technology used (plain film vs digital), criteria for recall and biopsy recommendations, skill level, work load, and operating point of the radiologist, and differences in the underlying epidemiology of breast cancer itself. Moreover, the benefits of screening also vary with the range of available treatments and their accessibility to the population under study. It is therefore advisable to specify the components of the intervention in detail so that users can determine how well the analysis reflects their situations. Health outcomes of the model should be directly relevant to the question posed and might include number of cases of disease, number of deaths (or deaths averted by an intervention), life years gained, quality-adjusted life years (QALYs), and costs. The time horizon of the model should be long enough to capture relevant differences in outcomes across strategies; a lifetime time horizon is often required.

In order to make the appropriate choices on all these factors the modeling team should consult widely with clinical, epidemiologic, and health services experts and stakeholders to ensure that the model represents disease processes appropriately and adequately addresses the decision problem.

Once the problem has been clearly conceptualized, conceptualizing the model is the next step. To convert the problem conceptualization into an appropriate model structure, ensuring it reflects current disease knowledge and the process modeled, several methods might be used (expert consultations, influence diagrams, concept mapping). Several problem characteristics should be considered to decide which modeling method is most appropriate: Will the model represent individuals or groups, are there interactions among individuals, what time horizon is appropriate, should time be represented as continuous or discrete, do events occur more than once, and are resource constraints to be considered?

Another dimension is how complex a model should be. The appropriate level of model complexity depends on the disease process, the scientific questions to be addressed by the model, and data available to inform model parameters. There is a tension between the simplicity of a model and the complexity of the disease process. Simpler models include fewer parameters making it more likely that model parameters can be estimated using observed data. Simpler models are easier to describe, may entail fewer assumptions, and are less likely to contain hidden errors, making them more transparent. However, more complex models can be used to address a wider range of scientific questions. One approach is to begin with relatively simple models, extending these as needed to address specific research questions.[7]

Once the model conceptualization has been finalized, parameter estimation can begin. All models have parameters that must be estimated. In doing so, when possible, analysts should conform to evidence-based medicine principles; for example, seek to consider all evidence, rather than selectively picking values that best accord with the modeler's preferences; use best-practice methods to avoid potential biases, as when estimating treatment effectiveness from observational sources; and employ formal evidence synthesis techniques.[32]

Some parameters might be estimated from observed data using various analytical techniques to produce a result that will be used as a direct model input. For example, data on treatment efficacy might be used by combining results from several trials on treatment effects, and using the obtained hazard rate reduction directly in the model.

Often, other parameters have to be estimated using the model itself. Typically, unknown model parameters are estimated by optimizing the fit between simulated and observed data, using, for example, least-squares, minimum chi-square, or maximum-likelihood methods. This process is usually referred to as calibration. Typically this process is used for model parameters that quantify unobservable aspects of the process being modeled. For example, a model might include the mammographic detection probability of a preclinical tumor. Such a parameter might be estimated by optimizing fit between simulation output and observed rates of incidence of screen-detected and interval (ie, between scheduled mammograms) cancers in a clinical trial. Fitting to data is well defined when a model is built for a particular intervention, and there are one or more randomized trials in which the effects of the intervention are reported in terms of end results and intermediate outcomes, which can be compared with model predictions. When observed data comes from multiple studies and disease registries, expert judgment is required for assessing data quality and prioritizing data for their importance in fitting.[33]

VALIDATION

Evaluation and optimization of cancer screening programs or scenarios using modeling is only useful if the estimated harms and benefits of screening are reasonably accurate. Testing the accuracy of models, that is, model validation, is, therefore, a crucial step in any modeling study.

Previously, five main types of validation have been distinguished: face validity, verification (or internal validity), cross validity, external validity, and predictive validity.[34] Face validity is the extent to which a model and its assumptions and applications correspond to current science and evidence, as judged by people who have expertise in the problem.[34] In other words, face validity exists when a plain explanation of the model structure and assumptions appears reasonable to a critical audience.[33]

Verification (or internal validity) addresses whether the model's parts behave as intended and the model has been implemented correctly.[34] This can, for example, be tested by assessing whether the model responds as expected in simplistic boundary conditions such as zero incidence, no other-cause mortality, no benefit from screening or treatment, and other (typically contrived) sets of input parameters where expected model results can be determined beforehand.[17]

Cross validation involves comparing a model with others and determining the extent to which they calculate similar results. If similar results are calculated by models using different methods, confidence in the results increases, especially if the models have been developed independently.[34]

In external validation, a model is used to simulate a real scenario, such as a clinical trial, and the predicted outcomes are compared with the real-world ones.[34] Ideally, external validation tests the model's ability to reproduce observed results in a validation data set that was not used as a source of parameter estimates or calibration while building the model. Given, however, that breast cancer screening models typically include parameters that vary from setting to setting, or among subpopulation groups, some of them not directly observable, it is usually difficult to completely avoid some degree of reliance on the validation data. Completely independent external validation requires that the variable aspects of screening, natural history of disease, and treatment noted in the previous section are the same as those which prevailed for the data sources from which the model was built. For this reason, external model validation of breast cancer screening models is typically imperfect. In addition, even a fully independent external validation in a single data set, or a small number of them, should not, by itself, be taken as a definitive endorsement of the model: the number of "degrees of freedom" in any model complex enough to approach a realistic data generating mechanism will always be too large for one or a handful of fits to data to confirm.

Predictive validity involves using a model to forecast events and, after some time, comparing the forecasted outcomes to the actual ones. On the one hand, predictive validation is the most desirable type of validation, as it corresponds best to the purpose of most models, which is predicting what will happen. On the other hand, the observations are by definition in the future, making it often difficult to test a models predictive validity[34] in a sufficiently timely manner to make practical use of its results. Predictive validity can sometimes be estimated by observing the model's performance in simulating the results of somewhat similar events in existing data sets. For example, if the question of interest concerns the outcomes associated with different intensities of screening, it may be relevant to check how well the model can reproduce the changes in incidence and mortality that occurred during a time when a similar population introduced screening and its use disseminated.

ROLE OF MODELING

Well done randomized controlled trials (RCTs) provide the strongest possible evidence regarding the effectiveness of interventions, and high quality observational studies are the second tier. But the available evidence at any time typically leaves some important questions unanswered. Moreover, some questions cannot, in practice, be approached with these methods. RCTs may include inadequate numbers of women in age groups of interest to policy makers. The populations studied may not be sufficiently similar to those of interest to the decision maker. RCTs typically study only one or small number of protocols for screening, whereas policy makers may wish to choose among many options. The duration of follow-up is limited, so projection of long-term outcomes requires other methods. If carried out in settings where mammography is available outside of the study, the control groups may be "contaminated," which may result in underestimation of screening effects compared to what would happen with the de novo introduction of screening. The results of an RCT may be of limited relevance if new mammographic technologies have been introduced since the trial concluded, or if the spectrum of available treatments has changed. Findings regarding subpopulations of special interest for policy may be nonexistent or underpowered.

By synthesizing the results of relevant RCTs and observational evidence, and supporting the projection of outcomes of hypothetical screening programs, models can overcome some of these limitations of RCTs and provide policy makers with information that covers a wider range of possibilities and may be more closely tailored to the prevailing circumstances in which the decision maker finds him/herself.

In the following sections, we will provide an overview of the different roles microsimulation models have had in evaluating the effects of breast cancer screening. Each category is explained and highlighted by selected examples.

INTERPRETATION

The interpretation of observational studies, and sometimes that of clinical trials, is made difficult by the fact that in the real world, influential factors other than the object of study are often changing too. For example, during the same period that mammography screening became widely available and widely used in the United States, new forms of adjuvant therapy for breast cancer were also introduced, and the use of adjuvant chemotherapy became more common. When systematic screening programs are introduced, changes in incidence and mortality may also be influenced by concurrent changes in risk factor prevalence or treatment patterns. Differences in breast cancer outcomes between different populations can seldom be ascribed to a single cause: typically the prevalences of different risk factors, utilization and implementation of screening, and treatment patterns will all differ. Ordinary statistical analyses, such as regression equations, have at best limited ability to accommodate such confounding variables. Simulation models, however, because they can represent complicated and multifaceted data generating processes, can disentangle the concurrent effects and support attribution of portions of the observed effects to each cause by providing projections of the expected outcomes under both real and counterfactual combinations of these factors.

Trials

Several RCTs have been performed to evaluate the effects of breast cancer screening, reporting significant mortality reductions for women aged 50–69 years.[35–37] For women younger than 50 years, breast cancer mortality reduction rates of 10–13% were published.[38,39] However, some women in the age group under 50 were also screened when they were 50 years old or older. Part of the observed mortality reduction in these women is likely to have been a result of detecting the cancer earlier in later rounds when the women were 50 years old or older. It is, however, not directly observable how large this proportion is. Therefore, a modeling study estimated what percentage of the observed mortality reduction for women aged 40–49 years at entry into the five Swedish screening trials might be attributable to screening these women at 50 years of age or older.[40] By simulating all Swedish trials, taking into account important trial characteristics, such as age distribution, attendance, and screening interval, it was estimated that around 70% of the 10% reduction in breast cancer mortality observed for women in their forties might be attributable to screening these women after they reach age 50.

Another example of dissecting the results of a clinical trial is Van Ravesteyn et al. applying the MISCAN model to simulate the UK Breast Screening Frequency Trial.[41] That trial directly compared annual and triennial screening intervals. The investigators found that the difference in breast cancer mortality between the two arms was not statistically significant (RR 0.93, 9% CI 0.63–1.37), a surprising result. The trial simulation replicated the findings of the actual trial, although it produced a slightly more favorable result. The original trial followed women for 36 months. The microsimulation was used to project lifetime mortality, with no material effect on the predicted relative risk of death. However, the projected relative risk became more favorable to annual screening if full attendance of all invitees was simulated and a higher mammogram sensitivity were achieved. The investigators concluded that given actual screening conditions that prevailed during the trial, the trialists' original expectation of a 25% breast cancer mortality reduction was overly optimistic, and consequently the study was substantially underpowered to detect the actually achievable reduction. They noted that measures to increase the sensitivity of mammography and obtain better adherence to the assigned screening schedules would have enhanced the power of the trial.

Observational data: trends

US breast cancer mortality in women aged 30–79 year decreased by 24% from 1989 to 2000. The decline was hypothesized to be due to the dissemination of screening mammography, adjuvant therapies for breast cancer, or both. Because both interventions were disseminated over approximately the same time period, it was not possible to separate the contributions of each to the mortality decline using standard techniques. Using modeling, an analysis with seven independently developed models using common inputs on utilization patterns of mammography and adjuvant therapy was conducted.[42] This analysis was one of the first that used multiple models that shared key inputs to address the same research question. The models first calibrated their inputs and parameters to provide a reasonable approximation to SEER incidence and mortality from 1975 through 2000. They then reran the simulations, once with the screening portions of the models "turned off," again with the adjuvant treatment portions turned off, and finally with both the screening and adjuvant treatment portions turned off. This made it possible to discern the separate impacts of screening and adjuvant treatment on modeled incidence and mortality. All models found that both screening and treatment reduced breast cancer mortality (thus, the observed reduction in breast cancer mortality could not be attributed to either factor alone), and each contributed about equally to the decline observed by 2000. Moreover, the effects were roughly additive: there was neither synergy nor interference between screening benefits and treatment improvements. The range of mortality reductions due to screening and adjuvant treatment was somewhat narrower for treatment than for screening, reflecting that the underlying evidence regarding treatment efficacy is more consistent. The approach used is illustrated in Fig. 5.1, where a recently updated version of one model's results is shown. Note that the mortality curves for adjuvant treatment but no screening and for screening but no adjuvant treatment diverge after 2000. This reflects the adoption of more effective forms of adjuvant chemotherapy introduced around the turn of the century. Although there have been technological improvements in breast cancer screening as well, their impact

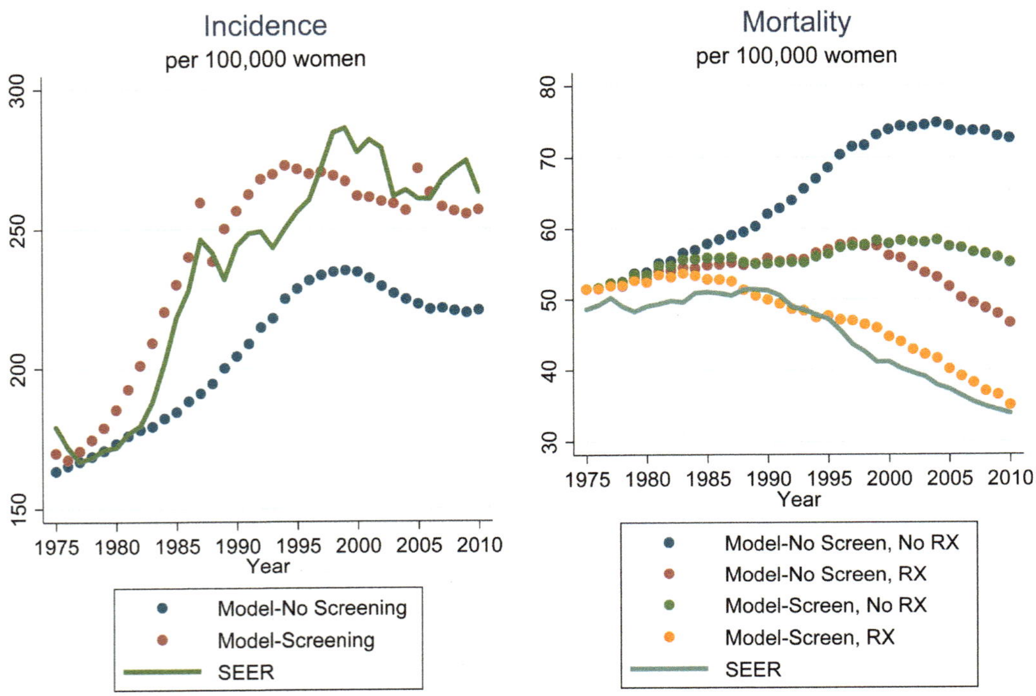

Age-adjusted to 2000 US Census

FIGURE 5.1

CISNET Model GE simulation of the impact of screening and adjuvant treatment on breast cancer incidence and mortality, 1975–2010.

on mortality is smaller and does not appear until 2005. For this model, at least, the conclusion that screening and adjuvant treatment contribute equally to mortality reduction does not apply after 2000.

Refining the question further, six of the same seven models more recently estimated the contributions to breast cancer mortality reduction of screening in treatment separately for estrogen-receptor (ER) positive and ER negative tumors. It had long been known that ER positive and negative tumors respond differently to chemotherapy and hormonal treatments. Less widely appreciated was the difference in the rates at which these tumors grow. The interaction of these differences in treatment responsiveness and susceptibility to screen detection had not previously been examined. The models found that whereas screening and adjuvant treatment played approximately equal roles in mortality reduction from ER negative breast cancer, reduction in mortality from ER positive tumors was more attributable to adjuvant treatment. Other ER specific differences were also noted. ER negative tumors are less likely to be screen detected than ER positive tumors, but when screen detected, they attain a greater survival benefit. As a corollary, when comparing annual to biennial mammography, the incremental benefit of annual screening is predominantly seen in ER negative tumors.[43]

An interesting problem also approached by modeling is the paradox of increased breast cancer mortality in the face of decreased incidence in African-Americans compared to United States (US) Whites. Two CISNET models undertook an investigation. Race-specific model inputs were developed that reflected known differences in age-specific incidence, distribution of biomarkers, and utilization of screening and treatment, finding that, while each of these factors contributes substantially to the observed difference in mortality, between 38% and 46% of the difference could not be explained.[44]

Obesity impacts with breast cancer in complicated ways. Premenopausally, obesity reduces the risk of breast cancer, but postmenopausally it confers greater risk.[45–49] Obese women tend to have lower breast density, and thus mammography may have higher sensitivity in this subpopulation,[50,51] although this finding has been disputed.[52] There is a tendency for oncologists to reduce dosages of adjuvant chemotherapy produced by standard formulas relying on body surface area or body weight because the recommended doses appears to be very high. Consequently the effectiveness of adjuvant chemotherapy in obese women appears to be reduced.[53,54] Finally, obesity may be associated with increased mortality from other causes.[55,56] Some of these associations are further confounded with racial differences, and it is natural to wonder to what extent the higher prevalence of obesity among Black women accounts for the increased breast cancer mortality they experience. These multiple influences of obesity on breast cancer, some working in opposing directions, cannot be disentangled impressionistically, and do not lend themselves to resolution through techniques such as meta-analysis of trials and observational studies. Direct simulation of the mechanisms driving breast cancer and the effects of screening and treatment offer the hope of understanding this complex situation. Chang and colleagues[57] applied two of the CISNET breast cancer models to this problem. They concluded that obesity as a whole accounts for only a small proportion of breast cancer incidence and mortality in both Blacks and Whites, and that none of the mortality difference between the races is attributable to the difference in prevalence of obesity. An interesting feature of modeling is that it is possible to simulate the results of strategies that could not be implemented in the real world. For example, nobody seriously believes that obesity can be eradicated. But knowing what the impact of a hypothetical obesity eradication on other health problems would be would provide an upper bound on what can be achieved with intensive efforts to reduce its prevalence. The Chang study concluded that elimination of obesity would prevent more breast cancer cases among both Black and White women than any other preventive measure except possibly widespread use of tamoxifen prophylaxis by high-risk women.

EXTRAPOLATION

The ability to extrapolate beyond available direct evidence is perhaps the most important attribute of simulation models. In general, when drawing up guidelines or setting policy, the available evidence does not quite fit with the situation at hand. This is particularly true of breast cancer screening. The earliest clinical trial of mammography began in 1963, and even the more recent ones were mostly carried out in the 1990s. Since then plain film mammography technique evolved, and, more recently, new technologies were introduced. In addition, even considering all of the trials together, only a handful of different screening schedules have been actually tested. The trials, large as they were, could not focus on particular subpopulations. The trials had a limited duration: none followed patients for life, and even in those with long-term follow-up there has often been substantial uptake of screening in what was originally the control group. For all these reasons, the applicability of clinical trial results to current decisions about breast cancer screening is limited. Habbema and colleagues[58] have noted that models will be most valuable in situations where the evidence base is substantial enough that credible models can be built based on it, but where the kind of gaps noted here remain.

Simulation models have the ability, by specifying some parameters differently, to project the outcomes that might have been seen had the circumstances of the trials been a closer match to what we currently face. While assuming that the natural history of the disease, and the mechanism of screen detection remain the same, a simulation model can examine the impact of varying starting and stopping ages, and intervals between consecutive screenings. The impact of different screening schedules in women at different levels of risk can be explored. And by modifying the assumptions about tumor sojourn times or test sensitivity, the implications of different technologies can be estimated. It is clear that it would be infeasible to study all of these issues in clinical trials.

Other protocols (screening ages, intervals)

Early clinical trials of breast cancer screening generally enrolled women past the age of 50 years. Elderly women, if not specifically excluded by protocol, participated only in small numbers. As a result, when breast cancer screening programs were adopted in Europe, and as the technology disseminated in the United States, there was variation in the starting and stopping ages recommended or implemented.

The Netherlands' program began in 1988 with biennial screening between ages 50 and 70.[59] By 1995, the question of raising the stopping age, which was felt not to be firmly based in evidence, arose.[60] Using the MISCAN model, the investigators concluded that extending screening to age 80 would make sense based solely on the balance of harms and benefits, although the incremental cost-effectiveness ratio was higher than was considered proportionate at that time (£36,000/QALY).

Interest in the appropriate stopping age for mammography has remained, and little new direct evidence of the effects of screening older women has become available since then. It is clear that the major concern is that the higher competing mortality in older women puts them at increased risk for overdiagnosis. Additional concerns are the perception that breast cancer is less aggressive in older women, and that they may be at increased risk for complications from treatment. Although the last of these factors has not been explored in models, more recent modeling efforts have incorporated age-varying breast cancer natural history, and have also examined competing mortality rates that are conditional on the extent of comorbidity. Lansdorp-Vogelaar and colleagues[61] performed a wide ranging investigation of appropriate comorbidity-dependent screening cessation ages for mammography, prostate-specific antigen testing for prostate cancer, and fecal immunochemical screening for colon cancer using several CISNET models. Interestingly, despite considerable differences in the actual levels of harms and benefits for these three cancer sites, age and comorbidity-specific harm to benefit ratios showed a remarkable level of consistency. For all three cancers, the US Preventive Services Task Force recommends ending screening, irrespective of comorbidity, at age 74. The investigators found that the same harm-benefit ratios could be obtained by stopping screening at age 66 in women with severe comorbidity, and by extending screening to age 76 in women with no comorbidity at all. (The average woman in this age range has mild comorbidity under the classification used in this study.)

An investigation using the same two breast cancer models as the Lansdorp-Vogelaar study, but with somewhat updated assumptions about screening operating characteristics and breast cancer natural history was presented to the US Preventive Services Task Force (USPSTF) for consideration, and the same conclusions were reached.[62] The USPSTF did not, however, choose to modify its current general recommendation to stop breast cancer screening at age 74.

If the question of when to stop screening was among the first raised, the question of when to start remains the most controversial. The USPSTF reviewed its recommendations for breast cancer screening in 2009. In addition to a conventional systematic evidence review,[63] they also considered output prepared by the CISNET models.[64] The point of the latter was primarily to try to provide more refined recommendations about screening interval (annual vs biennial) and the consequences of screening women between ages 40 and 49. The models reviewed all estimated that biennial screening provided approximately 80% of the breast cancer mortality reduction that could be achieved with annual screening, but with about half of the associated harms. The model outputs provided direct comparison of harm-benefit ratios (using various types of harms and benefits) for a wide range of screening schedules. The USPSTF ended up reiterating support for biennial screening in all women ages 50–74, while recommending that screening decisions for women 40–49 be based on an individual weighing of the risks and benefits. These recommendations proved controversial. Among the criticisms raised were that the Task Force based its recommendations on evidence obtained using plain-film mammography, which by then was being rapidly displaced by digital mammography, and failed to consider more aggressive screening schedules in high-risk women.

For its 2015 review of breast cancer screening recommendations, the Task Force again obtained a structured evidence review[65] as well as new modeling results.[62] The CISNET models previously used were updated to reflect the operating characteristics of digital mammography, and were also modified to examine subpopulations with high (heterogeneously dense or extremely dense on the BIRADS scale) and low (entirely fatty or scattered fibroglandular densities on the BIRADS scale) breast density, further substratified by level of breast cancer risk due to conventional breast cancer risk factors. This demonstrates the level of complexity that can be handled by microsimulation modeling using computing resources that are now widely available. For example, high breast density both increases the risk of breast cancer and reduces the sensitivity of mammography. The other breast cancer risk factors, however, affect breast cancer risk without large changes in the accuracy of mammograms. Moreover, breast density tends to decline with age, whereas other risk factors remain relatively constant or may increase (eg, family history or personal history of benign breast biopsy). Attempting to determine the net effects of these conflicting influences from an impressionistic review of clinical trials would be challenging at best. The use of models provided clearer answers than could otherwise be obtained, and, in particular, highlighted where these effects would sufficiently alter the harm-benefit ratios of different screening schedules to support alternative recommendations for a targeted subgroup.

Other screening modalities

During the first decade of this century, digital mammography has largely replaced plain film mammography. Enthusiasm for digital mammography was enhanced by the Digital Mammographic Imaging Screening Trial (DMIST), which found that digital mammography had similar accuracy as film mammography overall and offered increased sensitivity for women with heterogeneously or extremely dense breasts, women under age 50, and premenopausal women.[66] This enthusiasm in the clinical community was not tempered by the concurrent findings of no improvement in specificity. Nor, apparently was it tempered by the finding that switch from film to digital mammography would cost $331,000 per QALY gained.[67] Although it is unclear if the actual cost of producing, interpreting, and archiving a digital mammogram differs greatly from that of a plain film study, insurers, including the US government's Medicare program, generally provide higher reimbursements for the digital procedure. A comprehensive analysis of the costs of the transition from plain film to digital mammography in the United States was undertaken by Stout and colleagues.[68] Four of the CISNET population models were used collaboratively to provide quantitative estimates of the full impact of the switch to digital mammography. They concluded that replacing plain film mammography with digital has led to increased costs with small added health benefits (extending life expectancy by 0.73 days). In an associated cost-utility analysis they concluded that the cost-effectiveness of using digital in place of plain film is sensitive to the disutility a woman places on false-positive diagnoses. A similar analysis by De Gelder et al.[69] led to estimates that conversion to digital mammography in the Netherlands would lead to between 14% and 43% increase in overdiagnosis, depending on the assumptions made about the natural history of DCIS.

Although US health policy often is made without regard to costs, two of the CISNET models collaborated with representatives of the Centers for Disease Control and Prevention's National Breast and Cervical Cancer Early Detection Program (NBCCEDP) to evaluate the impact of the transition to digital mammography on that program.[70] The NBCCEDP operates under a constrained budget to provide mammograms and cervical Pap smears to low-income uninsured women aged 40–64. Because digital mammograms are more expensive, the program was faced with the possibilities of serving fewer women or providing its existing clients with less frequent screening. The guidance of the models was sought to determine how to allocate their resources so as to maximize the health benefits achieved. The study concluded that for those women screened, digital mammography led to 2–4% more life years gained. But this gain was erased and overwhelmed by the reduction in the number of women screened that the higher cost of digital necessitated, a net decrease of 22–24% fewer life years gained. However, this net loss could, in turn, be reversed by restricting screening to 2-year intervals, resulting in a net 8–13% increase in life years gained by mammography.

As mentioned above, women with high density breasts are at increased risk of developing breast cancer, and also at greater risk for false-negative mammograms. While the situation is somewhat better with digital than plain film mammography, concern remains over the adequacy of mammographic screening in these women. Recently, the notion that supplementary screening with hand-held ultrasound might improve the outlook for these women has gained popularity. Enthusiasm for this idea is sufficiently intense that at least 24 states in the United States, covering more than half the US population, have passed laws requiring that women be specifically informed if they are found to have dense breasts, and suggesting that they discuss the option of supplemental screening with their providers. Due to its widespread availability and relatively low cost, hand-held ultrasound (HHUS) is the most frequently proposed technology for supplemental screening. Sprague and colleagues[71] applied three of the CISNET models to gain an understanding of the economic and health implications if the use of hand-held ultrasound for supplemental screening of women with dense breasts became widespread. This modeling posed some unique challenges. There are no clinical trials to demonstrate the effectiveness of HHUS in this application, so a wide range of assumptions about sensitivity and specificity of ultrasound had to be considered. Furthermore, it was not possible to assume that the sensitivity and specificity of HHUS are independent of mammographic outcome because HHUS detection of breast cancers relies on different physical properties of tumors. Consequently, the models needed to develop and calibrate an entirely independent approach to sonographic detection for these studies. The models concluded that supplemental HHUS screening of biennially screened women aged 50–74 with heterogeneously or extremely dense breasts (BIRADS c or d) after negative mammograms would gain 1.7 QALYs per 1000 women. It would also entail an additional 354 biopsies following false-positive HHUS results, and substantially raise costs. The incremental cost-effectiveness ratio was $325,000 per

QALY. Restricting supplemental screening to women with extremely dense breasts (BIRADS d only) reduces this ratio to $246,000 per QALY, which is still beyond the range of widely accepted clinical preventive services.

Another approach to supplemental screening for women with dense breasts is digital breast tomosynthesis. This is an emerging technology, with two devices having so far been approved by the FDA. Early studies of this technology have indicated that the use of tomosynthesis increases detection of cancers while also reducing recalls for biopsies or further imaging.[72–74] Tomography's separation of shadows arising in different tissue planes, which may overlap and appear to be lesions or can overlap in ways that obscure lesions in mammograms, seems to be almost ideally suited to solve the problems that mammography faces in dense breasts. Lee and colleagues[75] applied one of the CISNET models to study this in women age 50–74 with extremely dense breasts (BIRADS d). Because of the limited data on the performance of tomosynthesis in combination with digital mammography, a wide range of assumptions was tested in sensitivity analysis. They concluded that supplemental digital tomography gained 5.5 QALY per 1000 women at a cost of $70,500 per QALY. In addition they projected a 32% reduction in false-positive findings. The rather favorable ICER result was fairly robust to changes in assumptions about the performance of digital tomosynthesis. In particular, only when digital tomosynthesis is assumed to be only minimally more sensitive or specific than digital mammography does the ICER climb above $100,000 per QALY. The factor with most influence on the ICER is the actual cost of digital tomosynthesis. Their base case assumption was that a supplemental tomosynthesis procedure would cost $50. (For comparison they assumed $139 for a digital mammogram alone). Of additional interest, the ICER is only minimally dependent on the disutility that women attach to undergoing mammography and diagnostic follow-up testing. Even with pessimistic assumptions about this, the ICER remains under $90,000 per QALY.

Impact of changes in other aspects of breast cancer on screening effectiveness

The applications of modeling in the preceding subsections focused on extrapolating from available screening data to predict the impact of changes in screening schedules or technology. We turn now to an application in which the impact of changes in other aspects of breast cancer on screening effectiveness were modeled. Mandelblatt and colleagues[76] building on earlier work[57] about the impact of obesity trends on breast cancer epidemiology, sought to compare the effectiveness of three general approaches to breast cancer mortality reduction going forward: (1) increased screening frequency, (2) reducing undertreatment of obese women, and (3) elimination of obesity. Although the same two models had previously concluded that elimination of obesity would be an effective approach to primary prevention of breast cancer[57] (also see section Observational data: trends), the current investigation projected that the greatest breast cancer mortality reduction for obese women would come from assuring that all received maximal chemotherapy (though this would come at the expense of increased chemotherapy toxicity). Annual screening from ages 40 through 54 and biennial screening from 55 until death in 90% of obese women would also have a substantial, but lesser, impact on breast cancer mortality. (see Fig. 5.2.)

COST-EFFECTIVENESS ANALYSIS

Estimating cost-effectiveness of a breast cancer screening program should, ideally, incorporate all events that arise during the lifetimes of affected women with or without screening. Once screening programs are established, direct evidence about the consequences of not-screening will be minimal to

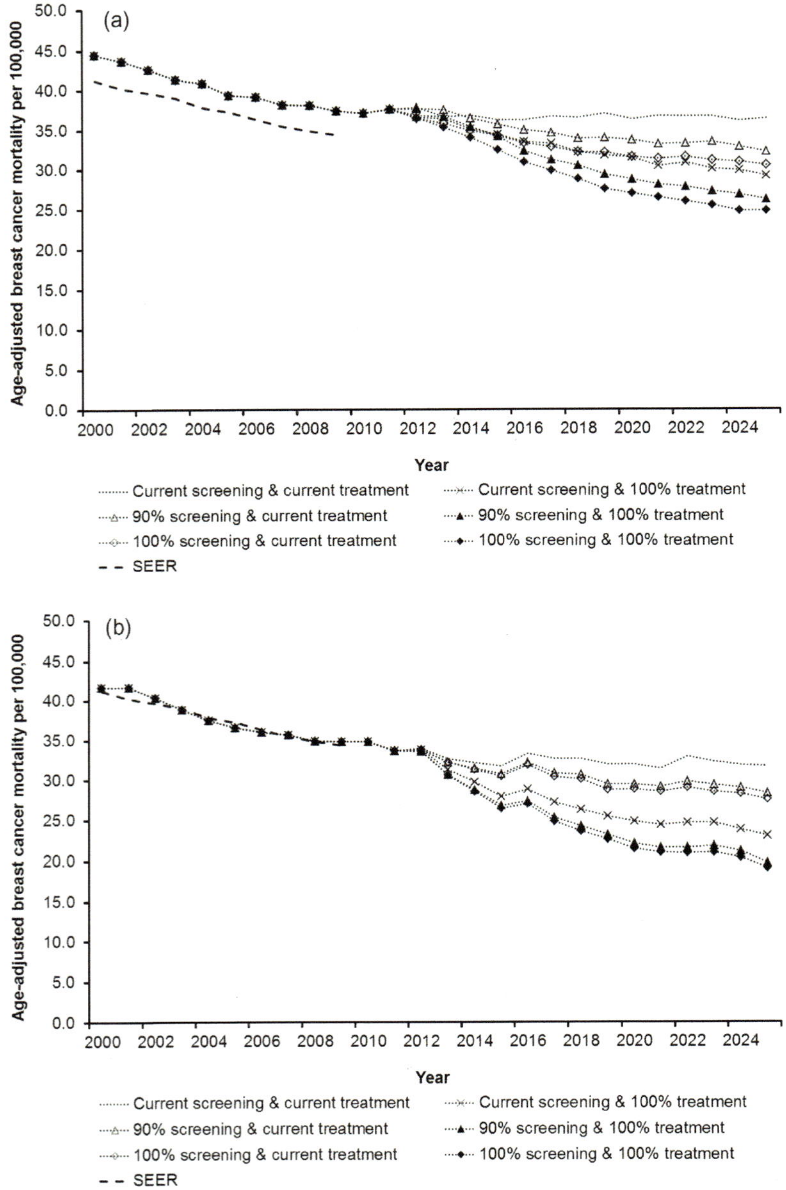

FIGURE 5.2

Projected impact on breast cancer mortality of enhanced screening and adjuvant treatment strategies. (a) SPECTRUM model and (b) MISCAN model.

Reproduced from Ref. 76 with permission of the publisher.

nonexistent. On the other hand, even the longest established screening programs have yet to achieve lifetime follow-up of even their initial participants. Simulation models can fill this gap by providing credible estimates of these unobserved events. In addition, they can provide estimates of cost-effectiveness of screening in defined subpopulations, or under alternative screening scenarios.

Cost-effectiveness of mammography as practiced, and under alternative approaches

Stout et al.[77] examined the cost-effectiveness of mammography screening, as used in the United States between 1990 and 2000 by women age 40 and over, and estimated that the US population had gained 1.7 million QALYs from its utilization of mammography, at a cost of approximately $37,000 each, if no disutility is attached to the additional evaluation of false-positive results. They also identified several screening schedules that could achieve additional gains in QALYs at modest cost, provided they could be achieved without large recruitment costs. The costs of recruiting women into additional screening, however, can reverse these conclusions, as was pointed out by Mandelblatt et al.[78] using a microsimulation model that is ancestral to the CISNET "Spectrum" model.[79]

Tosteson et al.[67] provided an early cost-effectiveness analysis of the conversion from plain-film to digital mammography. They concluded that universal replacement of plain film by digital mammography would both increase costs and decrease QALYs, but that targeting digital mammography to women under age 50 would be associated with a very acceptable incremental cost-effectiveness ratio of $26,500 per QALY. A somewhat higher, but still generally acceptable cost-effectiveness ratio would also be obtained targeting digital mammography to women who are either under age 50 or have dense breasts. See also the discussion of digital versus plain film mammography comparisons in Section "Other screening modalities."

Still more recently, Schousboe and colleagues[80] revisited the cost-effectiveness of mammography overall, and were the first to examine the joint effects of age, breast density, and other breast cancer risk factors on cost-effectiveness and the optimal screening schedule. They recommended deferring the onset of mammography to 50 years of age for women with breasts that are almost entirely fat breasts or with scattered fibroglandular densities (BIRADS a or b), but starting at age 40 for women with heterogeneously or extremely dense breasts (BIRADS c or d). Their analysis is of additional interest in that they also model scenarios in which women might reassess their mammography screening intervals to account for possibly declining breast density at ages 60 and 70, with reduction to every 3 or 4 years in women with breasts that are almost entirely fat (BIRADS a) and no other breast cancer risk factors.

STRENGTHS AND WEAKNESSES ("OPPORTUNITIES AND DRAWBACKS")

UNCERTAINTY

Whereas accepted standards of best practice in the design and implementation of clinical trials and cost-effectiveness analyses were developed several decades ago, the more recent acceptance of simulation modeling as an additional tool in the search for knowledge and understanding did not spur the promulgation of such standards until 2012.[30,32,34,81–84] As with the standards for the earlier methods, full implementation is sometimes infeasible or impractical. Even if such standards are sometimes "honored in the breach" they still provide a goal toward which the research community strives, and a benchmark against which researchers and clinicians can judge the quality of published studies.

Given that the standards proposed for modeling are relatively new, it will take some time before their effectiveness in improving the quality of modeling studies can be assessed. The standards should, in principle, increase confidence in the results of modeling. It is beyond the scope of this chapter to review these best practices. Instead, we summarize here three major categories of uncertainty in model results and approaches to understanding them, and reducing them.

Model results incorporate uncertainty from numerous sources: uncertainty in model structure, uncertainty in the values of model inputs and parameters, and sampling (Monte Carlo) error. The first two are important to understand for any particular model, though they may be difficult to assess in practice. The third can be reduced to acceptably small levels by choosing a sufficiently large sample size, and is, for this and other reasons, the least important source of uncertainty.

Structural uncertainty

All models, in the name of computational feasibility, are oversimplifications of reality. Most often simplifying assumptions are made for lack of knowledge of the real state; sometimes, though, verisimilitude is intentionally sacrificed to accommodate the constraints of programmability and computational burden. Such simplifying assumptions must be viewed critically as part of the assessment of a model's face validity. But even face validity, dependent as it is on prevailing understandings of mechanisms of disease, may in time prove wrong as the prevailing wisdom comes to need revision. The best assessment of the uncertainty associated with model structure is a sensitivity analysis in which other plausible model structures are tried and the results compared. For minor structural assumptions, this type of test may be accomplished directly. However, it may not be feasible to build alternative structural assumptions about a particular aspect of the process under study into an existing model: the programming task associated with doing so may be equal to or even greater than building a new model from scratch. One of the strengths of collaborative modeling, such as that undertaken by the CISNET consortium, is that the combined results of the different modeling groups constitute such a sensitivity analysis.[58,85] The different models use identical, or equivalent inputs and parameter estimates, but incorporate different structural assumptions into their modeling.

Model input uncertainty

The inputs used in modeling may arise from clinical trials or observational studies, or syntheses of these. Those sources, in turn, have uncertainty associated with them, and that uncertainty is then propagated into the results of the model. As with structural uncertainty, the best assessment arises from sensitivity analysis. For sufficiently small models, the state of the art is to carry out Monte Carlo (probabilistic) sensitivity analysis over reasonable prior distributions for all inputs that are not certain and estimate the expected value of perfect information.[32] There are, however, conceptual and practical obstacles to doing this. The uncertain parameters often correspond to unobservable quantities, which may or may not be independent of each other and of the observable inputs. Posing a credible prior distribution can, therefore, be quite difficult. Moreover, most breast cancer screening models are complicated simulations and are run with large sample sizes, making the testing of even a small number of combinations of inputs and parameters a computationally intensive challenge. It may be possible to abbreviate the process by carefully selecting key combinations of input assumptions, simulating the corresponding outputs, and then fitting a "meta-model" response surface to those results. This approach, however, presumes some known parametric or semiparametric form for the response surface, replacing the original model input uncertainty with a new structural uncertainty that may be even more resistant to verification.

It should be noted that the distinction between structural uncertainty and input uncertainty is not a sharp one. For example, a model might, in its code, incorporate the uncertain assumption that the sojourn time distribution for breast cancers, conditional on age and biomarkers, is exponential, with the single rate-parameter for that distribution an uncertain input. An alternative structure might use a different family of distributions, such as gamma, or Weibull instead. But note that this structural variation could also be captured by assuming a broad family of distributions, such as the generalized gamma distribution, which includes exponential, gamma, and Weibull. Were that approach taken, the "structural" uncertainty about the form of the distribution would become uncertainty about the values of three parameters of the generalized gamma, which would typically be inputs rather than embedded in the simulation code. The distinction, thus, may rest on which assumptions are represented in computer code and which in input data. It is usually easier to modify input data than revise code, so incorporating structural assumptions into input data rather than code facilitates both flexibility and assessment of uncertainty. (For example, the current version of CISNET's Model GE is relatively lean at 4350 lines of C++ code, but a complete set of input data spans 17.7 megabytes.)

Sampling (Monte Carlo) uncertainty

Although there are deterministic models of breast cancer screening at the population level, most existing models are stochastic microsimulations of individual women. For such models, the number of women simulated will influence the precision with which simulation output approaches the actual distribution of outcomes that is implied by all the structural assumptions and inputs to the model. This is analogous to the way the sample size in a clinical trial influences sampling error and the precision with which its outcomes are estimated. In principle, one can appeal to the Central Limit Theorem to prove that this type of uncertainty can be made arbitrarily small with probability arbitrarily close to 1 by choosing a sufficiently large sample size.

Indeed, the sample sizes that modelers choose when running their simulations may be the result of either formal or impressionistic assessments of what is needed to obtain a desired level of precision in the output. In fact, if one takes the perspective that the results of clinical trials, observational studies, and even tumor registry data are themselves random samples whose aggregate statistics include sampling error, one of the advantages of models is that the sample size, and the associated precision, are limited only by the computational resources and patience of the modeler. In particular, it is common for simulated results to be based on a larger sample size than the actual size of the target population being simulated. This can be seen, among other ways, when graphical time series of simulation output are superimposed on the corresponding real world data, and the former are substantially less "noisy."

While the magnitude of sampling uncertainty can be made arbitrarily small by increasing the sample size, with large sample sizes it becomes more difficult to provide an estimate of the precision achieved. The reason is that the estimation of standard errors of output statistics requires either a substantial number of replications of the simulation (with different starting points for the random number generators), or requires outputting aggregated statistics from numerous small subsets of the original sample. The former approach may exceed the computational resources reasonably available, and the latter may result in output files that are unmanageably large given available infrastructure.

Finally, it should be borne in mind that if the simulated sample size needed to provide sufficient precision to adequately answer a policy question for a population is a very large multiple of that population's actual size, then it seems reasonable to conclude that the policy issue in question does not actually have empirically realizable consequences in that population.

Strength from weakness: identify gaps in knowledge

An underappreciated aspect of exploring uncertainty in models is the ability to identify knowledge gaps that are in need of additional research. A key example of this relates to the extent of overdiagnosis that results from breast cancer screening. A necessary concomitant of early detection is that some women will die of unrelated causes during their lead time. This is particularly true for elderly women, but can occur at any age. Such a woman has not benefited from early detection: the breast cancer she learned of would never have surfaced in her lifetime had she not been screened. This situation is referred to as overdiagnosis. If, moreover, there are nonprogressive breast cancers that never surface clinically but are mammographically detectable, detection of any such lesion is an instance of overdiagnosis.

Note that it is not possible to identify individual women who have been overdiagnosed: once her lesion is screen detected, there is no way to know when, if ever, it would have surfaced clinically in the absence of screening. But that is not to say that overdiagnosis has no observable consequences. If we imagine a cohort of women living in two parallel universes, one of which provides a screening program and the other does not, overdiagnosis will be manifested as an increase in the lifetime incidence of breast cancer in the screened cohort: not only are all the lesions that would emerge without screening ultimately found, but additional lesions turn up as well.

There is considerable divergence among published estimates of overdiagnosis derived from clinical trials and observational studies. De Gelder et al.[86] note that some of this divergence is due to different denominators (women in population, women screened, all cancers among screened women, all cancers among unscreened women, or screen-detected lesions) used in calculating the rate. Moreover, other methodological issues arise: in estimating overdiagnosis from clinical trial data with short follow-up, or using observational data where screening utilization is not in a steady state, the extent of overdiagnosis will necessarily be overestimated.

Within breast cancer screening models, overdiagnosis is typically not explicitly modeled, but rather emerges as a consequence of whatever is assumed about the incidence of breast cancer in the absence of screening, the proportion of breast cancers that do not progress, the distribution of tumor sojourn times, and mortality from competing causes. Except for the last, none of these parameters is observable. While not all combinations of assumptions about these model inputs will be compatible with observed incidence and mortality data (whether from clinical trials or population data sources), the possibilities are narrowed by constraining the model to reasonably fitting the data. Still, there is no assurance that the incidence and mortality constraints are sufficient to identify uniquely all of these unobservable parameter distributions. And, indeed, De Gelder et al. were able to fit three rather different models equally well to data from the Dutch national screening program.[69] Crucially, these different models produced a range of estimates of overdiagnosis ratio (overdiagnosed breast cancers per 100 breast cancers that would be seen without screening) between 2.8 and 9.7. This greater than threefold difference in estimates could not be resolved within their model without imposing additional, untestable, ad hoc constraints.

This experience identifies overdiagnosis as an important topic for additional research. Clearly, being treated for a breast cancer that would never have become symptomatic is a substantial harm to a woman—the most substantial harm possible from a breast cancer screening program. (Despite this, because we cannot identify individual cases, the overdiagnosed women are likely to perceive themselves as having had their lives saved and be among mammography's most "satisfied customers.")

Based on the experience of De Gelder et al., and similar unpublished findings of some of the other CISNET modelers, advances in modeling are unlikely to resolve this problem. Rather, it would seem important to try to develop methods to distinguish progressive from nonprogressive tumors in biopsy specimens (or, better still, noninvasively), so as to avoid harmful treatment without offsetting benefits.

TRANSPARENCY

Transparency may be the most vexatious limitation of simulation models. Just as one must understand the methods used in designing and carrying out a clinical trial in order to interpret its results, one must understand the design and implementation of a model to have a secure understanding of its results. Whereas there are well established principles of study design and implementation, and these are widely known by and accessible to policy makers and the clinical community, the creation of computer micro-simulations is an arcane art, practiced and understood only by a small minority of policy makers and clinicians. Moreover, different modelers and different models may be constructed in different software packages or even hand coded in different low-level programming languages. As such, one modeler may find it difficult or impossible to actually read another's model code and understand how it works. There are general guidelines for program development and documentation developed by the computer science community, but adhering to them is sometimes difficult and time-consuming.[87] Shortcuts are frequently taken, leading to code that is insufficiently documented and may be difficult to read, understand, maintain, or modify, even by the person(s) who originally created it. And even extensive documentation of code may be unhelpful if the actual code is implemented differently from what the documentation states. It may be fair to state that most models are *fully* understood only by the programmer(s) who coded them.

Nevertheless, most clinicians do not have a complete understanding of how all the treatments they use in practice work, and this does not preclude their effective use of them. Similarly, although a policy maker is unlikely to have a complete understanding of the workings of a model whose output is being considered, if sufficient evidence of validity relevant to the questions at hand is available, a detailed understanding is not a prerequisite for effective use of the results.

To maximize transparency, model developers should document their code extensively (with comments as well as in documentation accessible to nonprogrammer users). They should adhere to accepted programming practices that simplify coding and reduce complexity and errors (eg, object oriented programming or structured programming). If the simulation is large enough to require multiple programmers to develop, an appropriate structure to manage and coordinate their activities should be in place, and internal validation should include tests of the consistency of handling of the same data elements and constructs by all parts of the code. Documentation accessible to nonprogrammers is critical to transparency. Such documentation should explain in reasonably nontechnical language how each component (which may be a module of code, or a class in an object-oriented language, or a procedure) of the model works. Equations for key relationships should be given if they cannot be satisfactorily explained in a few words. Diagrams showing how different parts of the model interact with each other are often extremely helpful. Finally, the end user should have the opportunity, if needed and desired, to have the model code itself and all input files reviewed independently by an independent person with suitable expertise.

COLLABORATIVE MODELING

Collaborative modeling[85] is a process where several modeling groups work together to create models with different underlying structure, but use common (or equivalent) inputs and parameter estimates, and then present their results together. In the process of doing this, the modeling groups, or representatives from them, meet periodically to share interim results, to critique each others' assumptions and methods, and to interpret their joint findings.

One strong advantage of the collaborative modeling approach is that it provides a sensitivity analysis for structural assumptions of all of the models involved. Findings which are common to all of the models have a level of support that is then independent of the particular structural assumptions of any of the models, and policy decisions based on such findings are likely to be robust. Nearly as important, findings which diverge across models are thereby identified as dependent on particular assumptions. Such findings may point to new research directions for clarifying which model's assumptions (if any) can be best verified through empirical investigation. Even when no verification of underlying assumptions is possible, the extent to which the models' findings diverge gives an estimate of the uncertainty attributable to those particular assumptions.

The ongoing exchanges and interactions among the modeling groups as the models are developed also mitigate errors in modeling, as assumptions and methods may be subjected to scrutiny and criticism before they are implemented. In addition, coding or other modeling errors may be uncovered when the modelers share initial results and one model is seen to diverge from a clear consensus of the others. Such divergence may represent dependence of an outcome on a structural assumption, but investigation of all such divergences sometimes leads to the discovery of coding errors, or mis-specified inputs, that are then corrected before results are released to interested parties or published. This type of review is more insightful, relevant, penetrating, and directly useful than is normally obtained with peer review of a single model during the publication process.[85] The level of focus and energy that modelers of each group applied to reviewing the work of all the others was greater than would be seen in a single-model effort that recruited the same people to serve on an advisory committee. There are also gains in the efficiency of the research process with collaborative modeling, in that the creation and use of common inputs avoids duplication of effort. Moreover, the size of the combined group and its influential publications also facilitated the development of partnerships.

Collaborative modeling is, in some ways, counter to the competitive culture of grant funded research. But the CISNET collaboration has proved that it can be done. Developing and maintaining a supportive group process is one of the keys to success. Support by the funding agency for the collaborative approach, and continuous engagement of the funder with the modeling collaborative is another.[85]

FUTURE DIRECTIONS

The authors have no crystal ball. But we would like to conclude this chapter by noting three emerging areas for the application of microsimulation models.

PLANNING CLINICAL TRIALS

In one sense, mathematical models have been used to plan clinical trials for decades. A prospective statistical power analysis is a statistical model of the process that the investigators believe will generate the data from a trial. That model is explored to determine a sufficient sample size to justify believing that the trial will likely provide an answer to its research questions. In general, these statistical models do not involve microsimulation, but for some complicated study designs, simulation is used to estimate statistical power.

Microsimulation models have the potential to do more than just estimate statistical power for a study design; they can be used to inform the design itself from the very beginning. For example, currently available treatments for early stage breast cancer are highly effective. In this context, it becomes difficult to study the effects of proposed improvements. Clinical trials might need to be extremely large in terms of both sample size and duration of follow-up in order to detect the small incremental benefits that potentially remain. Microsimulation models can be used to simulate various approaches to study design, going beyond sample size to include different outcomes, restriction to patient subpopulations, and alternative study designs. The microsimulation models can also simulate the study recruitment process. In the United States, the National Cancer Institute has recently funded a small pilot project to test the usefulness of microsimulations in this way. A clinical trial under consideration for implementation was identified, and two of the CISNET models will be adapted to project the results of implementing it in different ways. The modelers will be collaborating with clinical trials experts at NCI to identify and obtain results from relevant earlier clinical trials that can serve as a starting point to develop the microsimulation model and its inputs.

MULTILEVEL MODELING ("BRIDGING THE GAP")

The applications of microsimulation to breast cancer referred to in this chapter are all population-level models. Although most of these models contain explicit representations of the natural history of breast cancer, those representations are in terms of population-level phenomena such as population distributions of tumor growth rates or sojourn times. None of these models incorporates explicit representations of phenomena at the cellular level or below. From a reductionist perspective, ultimately these population-level natural history phenomena are the consequences of biological processes. In 2013, the United States' National Cancer Institute issued a program announcement to sponsor multiscale modeling of cancer, in which population phenomena would be modeled in terms of biological phenomena, so that observations at each scale could constrain the models at both scales. The purpose of the funding opportunity is described as follows:

> By incorporating insights and data from one end of the cancer research spectrum into the framework of the other, projects should be able to cross-validate data gathered at different scales, and explore links between basic biology, population science, and potential health applications in treatment, prevention, diagnosis, and/or screening. Proposed projects should pose a challenging cancer research question that can be addressed by connecting these two ends of the research spectrum that would be difficult to address or explain through biological or epidemiological investigation alone.[88]

Five separate projects have so far been funded under this program announcement, two of them relating to breast cancer.[89] One of these projects (Denis GV, PI) seeks to model the impact of obesity on breast cancer in African-American women by relating it to the metabolic effects associated with obesity. The other (Esserman LJ, PI) seeks to explain the possible effects of targeting adjuvant breast cancer treatment based on detailed molecular tumor subtypes at the population level. Both of these projects commenced in 2014 and results are not yet available. But work like this will test the potential of simulation models to allow population-level data to inform our understanding of biologic mechanisms in cancer, and vice versa.

METHODOLOGICAL ADVANCES

Eddy[90] has commented on the severe limitations of Markov process modeling for many clinical situations, among them the difficulty of representing factors that exhibit variability over the course of a person's lifetime. While the microsimulation models we have discussed here are not, strictly speaking, Markov processes, this limitation also applies to these models. For example, in the applications in which breast density was taken into account, the CISNET models began with a probability distribution for breast density at age 40 and then assumed that it could only change at ages 50 and 65, and that the only breast density transitions allowed at those ages were to remain the same or decrease by a single BIRADS level. Eddy's approach to overcoming this kind of limitation is to abandon discrete state modeling altogether and to represent each life history with differential equations that can be solved numerically; he has implemented this approach in the Archimedes model.[90] This new approach has been successfully applied to diabetes mellitus.[91,92] To date, there are no publications applying this type of modeling to breast cancer screening, but risk factors such as breast density and endogenous or exogenous exposure to estrogens and related hormones exhibit the kind of variation over time that Archimedes is designed to address. It may represent a future direction in breast cancer screening microsimulation models.

CONCLUSION

In the past three decades, spurred by the exponentially increasing availability of computational resources, mathematical models in general, and microsimulation models in particular have taken on an increasingly prominent place in the health literature. They continue to gain acceptance as tools for obtaining insight into the epidemiology of diseases and the effectiveness of health policy choices. They now play an important adjunctive role in the design, analysis, and implementation of breast cancer screening programs. Their ability to make credible predictions of outcomes in counterfactual conditions give the policy analyst more confidence to plan, initiate, and modify programs, while also highlighting areas needing further basic or clinical research.

Models are complex entities. They are vulnerable to several different types of error. Reliance on a model's output without a clear understanding of and confidence in how it works is risky. Concordance of results under sensitivity analysis and across several models with different structures enhance confidence in findings: decisions relying on robust results are most likely to prove effective in practice.

It is a by now almost a cliché to note George Box's observation that "Essentially, all models are wrong, but some are useful."[93] Microsimulation models in health care have now come of age to the extent that the intense skepticism that prevailed 40 years ago has receded and been replaced by recognition that the kind of models we can build today are among the useful ones.[94]

GLOSSARY

Markov process a model of a system that transitions through different states over time. The Markovian property is that the probability of next transitioning into a given state depends only on the state the system is currently in, independent of the history before the current state.

Overdiagnosis the detection during a screening program of lesions which would never have surfaced clinically in the absence of screening. Overdiagnosis is a necessary concomitant of early detection as some people die of unrelated causes while a still presymptomatic cancer is growing. In addition, if some cancers regress, or simply fail to progress, these lesions, which are destined never to be symptomatic, may be detected in a screening program.

Sojourn time the duration of the interval beginning with the first moment a lesion could possibly be detected by a screening test and ending when the lesion surfaces clinically.

Lead time the duration of the interval between screen detection of a lesion and the time when it would have surfaced clinically in the absence of screening. It is the formal term for the "earliness" of detection that results from screening. Note that the endpoints of this interval arise in mutually exclusive conditions, so that lead time is inherently unobservable. A person who is screened and dies during the lead time interval has been overdiagnosed (see above). The lead time for a lesion that would never progress to clinical recognition, even in the absence of competing mortality, is infinite.

LIST OF ABBREVIATIONS

MISCAN MIcrosimulation SCreening ANalysis (a cancer microsimulation model developed, maintained, and used by investigators at Erasmus Medical Center)
CISNET Cancer Intervention and Surveillance Modeling Network
RCT Randomized Controlled Trial
ER Estrogen receptor
US United States
QALY Quality adjusted life year
USPSTF United States Preventive Services Task Force
BIRADS Breast Imaging-Reporting and Data System. This system provides guidance to radiologists on the interpretation of breast images, and provides specific criteria for classifying breast density, among other things
DMIST Digital Mammographic Imaging Screening Trial. This was a randomized controlled trial comparing digital and plain film mammography
DCIS ductal carcinoma *in situ*

REFERENCES

1. Orcutt GH. A new type of socio-economic system. *Rev Econ Stat* 1957;**39**(2):116–23. Also available at *International Journal Microsimulation* 2007;**1**(1):3–9.
2. Fone D, Hollinghurst S, Temple M, Round A, Lester N, Weightman A, et al. Systematic review of the use and value of computer simulation modelling in population health and health care delivery. *J Pub Health* 2003;**25**(4):325–35.
3. Shwartz M. An analysis of the benefits of serial screening for breast cancer based upon a mathematical model of the disease. *Cancer* 1978;**41**(4):1550–64.
4. Shwartz M. A mathematical model used to analyze breast cancer screening strategies. *Oper Res* 1978;**26**(6):937–55.
5. Walter SD, Day NE. Estimation of the duration of a pre-clinical disease state using screening data. *Am J Epidemiol* 1983;**118**(6):865–86.
6. Eddy DM, Hasselblad V, McGivney W, Hendee W. The value of mammography screening in women under age 50 years. *J Am Med Assoc* 1988;**259**:1512–9.
7. Rutter CM, Zaslavsky AM, Feuer EJ. Dynamic microsimulation models for health outcomes: a review. *Med Decis Making* 2011;**31**(1):10–18.

8. Wikipedia Foundation. Microsimulation. <https://en.wikipedia.org/wiki/Microsimulation>; [accessed 03.09.15].
9. Eddy DM. *Screening for cancer: theory, analysis and design.* Englewood Cliffs: Prentice-Hall International; 1980.
10. Habbema JDF, Van Oortmarssen GJ, Lubbe JTN, Van der Maas PJ. The MISCAN simulation program for the evaluation of screening for disease. *Comp Methods Programs Biomed* 1985;**20**(1):79–93.
11. Van Oortmarssen GJ, Habbema JDF, Van Der Maas PJ, De Koning HJ, Collette HJ, Verbeek AL, et al. A model for breast cancer screening. *Cancer* 1990;**66**(7):1601–12.
12. Habbema JDF, Van Oortmarssen GJ, Lubbe JTN, Van der Maas PJ. Model building on the basis of Dutch cervical cancer screening data. *Maturitas* 1985;**7**(1):11–20.
13. Draisma G, Boer R, Otto SJ, Van der Cruijsen IW, Damhuis RA, Schröder FH, et al. Lead times and overdetection due to prostate-specific antigen screening: estimates from the European Randomized Study of Screening for Prostate Cancer. *J Natl Cancer Inst* 2003;**95**(12):868–78.
14. Loeve F, Boer R, Van Oortmarssen GJ, Van Ballegooijen M, Habbema JD. The MISCAN-COLON simulation model for the evaluation of colorectal cancer screening. *Comput Biomed Res* 1999;**32**(1):13–33.
15. Feuer EJ. Modeling the impact of adjuvant therapy and screening mammography on US breast cancer mortality between 1975 and 2000: introduction to the problem. *J Natl Cancer Inst Monogr* 2005;**36**:2–6.
16. Boer R, Plevritis S, Clarke L. Diversity of model approaches for breast cancer screening: a review of model assumptions by the Cancer Intervention and Surveillance Network (CISNET) Breast Cancer Groups. *Stat Methods Med Res* 2004;**13**(6):525–38.
17. Clarke LD, Plevritis SK, Boer R, Cronin KA, Feuer EJ. A comparative review of CISNET breast models used to analyze US breast cancer incidence and mortality trends. *J Natl Cancer Inst Monogr* 2005(36):96–105.
18. Plevritis SK, Sigal BM, Salzman P, Rosenberg J, Glynn P. A stochastic simulation model of US breast cancer mortality trends from 1975 to 2000. *J Natl Cancer Inst Monogr* 2006(36):86.
19. Szeto KL, Devlin NJ. The cost-effectiveness of mammography screening: evidence from a microsimulation model for New Zealand. *Health Policy* 1996;**38**(2):101–15.
20. Rojnik K, Naveršnik K, Mateović-Rojnik T, PrimicŽakelj M. Probabilistic cost-effectiveness modeling of different breast cancer screening policies in Slovenia. *Value Health* 2008;**11**(2):139–48.
21. Lee S, Zelen M. A stochastic model for predicting the mortality of breast cancer. *J Natl Cancer Inst Monogr* 2005;**36**:79–86.
22. Martinez-Alonso M, Vilaprinyo E, Marcos-Gragera R, Rue M. Breast cancer incidence and overdiagnosis in Catalonia (Spain). *Breast Cancer Res* 2010;**12**(4):R58.
23. Vilaprinyo E, Forne C, Carles M, Sala M, Pla R, Castells X, et al. Cost-effectiveness and harm-benefit analyses of risk-based screening strategies for breast cancer. *PloS One* 2014;**9**(2).
24. Comas M, Arrospide A, Mar J, Sala M, Vilaprinyó E, Hernández C, et al. Budget impact analysis of switching to digital mammography in a population-based breast cancer screening program: a discrete event simulation model. 2014.
25. Lee SY, Jeong SH, Kim YN, Kim J, Kang DR, Kim HC, et al. Cost-effective mammography screening in Korea: high incidence of breast cancer in young women. *Cancer Sci* 2009;**100**(6):1105–11.
26. Seigneurin A, François O, Labarère J, Oudeville P, Monlong J, Colonna M. Overdiagnosis from non-progressive cancer detected by screening mammography: stochastic simulation study with calibration to population based registry data. *Br Med J* 2011:343.
27. Olsen AH, Agbaje OF, Myles JP, Lynge E, Duffy SW. Overdiagnosis, sojourn time, and sensitivity in the Copenhagen mammography screening program. *Breast J* 2006;**12**(4):338–42.
28. Duffy SW, Tabar L, Olsen AH, Vitak B, Allgood PC, Chen TH, et al. Absolute numbers of lives saved and overdiagnosis in breast cancer screening, from a randomized trial and from the Breast Screening Programme in England. *J Med Screen* 2010;**17**(1):25–30.
29. Gunsoy NB, Garcia-Closas M, Moss SM. Modelling the overdiagnosis of breast cancer due to mammography screening in women aged 40 to 49 in the United Kingdom. *Breast Cancer Res* 2012;**14**(6):R152.

30. Roberts M, Russell LB, Paltiel AD, Chambers M, McEwan P, Krahn M. Conceptualizing a Model A Report of the ISPOR-SMDM Modeling Good Research Practices Task Force-2. *Med Decis Making* 2012;**32**(5): 678–89.
31. Philips Z, Ginnelly L, Sculpher M, Claxton K, Golder S, Riemsma R, et al. Review of guidelines for good practice in decision-analytic modelling in health technology assessment. *Health Technol Assess* 2004;**8**:1–158.
32. Briggs AH, Weinstein MC, Fenwick EA, Karnon J, Sculpher MJ, Paltiel AD, ISPOR-SMDM Modeling Good Research Practices Task Force. Model parameter estimation and uncertainty analysis: a report of the ISPOR-SMDM Modeling Good Research Practices Task Force Working Group-6. *Med Decis Making* 2012;**32**:722–32.
33. Habbema JDF, Boer R, Barendregt JJ. Chronic disease modeling. In: Heggenhougen K, Quah S, editors. *International encyclopedia of public health*, **vol. 1**. San Diego: Academic Press; 2008. p. 704–9.
34. Eddy DM, Hollingworth W, Caro JJ, Tsevat J, McDonald KM, Wong JB. Model transparency and validation a report of the ISPOR-SMDM Modeling Good Research Practices Task Force-7. *Med Decis Making* 2012;**32**(5):733–43.
35. Shapiro S. Evidence on screening for breast cancer from a randomized trial. *Cancer* 1977;**39**(6):2772–82.
36. Tabàr L, Vitak B, Chen HH, Duffy SW, Yen MFL, Chiang CF, et al. The Swedish two-county trial twenty years later. Updated mortality results and new insights from long-term follow-up. *Radiol Clin North Am* 2000;**38**(4):625–51.
37. Nystrom L, Andersson I, Bjurstam N, Frisell J, Nordenskjöld B, Rutqvist LE. Long-term effects of mammography screening: updated overview of the Swedish randomised trials. *Lancet* 2002;**359**:909–19.
38. Moss SM, Cuckle H, Evans A, Johns L, Waller M, Bobrow L. Effect of mammographic screening from age 40 years on breast cancer mortality at 10 years' follow-up: a randomised controlled trial. *Lancet* 2006;**368**(9552):2053–60.
39. Moss SM, Wale C, Smith R, Evans A, Cuckle H, Duffy SW. Effect of mammographic screening from age 40 years on breast cancer mortality in the UK Age trial at 17 years' follow-up: a randomised controlled trial. *Lancet Oncol* 2015;**16**(9):1123–32.
40. De Koning HJ, Boer R, Warmerdam PG, Bewemsterboer PM, Van der Maas PJ. Quantitative interpretation of age-specific mortality reductions from the Swedish breast cancer-screening trials. *J Natl Cancer Inst* 1995;**87**(16):1217–23.
41. Van Ravesteyn NT, Heijnsdijk EAM, Draisma G, De Koning HJ. Prediction of higher mortality reduction for the UK Breast Screening Frequency Trial: a model-based approach on screening intervals. *Br J Cancer* 2011;**105**:1082–8.
42. Berry DA, Cronin KA, Plevritis SK, Fryback DG, Clarke L, Zelen M, et al. Effect of screening and adjuvant therapy on mortality from breast cancer. *N Engl J Med* 2005;**353**(17):1784–92.
43. Munoz D, Near AM, Van Ravesteyn NT, Lee SJ, Schechter CB, Alagoz O, et al. Effects of screening and adjuvant therapy on specific US breast cancer mortality by estrogen receptor status. *J Natl Cancer Inst* 2014;**106**(8):dju289.
44. Van Ravesteyn NT, Schechter CB, Near AM, Heijnsdijk EA, Stoto MA, Draisma G, et al. Race-specific impact of natural history, mammography screening, and adjuvant treatment on breast cancer mortality rates in the United States. *Cancer Epidemiol Biomarkers Prev* 2011;**20**(1):112–22.
45. Carmichael AR, Bates T. Obesity and breast cancer: a review of the literature. *Breast* 2004;**13**(2):85–92.
46. Van den Brandt PA, Spiegelman D, Yaun SS, Adami HO, Beeson L, Folsom AR, et al. Pooled analysis of prospective cohort studies on height, weight, and breast cancer risk. *Am J Epidemiol* 2000;**152**(6):514–27.
47. Michels KB, Terry KL, Willett WC. Longitudinal study on the role of body size in premenopausal breast cancer. *Arch Intern Med* 2006;**166**(21):2395–402.
48. Yang XR, Chang-Claude J, Goode EL, Couch FJ, Nevanlinna H, Milne RL, et al. Associations of breast cancer risk factors with tumor subtypes: a pooled analysis from the Breast Cancer Association Consortium studies. *J Natl Cancer Inst* 2011;**103**(3):250–63.

49. Canchola AJ, Anton-Culver H, Bernstein L, Clarke CA, Henderson K, Ma H, et al. Body size and the risk of postmenopausal breast cancer subtypes in the California Teachers Study cohort. *Cancer Causes Control* 2012;**23**(3):473–85.
50. Banks E, Reeves G, Beral V, Bull D, Crossley B, Simmonds M, et al. Influence of personal characteristics of individual women on sensitivity and specificity of mammography in the Million Women Study: cohort study. *Br Med J* 2004;**329**(7464):477.
51. Kerlikowske K, Walker R, Miglioretti DL, Desai A, Ballard-Barbash R, Buist DS. Obesity, mammography use and accuracy, and advanced breast cancer risk. *J Natl Cancer Inst* 2008;**100**(23):1724–33.
52. Elmore JG, Carney PA, Abraham LA, Barlow WE, Egger JR, Fosse JS, et al. The association between obesity and screening mammography accuracy. *Arch Intern Med* 2004;**164**(10):1140–7.
53. Rosner GL, Hargis JB, Hollis DR, Budman DR, Weiss RB, Henderson IC, et al. Relationship between toxicity and obesity in women receiving adjuvant chemotherapy for breast cancer: results from cancer and leukemia group B study 8541. *J Clin Oncol* 1996;**14**(11):3000–8.
54. Colleoni M, Li S, Gelber RD, Price KN, Coates AS, Castiglione-Gertsch M, et al. Relation between chemotherapy dose, oestrogen receptor expression, and body-mass index. *Lancet* 2005;**366**(9491):1108–10.
55. Peeters A, Barendregt JJ, Willekens F, Mackenbach JP, Al Mamum A, Bonneux L. Obesity in adulthood and its consequences for life expectancy: a life-table analysis. *Ann Intern Med* 2003;**138**(1):24–32.
56. Flegal KM, Graubard BI, Williamson DF, Gail MH. Cause-specific excess deaths associated with underweight, overweight, and obesity. *J Am Med Assoc* 2007;**298**(17):2028–37.
57. Chang Y, Schechter CB, Van Ravesteyn NT, Near AM, Heijnsdijk EA, Adams-Campbell L, et al. Collaborative modeling of the impact of obesity on race-specific breast cancer incidence and mortality. *Breast Cancer Res Treat* 2012;**136**(3):823–35.
58. Habbema JDF, Wilt TJ, Etzioni R, Nelson HD, Schechter CB, Lawrence WF, et al. Models in the development of clinical practice guidelines. *Ann Intern Med* 2014;**161**:812–8.
59. De Koning HJ, Fracheboud J, Boer R, Verbeek AL, Collette HJ, Hendriks JH, et al. Nation-wide breast cancer screening in The Netherlands: support for breast-cancer mortality reduction. National Evaluation Team for Breast Cancer Screening (NETB). *Int J Cancer* 1995;**60**(6):777–80.
60. Boer R, De Koning HJ, Van Oortmarssen GJ, Van der Maas PJ. In search of the best upper age limit for breast cancer screening. *Eur J Cancer* 1995;**31A**(12):2040–3.
61. Lansdorp-Vogelaar I, Gulati R, Mariotto AB, Schechter CB, De Carvalho TM, Knudsen AB, et al. Personalizing age of cancer screening cessation based on comorbid conditions: model estimates of harms and benefits. *Ann Intern Med* 2014;**161**(2):104–12.
62. Mandelblatt JS, Cronin K, De Koning H, Miglioretti DL, Schechter C, Stout N. *Collaborative modeling of U.S. breast cancer screening strategies*. Rockville, MD: Agency for Health Care Quality and Research; 2015. AHRQ Publication No. 14-05201-EF-4.
63. Nelson HD, Tyne K, Naik A, Bougatsos C, Chan BK, Humphrey L. Screening for breast cancer: an update for the US Preventive Services Task Force. *Ann Intern Med* 2009;**151**(10):727–37.
64. Mandelblatt JS, Cronin KA, Bailey S, Berry DA, De Koning HJ, Draisma G, et al. Effects of mammography screening under different screening schedules: model estimates of potential benefits and harms. *Ann Intern Med* 2009;**151**(10):738–47.
65. Nelson HD, Cantor A, Humphrey L, Fu R, Pappas M, Daeges M, et al. *Screening for Breast Cancer: a systematic review to update the 2009 U.S. Preventive Services Task Force recommendation*. Rockville, MD: Agency for Health Care Quality and Research; 2015. AHRQ Publication No. 14-05201-EF-1.
66. Pisano ED, Gatsonis C, Hendrick E, Yaffe M, Baum JK, Acharyya S, et al. Diagnostic performance of digital versus film mammography for breast-cancer screening. *N Engl J Med* 2005;**353**(17):1773–83.
67. Tosteson ANA, Stout NK, Fryback DG, Suddhasatta A, Herman B, Hannah L, et al. Cost-effectiveness of digital mammography breast cancer screening: results from ACRIN DMIST. *Ann Intern Med* 2008;**148**(1):1–10.

68. Stout NK, Lee SJ, Schechter CB, Kerlikowske K, Alagoz O, Berry D, et al. Benefits, harms, and costs for breast cancer screening after US implementation of digital mammography. *J Natl Cancer Inst* 2014;**106**(6):dju092.
69. De Gelder R, Fracheboud J, Heijnsdijk EAM, den Heeten G, Verbeek AL, Broeders MJM, et al. Digital mammography screening: weighing reduced mortality against increased overdiagnosis. *Prev Med* 2011;**53**:134–40.
70. Van Ravesteyn NT, Van Lier L, Schechter CB, Ekwueme DU, Royalty J, Miller JW, et al. Transition from film to digital mammography: impact for breast cancer screening through the NBCCEDP. *Am J Prev Med* 2014;**48**(5):535–42.
71. Sprague BL, Stout NK, Schechter C, Van Ravesteyn NT, Cevik M, Alagoz O, et al. Benefits, harms, and cost-effectiveness of supplemental ultrasonography screening for women with dense breasts. *Ann Intern Med* 2014;**162**:157–66.
72. Ciatto S, Houssami N, Bernardi D, Caumo F, Pellegrini M, Brunelli S, et al. Integration of 3D digital mammography with tomosynthesis for population breast-cancer screening (STORM): a prospective comparison study. *Lancet Oncol* 2013;**14**(7):583–9.
73. Skaane P, Bandos AI, Gullien R, Eben EB, Ekseth U, Haakenaasen U, et al. Comparison of digital mammography alone and digital mammography plus tomosynthesis in a population-based screening program. *Radiology* 2013;**267**(1):47–56.
74. Friedewald SM, Rafferty EA, Rose SL, Durand MA, Plecha DM, Greenberg JS, et al. Breast cancer screening using tomosynthesis in combination with digital mammography. *J Am Med Assoc* 2014;**311**(24):2499–507.
75. Lee CI, Cevik M, Alagoz O, Sprague BL, Tosteson ANA, Miglioretti DL, et al. Comparative effectiveness of combined digital mammography and tomosynthesis screening for women with dense breasts. *Radiology* 2015;**274**(3):772–80.
76. Mandelblatt J, Van Ravesteyn N, Schechter C, Chang Y, Huang A-T, Near AM, et al. Which strategies reduce breast cancer mortality most? Collaborative modeling of optimal screening, treatment, and obesity prevention. *Cancer* 2013;**119**(14):2541–8.
77. Stout NK, Rosenberg MA, Trentham-Dietz A, Smith MA, Robinson SM, Fryback DG. Retrospective cost-effectiveness analysis of screening mammography. *J Natl Cancer Inst* 2006;**98**:774–82.
78. Mandelblatt JS, Schechter CB, Yabroff KR, Lawrence W, Dignam J, Muennig P, et al. Benefits and costs of interventions to improve breast cancer outcomes in African-American women. *J Clin Oncol* 2004;**22**:2554–66.
79. Mandelblatt J, Schechter CB, Lawrence W, Yi B, Cullen J. The SPECTRUM population model of the impact of screening and treatment on US breast cancer trends from 1975 to 2000: principles and practice of the model methods. *J Natl Cancer Inst Monogr* 2005;**36**:47–55.
80. Schousboe JT, Kerlikowske K, Loh A, Cummings CR. Personalizing mammography by breast density and other risk factors for breast cancer: analysis of health benefits and cost-effectiveness. *Ann Intern Med* 2011;**155**(1):10–20.
81. Caro JJ, Briggs AH, Siebert U, Kuntz KM. Modeling good research practices—overview: a report of the ISPOR-SMDM Modeling Good Research Practices Task Force-1. *Med Decis Making* 2012;**32**:667–77.
82. Siebert U, Alagoz O, Bayoumi AM, Jahn B, Owens DK, Cohen DJ, et al. State-transition modeling: a report of the ISPOR-SMDM Modeling Good Research Practices Task Force-3. *Med Decis Making* 2012;**32**:690–700.
83. Karnon J, Stahl J, Brennan A, Caro JJ, Mar J, Möller J. Modeling using discrete event simulation: a report of the ISPOR-SMDM Modeling Good Research Practices Task Force-4. *Med Decis Making* 2012;**32**:701–11.
84. Pitman R, Fisman D, Zaric GS, Postma M, Kretzschmar M, Edmunds J, et al. Dynamic transmission modeling: a report of the ISPOR-SMDM Modeling Good Research Practices Task Force Working Group-5. *Med Decis Making* 2012;**32**:712–21.
85. Habbema JD, Schechter CB, Cronin KA, Clarke LD, Feuer EJ. Modeling cancer natural history, epidemiology, and control: reflections on the CISNET breast group experience. *J Natl Cancer Inst Monogr* 2006(36):122.
86. De Gelder R, Heijnsdijk EAM, Van Ravesteyn NT, Fracheboud J, Draisma G, De Koning HJ. Interpreting overdiagnosis estimates in population-based mammography screening. *Epidemiol Rev* 2011;**33**:111–21.

87. Smith DJ, Wood KB. *Engineering quality software: a review of current practices, standards and guidelines including new methods and development tools*: Springer Science & Business Media; 2012.
88. National Institutes of Health, National Cancer Institute. *Program Announcement PAR 13-081: Bridging the gap between cancer mechanism and population science.* <http://www.grants.nih.gov/grants/guide/pa-files/PAR-13-081.html>; [accessed 02.09.15].
89. National Institutes of Health, National Cancer Institute. <http://projectreporter.nih.gov/reporter_searchresults.cfm>; [accessed 02.09.15].
90. Eddy D. Bringing health economic modeling to the 21st century. *Value Health* 2006;**9**(3):168–78.
91. Eddy DM, Schlessinger L. Archimedes: a trial-validated model of diabetes. *Diabetes Care* 2003;**26**:3093–101.
92. Eddy DM, Schlessinger L. Validation of the Archimedes diabetes model. *Diabetes Care* 2003;**26**:3102–10.
93. Box GEP, Draper NR. *Empirical model building and response surfaces*. New York: John Wiley & Sons; 1987. p. 424.
94. Mandelblatt J, Schechter C, Levy D, Zauber A, Chang Y, Etzioni R. Building better models: if we build them, will policy makers use them? Toward integrating modeling into health care decisions. *Med Decis Making* 2012;**32**(5):656–9.

CHAPTER

6

CHALLENGES IN UNDERSTANDING AND QUANTIFYING OVERDIAGNOSIS AND OVERTREATMENT

Alexandra L. Barratt and Gemma L. Jacklyn

School of Public Health, University of Sydney, Sydney, NSW, Australia

CHAPTER OUTLINE

Breast Cancer Screening. DOI: http://dx.doi.org/10.1016/B978-0-12-802209-2.00006-1

PLAIN LANGUAGE SUMMARY

Overdiagnosed breast cancer is breast cancer detected by screening that would not have caused any health problems had it been left undetected and untreated. Without screening, it would not ever have been detected. Overdiagnosed breast cancers are "real" cancers, in that they meet current professional standards for cancer diagnosis (ie, they are not false-positives), but detecting and treating these cancers does not improve health outcomes.

Over recent years, strong evidence that breast cancer overdiagnosis exists has been obtained from a range of sources, including three randomized controlled trials (RCTs). Furthermore the incidence of breast cancer (particularly ductal carcinoma in situ (DCIS) and early invasive breast cancer) increased strongly after screening mammography was introduced, while rates of advanced breast cancer declined only modestly or not at all. The excess incidence persists even after adjusting for other changes that increase breast cancer (such as use of hormone therapy, changing reproductive patterns, and increasing obesity). This pattern has been observed internationally, and is consistent with overdiagnosis.

Over the last 15 years, many ways to express overdiagnosis as a percentage have emerged; no single approach is "right." For providing information to women, the best way is to express overdiagnosis as the percentage of breast cancers diagnosed in a screened population of women during the years in which they participate in screening. Percentages which include (in the denominator) all breast cancers detected during women's lifetimes (ie, over long follow-up) may mislead because they dilute the estimate of overdiagnosis by including many cancers which have nothing to do with screening. Furthermore, including different time periods makes comparison between studies difficult.

We estimate that 15–30% of breast cancers that are detected in women who regularly participate in contemporary screening programs are overdiagnosed, based on results from randomized trials and well conducted observational studies. Lower estimates have been reported from studies with higher risks of bias.

Women who are overdiagnosed with breast cancer receive similar treatment as other women diagnosed with breast cancer, leading to overtreatment. Overtreatment resulting from overdiagnosis therefore affects 15–30% of women undergoing breast cancer treatment in a screened population. We cannot currently say with certainty whether an individual woman has been overdiagnosed, so this presents women and their doctors with difficult dilemmas about treatment choices. Overtreatment causes patient harm from side effects of treatment, and increases the costs and burdens of breast cancer for individual women and for the health care system.

Uncertainty remains about how much overdiagnosis has occurred since screening mammography was introduced, and this may never be known precisely. It is important to monitor the effects of new screening technologies (such as digital breast tomosynthesis) as these may result in incremental overdiagnosis compared to current practice. Future research should include randomized trials to assess new technologies within screening programs and studies to improve the evidence base about the harms and costs of overtreatment.

INTRODUCTION

Breast cancer is the most common cancer in women worldwide.[1] Its incidence increased in the 20th century, first in developed, and later in developing countries.[2,3] Changes in lifestyle-related risk factors contributed to rising incidence. These included changes in reproductive factors and choices, body mass index, use of hormone therapy and consumption of alcohol.[4] It is increasingly clear, however, that overdiagnosis—the detection by screening of breast cancers that would not cause harm and would not ever be found without screening—has also been a contributory factor.

During the last 30 years, the mortality from breast cancer has been falling due to advances in breast cancer treatment and screening.[5] Whilst this mortality benefit is important, to fully understand the value of breast cancer screening, readers must also consider its harms. In this chapter, we focus on, arguably, the most important harm of breast cancer screening—overdiagnosis. We discuss the challenge of understanding and quantifying breast cancer overdiagnosis and provide an up-to-date summary of the best quality research evidence.

DEFINING BREAST CANCER OVERDIAGNOSIS

- A patient perspective
- A statistical perspective
- A social perspective

The first challenge in understanding and quantifying breast cancer overdiagnosis is to define it,[6] as, without robust definition, valid quantification cannot proceed. Several approaches to this deceptively simple task have been used to date, and we outline these in this section.

A PATIENT PERSPECTIVE

The first, and widely used, definition is: *an overdiagnosed cancer is a cancer detected by screening that would not have presented clinically during that person's lifetime in the absence of screening.*[7] These preclinical cancers would never have caused symptoms or become life threatening.

An important concept implicit in this definition is the heterogeneity of breast cancer types and behaviors. Some breast cancers progress rapidly whereas others progress slowly, become static, or may even regress. This heterogeneity of cancer progression—from fast through slow to nonprogressive and regressive—is illustrated in Fig. 6.1. It leads to the possibility of overdiagnosis, through at least two major mechanisms (see Fig. 6.1).[7]

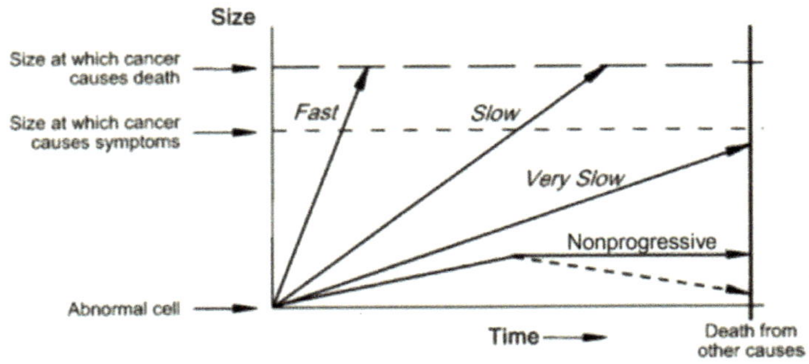

FIGURE 6.1

Heterogeneity in cancer progression.

Ref. 7, reproduced with permission.

One mechanism operates through the detection by screening of a preclinical cancer which, without screening, would have progressed to cause symptoms but the woman dies from a cause other than breast cancer. These cancers are labeled fast and slow in Fig. 6.1, and at some point would cause clinically apparent symptoms and disease. However, if women die from a cause other than breast cancer before the cancer would have caused symptoms, these cancers become overdiagnosed cancers, according to the definition earlier. Readers can think of this as overdiagnosis due to screen-detection of *progressive* preclinical cancer. This cause of overdiagnosis is an inevitable consequence of screening. The risk of overdiagnosis due to competing mortality increases steadily with age as the risk of death from other causes—such as heart disease—also increases.

The other important mechanism is through the detection of preclinical cancer which is nonprogressing (indolent) or even regressing. These cancers would never cause symptoms and disease no matter how long women had lived, yet may be readily detected by screening. Readers can think of this as overdiagnosis due to screen-detection of *nonprogressive preclinical cancer.*

The distinction between these two mechanisms of overdiagnosis is necessary to appreciate that some overdiagnosis, due to competing mortality, is inevitable in breast cancer screening. Unfortunately screening also has a tendency towards overdiagnosis due to the detection of preclinical cancer that is very slow or nonprogressive; this is the focus of most of this chapter. The distinction is also needed to understand the next definition.

A STATISTICAL PERSPECTIVE

Researchers who develop statistical models to estimate overdiagnosis in cancer screening may use a more technical definition: overdiagnosis *can be thought of as cases whose lead time exceeds their remaining years of life.*[8]

Lead time is the amount of time by which the diagnosis of cancer is advanced by screening. In other words, it is the period of time from screen-detection of a cancer to the clinical presentation of cancer (with symptoms) if screening had not occurred. As such, it is largely an unobservable phenomenon, and therefore has to be estimated.

Lead time is an important concept in this definition, and the definition is useful for modeling studies. However, Baker[9] points out that the concept lead time is not meaningful in relation to nonprogressive preclinical cancer[9] because, without screening, these cancers would *never* become symptomatic or diagnosed no matter how much lifetime remains.[9–11]

A SOCIAL PERSPECTIVE

Carter et al.[6] define overdiagnosis as occurring when

- Some patients are given a diagnosis of a condition
- The diagnosis meets current professional standards (it is not a false-positive)
- But the diagnosis carries an unfavorable benefit:harm ratio.

This definition makes the important point that overdiagnosis is different from a false-positive screening test result. An overdiagnosed breast cancer is a real breast cancer, meeting current professional, pathological criteria for cancer. But it does not behave and progress in ways that we have come to expect cancers to behave. This definition makes explicit that, because of this, overdiagnosis may lead patients to undergo medical and surgical intervention that are, at best, very unlikely to be beneficial but involve significant risk of psychological and physical harm (overtreatment). Furthermore, Carter et al. argue that overdiagnosis has inevitable social and ethical dimensions.[6] For example, social and ethical dimensions are involved when making a (value) judgment of no net benefit (unfavorable benefit:harm ratio), and in considering the best allocation of health care resources within societies.

These varying definitions begin to illustrate the complexity of quantifying overdiagnosis. Discussion of alternative definitions has unearthed important differences between perspectives, and uncovered that estimates of the frequency of overdiagnosis may hinge on researchers' choice of definition.

No matter which of these definitions is chosen, an overdiagnosed case is an intangible concept, which can only be perceived and quantified at a population level (a "view from space" if you will[12]). Currently, it is impossible to say with certainty whether any individual has been overdiagnosed or not. This reality lies at the heart of the conundrum of overdiagnosis and overtreatment, and presents policy makers, practitioners and patients with difficult dilemmas once screen-detected cancer is found, because at that point it is not possible to know whether the cancer detected is destined to be progressive or not.

HOW DO WE KNOW BREAST CANCER OVERDIAGNOSIS EXISTS?

Nonprogressive, harmless breast cancer, is a counterintuitive idea. Readers may wonder how we can be sure that overdiagnosis exists, if we cannot identify individual women who are overdiagnosed. To answer this question we need to consider the research evidence which has slowly accumulated since screening mammography was introduced in the 1960s. Taken as a whole it provides compelling evidence that breast cancer overdiagnosis exists and motivated investigators to conduct studies to try to quantify it.

THEORETICAL GROUNDS FOR EXPECTING OVERDIAGNOSIS

To understand the methods used to quantify overdiagnosis, an understanding of the effects of screening on breast cancer incidence is needed. An increase in incidence is expected with screening, especially after the first (prevalent) screening round. This "prevalence peak" occurs because cancers

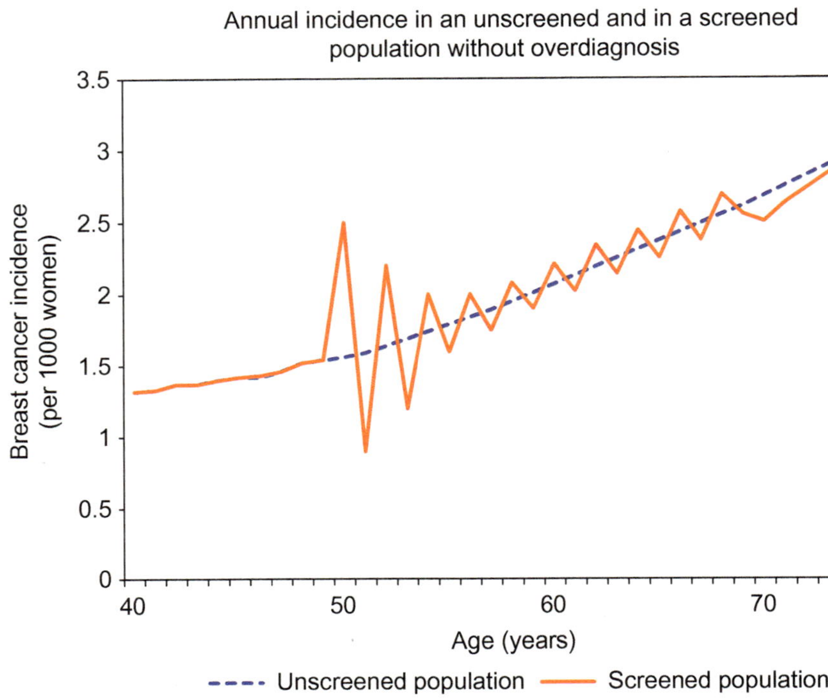

FIGURE 6.2

Illustration of the anticipated effect on incidence of the introduction of screening, hypothetical data.

Adapted from Ref. 13.

which were destined to present in subsequent years are detected earlier and so the age-specific incidence is augmented.[13] This pattern of increased incidence continues—to a lesser extent—following every subsequent screening round. In an ideal screening program without overdiagnosis, this excess of cancers during screening will be balanced by a deficit of cancers after screening ceases, because all the cancers that would have developed clinically by then will have already been diagnosed (see Fig. 6.2). This is necessary and desirable; without it the benefit of early detection could not be realized. However, when screening occurs with overdiagnosis, there is a residual excess incidence in the screened population, even many years after screening ends (Fig. 6.3).

Screening theory predicts overdiagnosis of nonprogressive or very slowly progressing breast cancer because screening will always have a higher probability of detecting slowly progressing cancer or nonprogressing cancer than of detecting rapidly progressing cancer, a phenomenon described as length bias, or prognostic selection[14] (Fig. 6.4).

The possibility that screening mammography might detect nonprogressing breast cancer was recognized early, for example by Feinleib and Zelen in 1969.[15] But their description of the tendency of screening to disproportionately detect low risk cancer was largely ignored. Forrest, in his influential

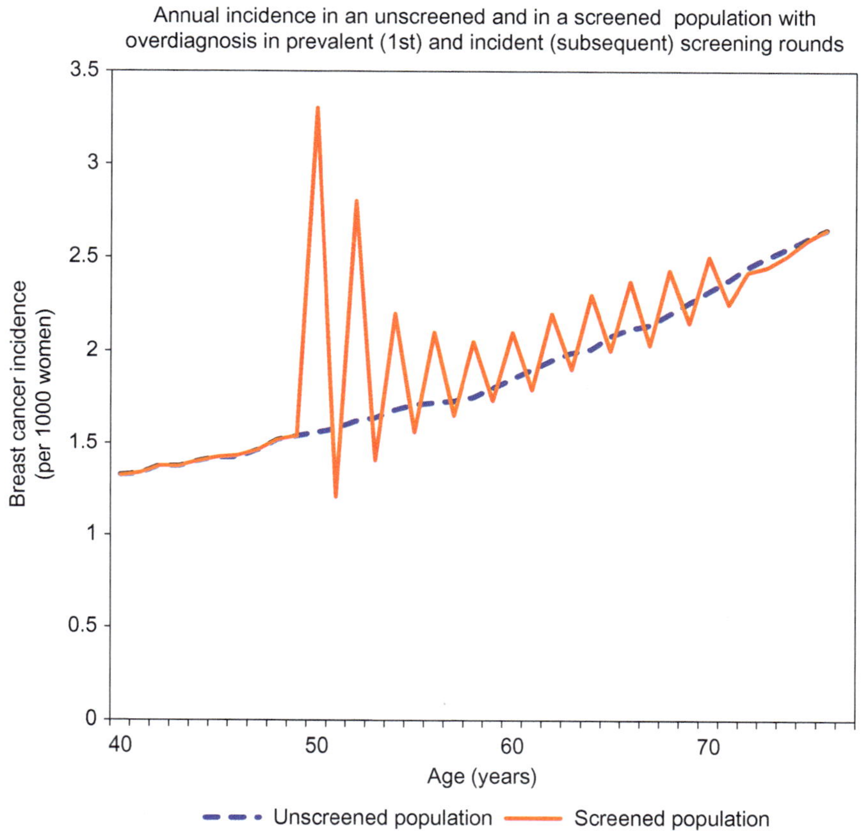

FIGURE 6.3

Illustration of the anticipated effect on incidence of the introduction of screening with overdiagnosis, hypothetical data.

Adapted from Ref. 13.

report on breast cancer screening for the UK health ministers in 1986, also mentioned the potential for overdiagnosis in breast cancer screening.[16]

EARLY EMPIRIC EVIDENCE OF OVERDIAGNOSIS

Large increases in incidence of early breast cancer have been widely observed, with first observations dating back to the 1970s, coinciding with the introduction of screening mammography in the US.[17] Later, the incidence of breast cancer among women 50–69 years rose between 2 and 10% per year, corresponding with the implementation of screening mammography in countries in Europe, the United Kingdom, North America, and Australia.[2,18] Studies in Sweden,[13] Norway,[19] Denmark,[20] the United States,[12] Canada,[21] and Australia[22] have shown marked increases in breast cancer incidence with the introduction of screening, even after breast cancer risk factors (reproductive factors, BMI, use of hormone therapy, and alcohol consumption) have been

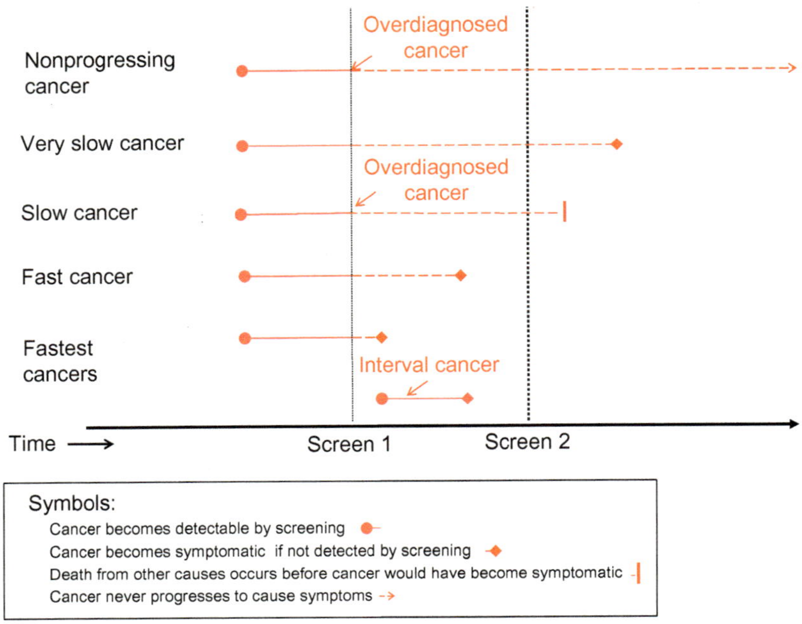

FIGURE 6.4

Length (overdiagnosis) bias: A screening episode (represented by the dashed line) will pick up more preclinical cancers that are progressing slowly, and so remain detectable but asymptomatic, for longer. Preclinical cancers that are more rapidly progressing may present with symptoms before the next screening round, as interval cancers. This is why screening can always be expected to detect proportionally more slowly progressing, good prognosis cancers than rapidly progressing cancers, a phenomenon known as length bias (also called prognostic selection bias or overdiagnosis bias). In this hypothetical example, screening detects three slowly progressing cancers (two of which are overdiagnosed), two fast cancers, and misses one interval (fastest) cancers. Note that very slow growing cancers remain asymptomatic for so long that they may still "available" to be detected at the next round, even if missed at the initial screening round.

taken into account. These rises in incidence led Fox,[17] and many others subsequently, to consider whether screening mammography itself could be driving up the incidence of breast cancer.

Arguably, more important than simply observing increasing incidence are changes in incidence patterns of early and advanced breast cancer. In an optimal screening scenario, as described by Esserman,[23] rates of advanced cancer should drop in response to increased detection (and treatment) of early stage disease. In turn, this drop in rates of advanced cancer should be a precursor to declining cancer mortality, and both are markers of an effective cancer screening intervention which improves health outcomes. Esserman,[23] however, also described worst-case and intermediate-case scenarios. In a worst-case scenario, the incidence of early cancer rises with the introduction of screening but with no subsequent reduction in advanced stage cancer. Such a pattern, if observed, would strongly suggest overdiagnosis. For a visual representation of Esserman's optimal, intermediate and worst-case screening scenarios (see Reference 23).[23]

Patterns consistent with an intermediate case scenario (as described by Esserman) in relation to breast cancer have been observed in recent decades. Rates of advanced cancer have declined modestly, or not at all in regions where screening mammography has been implemented, while rates of early breast cancer have substantially increased.[2,12,19,24,25] More recently, in 1998, the upper age limit for screening mammography in the Netherlands was extended from 69 to 75 years; after this change the incidence of early breast cancer strongly increased between 1998 and 2011 with only a small decrease in advanced breast cancer rates.[26]

In particular, large increases in DCIS incidence have been observed, coincident with the introduction of screening mammography. For example, Kerlikowske documented a 500% increase in incidence of DCIS among women over 50 years of age between 1983 and 2003.[27] DCIS now accounts for 20–25% of screen-detected breast cancer.[18,27] Notably, despite more than 20 years of detection and treatment of DCIS, incidence rates of invasive breast cancer have not declined.[28] This suggests that DCIS may not be an inevitable precursor lesion of most invasive cancers as previously thought. Instead, it makes more sense to think of DCIS as a marker of risk for future invasive breast cancer.[29,30]

With hindsight, we can now characterize the changes which have occurred in recent decades as screening mammography has been implemented. These changes are outlined in Table 6.1 and suggest screening is detecting low risk or nonprogressing breast cancer, some of which would never have become life-threatening.

Table 6.1 Characteristics of Screening Mammography Implementation Which May Signal Overdiagnosis

Characteristic		Notes and Explanation	References
Wide uptake of a cancer screening test with potential for overdiagnosis	✓	Screening mammography has expanded steadily in western countries over the last three decades. Currently 72% of US women aged 50–74 years report being screened for breast cancer in the last 2 years.[31] Participation in regular (3 yearly) screening mammography is about 75% among women 50–70 years in the United Kingdom.[32]	31,32
Increased cancer incidence following introduction of screening	✓	Evidence in 35 countries of increased incidence in the years after the introduction of screening mammography.	3
Increased early stage cancer incidence without commensurate decrease in advanced cancer rates, and/or mortality	✓	In an ideal screening scenario (without overdiagnosis) increased detection of early stage cancer should reduce advanced cancer rates and mortality. In intermediate and worst-case scenarios (adversely affected by overdiagnosis), early stage cancer incidence increases strongly, while advanced cancer rates and/or mortality decline only modestly or not at all. Large increases in early breast cancer (DCIS and early invasive breast cancers) have been consistently observed, with only modest declines in advanced stage cancer rates. Breast cancer mortality rates are declining, however this is likely due to improvements in treatment, particularly the introduction of adjuvant therapy, as well as screening.	5,12,23–26,33,34

(Continued)

Table 6.1 Characteristics of Screening Mammography Implementation Which May Signal Overdiagnosis (Continued)

Characteristic		Notes and Explanation	References
Improved case-fatality rate and/or stable mortality rate	✓	Five-year survival figures steadily improved with uptake of screening mammography, and are now >90% for early breast cancer.	35,36
Evidence of increased treatment and treatment related harms	✓	Significant increases in the provision of breast cancer treatment (in absolute terms) have been observed in response to the increasing incidence. Breast surgery is provided to almost all women with screen-detected cancer, and increased rates of mastectomy have been observed in association with screening mammography and in response to increasing detection of DCIS. As a consequence of increased treatment provision, the absolute number of women experiencing short and long-term adverse effects of breast cancer treatment has also increased.	18,37–41

HOW CAN BREAST CANCER OVERDIAGNOSIS BE QUANTIFIED? (METHODS)

The current accepted view is that breast cancer overdiagnosis exists,[42,43] but how frequently it occurs remains unclear. To quantify breast cancer overdiagnosis, there are several preliminary considerations. The first is: how should we numerically express overdiagnosis so that an estimate of its frequency is comprehensible, useful, and consistently expressed between studies? Other essential considerations are: given we cannot (yet) identify overdiagnosed individuals, what types of studies can we use to quantify it? And what kind of biases may affect them? We consider these issues now, before moving to consider the results of the studies to date in the next section.

HOW IS OVERDIAGNOSIS EXPRESSED?

There are several ways of expressing overdiagnosis in numeric terms, as described by Marmot,[18] Etzioni,[44] de Gelder,[45] and Welch.[7] Understanding the differences in these expressions is necessary to be able to accurately interpret and apply the results of studies that quantify overdiagnosis. Variations chiefly relate to choice of denominator.

Different expressions of overdiagnosis can be illustrated by reference to the data shown in Table 6.2, from the Malmö trial, a large randomized trial of screening mammography conducted in Sweden from 1976.[46] In this trial, women aged 45–69 at randomization were invited to screening every 18–24 months between 1976 and 1990. After the active intervention phase (screening period), screening was still offered to the younger women (aged 45–54 years at randomization), but not to the older women (aged 55–69 years at randomization). Follow-up of all women continued up to December 2001. As most of the screening mammography RCTs invited the control group to screen after the intervention period, this unusual trial design provides a rare opportunity to observe incidence changes during and *after screening* within the context of a randomized trial. At the end of the screening period of the trial, there were more cancers in the invited group (438 vs 324), an excess of 114 cancers (see Table 6.2) among the population of older

Table 6.2 Data From Malmö I Trial for Women Aged 55–69 Years (ie, Born 1908–22): 10 Years of Screening and an Average of 15 Years Follow-Up

	Cumulative Number of Cancers in the Invited to Screening Mammography Arm (N = 20,695)	Cumulative Number of Cancers in the Control Arm (N = 20,783)	Difference
Years 1–10 (screening years: screening every 18–24 months)	438 282 (screen detected only, ie, excluding interval cancers)	324	114
Years 1–15 (ie, screening years plus 5 years follow-up past the end of screening)	780	698	82

Data from Ref. 46.

women. This is expected because screening detects cancers earlier than they would have been diagnosed in the absence of screening due to lead time (see "How Do We Know Breast Cancer Overdiagnosis Exists?" section). Once screening ends, the rate of detection of cancers in the previously screened group should slow compared to the control group, compensating for the earlier increased incidence. This is called the "compensatory drop" in the invited group (or sometimes "catch-up" by the control group). This "compensatory drop" in the invited group can be observed in the Malmö I trial data shown in Table 6.2: 5 years after the end of screening, the excess incidence in the invited group compared to the control group has been reduced from 114 extra cancers to 82 extra cancers.

This excess of 82 cancers therefore represents the overdiagnosed cancers, once lead time (compensatory drop) is allowed for. Any method that attempts to measure the percentage of overdiagnosis attributable to screening mammography should use the excess cancers allowing for lead time in the *numerator* of the percentage calculation.

The choice of *denominator* depends on the desired perspective. For example, the overdiagnosed cancers (allowing for lead time), $N = 82$, can be expressed as a percentage of *all cancers diagnosed during the screening period.* This expression is the method preferred and recommended by the Independent UK Panel on Breast Cancer Screening as the clearest and most intuitive way of providing information to women about the risk of overdiagnosis from screening mammography (Method C from the Independent UK Panel on Breast Cancer Screening).[42] In this example its numeric value is 82/438 or 18.7% and is interpreted as 18.7% of all cancers diagnosed during the period of screening were overdiagnosed. Alternatively, the same excess of 82 cancers can be expressed as 82/282, that is, 29% of *screen-detected* cancers (Method D from the Independent UK Panel on Breast Cancer Screening).

Other expressions of the percentage of overdiagnosis are also possible, for other purposes. For example, if you prefer to express the overdiagnosed cancers as a percentage of all the cancers diagnosed during women's lifetimes, then all cancers to the age of 84 (or some other long period of follow-up) may be the best denominator. As an example of this expression, the data from the Canadian National Breast Screening Study can be used as this trial continued to collect follow-up information for many years. The Canadian National Breast Screening Study provided 5 years of annual screening, and follow-up continued for 20 years after the end of the screening period without either group being invited to screening.[21] With long-term follow-up after the end of screening (ie, allowing for lead time),

Table 6.3 Data From Canadian National Breast Cancer Screening Study, Women Aged 40–59 Years; 5 Years of Screening and an Average of 25 Years of Follow-Up

	Cumulative Number of Cancers in the Screening Mammography Arm (N = 44,925)	Cumulative Number of Cancers in the Control Arm (N = 44,910)	Difference
Years 1–5 (screening years, 5 annual rounds)	666 484 (screen detected only, ie, excluding interval cancers)	524	142
Years 1–10 (ie, Screening years plus 5 years follow-up past the end of screening)	1180	1080	100
Years 1–25 (ie, screening years plus 20 years follow-up past the end of screening)	3250	3133	117

Data from Ref. 21.

there were 117 excess cancers in the invited group. These 117 extra are 3.6% of the 3250 cancers *ever* diagnosed in the invited group over *25 years* (see Table 6.3). Thus, this expression, which gives overdiagnosed cancers as a percentage of all cancers detected during screening *plus all subsequently diagnosed cancers no matter how long after screening they were found* (Method B from the Independent UK Panel), is much smaller than the overdiagnosed cancers as a percentage of all cancers found in the invited group *during the screening* period (117/666 = 17.6%). These calculations demonstrate that including all cancers diagnosed over long-term follow-up in the denominator greatly diminishes the apparent frequency of overdiagnosis. Some argue this is inappropriate because it dilutes the estimate of overdiagnosis by including in the denominator many cancers which have nothing at all to do with screening.[11,47,48] Furthermore, any estimate will vary depending on exactly how many years of follow-up after screening are included in the denominator, making it difficult to compare estimates from different studies.[11,47,48]

Expressions other than percentage risk of overdiagnosis are possible too,[42,45] (for example a relative risk of overdiagnosis [13,49–51]), but are less readily interpretable and not recommended by the Independent UK Panel. These will not be discussed further, but it may be useful for readers to bear in mind that there is no single "right" expression, as some may be useful for different purposes. Readers of studies that seek to quantify overdiagnosis, are advised to check carefully how estimates of overdiagnosis are expressed in any particular study.

GENERAL PRINCIPLES OF STUDY DESIGN FOR QUANTIFYING OVERDIAGNOSIS

As with the estimation of any other outcome of screening (eg, cancer mortality) general principles of study design apply. Ideally, investigators compare two populations—one screened (intervention group) and one not screened (control group)—to observe differences in outcomes over an appropriate time frame. When quantifying overdiagnosis—as distinct from quantifying the mortality benefit of screening—investigators compare the *incidence* of breast cancer in screened and unscreened populations, not the breast cancer mortality. As in all intervention studies, there is a risk of coming to the wrong conclusion due to random error (chance) or because of bias.[52] The main biases are selection bias, confounding, and measurement bias.[11,52] Selection bias and confounding may be avoided by well-designed and well-conducted randomized trials of screening.[11] Measurement bias may be minimized by blind assessment of key outcomes.[40] In screening studies we also have to contend with the possibility of length bias (as discussed in "How do we know breast cancer overdiagnosis exists?" Section) and lead time bias.

Allowing for lead time is essential in screening studies that measure the effectiveness (mortality benefit) of an invitation to screening (see chapters: Estimates of Screening Benefit: The Randomized Trials of Breast Cancer Screening, Weighing the Benefits and Harms: Screening Mammography in the Balance, and The Importance of Observational Evidence to Estimate and Monitor Mortality Reduction From Current Breast Cancer Screening). Lead time is also very relevant to studies that estimate overdiagnosis because it will cause a temporary increase in cancer incidence as outlined earlier. As such, studies that estimate overdiagnosis without allowing for lead time will overestimate overdiagnosis.[13,53,54] However, allowing appropriately for lead time in studies of overdiagnosis is complex and contested, especially in studies other than RCTs.[9,10,53–55]

There are a number of approaches to adjusting for lead time when estimating overdiagnosis, depending on the study design. These are outlined in the following discussion of different study designs that may be used to quantify overdiagnosis.

In summary, the general approach to quantifying overdiagnosis involves comparing the breast cancer incidence in the population invited to screening with that in the unscreened population, after allowing for (or "removing") the excess incidence which is due to lead time. Any remaining excess cancers represent overdiagnosis, as long as other biases (selection, confounding, and measurement) have been avoided.

WHAT TYPES OF STUDY CAN BE USED AND WHAT BIASES MAY AFFECT THEM?

Three main types of studies can be used to quantify overdiagnosis: RCTs, observational studies (including cohort, ecological, and case–control studies), and disease progression modeling studies. The strengths and limitations of these study types are summarized in Table 6.4.

RANDOMIZED CONTROLLED TRIALS

In empiric approaches with direct observation of populations invited to screening, the greatest problem is finding a reference population that has not been invited with the same breast cancer risk as the invited population to act as a control. This problem is best solved by well-designed and well conducted RCTs, which, by virtue of randomization, provide an unscreened control group with a similar underlying breast cancer risk to the intervention group, enabling a fair comparison of the impact of an invitation to screening on breast cancer incidence, and of overdiagnosis.

As discussed in chapter "Estimates of Screening Benefit: The Randomized Trials of Breast Cancer Screening", the main RCTs of screening mammography were conducted in the time period 1960–90.[40] With the exception of the UK Age Trial of UK women aged 40–41 years, trials were all conducted before contemporary breast cancer screening programs were established.

Although we could expect that these trials would have been protected from selection bias, confounding and measurement bias (in terms of recording incidence) by virtue of their randomized, prospective design, none were designed with the aim of measuring overdiagnosis, and only three have features which

Table 6.4 Summary of Main Strengths and Limitations of Study Types to Quantify Breast Cancer Overdiagnosis

Design	Strengths	Limitations
Randomized controlled trials	Avoid selection bias and confounding through randomized comparison groups, with complete ascertainment and analysis by intention to treat. Analysis and adjustment for lead time is relatively simple and transparent (if neither group is screened after the intervention period and follow-up is continued). May be useful for monitoring overdiagnosis with short term outcomes such as interval cancer rates.	Trials will not be able to measure overdiagnosis if population screening is introduced at the conclusion of the intervention period (screening years). Limited applicability as most of the trials were undertaken 30 years ago and used plain film X-ray.
Observational studies	Good applicability as they use contemporary data from screening programs in many countries. Some have good control populations for comparison, and these have lower risk of selection bias and confounding than other observational studies. May be useful for monitoring overdiagnosis.	Susceptible to selection bias, confounding and measurement bias. Allowing for lead time is more complex than in appropriately designed randomized trials due to use of dynamic populations.
Modeling studies	Good applicability as they use contemporary data. Can model any screening policy. May avoid selection bias and confounding. if based on high quality data.	May include complex and nontransparent methods May rely on untested (or untestable) assumptions. Not easily validated

allowed them to adjust for lead time. These three trials were the Malmö I trial of women aged 55–69 years, and the two parts of the Canadian National Breast Screen Study (which we used to illustrate several ways of expressing overdiagnosis in the "How is overdiagnosis expressed?" section). In these three trials, neither the intervention nor control group were invited to screening at the end of the screening period, but there was long term follow-up of women. This enables an estimate of excess breast cancer incidence to be obtained after the "compensatory drop" period as demonstrated in Table 6.2 and Table 6.3 (ie, after allowing for lead time), so they can be used to estimate overdiagnosis directly.[11,18]

While in principle randomized trials provide high quality evidence, they have limitations. They may still be subject to important bias.[40] There are also time and financial constraints. By the time large trials have screened and adequately followed-up their participants, the results may no longer be applicable to contemporary screening programs, because, either the screening technology or the treatment context has changed. Whereas the Independent UK Panel chose to rely on the (now old) randomized trials, Carter et al. recommend that well conducted observational studies may be more efficient and useful for measuring and monitoring overdiagnosis in contemporary cancer screening.[11]

OBSERVATIONAL STUDIES

Many observational studies (comprising ecological and cohort studies) have estimated breast cancer overdiagnosis. In general they have used approaches which were similar in concept to the randomized trials; that is, they compared incidence in women invited to screening to those not offered screening. These studies generally made use of data routinely collected by screening programs or national registries to compare populations invited to screening against a group not invited, such as geographical areas with and without screening programs. Without randomized comparison groups, these studies were more susceptible to selection bias and confounding. As differences in breast cancer risk in the populations who were invited and not invited cannot be excluded, it could be these differences, rather than overdiagnosis, which explain any observed excess incidence (confounding).

Furthermore, observational studies still have to allow for lead time, and this is not straightforward to achieve as it is in appropriately designed randomized trials. Allowing for lead time in observational studies requires one of the following approaches: (1) Some years of follow-up after the end of screening in the population invited to screening may be undertaken to allow investigator to use the "compensatory drop" method (ie, the same approach we illustrated with data from the Malmö I and Canadian trials); (2) A statistical adjustment for lead time on breast cancer incidence may be used[11,44,54]; or (3) Comparison of incidence in invited and control populations once screening is in "steady state" may be undertaken, that is, once the number of women entering the population (because they become old enough to participate in screening, eg, at 50 years of age) is approximately equal to the number of women exiting screening (eg, at 70 or 75 years). Because women usually participate in screening for 20–30 years (eg, from age 50 to age 75), steady state analyses can only be done once screening has been widely adopted in a country or region for approximately three decades. Estimates of lead time from modeling studies (Modeling studies) are sometimes used in observational studies as the basis for the statistical adjustment for lead time (limitations of this approach are similar to those described below for modeling studies). A new approach has been to estimate lead time among interval cancers only in a population invited to screening, and then use this estimate to adjust for lead time in an observational study.[56] In the one study in which it has been used to date,[56] this approach obtained a much shorter estimate of lead time, closer to earlier estimates made prior to wide introduction of highly sensitive screening mammography.[15,57,58]

A case–control study design was recently used as a novel approach to estimate overdiagnosis.[59] While the case–control study design has been used extensively to assess the mortality benefit of breast cancer screening, until this study it not been used to estimate overdiagnosis and it remains unclear how susceptible to bias such a study design may be when used for this purpose.[60]

MODELING STUDIES

Another approach is to build a statistical model, and use it to estimate the frequency of outcomes that we are interested in, including overdiagnosis. Different models may use different approaches, structures, and assumptions but generally aim to model cancer progression with and without screening. Modelers may obtain data on cancer incidence (and mortality, and other screening variables) from a population with or without screening interventions and use it to build (infer) a model of breast cancer-related events. For example, they may model stage-specific breast cancer incidence and mortality with and without a screening intervention, including estimates of lead time and the frequency of overdiagnosis.[44,57,61,62] Models may develop complex structures based on cancer biology, modeling the natural progression of breast cancer from early preclinical disease through to detection by screening or clinical diagnosis and beyond (eg, MISCAN model[45,58]). Like the other methods described above, models need an estimate of incidence without screening, and obtaining appropriate estimates is challenging unless data from an applicable randomized trial are available (as, eg, used by van Oortmarssen et al.[58] and Duffy et al.[63]).

Ideally models are validated by comparing modeled estimates with data from populations other than those which provided the data for model development and calibration.[11]

A strength of modeling is that investigators can model various screening scenarios to answer policy questions about the outcomes that are likely to be achieved by a population based screening program with any given set of characteristics (eg, age groups to be invited, screening interval, screening technology used) over many screening rounds. They can be used to model all screening outcomes, including deaths from breast cancer (and the mortality benefit of screening), false-positives, and the number of overdiagnosed cancers. In the past, they have most often been used to estimate the mortality benefits of screening, rather than to quantify overdiagnosis.

When using models to estimate overdiagnosis, one of the main uncertainties involves the proportion of preclinical cancers which are nonprogressive and the duration and distribution of lead time. As lead time is unobservable in practice, assumptions have to be made, without ever being able to fully validate them. Criticisms of models include that they have not allowed adequately for nonprogressive preclinical cancer[9,10] and rely on assumptions about the duration and distribution of lead time.[11,48] Unfortunately, we do not currently know the proportions of preclinical breast cancers (of different tumor types) which are nonprogressive and therefore models must rely on estimates, assumptions and sensitivity analyses to explore the range of possible outcomes.[8,9,44,62]

In summary, breast cancer overdiagnosis can be quantified using several methodologies, which have important differences. Understanding the methodology can be a challenge in itself. It is important to look for biases unique to screening, as well biases applicable to each study design.

HOW MUCH OVERDIAGNOSIS IS THERE? WHAT STUDIES HAVE BEEN DONE, AND WHAT DO THEY SHOW?

In this section we consider studies that have aimed to draw conclusions about how frequently overdiagnosis occurs. We consider reviews, RCTs, observational studies and modeling studies.

REVIEWS

Several reviews of studies to estimate breast cancer overdiagnosis have been published over the last 10 years.[13,40,44,50,54] In 2012, Cancer Research UK and the Department of Health (England) commissioned a review, to be conducted by expert methodologists who had no history of research in breast cancer screening.[42] In 2015, in a brief statement, the International Agency for Research on Cancer (IARC) reported on its updated review on the benefits and harms of screening mammography, and included estimates of overdiagnosis.[43] A full report of their methodology and results, however, is not yet available.[43] The US Preventive Services Task Force (USPSTF) has also completed an updated evidence review of the benefits and harms of screening mammography, including overdiagnosis.[37] While these reviews addressed mortality benefits of screening mammography, all three included studies that estimated overdiagnosis as well.

The only comprehensive, systematic review of cancer overdiagnosis published to date is that of Carter.[11] This review had several strengths relevant to our purpose: it focused on the outcome of overdiagnosis (rather than mortality benefit), it considered all study types and searched for all published estimates of breast cancer overdiagnosis, and carefully and objectively rated the methodology of each study with the aim of ascertaining the best method for quantifying overdiagnosis. In relation to breast cancer, they identified 3 RCTs (the Malmö I trial, and the two component trials of the Canadian National Breast Screening Study), 18 observational studies, and 7 unique models used to quantify overdiagnosis in breast cancer screening. Each study was assessed for risk of bias in relation to its study design, quality of analysis, calculation and expression of overdiagnosis. For each set of studies, the strength of evidence was assessed, as recommended by GRADE.[64]

We used the Carter systematic review as our starting point, and considered individual studies and reviews published subsequently. As Carter did not pool the results of studies, we also included the pooled estimate of overdiagnosis in randomized trials provided by the Independent UK Panel. We note that no reviews have been able to obtain a precise, pooled estimate of overdiagnosis from all studies because of the heterogeneity in study designs, methods, and contexts.

RANDOMIZED CONTROLLED TRIALS

Overdiagnosed cancers accounted for 15% and 22% of cancers diagnosed during the screening period in women in the screening intervention arms of the Malmö and Canadian trials respectively, after allowing for lead time.[11] Looking at the trials in more detail, the percentages of overdiagnosed cancers were 18.7% in Malmö I (women 55–69 years), 22.7% for Canada I (women 40–49 years), and 16.0% for Canada II (women 50–59 years).[18] Metaanalysis of these trials by the UK panel produced a combined risk of overdiagnosis of 19% (95% CI (confidence interval) 15.2–22.7). These studies and the pooled estimate are shown in Table 6.5.

Subsequently one more trial has published estimates of overdiagnosis. The UK Age Trial randomized women aged 39–41 years to be invited to annual screening for 8 years or no screening.[66] Like most of the earlier RCTs, both groups were invited to the national breast screening program at the end of the screening period of the trial. This trial is not designed to measure overdiagnosis as it does not allow for "catch up" of the control group. Therefore, we have not included it in Table 6.5, for the same reason that we have not included any of the other trials characterized by this design feature. At the end of the intervention period, there was a significant excess of DCIS diagnosed among invited women (compared to the control group), but no excess of invasive breast cancer. This result suggests little or no overdiagnosis of invasive breast cancer, but significant overdiagnosis of DCIS.

OBSERVATIONAL STUDIES

Carter identified 18 observational studies that have attempted to quantify overdiagnosis. They assessed these studies for their risk of bias, the appropriateness of the calculation and expression of overdiagnosis, and the way they handled lead time.

Many of these studies were significantly affected by selection bias and confounding. Furthermore, many had not analyzed their data in ways that meaningfully quantify overdiagnosis nor handled lead time well. Of those using the compensatory drop or catch up approach, few studies had obtained enough follow-up after the end of screening to adequately allow for lead time. Of those that used statistical adjustment, some used lead time estimates from models, and others used simple adjustments involving assumptions such as average lead time equaling 2 or 5 years. Carter et al. rated poorly all observational studies that used a statistical approach to adjust for lead time because of lack of transparency and/or unverifiable assumptions about lead time distribution. Due to their susceptibility to bias, observational

Table 6.5 Results From Best Quality Randomized Trials[1] and Observational Studies[2,3,4]

	Method of Allowing for Lead Time	Estimate of Overdiagnosis (%)[a]	95% CI
Randomized Controlled Trials			
Malmö I (55–69 years)	Follow-up for at least 5 years past end of screening	18.7	15.1–22.4
Canadian National Breast Screening Study	Follow-up for at least 5 years past end of screening		
I (40–49 years)		22.7	18.4–27.0
II (50–59 years)		16.0	12.5–19.5
Malmö I and Canada I and II combined by Marmot (2013)		19.0	15.2–22.7
Observational Studies			
Bleyer[2]	Steady-state screening, more than 20 years of screening implementation	31	
Jorgensen (2009) (pooled estimate obtained from United Kingdom, Canada, Australia, Sweden, and Norway data)[2]	Follow-up for 7 years past end of screening	52	46–58
Jorgensen (2009) (Denmark)[2]	Follow-up for 10–12 years past end of screening	33	
Zahl (2004) (Sweden)[2]	Follow-up for up to 14 years past end of screening	45	41–49
Zahl (2012) (Norway)[2]	Follow-up for up to 14 years past end of screening	50	
Beckmann (2015)[3]	Based on lead time estimated from interval cancers		
50–59 years		16.2	8.5–20.6
60–69 years		16.9	4.9–24.6
Ripping (2015)[4]	Follow-up for 5 years past end of screening	22	

[1]Ref. 18, [2]Ref. 11, [3]Ref. 56, [4]Ref. 65.
[a]Overdiagnosis expressed as excess breast cancers (invasive and DCIS) after allowing for lead time as a % of all breast cancers detected in population invited to screening during screening period.

studies were considered, but not relied on, by the Independent UK Panel[18] which rated RCTs as providing more valid information.

Despite their shortcomings, Carter et al. considered that some observational studies had addressed the potential biases in acceptable ways and provided useful evidence. Accordingly the findings from the best quality observational studies are presented in Table 6.5, along with the results of the randomized trials described earlier.

The best observational studies are those that had:

- a low risk of selection bias and confounding by choosing suitable control populations (often multiple control populations) and adjusting for important risk factors such as use of hormone therapy and differences in breast cancer incidence trends;
- analyzed their data appropriately and expressed their estimates of overdiagnosis over appropriate timeframes, thus avoiding dilution of their estimates by including cancers diagnosed long after screening ends in the denominator; and
- managed lead time in acceptable ways, such as including time for the "compensatory drop" after screening ends, or using data over a long time period such as 30 years when breast screening is in "steady-state."

We identified four additional observational studies that aimed to quantify overdiagnosis published since Carter's systematic review.[51,56,59,65] We rated these using the same criteria as Carter et al. We rated Beckmann[59] and Heinavaara[51] as being affected by significant limitations, including inadequate control of selection bias and confounding, and calculating and expressing overdiagnosis in ways that dilute it by including age groups that lack the potential to be overdiagnosed. We rated Ripping[65] and Beckmann[56] as stronger studies. Both compared breast cancer incidence in populations invited to screening with incidence expected without screening by modeling incidence in ways that attempted to control for confounding by variables such as hormone use, age, and temporal trends. Both included in their analyses expressions of overdiagnosis as excess cancers as a percentage of expected cases during screening, and both have dealt with lead time in reasonable (though very different) ways. These studies are therefore also included in Table 6.5.

MODELING STUDIES

Carter et al. identified seven unique breast cancer models that have been used to quantify breast cancer overdiagnosis attributable to screening mammography in the United Kingdom and Europe (the Netherlands, Sweden, Spain, Denmark, and France). They rated the risk of bias in the studies in relation to the clarity and transparency of assumptions made in the model, the extent to which assumptions were supported by systematically reviewed evidence, the probability of bias in the model data sources, control of confounding, and inclusion of sensitivity analyses and external validation (validation against a different population from the one used to calibrate the model).[11]

No study provided a table of assumptions or discussed potential biases in their data sources. None were supported by systematically reviewed evidence. Four studies were rated as having high risk of bias and three studies as having moderate risk of bias. Most undertook some sensitivity analyses but only three varied the estimate of lead time, with large effects on the results. No model was validated externally against another population from the one in which the model was developed. All studies modeled lead time using incidence data that included overdiagnosed cases in the calculation, therefore obtaining prolonged estimates of lead time and likely leading to underestimation of overdiagnosis. Furthermore, three did not include competing mortality and therefore underestimate overdiagnosis. Due to the high risk of bias in these studies, and their largely unexplored sensitivity to important assumptions, in line with Carter et al. and Marmot et al, we have not included them in Table 6.5, but briefly summarize the results: Of the six modeling studies that presented estimates of overdiagnosis as percentage of screen-detected cancers, estimates were generally low; four estimated overdiagnosis less than 10% (invasive and DCIS), one study estimated overdiagnosis as 8.9–15.2% for steady state screening (invasive and DCIS), and one estimated overdiagnosis of DCIS at 31.9% and invasive cancer 3.3%.[11] As these models have been developed over the last 20 (or more) years, they model the impact of screening using film mammography.

Subsequently the Breast Cancer Working Group of CISNET reported results from six unique models to evaluate *digital* screening mammography, under eight different scenarios to inform the 2015 breast cancer screening guidelines.[62] Digital mammography has been incrementally incorporated into screening mammography, replacing film mammography over the last 15 years in most countries. Of the six models, five modeled DCIS and invasive cancer. Four models, Model D (Dana-Farber Cancer Institute), Model E (Erasmus Medical Center), Model GE (Georgetown University Medical Center, and Model W (University of Wisconsin) allowed for nonprogressing preclinical DCIS, but only one (Model W) allowed some nonprogressing invasive breast cancer as well. Model M (M.D. Anderson Cancer Center) is a Bayesian model which made no assumptions about the natural history of breast cancer. Model S (Stanford University) did not include DCIS and assumed all invasive cancers are progressive. All models provided information about their assumptions and data sources, were calibrated against US breast cancer incidence trends, and were validated against mortality reductions observed in the UK Age Trial. In terms of estimating overdiagnosis, major assumptions were in relation to the incidence increase in the absence of a screening intervention and the proportions of nonprogressive preclinical disease. Overdiagnosis was expressed as both an absolute rate and a percentage of all cancers diagnosed, but the denominator for the percentage overdiagnosed included all cancers diagnosed in the group that received a screening intervention from age 40 to death, which dilutes the estimated percentage of overdiagnosed cancers. For these reasons we have not included these studies in Table 6.5, but note that for biennial screening from 50–74 years of age the modeled estimates ranged 8–22%.

Overdiagnosis estimates from three of the models were published in a separate study.[67] As in the CISNET review, Model W allowed for a proportion of invasive breast cancer and DCIS to be nonprogressive while the other two models (Model E and Model G-E) only allowed for nonprogressive DCIS. In this paper, overdiagnosis was expressed in several ways, including as a percentage of breast cancers diagnosed during a biennial screening period from age 50 to 74 years. Model G-E and Model E estimated 6% and 11% respectively of breast cancers (DCIS and invasive) during the screening period would be overdiagnosed, and Model W estimated 27% of breast cancers would be overdiagnosed.

Quantifying breast cancer overdiagnosis is challenging. It is not possible to make a precise conclusion about how frequently it occurs. From the best available evidence of randomized trials and the best quality observational study[11,12] (presented in Table 6.5) we conclude that for women aged 50–70 years it is likely that 15–30% of breast cancers among women regularly screened are overdiagnosed cancers.

WHY DO STUDIES COME TO SUCH DIFFERENT CONCLUSIONS?

METHODOLOGY

Earlier sections have highlighted how the choice of study design may account for some of the diversity in estimates. The literature review by Puliti et al.[54] for the Euroscreen working group relied heavily on modeling and observational studies that used statistical adjustment for lead time, which they considered the most appropriate means of dealing with lead time. They concluded that "The most plausible estimates of overdiagnosis range from 1% to 10%." and that "Substantially higher estimates of overdiagnosis reported in the literature are due to lack of adjustment for breast cancer risk/and or lead time." The recent viewpoint statement by IARC appears to rely on the Euroscreen review, however further details are not yet available as to date their full report has not been published.[43]

In contrast the Independent UK Panel's "judgment is that the best estimates will come from long term follow-up of RCTs" and that observational and modeling studies involve assumptions which can greatly affect the results and generally are not verifiable.[18] They reported they were not persuaded that such approaches could be relied upon to estimate overdiagnosis.

As described earlier, the systematic review by Carter carefully considered biases that may affect RCTs, observational studies and modeling studies and came to the conclusion that the RCTs now lack external validity, modeling studies require unverifiable assumptions about cancer progression, and that observational studies "when performed well can provide a more valid and reliable estimate of overdiagnosis."[11] Transparent and internationally agreed criteria for rating the methodological quality of studies of overdiagnosis for use in future systematic reviews would be very helpful.

CONTEXTUAL FACTORS

Etzioni has noted that context may be another influential feature in so far as the extent of overdiagnosis will depend on the mammography technology used, the frequency of screening (1, 2, or 3 yearly) and the proportion of the population that participates in screening.[44]

CONFLICT OF INTEREST

Others have written about the potential for financial, intellectual and reputational conflicts of interest to impact on disease definitions, the use of certain estimates in reviews and recommendations made by guideline panels.[68,69] Within the breast cancer overdiagnosis debate, researchers hold strong views about methods for quantifying overdiagnosis. It was for this reason that, in the United Kingdom, Professor Sir Michael Marmot was asked to chair an independent panel to look at the evidence about breast cancer screening. In contrast to all other reviews, panel members could not have published in breast cancer screening.[42]

It seems clear therefore that future evidence reviews about overdiagnosis must attend carefully to the potential for conflicts of interest of all kinds, not just financial. Furthermore it seems wise to take up the suggestion by Guyatt et al.[68] of separating the process of evidence review from the process of developing recommendations.

WHY BREAST CANCER OVERDIAGNOSIS MATTERS: OVERTREATMENT

All women diagnosed with breast cancer, including DCIS, in a screened population are offered treatment. This is because health professionals are currently unable to differentiate between or predict which breast cancers will be nonprogressive and which ones will progress due to the lack of accurate prognostic markers. As some of these women have been overdiagnosed, they will also be overtreated as a result, that is receive treatments which will not, by definition, provide benefit but carry risks of adverse effects. In this section, we consider how we might quantify overtreatment, and its impact on women and societies (see also chapters: Treatment of Screen-Detected Breast Cancer: Can We Avoid or Minimize Overtreatment? and Informed and Shared Decision-Making in Breast Screening).

QUANTIFYING OVERTREATMENT

We can attempt to quantify overtreatment in a screened population by apportioning all treatment into treatment and overtreatment. Thus, if we are fairly confident that 15–30% of all breast cancers diagnosed in a screened population represent overdiagnosis, then we can be fairly confident that approximately 15–30% of all breast cancer treatment in a screened population represents overtreatment. Others have used this approach to describe the likely extent of overtreatment in a screened population[18] and to quantify its economic cost.[70] An assessment of the magnitude and severity of overtreatment at a population level may also be informed by the distribution of breast cancer stage, size, grade, and tumor type in the population. So, while overtreatment may occur in about 15–30% of women diagnosed with breast cancer in a screened population overall, women with screen-detected DCIS and small, screen-detected early-stage breast cancer are more likely to experience overtreatment than women with more advanced cancer. A detailed study to quantify overtreatment in this way has not been done yet to our knowledge.

When treating individual women, however, a population perspective is not very useful. Clinicians have to consider the risk of overdiagnosis in each patient on a spectrum of probability, as we are currently unable to identify overdiagnosed cancers and thus overtreated women. How should they proceed?

For women for whom the risk of having been overdiagnosed is low, the probability of benefiting from breast cancer treatment is high. (See Fig. 6.5, top left of treatment benefit line.) For example, a woman who has an interval cancer has a zero probability of being overdiagnosed. For her, there is a high probability of benefiting from treatment. Conversely, for women for whom the probability of having been overdiagnosed is high—for example, women with screen-detected, low risk DCIS—the probability of benefiting from cancer treatment is much lower, perhaps even approaching zero. At the hypothetical point at which the probability of overdiagnosis is 100%, there is no probability of benefiting from treatment. At this point, all treatment provided is overtreatment.

Furthermore, when the probability of overdiagnosis is high, and the probability of benefiting from treatment is low, there should be a much lower threshold of acceptable treatment harms. Again at the hypothetical extreme of the probability of overdiagnosis being 100%, no amount of treatment harm is acceptable because treatment cannot result in benefit. In some cases, the provision of some forms of treatment may be likely to represent overtreatment; routine radiotherapy for completely excised, screen-detected, low grade DCIS for example,[30] but most of the time, where the boundaries of possible overtreatment lie will depend on a mix of the woman's tumor characteristics, her overall health, age, life expectancy and on her treatment preferences.

At present the best we can do to estimate the probability of overdiagnosis is to consider the probability of the cancer being a progressive cancer, capable of causing symptoms and becoming life threatening within the remaining life-expectancy of the individual woman. This assessment will, at present, be based on histopathological features such as stage, size, grade, tumor type, and other features, such as mode of detection, results of molecular tests, and the remaining life-expectancy of the woman. For example, screen-detected cancers often have good prognostic features,[71,72] and tubular cancers in particular have excellent prognosis.[73]

In the next section, we consider the impacts of breast cancer diagnosis and treatment on women's lives from the point of view of someone who has been overdiagnosed, and who therefore cannot benefit from the treatment (as shown in the bottom right of Fig. 6.5), even though we cannot identify these

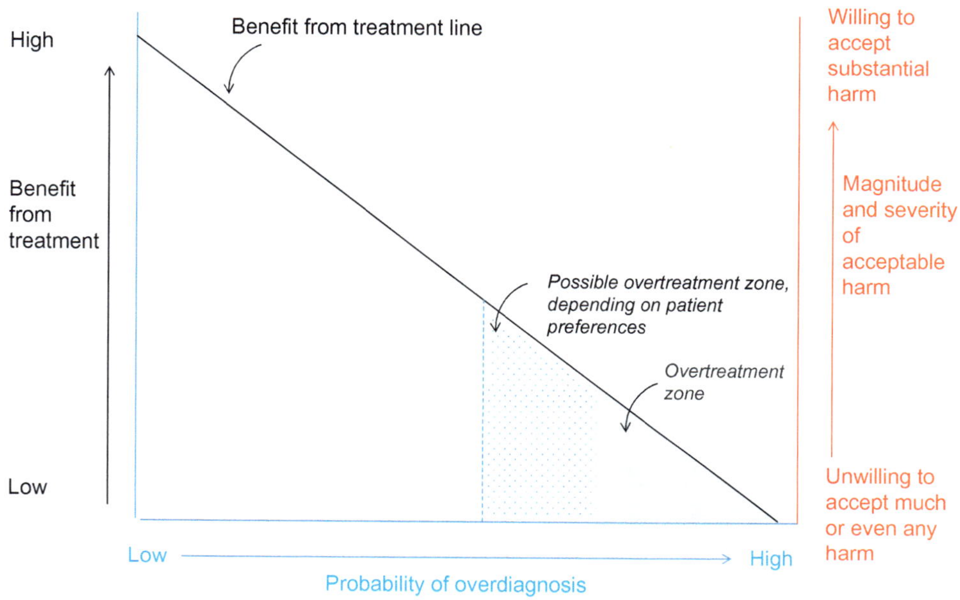

FIGURE 6.5

Relationship between probability of overdiagnosis, benefit:harm ratio of treatment and risk of overtreatment (overtreatment zone).

women. We recognize that for women who are *not* overdiagnosed, these treatments are potentially life-saving and extremely valuable, and valued by them and their families.

LABELING: BEING TOLD YOU HAVE BREAST CANCER

Before considering physical harms, we must not neglect the psycho-social impact of being told you have breast cancer. This is a significant life event, with immediate and long term psycho-social impacts in its own right.[74] Depression and anxiety are common experiences in the years following a cancer diagnosis.[75] Furthermore the awareness or perception of increased cancer risk in the family affects people other than the woman diagnosed, including her children, siblings, and other family members. Relationships within families and with friends are affected, as individual resilience and social support resources are tested. The effects begin immediately after diagnosis and, while many women cope well with treatment and the psycho-social adjustment required, some long-term breast cancer survivors may continue to have difficulties with emotional adjustment (fear of recurrence, feelings of vulnerability) for many years.[74,76]

OVERTREATMENT OF DCIS

Although not a life-threatening condition itself, DCIS is currently treated similarly to invasive breast cancer.[27,77] In the United States, women with DCIS (Stage 0 breast cancer) are treated with surgery (mastectomy or lumpectomy).[37] Radiotherapy may be added to lumpectomy, and endocrine therapy may be offered according to hormone receptor status.

This situation is complicated by the considerable uncertainty about the probability of subsequent invasive breast cancer after a DCIS diagnosis, if left untreated, as, in practice, this rarely happens.[78] The cumulative probability of invasive breast cancer after treatment for DCIS appears to be about 5–10% over 5 years,[79,80] and 5–20% over 20 years.[29,80] A large, observational study of 108,196 women diagnosed with DCIS has confirmed a low risk of breast cancer mortality after a diagnosis of DCIS for women aged 40 and over.[29] The 20-year risk of breast cancer mortality was 3.0% (95% CI 3.0–3.6) for women diagnosed with DCIS between age 40 and 59 years. Prior to screening, DCIS accounted for 2–3% of all breast cancer diagnoses, whereas it now accounts for about 20% of screen-detected cancers, and most DCIS is detected by screening.[30] Consistent with earlier research showing increasing rates of invasive breast cancer despite many years of detection and treatment of DCIS,[12,28] these data support a reexamination of the necessity to treat all screen-detected DCIS. Instead, thinking about DCIS as a risk factor for invasive breast cancer may be more useful, with consideration of lifestyle modification and endocrine therapy to reduce risk.[30]

OVERTREATMENT OF EARLY, INVASIVE SCREEN-DETECTED BREAST CANCER

Treatment includes surgery, radiotherapy, adjuvant endocrine therapy, and chemotherapy,[18,37] according to local clinical guidelines and practice for the stage and grade of cancer, overall clinical status and personal preferences.[37] In the United States, most patients with early invasive breast cancer undergo surgery, radiation therapy and 5–10 years of endocrine therapy for women with ER + cancers.[37] In the NHS screening programs, 99% of women with screen-detected breast cancer (DCIS and invasive breast cancer) undergo surgery, and approximately 70% have adjuvant radiotherapy and hormone therapy.[18] As we have shown, a sizeable proportion of this treatment provision represents overtreatment.

While the proportion of women with early breast cancer treated with mastectomy decreased in the 1980s and early 1990s with increasing use of breast conserving surgery,[81] recent analyses from the United States show that surgical treatment for early breast cancer appears to be expanding. More women are choosing mastectomy over breast conserving surgery, with the greatest increase among women diagnosed with DCIS.[38] Furthermore 20% of women diagnosed with early breast cancer are considering and 7% are receiving contralateral prophylactic mastectomy.[82] Risk of death from breast cancer surgery is small in the short-term, for example, even with extensive surgery the risk of death is less than 0.3%.[18] Complications of mastectomy include pain, infection, scarring, seroma, and lymphedema.[83] While these risks are relatively low for individual women (10–20%[84]), they are increased with bilateral mastectomy.[85,86]

There are short and longer term risks of radiotherapy, especially for women with a left sided breast cancer, with the increased risk apparent within 5 years of radiotherapy.[39] Radiotherapy also increases the risk of developing other cancers, primarily lung cancer, with the risk of incidence and mortality from lung cancer approximately doubled over 15 years.[34]

In a large adjuvant treatment trial, adjuvant hormone therapy resulted in hot flushes (30% of women), trouble sleeping (20%), weight gain (20%), loss of interest in sex (8–16%), and lack of energy (16–20%).[87] Chemotherapy is generally used for high risk or advanced invasive cancer, but, to the extent that it may be used for early stage invasive cancer, it is possible that chemotherapy (which has many side effects) may contribute to overtreatment (see also chapter: Treatment of Screen-Detected Breast Cancer: Can We Avoid or Minimize Overtreatment?).

COSTS, RESOURCE IMPLICATIONS, AND OPPORTUNITY COSTS FROM OVERDIAGNOSIS AND OVERTREATMENT

We close this section by noting that this substantial burden of overtreatment contributes to increasing costs to the healthcare system, as well as the pressure on healthcare staff and infrastructure resources within it. A recent estimate of annual costs of breast cancer overdiagnosis due to screening in the United States among women aged 40–59 years was $1.2 billion.[70] Average expenditures were $52,000 and $12,000 per woman overdiagnosed with invasive breast cancer and DCSI, respectively, in the 12 months following diagnosis. These are underestimates of the true costs of overdiagnosis, as flow-on costs accrued after 12 months (eg, ongoing monitoring, hormonal treatment, and health care consultations) were not included. Women, as well as health service systems and providers, may experience costs from higher insurance premiums and loss of income[88,89] as well as out-of-pocket expenses for treatment.[70]

As overdiagnosis and overtreatment adversely affect the benefit:harm ratio of early detection and treatment (as shown in Fig. 6.5), they reduce the cost-effectiveness of screening as an intervention. The Independent UK Panel recommended a reassessment of cost-effectiveness of screening mammography.[42] A subsequent cost-effectiveness analysis, with inclusion of the costs of overdiagnosis, found that there is only a moderate probability of screening mammography remaining cost-effective at a standard threshold (£20,000 per QALY),[90] and that risk-based, individualized screening may be more efficient and provide better benefit:harm ratios than uniform screening policies.[91] Further research is needed to better quantify the costs (including flow-on costs and opportunity costs) and impacts on cost-effectiveness of overdiagnosis and overtreatment in screening mammography.

In summary, while we cannot precisely identify individual women who are overdiagnosed and overtreated it is likely that about 15–30% of women who receive treatment for breast cancer in a screened population are overtreated thereby exposing women to risk of harm, without delivering benefit. Furthermore, once found it is very difficult, if not impossible, not to treat early breast cancer. In this way, overdiagnosis caused by screening mammography inadvertently turns some well women into patients who are exposed to the harms and risks of cancer therapies.[18] Thus taking steps to minimize overdiagnosis and overtreatment is very important (see also chapter: Treatment of Screen-Detected Breast Cancer: Can We Avoid or Minimize Overtreatment?). Finally we note the opportunity cost of overtreatment, as overtreatment of some individuals risks under treatment of others in a health system with constrained resources. Overtreatment is a form of very low value—or zero value—healthcare, and as with all low value care it may divert resources away from the provision of interventions that are more beneficial, safe, and cost-effective.[92,93]

MONITORING OVERDIAGNOSIS IN ESTABLISHED SCREENING PROGRAMS

MONITORING THE IMPACT OF NEW SCREENING TECHNOLOGY

Due to the limitations in the evidence base described in this chapter, we may never know precisely how frequently overdiagnosis has occurred since the introduction of screening mammography. In principle, RCTs provide the highest quality information, but the trials of screening mammography are old and cannot reliably be applied to contemporary screening. The most urgent question now is, given screening mammography is well established with some level of overdiagnosis occurring, how can we effectively monitor increases or decreases (incremental change) in overdiagnosis as new breast screening technologies become available?

New technology holds potential for augmenting the benefits of early detection of breast cancer if it can increase the early detection of *progressive* preclinical cancer. Increased detection of nonprogressive preclinical cancer, however, will adversely affect the benefit:harm ratio of breast cancer screening by increasing overdiagnosis. Evidence of improved benefit in terms of important short term outcomes—such as reduced interval cancer rates—and long term outcomes such as reduced mortality, is needed and cannot simply be assumed to flow from increased detection rates at screening.[94] Obtaining this evidence requires implementing promising new technologies in RCTs embedded within screening programs.[95]

Although we recognize there are professional and diagnostic benefits of digital mammography,[96,97] it was widely adopted into screening practice with little to no RCT evidence[98] of reduced mortality or its contribution to overdiagnosis, and likely represents a missed opportunity to estimate incremental benefit and harm from its introduction. Early data suggest digital breast tomosynthesis increases breast cancer detection at screening in some groups of women, but whether this will translate into improved mortality or incremental overdiagnosis is, as yet, unknown.[99,100] (see also chapter: Evolution of Mammography Screening: From Film Screen to Digital Breast Tomosynthesis.)

MONITORING THE IMPACT OF CHANGING SCREENING POLICY

There is strong promotion of screening in Western countries,[101] and little public and professional understanding of the risks of overdiagnosis.[102,103] Thus, it may be tempting to many people to think that if screening is a public good, then more screening should be better and deliver more benefit. As a result, overscreening may occur readily, for example, by screening too frequently (annual vs 2 yearly screening) or by screening older women with short life-expectancies.[104,105] However, as with introducing new technology, we should not assume that screening more often, or for longer, will positively impact the ratio of benefit to harm. A 10-year evaluation of the impact of extending the upper age limit for screening mammography in the Netherlands from 69 to 75 years does not appear to have improved health outcomes. The authors reported that the incidence of early breast cancer increased strongly, but there was little reduction in advanced cancer rates.[26] Overdiagnosis in older women who continue (or cease) screening could readily be monitored if changes like this were implemented via RCTs within screening services, as in the UK Age Extension Trial https://clinicaltrials.gov/ct2/show/NCT01081288 (see also chapter: Breast Cancer Screening in the Older Woman).

CONCLUSION

Understanding and quantifying breast cancer overdiagnosis and overtreatment is extremely challenging. A consistent body evidence has demonstrated large increases in breast cancer incidence, and especially incidence of DCIS and early invasive breast cancer, following implementation of screening mammography around the world. In the last 15 years, randomized trials, observational studies, and modeling studies have been used to quantify overdiagnosis. Each of these approaches has strengths, but also important weaknesses and limitations. From our review of this evidence, we conclude that for women aged 50–70 years it is likely that 15–30% of cancers among women regularly screened are overdiagnosed based on the results of randomized trials in women of this age, and the best quality observational studies. Overdiagnosis could be more frequent in contemporary screening programs, because of increasing sensitivity of new screening technology.

Consequently we estimate that 15–30% of women in a screened population who undergo breast cancer treatment are overtreated. In this way screening mammography inadvertently converts some healthy women into breast cancer patients, with potential for short- and long-term adverse consequences from cancer treatment. While women experience the consequences overdiagnosis and overtreatment, it is not possible to say with certainty whether an individual woman has been overdiagnosed or not as we do not yet have tests to distinguish progressive from nonprogressive breast cancer. This presents a difficult dilemma for women and clinicians, whereby they must try to optimize treatment based on the probability of overdiagnosis in the individual, based on the cancer stage and histopathology. As well as causing harm to patients, overtreatment increases the cost and burden of breast cancer for individual women, their families and for the health care system.

It may not be possible in the foreseeable future to more accurately quantify the risk of overdiagnosis and overtreatment attributable to an invitation to screening mammography. Rather, the methodological advances of the past 10 years will help monitor incremental overdiagnosis that may accompany the introduction of new screening technologies.

Breast cancer overdiagnosis and overtreatment are important downsides of screening mammography. Along with the impact of false-positive results, the consequences of overdiagnosis—for individual women and for societies—need to be weighed against the benefits of screening mammography outlined in other sections. Whether the balance of mortality benefit outweighs the harms of overdiagnosis is a value judgment and varies widely between individuals.[106] Awareness of overdiagnosis as a risk of breast cancer screening is poor in the community.[102,103] Women, even when carefully informed, find it challenging to understand.[107–111] With increasing research evidence about overdiagnosis and overtreatment however, there is a growing need to move away from promotional information about screening mammography and towards balanced information that better informs women of the benefit and the harms of screening and supports their autonomy and right to make their own informed choices.[42,92,109,111–113]

REFERENCES

1. Ferlay J, Soerjomataram I, Dikshit R, Eser S, Mathers C, Rebelo M, et al. Cancer incidence and mortality worldwide: sources, methods and major patterns in GLOBOCAN 2012. *Int J Cancer* 2015;**136**(5):E359–86.
2. Hery C, Ferlay J, Boniol M, Autier P. Changes in breast cancer incidence and mortality in middle-aged and elderly women in 28 countries with Caucasian majority populations. *Ann Oncol* 2008;**19**(5):1009–18.
3. Hery C, Ferlay J, Boniol M, Autier P. Quantification of changes in breast cancer incidence and mortality since 1990 in 35 countries with Caucasian-majority populations. *Ann Oncol* 2008;**19**(6):1187–94.
4. Bray F, McCarron P, Parkin DM. The changing global patterns of female breast cancer incidence and mortality. *Breast Cancer Res* 2004;**6**(6):229–39.
5. Berry DA, Cronin KA, Plevritis SK, Fryback DG, Clarke L, Zelen M, et al. Effect of screening and adjuvant therapy on mortality from breast cancer. *N Engl J Med* 2005;**353**(17):1784–92.
6. Carter SM, Rogers W, Heath I, Degeling C, Doust J, Barratt A. The challenge of overdiagnosis begins with its definition. *BMJ* 2015;**350**:h869.
7. Welch HG, Black WC. Overdiagnosis in cancer. *J Natl Cancer Inst* 2010;**102**(9):605–13.

8. Duffy SW, Parmar D. Overdiagnosis in breast cancer screening: the importance of length of observation period and lead time. *Breast Cancer Res* 2013;**15**(3):R41.
9. Baker SG, Prorok PC, Kramer BS. Lead time and overdiagnosis. *J Natl Cancer Inst* 2014;**106**(12).
10. Zahl PH, Jorgensen KJ, Gotzsche PC. Lead-time models should not be used to estimate overdiagnosis in cancer screening. *J Gen Intern Med* 2014;**29**(9):1283–6.
11. Carter JL, Coletti RJ, Harris RP. Quantifying and monitoring overdiagnosis in cancer screening: a systematic review of methods. *BMJ* 2015;**350**:g7773.
12. Bleyer A, Welch HG. Effect of three decades of screening mammography on breast-cancer incidence. *N Engl J Med* 2012;**367**(21):1998–2005.
13. Biesheuvel C, Barratt A, Howard K, Houssami N, Irwig L. Effects of study methods and biases on estimates of invasive breast cancer overdetection with mammography screening: a systematic review. *Lancet Oncol* 2007;**8**(12):1129–38.
14. Morrison AS. *Screening in chronic disease*. New York, NY: Oxford University Press; 1992.
15. Feinleib M, Zelen M. Some pitfalls in the evaluation of screening programs. *Arch Environ Health* 1969;**19**(3):412–5.
16. Forrest P, Chamberlain J, Elton A, Evan K, Gravelle H, Hayes D, et al. *Breast cancer screening report to the Health Ministers of England, Wales, Scotland & Northern Ireland*. Department of Health and Social Science; 1986.
17. Fox MS. On the diagnosis and treatment of breast cancer. *JAMA* 1979;**241**(5):489–94.
18. Marmot MG, Altman DG, Cameron DA, Dewar JA, Thompson SG, Wilcox M. The benefits and harms of breast cancer screening: an independent review. *Br J Cancer* 2013;**108**(11):2205–40.
19. Kalager M, Adami HO, Bretthauer M, Tamimi RM. Overdiagnosis of invasive breast cancer due to mammography screening: results from the Norwegian screening program. *Ann Intern Med* 2012;**156**(7):491–9.
20. Jorgensen KJ, Gotzsche PC. Overdiagnosis in publicly organised mammography screening programmes: systematic review of incidence trends. *BMJ* 2009;**339**:b2587.
21. Miller AB, Wall C, Baines CJ, Sun P, To T, Narod SA. Twenty five year follow-up for breast cancer incidence and mortality of the Canadian National Breast Screening Study: randomised screening trial. *BMJ* 2014;**348**:g366.
22. Morrell S, Barratt A, Irwig L, Howard K, Biesheuvel C, Armstrong B. Estimates of overdiagnosis of invasive breast cancer associated with screening mammography. *Cancer Causes Control* 2010;**21**(2):275–82.
23. Esserman L, Shieh Y, Thompson I. Rethinking screening for breast cancer and prostate cancer. *JAMA* 2009;**302**(15):1685–92.
24. Hofvind S, Lee CI, Elmore JG. Stage-specific breast cancer incidence rates among participants and non-participants of a population-based mammographic screening program. *Breast Cancer Res Treat* 2012;**135**(1):291–9.
25. Autier P, Boniol M, Middleton R, Dore JF, Hery C, Zheng T, et al. Advanced breast cancer incidence following population-based mammographic screening. *Ann Oncol* 2011;**22**(8):1726–35.
26. de Glas NA, de Craen AJ, Bastiaannet E, Op 't Land EG, Kiderlen M, van de Water W, et al. Effect of implementation of the mass breast cancer screening programme in older women in the Netherlands: population based study. *BMJ* 2014;**349**:g5410.
27. Kerlikowske K. Epidemiology of ductal carcinoma in situ. *J Natl Cancer Inst Monogr* 2010;**2010**(41): 139–41.
28. Ozanne EM, Shieh Y, Barnes J, Bouzan C, Hwang ES, Esserman LJ. Characterizing the impact of 25 years of DCIS treatment. *Breast Cancer Res Treat* 2011;**129**(1):165–73.
29. Narod SA, Iqbal J, Giannakeas V, Sopik V, Sun P. Breast cancer mortality after a diagnosis of ductal carcinoma in situ. *JAMA Oncol* 2015;**1**(7):888–96.
30. Esserman L, Yau C. Rethinking the standard for ductal carcinoma in situ treatment. *JAMA Oncol* 2015;**1**(7):881–3.
31. Centers for Disease Control and Prevention. *Cancer screening—United States, 2010*. Centers for Disease Control and Prevention; 2012.

32. Cancer Research UK. *Breast screening statistics—Breast cancer screening trends over time.* <http://www.cancerresearchuk.org/health-professional/cancer-statistics/statistics-by-cancer-type/breast-cancer/screening#heading-Four> [accessed 12.08.15].
33. Early Breast Cancer Trialists' Collaborative Group (EBCTCG) Comparisons between different polychemotherapy regimens for early breast cancer: meta-analyses of long-term outcome among 100,000 women in 123 randomised trials. *Lancet* 2012;**379**(9814):432–44.
34. Early Breast Cancer Trialists' Collaborative G Effects of radiotherapy and of differences in the extent of surgery for early breast cancer on local recurrence and 15-year survival: an overview of the randomised trials. *Lancet* 2005;**366**(9503):2087–106.
35. Susan G. Komen. *Survival after breast cancer.* <http://ww5.komen.org/BreastCancer/LivingwithBreastCancerIntroduction.html> [accessed 12.08.15].
36. Walters S, Maringe C, Butler J, Rachet B, Barrett-Lee P, Bergh J, et al. Breast cancer survival and stage at diagnosis in Australia, Canada, Denmark, Norway, Sweden and the UK, 2000-2007: a population-based study. *Br J Cancer* 2013;**108**(5):1195–208.
37. Nelson HD, Pappas M, Cantor A, Griffin J, Daeges M, Humphrey L. Harms of breast cancer screening: Systematic review to update the 2009 U.S. preventive services task force recommendation. *Ann Intern Med* 2016 [Published online 12 January 2016. Available from: http://dx.doi.org/10.7326/M15-0970].
38. Kummerow KL, Du L, Penson DF, Shyr Y, Hooks MA. Nationwide trends in mastectomy for early-stage breast cancer. *JAMA Surg* 2014;**150**(1):9–16.
39. Darby SC, Ewertz M, McGale P, Bennet AM, Blom-Goldman U, Bronnum D, et al. Risk of ischemic heart disease in women after radiotherapy for breast cancer. *N Engl J Med* 2013;**368**(11):987–98.
40. Gotzsche PC, Jorgensen KJ. Screening for breast cancer with mammography. *The Cochrane database of systematic reviews* 2013;**6**:CD001877.
41. Vaidya JS, Wenz F, Bulsara M, Tobias JS, Joseph DJ, Keshtgar M, et al. Risk-adapted targeted intraoperative radiotherapy versus whole-breast radiotherapy for breast cancer: 5-year results for local control and overall survival from the TARGIT-A randomised trial. *Lancet* 2014;**383**(9917):603–13.
42. Independent UK Panel on Breast Cancer Screening The benefits and harms of breast cancer screening: an independent review. *Lancet* 2012;**380**(9855):1778–86.
43. Lauby-Secretan B, Scoccianti C, Loomis D, Benbrahim-Tallaa L, Bouvard V, Bianchini F, et al. Breast-cancer screening—viewpoint of the IARC Working Group. *N Engl J Med* 2015;**372**(24):2353–8.
44. Etzioni R, Gulati R, Mallinger L, Mandelblatt J. Influence of study features and methods on overdiagnosis estimates in breast and prostate cancer screening. *Ann Intern Med* 2013;**158**(11):831–8.
45. de Gelder R, Heijnsdijk EA, van Ravesteyn NT, Fracheboud J, Draisma G, de Koning HJ. Interpreting overdiagnosis estimates in population-based mammography screening. *Epidemiol Rev* 2011;**33**(1):111–21.
46. Zackrisson S, Andersson I, Janzon L, Manjer J, Garne JP. Rate of over-diagnosis of breast cancer 15 years after end of Malmo mammographic screening trial: follow-up study. *BMJ* 2006;**332**(7543):689–92.
47. Zahl P-H, Jørgensen KJ, Mæhlen J, Gøtzsche PC. Biases in estimates of overdetection due to mammography screening. *Lancet Oncol* 2008;**9**(3):199–201.
48. Zahl PH, Jorgensen KJ, Gotzsche PC. Overestimated lead times in cancer screening has led to substantial underestimation of overdiagnosis. *Br J Cancer* 2013;**109**(7):2014–9.
49. Gotzsche PC. On the benefits and harms of screening for breast cancer. *Int J Epidemiol* 2004;**33**(1):56–64. discussion 9–73.
50. Moss S. Overdiagnosis and overtreatment of breast cancer: overdiagnosis in randomised controlled trials of breast cancer screening. *Breast Cancer Res* 2005;**7**(5):230–4.
51. Heinavaara S, Sarkeala T, Anttila A. Overdiagnosis due to breast cancer screening: updated estimates of the Helsinki service study in Finland. *Br J Cancer* 2014;**111**(7):1463–8.
52. Guyatt G, Rennie D, Meade M, Cook D, American Medical A *Users' guides to the medical literature: a manual for evidence-based clinical practice.* New York, NY: McGraw-Hill Education; 2015.

53. Duffy SW, Lynge E, Jonsson H, Ayyaz S, Olsen AH. Complexities in the estimation of overdiagnosis in breast cancer screening. *Br J Cancer* 2008;**99**(7):1176–8.
54. Puliti D, Duffy SW, Miccinesi G, de Koning H, Lynge E, Zappa M, et al. Overdiagnosis in mammographic screening for breast cancer in Europe: a literature review. *J Med Screen* 2012;**19**(Suppl. 1):42–56.
55. Etzioni R, Gulati R. Oversimplifying overdiagnosis. *J Gen Intern Med* 2014;**29**(9):1218–20.
56. Beckmann K, Duffy SW, Lynch J, Hiller J, Farshid G, Roder D. Estimates of over-diagnosis of breast cancer due to population-based mammography screening in South Australia after adjustment for lead time effects. *J Med Screen* 2015;**22**(3):127–35.
57. Walter SD, Day NE. Estimation of the duration of preclinical disease state using screening data. *Am J Epidemiol* 1983;**118**(6):865–86.
58. van Oortmarssen GJ, Habbema JD, Lubbe JT, van der Maas PJ. A model-based analysis of the HIP project for breast cancer screening. *Int J Cancer* 1990;**46**(2):207–13.
59. Beckmann KR, Lynch JW, Hiller JE, Farshid G, Houssami N, Duffy SW, et al. A novel case-control design to estimate the extent of over-diagnosis of breast cancer due to organised population-based mammography screening. *Int J Cancer* 2015;**136**(6):1411–21.
60. Barratt A, Irwig L, Glasziou P. A novel case-control design to estimate the extent of over-diagnosis of breast cancer due to organised population-based mammography screening. *Int J Cancer* 2014;**136**(10):2486.
61. National Cancer Institute at the National Institutes of Health. *CISNET Model Registry—A comparative overview of CISNET population models.* <https://resources.cisnet.cancer.gov/registry/site-summary/breast/>; 2015 [accessed 20.08.15].
62. Mandelblatt JS, Stout NK, Schechter CB, van den Broek JJ, Miglioretti DL, Krapcho M, et al. Collaborative modeling of the benefits and harms associated with different U.S. breast cancer screening strategies. *Ann Intern Med* 2016 [Published online 12 January 2016. Available from: http://dx.doi.org/10.7326/M15-1536].
63. Duffy SW, Agbaje O, Tabar L, Vitak B, Bjurstam N, Bjorneld L, et al. Overdiagnosis and overtreatment of breast cancer: estimates of overdiagnosis from two trials of mammographic screening for breast cancer. *Breast Cancer Res* 2005;**7**(6):258–65.
64. Grade WG. Grading quality of evidence and strength of recommendations. *BMJ* 2004;**328**:1490–7.
65. Ripping TM, Verbeek AL, Fracheboud J, de Koning HJ, van Ravesteyn NT, Broeders MJ. Overdiagnosis by mammographic screening for breast cancer studied in birth cohorts in The Netherlands. *Int J Cancer* 2015;**137**(4):921–9.
66. Moss SM, Wale C, Smith R, Evans A, Cuckle H, Duffy SW. Effect of mammographic screening from age 40 years on breast cancer mortality in the UK Age trial at 17 years' follow-up: a randomised controlled trial. *Lancet Oncol* 2015;**16**(9):1123–32.
67. van Ravesteyn NT, Stout NK, Schechter CB, Heijnsdijk EA, Alagoz O, Trentham-Dietz A, et al. Benefits and harms of mammography screening after age 74 years: model estimates of overdiagnosis. *J Natl Cancer Inst* 2015;**107**(7). Available online <http://jnci.oxfordjournals.org/content/107/7/djv103.short>.
68. Guyatt G, Akl EA, Hirsh J, Kearon C, Crowther M, Gutterman D, et al. The vexing problem of guidelines and conflict of interest: a potential solution. *Ann Intern Med* 2010;**152**(11):738–41.
69. Moynihan RN, Cooke GP, Doust JA, Bero L, Hill S, Glasziou PP. Expanding disease definitions in guidelines and expert panel ties to industry: a cross-sectional study of common conditions in the United States. *PLoS Med* 2013;**10**(8):e1001500.
70. Ong MS, Mandl KD. National expenditure for false-positive mammograms and breast cancer overdiagnoses estimated at $4 billion a year. *Health Aff (Millwood)* 2015;**34**(4):576–83.
71. Nagtegaal ID, Allgood PC, Duffy SW, Kearins O, Sullivan EO, Tappenden N, et al. Prognosis and pathology of screen-detected carcinomas: how different are they? *Cancer* 2011;**117**(7):1360–8.
72. Sagara Y, Mallory MA, Wong S, Aydogan F, DeSantis S, Barry WT, et al. Survival benefit of breast surgery for low-grade ductal carcinoma in situ: a population-based cohort study. *JAMA Surg* 2015;**150**(8):739–45.

73. Rakha EA, Lee AH, Evans AJ, Menon S, Assad NY, Hodi Z, et al. Tubular carcinoma of the breast: further evidence to support its excellent prognosis. *J Clin Oncol* 2010;**28**(1):99–104.
74. Ganz PA. Psychological and social aspects of breast cancer. *Oncology (Williston Park)* 2008;**22**(6):642–6. 650; discussion 650, 653.
75. Mitchell AJ, Chan M, Bhatti H, Halton M, Grassi L, Johansen C, et al. Prevalence of depression, anxiety, and adjustment disorder in oncological, haematological, and palliative-care settings: a meta-analysis of 94 interview-based studies. *Lancet Oncol* 2011;**12**(2):160–74.
76. Ganz PA, Desmond KA, Leedham B, Rowland JH, Meyerowitz BE, Belin TR. Quality of life in long-term, disease-free survivors of breast cancer: a follow-up study. *J Natl Cancer Inst* 2002;**94**(1):39–49.
77. Total Health. *New UK DCIS trial aims to help women avoid unnecessary breast operations*. <http://www.total-health.co.uk/blog/new-uk-dcis-trial-aims-help-women-avoid-unnecessary-breast-operations>; December 11, 2013 [accessed 27.08.15].
78. Erbas B, Provenzano E, Armes J, Gertig D. The natural history of ductal carcinoma in situ of the breast: a review. *Breast Cancer Res Treat* 2006;**97**(2):135–44.
79. Fisher B, Dignam J, Wolmark N, Wickerham DL, Fisher ER, Mamounas E, et al. Tamoxifen in treatment of intraductal breast cancer: National Surgical Adjuvant Breast and Bowel Project B-24 randomised controlled trial. *Lancet* 1999;**353**(9169):1993–2000.
80. To T, Wall C, Baines CJ, Miller AB. Is carcinoma in situ a precursor lesion of invasive breast cancer? *Int J Cancer* 2014;**135**(7):1646–52.
81. Ernster V, Barclay J, Kerlikowske K, Grady D, Henderson I. Incidence of and treatment for ductal carcinoma in situ of the breast. *JAMA* 1996;**275**(12):913–8.
82. Hawley ST, Jagsi R, Morrow M, Janz NK, Hamilton A, Graff JJ, et al. Social and clinical determinants of contralateral prophylactic mastectomy. *JAMA Surg* 2014;**149**(6):582–9.
83. DiSipio T, Rye S, Newman B, Hayes S. Incidence of unilateral arm lymphoedema after breast cancer: a systematic review and meta-analysis. *Lancet Oncol* 2013;**14**(6):500–15.
84. Vitug AF, Newman LA. Complications in breast surgery. *Surg Clin North Am* 2007;**87**(2) 431–51, x.
85. Barton MB, West CN, Liu IL, Harris EL, Rolnick SJ, Elmore JG, et al. Complications following bilateral prophylactic mastectomy. *J Natl Cancer Inst Monogr* 2005;**35**:61–6.
86. Osman F, Saleh F, Jackson TD, Corrigan MA, Cil T. Increased postoperative complications in bilateral mastectomy patients compared to unilateral mastectomy: an analysis of the NSQIP database. *Ann Surg Oncol* 2013;**20**(10):3212–7.
87. Fallowfield L, Cella D, Cuzick J, Francis S, Locker G, Howell A. Quality of life of postmenopausal women in the Arimidex, Tamoxifen, Alone or in Combination (ATAC) Adjuvant Breast Cancer Trial. *J Clin Oncol* 2004;**22**(21):4261–71.
88. Jagsi R, Hawley ST, Abrahamse P, Li Y, Janz NK, Griggs JJ, et al. Impact of adjuvant chemotherapy on long-term employment of survivors of early-stage breast cancer. *Cancer* 2014;**120**(12):1854–62.
89. Lauzier S, Maunsell E, Drolet M, Coyle D, Hebert-Croteau N, Brisson J, et al. Wage losses in the year after breast cancer: extent and determinants among Canadian women. *J Natl Cancer Inst* 2008;**100**(5):321–32.
90. Pharoah PD, Sewell B, Fitzsimmons D, Bennett HS, Pashayan N. Cost effectiveness of the NHS breast screening programme: life table model. *BMJ* 2013;**346**:f2618.
91. Vilaprinyo E, Forne C, Carles M, Sala M, Pla R, Castells X, et al. Cost-effectiveness and harm-benefit analyses of risk-based screening strategies for breast cancer. *PLoS One* 2014;**9**(2):e86858.
92. Heath I. Overdiagnosis: when good intentions meet vested interests—an essay by Iona Heath. *BMJ* 2013;**347**:f6361.
93. Elshaug AG, McWilliams J, Landon B. The value of low-value lists. *JAMA* 2013;**309**:775–6.
94. Irwig L, Houssami N, Armstrong B, Glasziou P. Evaluating new screening tests for breast cancer. *BMJ* 2006;**332**(7543):678–9.

95. Bell KJ, Bossuyt P, Glasziou P, Irwig L. Assessment of changes to screening programmes: why randomisation is important. *BMJ* 2015;**350**:h1566.
96. Pisano ED, Gatsonis C, Hendrick E, Yaffe M, Baum JK, Acharyya S, et al. Diagnostic performance of digital versus film mammography for breast-cancer screening. *N Engl J Med* 2005;**353**(17):1773–83.
97. Pisano ED, Hendrick RE, Yaffe MJ, Baum JK, Acharyya S, Cormack JB, et al. Diagnostic accuracy of digital versus film mammography: exploratory analysis of selected population subgroups in DMIST. *Radiology* 2008;**246**(2):376–83.
98. Skaane P, Hofvind S, Skjennald A. Randomized trial of screen-film versus full-field digital mammography with soft-copy reading in population-based screening program: follow-up and final results of Oslo II study. *Radiology* 2007;**244**(3):708–17.
99. Ciatto S, Houssami N, Bernardi D, Caumo F, Pellegrini M, Brunelli S, et al. Integration of 3D digital mammography with tomosynthesis for population breast-cancer screening (STORM): a prospective comparison study. *Lancet Oncol* 2013;**14**(7):583–9.
100. Houssami N, Macaskill P, Bernardi D, Caumo F, Pellegrini M, Brunelli S, et al. Breast screening using 2D-mammography or integrating digital breast tomosynthesis (3D-mammography) for single-reading or double-reading—evidence to guide future screening strategies. *Eur J Cancer* 2014;**50**(10):1799–807.
101. Woloshin S, Schwartz LM. How a charity oversells mammography. *BMJ* 2012;**345**:e5132.
102. Wegwarth O, Gigerenzer G. Less is more: overdiagnosis and overtreatment: evaluation of what physicians tell their patients about screening harms. *JAMA Intern Med* 2013;**173**(22):2086–7.
103. Moynihan R, Nickel B, Hersch J, Beller E, Doust J, Compton S, et al. Public opinions about overdiagnosis: a national community survey. *PLoS One* 2015;**10**(5):e0125165.
104. Walter LC, Schonberg MA. Screening mammography in older women: a review. *JAMA* 2014;**311**(13): 1336–47.
105. Royce TJ, Hendrix LH, Stokes WA, Allen IM, Chen RC. Cancer screening rates in individuals with different life expectancies. *JAMA Intern Med* 2014;**174**(10):1558–65.
106. Van den Bruel A, Jones C, Yang Y, Oke J, Hewitson P. People's willingness to accept overdetection in cancer screening: population survey. *BMJ* 2015;**350**:h980.
107. Hersch J, Jansen J, Barratt A, Irwig L, Houssami N, Howard K, et al. Women's views on overdiagnosis in breast cancer screening: a qualitative study. *BMJ* 2013;**346**:f158.
108. Waller J, Whitaker KL, Winstanley K, Power E, Wardle J. A survey study of women's responses to information about overdiagnosis in breast cancer screening in Britain. *Br J Cancer* 2014;**111**(9):1831–5.
109. Hersch J, Barratt A, Jansen J, Irwig L, McGeechan K, Jacklyn G, et al. Use of a decision aid including information on overdetection to support informed choice about breast cancer screening: a randomised controlled trial. *Lancet* 2015;**385**(9978):1642–52.
110. Biller-Andorno N, Juni P. Abolishing mammography screening programs? A view from the Swiss Medical Board. *N Engl J Med* 2014;**370**(21):1965–7.
111. Gigerenzer G. Towards a paradigm shift in cancer screening: informed citizens instead of greater participation. *BMJ* 2015;**350**:h2175.
112. Esserman LJ, Thompson Jr. IM, Reid B. Overdiagnosis and overtreatment in cancer: an opportunity for improvement. *JAMA* 2013;**310**(8):797–8.
113. Elmore JG, Kramer BS. Breast cancer screening: toward informed decisions. *JAMA* 2014;**311**(13):1298–9.

CHAPTER

CHALLENGES AND OPPORTUNITIES IN THE IMPLEMENTATION OF RISK-BASED SCREENING FOR BREAST CANCER

7

D. Gareth Evans[1,2,3,6], Anthony Howell[1,3,5], Anthony J. Maxwell[1,3,4] and Susan Astley[1,3,4]

[1]Genesis Breast Cancer Prevention Centre and Nightingale Breast Screening Centre, University Hospital of South Manchester, Manchester, United Kingdom, [2]Genomic Medicine, Manchester Academic Health Sciences Centre, University of Manchester and Central Manchester Foundation Trust, Manchester, United Kingdom, [3]Manchester Academic Health Science Centre, University Hospital of South Manchester, The University of Manchester, Manchester, United Kingdom, [4]Centre for Imaging Sciences, Institute for Population Health, University of Manchester, Manchester, United Kingdom, [5]The Christie NHS Foundation Trust, Manchester, United Kingdom, [6]Consultant Clinical Geneticist, Genomic Medicine, MAHSC, St. Mary's Hospital, Manchester, United Kingdom

CHAPTER OUTLINE

Breast Cancer Screening. DOI: http://dx.doi.org/10.1016/B978-0-12-802209-2.00007-3

PLAIN LANGUAGE SUMMARY

There is widespread interest in trying to change the interval at which women undergo breast cancer screening based on their actual risk of breast cancer. This risk-based screening may improve the proportions of breast cancer detected early and possibly reduce the number of women who need to be screened with reduction in the associated harms of overdiagnosis. Risk factors are already used to determine screening: for example, age is used to determine who is eligible for screening and age of onset of screening may be reduced and screening frequency maybe increased in women with a family history. Women with *BRCA1* or *BRCA2* mutations are screened using MRI in addition to mammography because of the potential for missing cancers and the high risk of interval cancers in mutation positive women. The question arises whether such risk-adapted screening can improve the ability to detect breast cancers whilst reducing the number of women that are unnecessarily recalled for harmless changes on the mammogram. In general, incorporation of additional risk factors such as hormonal factors, the density of breast tissue on the mammogram, and genetic factors to age and family history improves the predictive accuracy of risk estimates. Additional screening modalities such as ultrasound, MRI, and digital breast tomosynthesis may increase detection rates and reduce cancers occurring between screens. However, it is not clear how these modalities and additional risk factors may be applied in breast screening and national programs, and whether this will be beneficial to the women screened. Here we discuss some of the challenges and potential opportunities of attempting to introduce risk-adapted screening.

INTRODUCTION

The use of mammography is first identified on PubMed in 1939[1] and population screening first referred to in 1968.[2] The introduction of population-based screening programs occurred in the late 1980s after the results of a number of important randomized controlled trials showed a reduction in mortality from 2-yearly mammography in women particularly over 50 years of age.[3] Most national screening programs and screening guidelines recommend annual or biennial two-view mammography, which has transitioned between 2005 and 2015 from film-screen to full field digital mammography. The UK opted for a screening interval of 3 years based on recommendations made in the Forrest Report in

1986.[4] The original aim was to offer mammography screening to all women aged 50–64 years of age. Women were invited dependent on their locality between ages 49 and 53 years (screening vans travel around each screening area) and then offered screening on a 3-yearly basis. The upper age limit was extended to 69 years in 2000 and there is currently an age extension trial[5,6] evaluating the effectiveness of an additional screen aged 47–49 years and another aged 71–73 years compared with the standard screening. Although currently screening ends at 70 (or 73 in age extension) women may self-refer for screening beyond this age. Most other countries with screening programs, including Scandinavia and the Netherlands, offer 2-yearly screening based on a period below the 30-month lead time. Countries with no screening programs, such as the USA, recommend annual screening in their guidelines.

Over the past two decades, deaths from breast cancer in most westernized countries have fallen by 30–40% in women <70 years. Some of this reduction has been attributed to mammographic screening. It is, however, difficult to distinguish the potential benefits of mammography from more widespread use of adjuvant systemic therapies and general improvements in overall care.[7,8] A recent review of the UK National Health Service Breast Screening Programme (NHSBSP) estimated that it reduced breast cancer mortality by 20%, thus saving 1300 lives annually.[9] The challenge is to improve the effectiveness of mammographic screening further. One approach is to assess the value of screening based on risk, where women at high risk are screened more frequently and earlier than those at low risk.

IMPROVING SCREENING BY BASING ITS APPLICATION ON RISK

One hypothesis, which remains to be tested is that screening based on risk will lead to improvements in breast cancer mortality. Screening is more efficient in subgroups with higher disease prevalence. Risk-based screening may increase benefits and decrease harms and costs associated with screening Risk may be used to adapt several aspects of screening strategies. First, women at high risk may benefit from starting screening at an earlier age and/or stopping screening at a later age. Second, women at high risk of a true interval cancer (ie, a fast growing tumor that develops and becomes symptomatic in between screens) may benefit from more frequent screening, and women at low risk or with slow growing tumors (eg, older women and women with fatty breasts) may avoid the harms of screening by being screened less frequently. Third, women at high risk of a missed cancer on mammography (eg, women at high risk and dense breast tissue) may benefit from supplemental screening with other modalities, such as tomosynthesis, ultrasound, or MRI. Last, women at high risk of a screening harm from mammography such as a false-positive result or radiation-induced breast cancer, may benefit from an alternative screening modality such as tomosynthesis for reducing false-positive recalls and ultrasound or MRI for avoiding ionizing radiation. These are separate but highly interrelated issues. For example, breast density increases risk of breast cancer but may also decrease the sensitivity for mammography, indicating a potential need for alternative or supplemental screening modalities. Family history in both first and to a lesser extent second degree relatives increases risk of breast cancer but is also associated with a greater incidence of interval cancers compared with women without a family history. The UK National Health Service Breast Screening Programme (NHSBSP) three-yearly screening may result in more interval cancers than programs that screen more frequently.[10] There is evidence that women at very high risk of breast cancer are more likely to develop interval cancers[11] and reduction of the screening interval or supplemental screening in this poor prognosis group may be indicated,[11,12] particularly as the cancers that do develop in women at very high risk tend to have faster doubling times than those in the general population. The Swedish two-county study showed that women with a positive family history of breast cancer were more likely to develop breast cancer between their biennial screening examinations than similar women with negative family histories.[10]

RISK FACTOR-ADAPTED MAMMOGRAPHIC SCREENING

Screening is already based on risk since age is a major breast cancer risk factor and all national screening programs and screening guidelines recommend starting screening at an age when breast cancer becomes more common. Some countries recommend younger women be screened more frequently given evidence they have more aggressive tumors. However a very recent paper suggests that menopausal status might be a better factor than age when considering screening interval.[13] Premenopausal women were more likely to be diagnosed with later stage disease with poorer prognostic characteristics when screened biennially versus annually. However, there was no difference for postmenopausal women. And no differences within age group. Biologically, this might make sense if hormones affects aggressiveness.

In some countries, the age of commencing screening is lower and screening more frequent when another major risk factor is taken into account, namely a family history of breast cancer, since the disease arises at a younger age and often more rapidly in this group. These two risk factors are important since they are used as criteria to improve the utility and cost of screening. However, women may have other risk factors which may add to family risk or be present in the absence of a family history and the question is whether these other factors improve risk estimation and, in turn, whether their application will result in further reductions of breast cancer mortality.

Women with a family history may be referred to genetics services by their family doctor. However, factors other than age and family history are either not well known by women or their family doctor to affect risk, such as age of first pregnancy, or are occult, such as mammographic density and single nucleotide polymorphisms (SNPs), and require further investigation for their estimation. Thus further questions arise concerning the number of risk factors we need to know in order to determine risk as precisely as possible, how this information may be collected, and how such information may be given to women and applied in national screening programs and screening guidelines.

HOW MANY RISK FACTORS?

If risk factor directed screening were tested in randomized trials versus standard screening, decisions would need to be made concerning the optimal methods for estimation of breast cancer risk. There may have to be a balance between what is desirable versus what is possible. A relatively simple approach is to ask women at screening for information concerning age, family history, and other factors such as age of first pregnancy. More difficult approaches include determination of mammographic density and measuring breast cancer risk SNPs and possibly adding this information to standard risk factors.

FAMILIAL RISK

Family history of breast cancer is one of the strongest risk factors for developing the disease. Early age at onset, bilaterality and multiple affected relatives, particularly on the same side of the family, increase breast cancer risk.[14,15] It is estimated that 27% of breast cancer is accounted for by hereditary factors although only 15–20% of women who develop breast cancer have a family history of the disease.[16] Approximately 10% of familial risk is associated with inheritance of mutations in high and moderate risk genes, and although important to individuals, screening for such gene mutations on a population basis is not currently practicable and is only relevant to a small proportion of women. Genome-wide association studies are likely to unravel much of the remaining "inherited component" in the next 5–10 years.[17–19] Except in very rare cases such as Cowden's disease,[20] there are no phenotypic clues that help to identify women who carry pathogenic mutations. Evaluation of the family history, therefore, remains necessary to assess the likelihood that a predisposing gene is present within a family. Women with a strong family history of breast cancer are also at increased risk before the age at which most mass screening programs and screening guidelines recommend starting screening.

Family history clinics have been set up around the developed world since the 1980s.[21] Evidence is emerging of the potential benefit of annual mammography in women with a first-degree family history in their forties[22] and there may also be benefit in the thirties for women with a strong family history.[23] For women at very high risk under age 50 years, MRI breast screening has been shown to be very effective at early detection, in particular in carriers of pathogenic mutations in *BRCA1* and *BRCA2*.[24–28] There is some evidence for a survival benefit,[29] but this is still not conclusive for *BRCA1* carriers[30] in whom mammography has a low sensitivity of <40% in a combined mammography and MRI-based screening program[24–28] and for whom there are very high rates of interval cancers with mammographic screening alone.[31] As a result of the strong evidence for high MRI screening sensitivity, this was recommended annually for women at very high risk of breast cancer (including *BRCA1/BRCA2/TP53* carriers) aged 30–49 years of age in 2006 by NICE in the UK[32] and also in 2007 for those at 25% or higher risk lifetime in the USA.[33] Updated NICE guidelines in 2013 also recommend annual mammography until aged 70 years in mutation carriers[34] (see also chapter: Screening for Breast Cancer in Women With Dense Breasts).

Other risk factors

Although family history is the most easily identified risk factor for breast cancer apart from age, even women with no family history may be at sufficient risk to consider earlier or more frequent screening or supplemental screening by virtue of combinations of other factors. Early menarche, late first full term pregnancy or nulliparity, current combined hormone replacement therapy (HRT) use after 50 years and postmenopausal obesity can all increase the risk of breast cancer by up to 20–50% over the average.[17,34] Mammographic breast density is one of the strongest risk factors, increasing risk by 4–6 fold between the bottom and top 20% of mammographic density in the population. High mammographic density also substantially increases the chances of developing interval breast cancers,[35,36] suggesting that density should be incorporated into risk models.[17,34–40] Stratification of screening frequency by risk is likely to be cost-effective.[41,42] Screening interval could be shorter for women at high-risk and longer for those at low-risk. A major challenge with such a policy is identification of an individual woman's breast cancer risk.

COMBINING STANDARD RISK FACTORS: RISK MODELS

Breast cancer risk is usually assessed using models which include family history of breast cancer and possibly other cancers (eg, ovarian), reproductive and hormonal history (age at first full term pregnancy, menarche, and menopause, and postmenopausal hormone therapy use), height and weight, and history of prior benign breast biopsies and their histology.[43–45] Models generally perform well for predicting risk in a population (eg, 1 in 4 lifetime risk) but not for individual risk ("am I the one to develop cancer or one of the three who will not").[17,34,37] For screening on a population basis this risk stratification is probably already sufficient. The Gail,[44] BCSC,[39] and Tyrer-Cuzick[43] models may be used to determine general risk whereas others, such as Claus, BRCAPRO, the Manchester Score, and BOADICEA, are currently used to predict the presence of mutations in high risk genes, such as *BRCA1* and *BRCA2*.

In the US, the Gail model is widely used. It is based on age, number of first degree relatives with breast cancer, number of surgical breast biopsies, and reproductive factors as above. In a comparison of models using UK data, it was demonstrated that for women with a family history of breast cancer, the Tyrer-Cuzick model performed better than the Gail model; similar results were reported in studies in the US.[43,44] The Tyrer-Cuzick model has a more extensive familial component, and includes HRT use, height and weight, and the histology of surgical biopsies.[42] The BCSC risk model also has better discriminatory accuracy that the Gail model. It includes breast density, age, race/ethnicity, first degree family history, and history of breast biopsy and was recently updated to include type of benign breast disease.[39,46] It has better discriminatory accuracy than the Gail model. Given it only includes five risk factors, it is easy to use in clinical practice.

ADDING MAMMOGRAPHIC DENSITY TO STANDARD MEASURES

Mammographic breast density is one of the strongest risk factors for breast cancer increasing risk by 4–6 fold between the bottom and top 20% of mammographic density in the population suggesting that density should be incorporated into risk models.[17,34,37,38,47] Density also has a substantial heritable component.[38,48] Some data indicate that stratification of screening frequency by risk may be more effective and likely to be cost effective[41,42] if density is included (see also chapter: Screening for Breast Cancer in Women with Dense Breasts).

There is evidence that incorporating density into the standard models can increase the model's predictive values when added to the Gail model irrespective of the method of density estimation (BIRADS, percent density, and volumetric assessment[49,50]) and to the BCSC model.[46] In the PROCAS (Predicting the Risk Of Cancer At Screening) study, percentage density was estimated by two radiologists for each of >50,000 women in the Manchester NHSBSP using a visual analog scale (VAS) and adjusted for age and body mass index. Fig. 7.1 shows a distribution of the odds ratio for the Tyrer-Cuzick model alone, adjusted visual density, and the combination of the two. The value of such analyses may be assessed by the increase in the proportion of women appearing in the high and low risk groups. Density modestly improved on the T-C model. However, when the two methods were combined, the proportion of women in the moderate risk group (5–8% 10-year risk) increased from 8.6% using the TC model to 12.3% when the T-C results were combined with adjusted visual density. In the high risk group (>8% 10-year risk) the proportion increased from 1.2% to 2.7% (Fig. 7.1).

In the PROCAS study density was also estimated using volumetric assessment of density (see below). The value of this method is that it may be estimated automatically making it more transferable to national screening programs.

The overall spread of risks can be seen in Fig. 7.2 from a combination of Gail and Tyrer-Cuzick incorporating mammographic density.

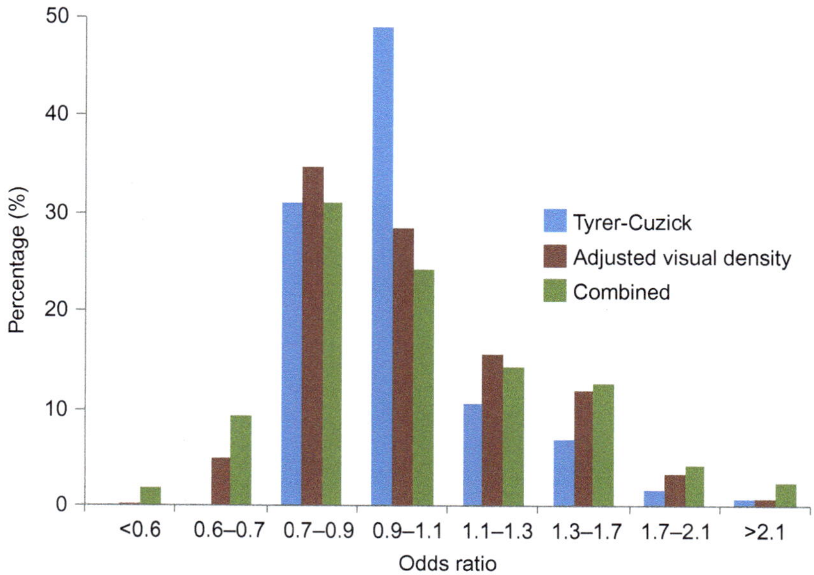

FIGURE 7.1

The percentage of women in the PROCAS study in each risk category and how this is changed when density is added to the Tyrer-Cuzick Risk model. Density was estimated visually and the value adjusted for age and body mass index (Adjusted visual density (Density Residual)). Adding density moved many women from average to higher or lower risk of developing breast cancer ($n \geq 50{,}000$ women). Odds ratio refers to the odds of developing breast cancer.

ADDING BREAST CANCER RISK ASSOCIATED SINGLE NUCLEOTIDE POLYMORPHISMS (SNPs)

Incorporating common genetic variants (SNPs) into risk assessment is also likely to improve the precision of risk assessments in women with and without a family history. Using 77 SNPs in 33,673 breast cancer cases and 33,381 control women of European origin a three-fold difference in lifetime risk between women in the lowest and highest quintiles of the Polygenic Risk Score (PRS)was reported[51] (5.2% (lowest) and 16.6% (highest) for a woman without family history, and 8.6% and 24.4% for a woman with a first-degree family history of breast cancer). Using a threshold of 2.4% for 10-year risk to commence screening 20% of the population would never reach that risk based on a PRS alone.[42]

There have been a small number of studies using fewer SNPs to assess how to improve the prediction of risk. On the whole the increase in risk prediction has been modest (summarized in Ref. 18).

In the PROCAS study salivary samples were collected from women in the study and the top 18 breast cancer risk SNPs estimated in 9346 of them (Fig. 7.3).

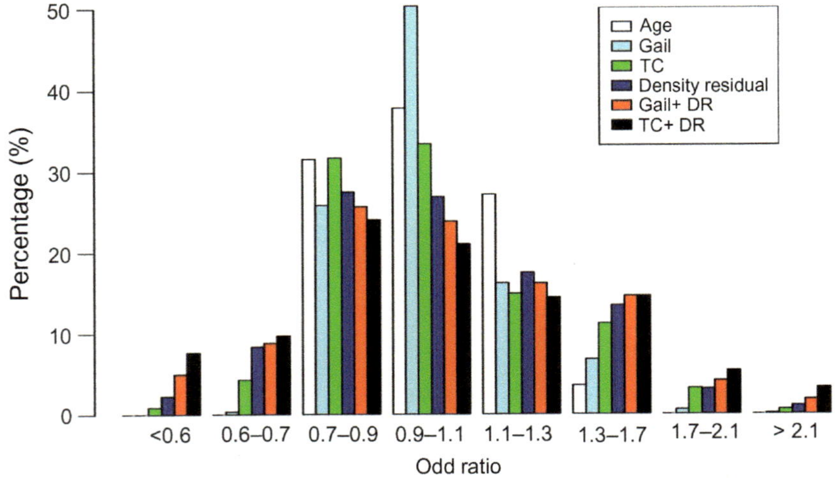

FIGURE 7.2

Observed risk distributions using fitted odds ratios (ORs) in the PROCAS study. Each odds ratio is scaled to be 1.0 for mean in the sample. DR-mammographic density assessed visually. The density residual is the observed density adjusted for age and body mass index. Adding the DR to the Gail and Tyrer-Cuzick models has the effect of changing the ORs so that more women were included in the high and low OR groups.

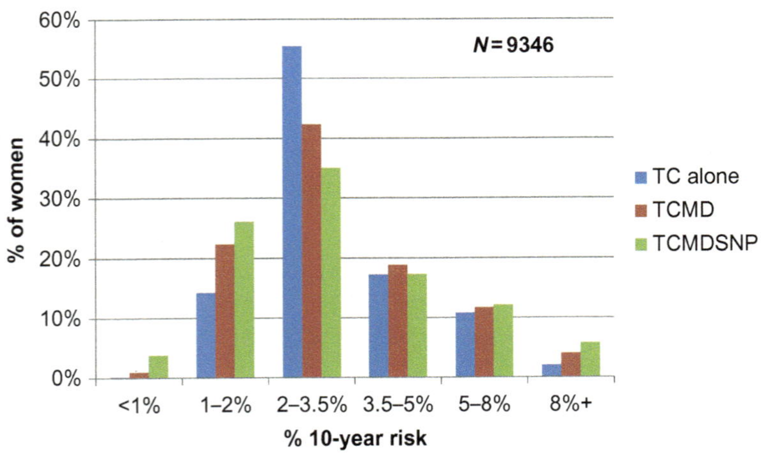

FIGURE 7.3

A subgroup of 10,000 women in the PROCAS study provided saliva specimens which were used to estimate the distribution of 18 single nucleotide polymorphisms (SNPs) associated with breast cancer risk. The effect of adding visually assessed density (TCMD) and SNPs (TCMDSNP) to the Tyrer-Cuzick model (TC alone) on the distribution of risk is illustrated. The numbers of women in the moderate and high risk groups increased from 12 to 18% when density and SNPs were added to the TC model. The proportion in the average risk group dropped from 55.5 to 35%.

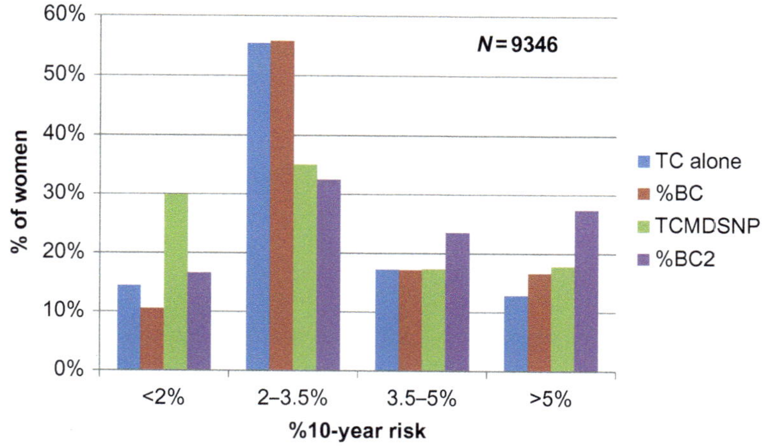

FIGURE 7.4

Distribution of 10 year breast cancer risks and 391 incident breast cancers using TC or TC and MD+ SNPs.

In this subgroup of women,(relative to the main study ($n \geq 50{,}000$)), the proportion of women in the moderate and high risk categories increased from 9% using the T-C model alone compared with 18% when density and SNP18 were added to TC.

The addition of SNPs and density also improved the precision of predicting cancers. Fig. 7.4 shows that over 50% of the cancers occurred in the 32% of the population at above average risk (>3.5% 10-year).

%BC—Percentage of total prospective breast cancers per risk for TC alone.

%BC2—Percentage of total prospective breast cancers per risk for TCMDSNP.

SCREENING BASED ON PREDICTION OF RISK OF MISSED AND OF INTERVAL CANCERS

Whilst tailoring screening interval according to individual risk of developing breast cancer would be an important first step, it is also important to realize the limitations of mammography as a tool for breast cancer screening, and to consider alternative screening modalities that could potentially be used to supplement mammography in a personalized screening program to identify those most at risk of an interval cancer.[35]

EFFECTIVENESS OF MAMMOGRAPHY

Mammographic sensitivity depends on a number of variables, including the density of the breasts, the woman's age, the nature of the cancers that occur, and factors influencing mammographic interpretation. It is important to realize the limitations of mammography and that the efficacy of mammography as a screening tool for breast cancer depends on the composition of a woman's breasts.[52]

The sensitivity of screening mammography (the number of cancers detected at mammography as a proportion of the sum of the screen detected cancers and those presenting as interval cancers in the following year) is approximately 90% for women with fatty breasts, but only 50–70% for those with dense breasts.[35,52,53] This is because of the masking effect caused by dense fibroglandular tissue. Whilst younger women in general have denser breasts than older women, there is some evidence to suggest that younger age is independently associated with poorer mammographic sensitivity, probably because the more aggressive cancers that tend to occur in younger women often grow rapidly, but also have mammographic features that are more difficult to distinguish from normal tissue than other cancers.[54,55] These are particular problems with the triple negative cancers that occur in women with *BRCA1* gene mutations.[56]

Review of the previous screening mammograms of women presenting with interval cancers or with cancers detected on incident screening shows that in around 25% of cases there is evidence of the cancer on the previous screening mammograms.[57–60] Double reading is used routinely in some screening programs, and this has been shown to increase the screening yield by 10–15%.[61,62] Single reading with computer aided detection (CAD) is also used, especially in the USA, although the high false prompt rate of CAD remains a problem[63] with no improvement in sensitivity in a large US study in community practice.[64]

Full field digital mammography (FFDM) has now largely replaced film-screen technology. The Digital Mammographic Imaging Screening Trial (DMIST) study from the USA demonstrated that digital mammography is significantly more sensitive than film-screen technology in women below the age of 50 and in those with dense breasts.[52] However, breast density remains a significant factor limiting sensitivity. Women with dense breasts are at a disadvantage in a one-size-fits-all screening program; not only are they at higher risk of developing cancer, but if a cancer is present it is less readily detected. Furthermore, with the exception of the fewer than 10% of women aged over 40 who have extremely dense breasts, composite densities due to the overlap of normal tissue are more common in those with denser breasts, resulting in a higher rate of false positive recall for further assessment.[35]

Despite these limitations, X-ray mammography has a number of advantages as a mass screening modality: it is relatively inexpensive, widely available, quick to perform, and able to detect microcalcification. Mammographic interpretation is well-established and there is a large pool of trained readers. Disadvantages of mammography, apart from the sensitivity and specificity issues noted above, include the use of ionizing radiation (although at a very low dose) and discomfort caused by the breast compression which can deter women from reattending.[65]

TOMOSYNTHESIS

One of the most exciting recent developments in screening technology is digital breast tomosynthesis (DBT), in which a series of very low dose mammograms taken over a limited angular range are reconstructed into a series of thin (usually 1 mm) contiguous slices. This can be done in the same breast compression as a conventional 2D digital mammogram and gives a similar radiation dose. Each DBT slice contains in-focus information at a particular depth along with an out-of-focus component from other depths. As the reader scrolls through the stack the reduction in the masking effect of overlapping tissues makes many cancers (particularly those associated with architectural distortion) conspicuous. It also allows composite glandular densities seen on the corresponding 2D mammogram to be resolved.

For several reasons, including microcalcification assessment and ease of comparison with serial examinations, 2D mammography has continued to be used in addition to DBT. However, in order to reduce the need for the additional radiation, synthetic 2D mammograms created from the DBT projection images have been developed and shown to be diagnostically equivalent to conventional 2D mammograms.[66,67]

Although there are no randomized trials comparing DBT with 2D mammography in the literature, a number of retrospective reader studies including the UK TOMMY study[66] and three prospective population screening studies examining the relative contributions of 2D mammography and DBT have been published.[68–70] In general these have shown a superior cancer detection performance of 2D+ DBT over 2D mammography alone (40% more invasive cancers in the largest series[68]) and a higher specificity. In-service retrospective studies show similar findings[71–73] (see also chapter: Evolution of Mammography Screening: From Film Screen to Digital Breast Tomosynthesis).

DBT appears to offer particular advantages for screening women with dense breasts. The TOMMY study [66] demonstrated a 93% sensitivity of DBT+2D in dense breasts compared to 86% for 2D only ($p = 0.03$). Specificity was also significantly higher at 69% (95% CI 67–71) compared with 58% (95% CI 56–60) for 2D only. A retrospective review from the USA[58] demonstrated that on multivariate analysis the greatest reductions in recall rates were seen in younger women (25% with 2D alone to 11% with DBT+2D in those below 40, 16.3% to 10.4% for those aged 40 to 49; $p < 0.01$) and those with dense breasts (adjusted odds ratios for heterogeneously dense and extremely dense compared to fatty of 2.17 and 1.56; $p < 0.001$).

Widespread implementation of screening with DBT is likely to be limited by a number of factors, including the capital cost of the mammography equipment, the need for additional digital image storage and, probably most importantly, the examination reading times which are approximately doubled.[68,70,74] Nonetheless, even in screening programs with limited additional capacity, selective screening with DBT of women in the first screening round and continuing for those with dense breasts and at increased risk may be cost-effective, particularly as these are the women in whom the reduction in recall rate with DBT is likely to be greatest. Further, the evidence on DBT is evolving rapidly, for example one study has shown that DBT population screening based on single-reading performs substantially better than double-reading of standard mammography,[75] and another study found that one-view DBT detected significantly more cancers than two-view mammography.[76] More details on DBT for population screening are included in chapter "Evolution of Mammography Screening: From Film Screen to Digital Breast Tomosynthesis".

MRI

Contrast enhanced Magnetic Resonance Imaging (MRI) has been shown to have higher sensitivity than mammography in women with a strong family history of breast cancer.[77] A particular advantage for young women and those with dense breasts is that it is not affected by breast density. It is, however, not as specific as mammography, and increased cost and use of contrast mean that it is only practical as a screening tool for a relatively small group of women[78]; in the UK it is used for screening young women

Table 7.1 NICE Guideline Recommendations Relating to Breast Surveillance in Women with a Family History of Breast Cancer

	Moderate risk Lifetime risk 17–29% 10-year risk 3–7.9% aged 40–49 years	High risk Lifetime risk 30% + 10-year risk 8% +	Gene carriers and 30–50% likelihood for TP53, BRCA1, BRCA2
Mammography	Annual aged 40–49	Annual aged 40–59	Annual aged 40–69 except TP53
MRI	N/a	N/a	Annual aged 30–49 25–59 for TP53

with a strong family history, with additional mammography from the age of 40 (Table 7.1).[34] Recently an abbreviated MRI scan protocol of approximately 3 min duration has been proposed as a means of reducing the cost of screening MRI,[79] although this has not, as yet, been widely adopted.

For women at very high risk under age 50 years MRI breast screening is the method of choice particularly for *BRCA1* and *BRCA2* mutation carriers.[24–29] Mammography in *BRCA1* carriers has low sensitivity (<40%[24–28]) and very high rates of interval cancers.[31]

ULTRASOUND

Whole breast ultrasound has been investigated as a supplemental screening method in women with mammographically dense breasts. In the ACRIN 6666 trial in the USA,[80] 2809 women underwent mammography and whole breast hand-held ultrasound by a physician. The combined modalities yielded 4.2 additional cancers per 1000 women screened (95% CI 1.1–7.2 per 1000) but at the cost of a large increase in the number of false positives with a Positive Predictive Value (PPV) of biopsy recommended by mammography combined with ultrasound of only 11.2% (95% CI 7.8–15.6%) compared with 22.6% (95% CI 14.2–33) for mammography alone.

The recent development of automated breast ultrasound (ABUS) allows a standardized examination in several planes to be performed by a technologist. The images can subsequently be reviewed by a radiologist on a diagnostic workstation. The SomoInsight study in the USA[81] examined over 15,000 women with dense breasts with mammography and ABUS and showed an increase in cancer detection with ABUS of 1.9 per 1000, 93% of which were invasive. Again there was a marked reduction in specificity, the recall rate increasing from 15% for mammography alone to over 28% with the addition of ABUS.

Using three microsimulation models, Sprague and colleagues[82] estimated that the cost-effectiveness ratio for supplemental ultrasound screening of women with heterogeneously and extremely dense breasts in the US was $325,000 per QALY, and even in only those with extremely dense breasts was $246,000.

Despite the increased sensitivity that supplemental ultrasound confers, its additional costs and high recall rate suggest that its role in a stratified screening regime would perhaps be limited to a group of women who do not qualify for MRI (or in whom MRI is contraindicated) and have dense breasts and are at moderate to high risk.

IMPROVEMENTS IN THE ESTIMATION OF MAMMOGRAPHIC DENSITY

Estimation of breast density is usually derived from a woman's mammograms. The most widely used method is visual assessment using the American College of Radiology BI-RADS system,[83] in which radiologists assign a mammogram to one of four categories (ref BI-RADS). This is widely used in the USA, more to provide women with an indication of the likely sensitivity of X-ray mammography than to inform them about cancer risk. BI-RADS is, however, subjective and lacks resolution,[84] which limits its usefulness as a means of stratification. Semi-automated methods such as Cumulus [85] have been extensively related to breast cancer risk,[86] but are impractical for population-based screening. The advent of FFDM has paved the way for fully automated analysis, and commercial software now exists that estimates volumes of fat and gland by modeling the physics of the imaging process.[87] These methods output separate estimates of the volumes of fat and fibroglandular tissue, which can be combined to generate a relative breast density score or interpreted individually. Volumes of gland are likely to be more robust to weight fluctuations, as the volume of fat is strongly correlated with Body Mass Index (BMI) whereas dense volume is only moderately correlated.[88] The main advantages of such methods are ease of use and reproducibility; accuracy of all methods is harder to assess because of lack of reliable ground truth regarding the actual composition of the breast. Mammographic density methods do, however, show a high degree of correlation with volumes segmented from MRI, which is often used as a comparator.[89] The prime disadvantage of breast density measures made from mammograms is the use of ionizing radiation in mammography. Whilst the dose is very low, the effectiveness of mammography is reduced in younger women and there is less justification for making an early assessment of density using this method, before the age at which screening would normally start (such as age 35) and with a view to stratifying from the very first screen.

It may be the case that local, area-based density measures are the most appropriate for assessing risk of masking, since a lesion may be masked by a small dense area in a breast which otherwise contains only a moderate amount of dense tissue, and would not be classified as high risk based purely on quantity or proportion of density. There is also some evidence that the pattern of density, measured automatically using computer-based texture analysis methods, is relevant for cancer risk estimation.[90,91] Whilst assessing density in younger women might identify women at increased risk who may benefit from screening this needs to be balanced against any earlier exposure to radiation for all women.

PREDICTING THE WOMEN WHO NEED SCREENING MODALITIES IN ADDITION TO MAMMOGRAPHY

Simple risk stratification does not necessarily identify those most at risk of aggressive interval cancers.[35] Nonetheless, higher breast density does predict those at higher risk of breast cancer as well as women with a greater risk of developing an interval cancer. The results of the Manchester PROCAS study indicate that there appears to be a group of women who are not only at high risk of breast cancer but this group have a significant trend to develop more aggressive breast cancers. Analysis of the study suggests, that for 70% of women, screening every three years is sufficient and cost-effective.[92] The data thus indicate that for 30% reduction of the screening interval will be beneficial. It might be that a subset of these would be at sufficient risk to justify MRI and at a lower risk ultrasound if mammographic density is a major component of their risk.

CHALLENGES OF RISK FACTOR-BASED SCREENING

Risk factor-based screening is already in place in several screening programs and recommended in many guidelines. Since facilities exist to assess the importance of family history in most countries and to offer mammography and MRI based on this risk factor. However, Family History Clinics are referral practices and provide face-to-face advice and further investigations. This is possible because there are relatively small numbers of younger women at moderate and high risk and even smaller numbers with major gene mutations. This situation may change with the rapid development of testing of panels of breast cancer genes that confer moderate and high risk and debates about population testing for *BRCA1* and *BRCA2*.[93] A great deal more research is required before many of the genes such as *NBN, RAD51, RAD51C, RAD51D*, and *BRIP1* have accurate risks ascribed to them and whether indeed the risks are sufficient for additional screening.[94]

Risk factor-based screening is different to selection on family history alone. The total population of screened women need to be approached in order to evaluate these risks which immediately raises logistical and a number of ethical issues which remain to be solved if risk factor-based screening is to be used on the population of women screened by mammography in national programs. Here we highlight a series of challenges that have to be faced.

COLLECTING RISK INFORMATION

If standard risk models, such as Gail, BCSC, and Tyrer-Cuzick, are to be used in screening programs, questionnaires need to be sent to women or made available online in order to provide information to populate the models. However, in countries without programs physicians can make risk assessments face-to-face. The offer of risk assessment may be sent at the time of the screening episode, but it may be best to send at the time women are informed of a normal mammogram. In a trial, informed consent is required but not if a program becomes standard of care.

ADDING OTHER RISK FACTORS

The results of the PROCAS and other studies suggest that other factors, such as density and SNPs, provide additional risk information over and above the standard models.[95,96] Estimation of density is important, not only is it a strong risk factor but also may be used to estimate risk and also to indicate the potential utility of adding additional screening modalities to digital mammography alone. In the USA density is assessed by radiologists using the BIRADs system and, in many states, it is mandatory to inform the screened woman of the result. In other parts of the world density is estimated as a percentage of dense versus nondense tissue. It is possible to introduce such a system, as shown in PROCAS[95,96] and KARMA,[97] but it seems unlikely that this method could be used in national screening programs unless made mandatory. However, it is possible to use automatic measures of area and volume of dense and nondense tissue using commercially available software such as Quantra and Volpara. More information is required to assess their utility versus visual estimations for giving risk information, but they have the great advantage of giving automated assessment of density from the digital mammogram. Thus, it is quite possible, to allow downloading of risk questionnaire data into models and to add density data automatically so that the readout can be sent to the screened woman with appropriate explanation. It will also be important to have measures in place to maintain confidentiality.

SNPs used alone give an indication of risk[51] but our own and the data of others[46] indicate they add risk information in addition to standard models and density. The KARMA, PROCAS, and other studies demonstrate that it is possible to collect saliva or blood samples in investigational studies but incorporation of SNP risk information is logistically difficult and expensive in the context of national screening programs. Further studies are required to determine how this might be accomplished but once SNP information is available it is relatively straight-forward to incorporate into risk algorithms.[96]

GIVING RISK INFORMATION

Risk is assessed with the strong implication that screened woman will be informed of the results. Because of the large numbers of women in screening programs there is no question that the majority of risk assessments cannot be given either face-to-face or on the telephone. Risks must be given via mail or, preferably, the internet. Explaining overall risk and potentially the components of risk from the model, density, and SNPs requires careful development of explanatory letters related to the degree of risk the screened woman has. It is customary in family history clinics to offer women with moderate and high risk an appointment. If this approach is implemented in family history clinics and Genetics Centers there will be a need to assess staffing levels with, potentially, considerable staffing implications and costs.

The evaluation of programs designed to communicate risk must consider the major harms and benefits that apply to women in the program. The main benefits of feedback consist of greater knowledge of risk and making more informed choices where offered different screening intervals, additional modalities of screening and chemoprevention and lifestyle choices. The main potential harms include increased anxiety and worry about cancer in women informed of high risks and false reassurance in women at low risk, resulting in lack of attendance at screening and poor attention to health related behaviors that not only reduce breast cancer risk but are implicated in many other common health conditions such as cardiovascular disease, diabetes and other cancers. There are few data with respect to screening programs but behavioral studies in other conditions suggest a small or no effect on risk-reducing behaviors and little evidence of elevated distress.[85] Given the low evidence base for the psychological effects of risk communication in screening programs further studies are necessary to assess risks and benefits.

ORGANIZATIONAL ISSUES FOR SCREENING PROGRAMS

Risk-based screening may indicate more frequent screening for some women and less frequent screening for others, the addition of supplemental screening modalities in women at high risk of missed or interval cancers, and use of alternative screening modalities for women at high risk of a false-positive recall from mammography. Given the current constant pressure of numbers in peripatetic and static sites, staffing issues, and pressure on radiologists and ancillary staff, introducing layers of complexity into screening programs will not be welcomed unless there is clear evidence of benefit to women in the program. However, in the UK, the NHSBSP has responded well to pressures of already mandated increased (annual) screening to some groups of women and the addition of MRI to women with mutations in the *BRCA1* and *BRCA2* genes or at equivalent genetic risk. This is also being developed in the Netherlands and Canada for those with very dense breasts.

COST-EFFECTIVENESS

All studies in this area must have mandatory economic analyses. The types of program described above appear expensive with respect to manpower and investigatory costs. This is particularly so with respect to SNP chip costs and, initially, the costs may have to be borne by the consumer until prices are reduced by increased use. Nonetheless favorable assessments have been published.[42]

EVIDENCE FOR EFFECTIVENESS

Given the controversy concerning the effectiveness of breast cancer screening, it is important to put the evidence base for risk factor-adapted screening on as sound a scientific footing as possible. It is not clear whether the fact that risk factor-adapted screening is already used in a limited way is useful or not to convince potential health service providers. We already have useful information (summarized above) that we can improve risk estimation and the definition of high risk groups by adding density and SNP information to the standard models. Also we know that ultrasound and tomosynthesis can add to mammography in high risk groups and that a combination of BI-RAD and Gail/BCSC can predict interval cancers.[35]

However, the ultimate criterion for assessing the value of risk factor-adapted screening is a reduction in breast cancer mortality. This is a long-term and, possibly not achievable, goal and a paucity of intermediate end points, although less common, may be required such as the reduction in frequency of large aggressive cancers, reduction of interval cancer rates, and reduction in mastectomies and the use of chemotherapy and radiotherapy.

Randomized trials will be very expensive and difficult to perform to include all risk factors including SNPs. Although a randomized trial of personalized risk versus annual usual screening is underway in the USA without SNPs (http://www.pcori.org/research-results/2015/enabling-paradigm-shift-preference-tolerant-rct-personalized-vs-annual). We favor comparisons of consecutive groups of screened women, one as a control and the next gene risk factor-adapted screening (about 8000 in each group) with acceptability to and uptake of chemoprevention and additional screening as end points.

OPPORTUNITIES OF RISK FACTOR-ADAPTED SCREENING

Although the outlook of women diagnosed with breast cancer has improved considerably over the past 25 years (nearly a halving of death rates) approximately 20% of women still die from the disease and all are subject to the psychological and physical trauma of its diagnosis and treatment. Nonetheless, if harms such as False Positives, overdiagnosis, overtreatment, and reduced radiation exposure could be obtained by reducing screening in those at low risk. Risk factor-adapted screening will not reduce rates of diagnosis (it will possibly increase them) but should result in improvements in early diagnosis of cancers likely to metastasize and in others smaller tumors where there may then be reductions in the need for aggressive treatments.

Also risk assessment programs may result in increase in uptake of risk reduction of breast cancer (chemoprevention) and the reduction of breast cancer (lifestyle change) which can be an exemplar for similar approaches in other cancers and other diseases. It may also provide platforms for testing new approaches to diagnosis and treatment which are under continual development worldwide.

FUTURE RESEARCH DIRECTIONS AND TRENDS

A great deal of further research is required to fully implement risk-adapted screening on a population basis. This will require research into how to incorporate new risk information such as that from SNPs and mammographic density, but also ways of automating the assessments. The practicalities of introducing such "risk-adapted" screening are outlined above, but the current state of knowledge would indicate that systems for assessing and communicating risk would have to be introduced into national screening programs. For population models, such as the Tyrer-Cuzick and BSCS, and assessing density this seems eminently possible. The greatest improvement in risk estimation was when SNP18 were added to T-C. Evaluating SNPs nationally would be a major undertaking and the evidence from our own calculations and those of others indicates that estimating all available breast "risk" SNPs would add additional expense. A SNP chip which analyzes all known polymorphisms would be a viable approach and more extensive use would reduce costs. Evaluation of risks of other diseases appears attractive but considerable work would be required in order to make this a safe and effective reality. Finally the impact of identifying women at high and moderate risk must also be undertaken before widespread implementation. This will need to include a cost-effectiveness analysis that balances the potential harms and benefits.

CONCLUSIONS

Risk-adapted screening is already taking place in many parts of the world based on family history. However, great strides are necessary before population-based programs could be introduced. There is no doubt that incorporation of genetic risk data from SNPs and mammographic density are substantially improving the precision of risk assessments and identifying those not only at greater risk of breast cancer, but of interval cancers. More work is required to assess how best to incorporate risk-adapted screening, whether it is cost-effective and whether it is acceptable to the great majority of women who will be affected by it.

LIST OF ACRONYMS AND ABBREVIATIONS

ABUS Automated breast ultrasound
BRCA1 BReastCAncer 1 gene
BRCA2 BReastCAncer 2 gene
DR Density Residual
FHC Family History Clinic

HRT	hormone replacement therapy
MD	Mammographic Density
MRI	Magnetic Resonance Imaging
NBN, RAD51, TP53, RAD51C, RAD51D and BRIP1	*Other* gene names
NHSBSP	National Health Service Breast Screening Programme
NICE	National Institute for Healthcare and Clinical Excellence
ORs	Odds ratios
PROCAS	Predicting the Risk of Cancer at Screening
SNPs	Single Nucleotide Polymorphisms
TC	Tyrer-Cuzick
VAS	Visual Assessment Scale

REFERENCES

1. Collins DC. The dangers of employing thorium dioxide solution in mammography. *Can Med Assoc J* 1939;**40**(5):440–2.
2. Hutchison GB, Shapiro S. Lead time gained by diagnostic screening for breast cancer. *Natl Cancer Inst* 1968;**41**(3):665–81.
3. Tabár L, Dean PB. The control of breast cancer through mammography screening. What is the evidence? *Radiol Clin North Am* 1987;**25**(5):993–1005.
4. <http://www.cancerscreening.nhs.uk/breastscreen/publications/forrest-report.html>.
5. <http://www.cancerscreening.nhs.uk/breastscreen/research-age-extension-full-rct-faqs.html>.
6. <http://www.isrctn.com/ISRCTN33292440>.
7. CR-UK, CancerStats Incidence – UK. Cancer Research UK. 2012, <www.cancerresearchuk.orghttp://info.cancerresearchuk.org/cancerstats/types/breast/index.htm?script=true> [accessed 01.05.15].
8. Parkin DM, Bray F, Ferlay J, Pisani P. Global cancer statistics, 2002. *CA Cancer J Clin* 2005;**55**:74–108.
9. Marmot MG, Altman DG, Cameron DA, Dewar JA, Thompson SG, Wilcox M. The benefits and harms of breast cancer screening: an independent review. *Br J Cancer* 2013;**108**(11):2205–40.
10. Bennett RL, Sellars SJ, Moss SM. Interval cancers in the NHS breast cancer screening programme in England, Wales and Northern Ireland. *Br J Cancer* 2011;**104**(4):571–7.
11. Nixon RM, Pharoah P, Tabar L, Krusemo UB, Duffy SW, Prevost TC, et al. Mammographic screening in women with a family history of breast cancer: some results from the Swedish two-county trial. *Rev Epidém et Santé Publ* 2000;**48**:325–31.
12. Porter GJ, Evans AJ, Burrell HC, Lee AH, Chakrabarti J. NHSBSP type 1 interval cancers: a scientifically valid grouping? *Clin Radiol* 2007;**62**(3):262–7.
13. Miglioretti DL, Zhu W, Kerlikowske K, Sprague BL, Onega T, Buist DSM, et al. Risk of less-favorable breast tumor characteristics with biennial versus annual mammography. *JAMA Oncol* 2015;**1**(8):1069–77.
14. Claus EB, Risch N, Thompson WD. Genetic analysis of breast cancer in the cancer and steroid hormone study. *Am J Hum Genet* 1991;**48**(2):232–42.
15. Newman B, Austin MA, Lee M, King M. Inheritance of human breast cancer: evidence for autosomal dominant transmission in high-risk families. *Proc Natl Acad Sci USA* 1988;**85**:3044–8.
16. Lichtenstein P, Holm NV, Verkasalo PK, Iliadou A, Kaprio J, Koskenvuo M, et al. Environmental and heritable factors in the causation of cancer – analyses of cohorts of twins from Sweden, Denmark, and Finland. *N Engl J Med* 2000;**343**(2):78–85.
17. Howell A, Anderson AS, Clarke RB, Duffy SW, Evans DG, et al. Risk determination and prevention of breast cancer. *Breast Cancer Res* 2014;**16**(5):446.

18. Mavaddat N, Antoniou AC, Easton DF, Garcia-Closas M. Genetic susceptibility to breast cancer. *Mol Oncol* 2010;**4**(3):174–91.
19. Michailidou K, Beesley J, Lindstrom S, Canisius S, Dennis J, Lush MJ, et al. Genome-wide association analysis of more than 120,000 individuals identifies 15 new susceptibility loci for breast cancer. *Nat Genet* 2015;**7**(4):373–80. Available from: http://dx.doi.org/10.1038/ng.3242.
20. Liaw D, Marsh DJ, Li J, Dahia PL, Wang SI, Zheng Z, et al. Germline mutations of the PTEN gene in Cowden disease, an inherited breast and thyroid cancer syndrome. *Nat Genet* 1997;**16**(1):64–7.
21. Evans DGR, Cuzick J, Howell A. Cancer genetics clinics. *Eur J Cancer* 1996;**32**:391–2.
22. FH01 collaborative teams. Mammographic surveillance in women younger than 50 years who have a family history of breast cancer: tumour characteristics and projected effect on mortality in the prospective, single-arm, FH01 study. *Lancet Oncol* 2010;**11**:1127–34.
23. Evans DG, Thomas S, Caunt J, Roberts L, Howell A, Wilson M, et al. Mammographic surveillance in women aged 35–39 at enhanced familial risk of breast cancer (FH02). *Fam Cancer* 2014;**13**(1):13–21.
24. Kuhl CK, Schrading S, Leutner CC, Morakkabati-Spitz N, Wardelmann E, Fimmers R, et al. Mammography, breast ultrasound, and magnetic resonance imaging for surveillance of women at high familial risk for breast cancer. *J Clin Oncol* 2005;**23**:8469–76.
25. Warner E, Plewes DB, Hill KA, Causer PA, Zubovits JT, Jong RA, et al. Surveillance of BRCA1 and BRCA2 mutation carriers with magnetic resonance imaging, ultrasound, mammography, and clinical breast examination. *J Am Med Assoc* 2004;**292**:1317–25.
26. MARIBS study group. Screening with magnetic resonance imaging and mammography of a UK population at high familial risk of breast cancer: a prospective multicentre cohort study (MARIBS). *Lancet* 2005;**365**:1769–78.
27. Sardanelli F, Podo F, D'Agnolo G, Verdecchia A, Santaguilani M, Musumeci R, et al. Multicenter comparative multimodality surveillance of women at genetic-familial high risk for breast cancer (HIBCRIT Study): interim results. *Radiology* 2007;**242**:698–715.
28. Hagen AI, Kvistad KA, Maehle L, Holmen MM, Aase H, Styr B, et al. Sensitivity of MRI versus conventional screening in diagnosis of BRCA-associated breast cancer in a national prospective series. *Breast* 2007;**16**(4):367–74.
29. Evans DG, Kesavan N, Lim Y, Gadde S, Hurley E, Massat NJ, et al. MRI breast screening in high-risk women: cancer detection and survival analysis. *Breast Cancer Res Treat* 2014;**145**(3):663–72.
30. Møller P, Stormorken A, Jonsrud C, Holmen MM, Hagen AI, Clark N, et al. Survival of patients with *BRCA*1-associated breast cancer diagnosed in an MRI-based surveillance program. *Breast Cancer Res Treat* 2013;**139**(1):155–61.
31. Tilanus-Linthorst M, Verhoog L, Obdeijn IM, Bartels K, Menke-Pluymers M, Eggermont A, et al. A BRCA1/2 mutation, high breast density and prominent pushing margins of a tumor independently contribute to a frequent false-negative mammography. *Int J Cancer* 2002:10291–5.
32a. McIntosh A, Shaw C, Evans G, Turnbull N, Bahar N, Barclay M, et al. *Clinical guidelines and evidence review for the classification and care of women at risk of familial breast cancer*. London: National Collaborating Centre for Primary Care/University of Sheffield; 2004 updated 2006. NICE guideline CG041. <www.nice.org.uk>.
32b. Ciatto S, et al. Breast density as a determinant of interval cancer at mammographic screening. *Brit J Cancer* 2004;**90**:393–6.
33. Saslow D, Boetes C, Burke W, Harms S, Leach MO, Lehman CD, et al. American Cancer Society guidelines for breast screening with MRI as an adjunct to mammography. *CA Cancer J Clin* 2007;**57**(2):75–89.
34. Evans DG, Graham J, O'Connell S, Arnold S, Fitzsimmons D. Familial breast cancer: summary of updated NICE guidance. *Br Med J* 2013;**346**:f3829. Available from: http://dx.doi.org/10.1136/bmj.f3829.
35. Kerlikowske K, Zhu W, Tosteson ANA, Sprague BL, Tice JA, Lehman CD, et al. Identifying women with dense breasts at high risk for interval cancer. *Ann Internal Med* 2015;**162**(10):673. Available from: http://dx.doi.org/10.7326/m14-1465.

36. Evans DG, Howell A. Can the breast screening appointment be used to provide risk assessment and prevention advice? *Breast Cancer Res* 2015.
37. Amir E, Freedman OC, Seruga B, Evans DG. Assessing women at high-risk of breast cancer: a review of risk assessment models. *J Natl Cancer Inst* 2010;**102**:680–91.
38. Boyd NF, Dite GS, Stone J, Gunasekara A, English DR, McCredie MRE, et al. Heritability of mammographic density, a risk factor for breast cancer. *N Engl J Med* 2002;**347**:886–94.
39. Tice JA, Cummings SR, Smith-Bindman R, Ichikawa L, Barlow WE, Kerlikowske K. Using clinical factors and mammographic breast density to estimate breast cancer risk: development and validation of a new predictive model. *Ann Intern Med* 2008;**148**(5):337–47.
40. Mandelson MT, Oestreicher N, Porter PL, White D, Finder CA, Taplin SH, et al. Breast density as a predictor of mammographic detection: comparison of interval- and screen-detected cancers. *J Natl Cancer Inst* 2000;**92**:1081–7.
41. Pharoah PD, Sewell B, Fitzsimmons D, Bennett HS, Pashayan N. Cost effectiveness of the NHS breast screening programme: life table model. *Br Med J* 2013;**346**:f2618.
42. Schousboe JT, Kerlokowske K, Loh A, Cummings SR. Personalizing mammography by breast density and other risk factors for breast cancer: analysis of health benefits and cost-effectiveness. *Ann Intern Med* 2011;**155**:10–20.
43. Tyrer J, Duffy SW, Cuzick J. A breast cancer prediction model incorporating familial and personal risk factors. *Stat Med* 2004;**23**:1111–30.
44. Gail MH, Brinton LA, Byar DP, Corle DK, Green SB, Schairer C, et al. Projecting individulized probabilities of developing breast cancer for white females who are being examined annually. *J Natl Cancer Inst* 1989;**81**:1879–86.
45. Costantino JP, Gail MH, Pee D, Anderson S, Redmond CK, Benichou J, et al. Validation studies for models projecting the risk of invasive and total breast cancer incidence. *J Natl Cancer Inst* 1999;**91**:1541–8.
46. Vachon CM, Pankratz VS, Scott CG, Haeberle L, Ziv E, Jensen MR, et al. The contributions of breast density and common genetic variation to breast cancer risk. *J Natl Cancer Inst* 2015;**107**(5).
47. Santen R, Boyd N, Chlebowski RT, Cummings S, Cuzick J, Dowsett M, et al. Critical assessment of new risk factors for breast cancer: considerations for development of an improved risk prediction model. *Endocr Relat Cancer* 2007;**14**:169–87.
48. Pankow JS, Vachon CM, Kuni CC, King RA, Arnett DK, Gabrick DM, et al. Genetic analysis of mammographic breast density in adult women: evidence of a gene effect. *J Natl Cancer Inst* 1997;**89**:549–56.
49. Barlow WE, White E, Ballard-Barbash R, Vacek PM, Titus-Ernstoff L, Carney PA, et al. Prospective breast cancer risk prediction model for women undergoing screening mammography. *J Natl Cancer Inst* 2006;**98**:1204–14.
50. Chen J, Pee D, Ayyagari R, Graubard B, Schairer C, Byrne C, et al. Projecting absolute invasive breast cancer risk in white women with a model that includes mammographic density. *J Natl Cancer Inst* 2006;**98**:1215–26.
51. Mavaddat N, Pharoah PD, Michailidou K, Tyrer J, Brook MN, Bolla MK, et al. Prediction of breast cancer risk based on profiling with common genetic variants. *J Natl Cancer Inst* 2015;**107**(5).
52. Pisano ED, Gatsonis C, Hendrick E, Yaffe M, Baum JK, Acharyya S, et al. Diagnostic performance of digital versus film mammography for breast-cancer screening. *N Engl J Med* 2005;**353**(17):1773–83.
53. Kolb TM, Lichy J, Newhouse JH. Comparison of the performance of screening mammography, physical examination, and breast US and evaluation of factors that influence them: an analysis of 27,825 patient evaluations. *Radiology* 2002;**225**:165–75.
54. Buist DSM, Porter PL, Lehman C, Taplin SH, White E. Factors contributing to mammography failure in women aged 40–49 years. *J Natl Cancer Inst* 2004;**96**:1432–40.
55. Ciatto S, Visioli C, Paci E, Zappa M. Breast density as a determinant of interval cancer at mammographic screening. *Br J Cancer* 2004;**90**:393–6.

56. Brekelmans CTM, Seynaeve C, Bartels CCM, Tilanus-Linthorst MM, Meijers-Heijboer EJ, Crepin CM, et al. Effectiveness of breast cancer surveillance in BRCA1/2 gene mutation carriers and women with high familial risk. *J ClinOncol* 2001;**19**:924–30.
57. Otten JDM, Karssemeijer N, Hendriks JHCL, Groenewoud JH, Fracheboud J, Verbeek ALM, et al. Effect of recall rate on earlier screen detection of breast cancers based on the Dutch performance indicators. *J Natl Cancer Inst* 2005;**97**(10):748–54.
58. Haas BM, Kalra V, Geisel J, Raghu M, Durand M, Philpotts LE. Comparison of tomosynthesis plus digital mammography and digital mammography alone for breast cancer screening. *Radiology* 2013;**269**:694–700. Available from: http://dx.doi.org/10.1148/radiol.13130307.
59. Daly CA, Apthorp L, Field S. Second round cancers: how many were visible on the first round of the UK National Breast Screening Programme, three years earlier? *Clin Radiol* 1998;**53**:25–8.
60. Sylvester PA, Kutt E, Baird A, Vipond MN, Webb AJ, Farndon JR. Rate and classification of interval cancers in the breast screening programme. *Ann R Coll Surg Engl* 1997;**79**:276–7.
61. Anderson EDC, Muir BB, Walsh JS, Kirkpatrick AE. The efficacy of double reading mammograms in breast screening. *Clin Radiol* 1994;**49**(4):248–51.
62. Thurfjell EL, Lernevall KA, Taube AAS. Benefit of independent double reading in a population-based mammography screening program. *Radiology* 1994;**191**:241–4.
63. Gilbert FJ, Astley SM, Gillan MGC, Agbaje OF, Wallis MG, James J, et al. Single reading with computer-aided detection for screening mammography. *N Engl J Med* 2008;**359**(16):1675–84.
64. Lehman C, Wellman RD, Buist DSM, Kerlikowske K, Tosteson ANA, Miglioretti DL. Diagnostic accuracy of digital screening mammography with and without computer-aided detection. *JAMA Intern Med* 2015;**175**(11): 1828–37.
65. Whelehan P, Evans AJ, Wells M, Macgillivray S. The effect of mammography pain on repeat participation in breast cancer screening: a systematic review. *Breast* 2013;**22**:389–94.
66. Gilbert FJ, Tucker L, Gillan MG, Cooke WJ, Duncan KA, Michell MJ, et al. The TOMMY trial: a comparison of TOMosynthesis with digital MammographY in the UK NHS Breast Screening Programme-a multicentre retrospective reading study comparing the diagnostic performance of digital breast tomosynthesis and digital mammography with digital mammography alone. *Health Technol Assess (Winchester, England)* 2015;**19**(4):1–136.
67. Skaane P, Bandos AI, Eben EB, Jebsen IN, Krager M, Haakenaasen U, et al. Two-View digital breast tomosynthesis screening with synthetically reconstructed projection images: comparison with digital breast tomosynthesis with full-field digital mammographic images. *Radiology* 2014;**271**:655–63.
68. Skaane P, Bandos AI, Gullien R, Eben EB, Ekseth U, Haakenaasen U, et al. Comparison of digital mammography alone and digital mammography plus tomosynthesis in a population-based screening program. *Radiology* 2013;**267**:47–56.
69. Ciatto S, Houssami N, Bernardi D, Caumo F, Pellegrini M, Brunelli S, et al. Integration of 3D digital mammography with tomosynthesis for population breast-cancer screening (STORM): a prospective comparison study. *Lancet Oncol* 2013;**14**:583–9.
70. Lång K, Andersson I, Rosso A, Tingberg A, Timberg P, Zackrisson S. Performance of one-view breast tomosynthesis as a stand-alone breast cancer screening modality: results from the Malmö Breast Tomosynthesis Screening Trial, a population-based study. *Eur Radiol Published Online First* 2016;**26**(1):184–90. Available from: http://dx.doi.org/10.1007/s00330-015-3803-3.
71. McCarthy AM, Kontos D, Synnestvedt M, Tan KS, Heitjan DF, Schnall M, et al. Screening outcomes following implementation of digital breast tomosynthesis in a general-population screening program. *J Natl Cancer Inst* 2014:106. Available from: http://dx.doi.org/10.1093/jnci/dju316.
72. Lourenco AP, Barry-Brooks M, Baird G, Tuttle A, Mainiero MB. Changes in recall type and patient treatment following implementation of screening digital breast tomosynthesis. *Radiology* 2014:140317. Available from: http://dx.doi.org/10.1148/radiol.14140317.

73. Durand MA, Haas BM, Yao X, Geisel JL, Raghu M, Hooley RJ, et al. Early clinical experience with digital breast tomosynthesis for screening mammography. *Radiology* 2015;**274**:85–92.
74. Bernardi D, Ciatto S, Pellegrini M, Anesi V, Burlon S, Cauli E, et al. Application of breast tomosynthesis in screening: incremental effect on mammography acquisition and reading time. *Br J Radiol* 2012;**85**:e1174–8.
75. Houssami N, Macaskill P, Bernardi D, Caumo F, Pellegrini M, Brunelli S, et al. Breast screening using 2D-mammography or integrating digital breast tomosynthesis (3D-mammography) for single-reading or double-reading – evidence to guide future screening strategies. *Eur J Cancer* 2014;**50**(10):1799–807.
76. Lång K, Andersson I, Rosso A, Tingberg A, Timberg P, Zackrisson S. Performance of one-view breast tomosynthesis as a stand-alone breast cancer screening modality: results from the Malmö Breast Tomosynthesis Screening Trial, a population-based study. *Eur Radiol* 2016;**26**(1):184–90. [Epub ahead of print].
77. Kriege M, Brekelmans CTM, Boetes C, Besnard PE, Zonderland HM, Obdeijn IM, et al. Efficacy of MRI and mammography for breast-cancer screening in women with a familial or genetic predisposition. *N Engl J Med* 2004;**351**(5):427–37.
78. Norman RP, Evans DG, Easton DF, Young KC. The cost-utility of magnetic resonance imaging for breast cancer in BRCA1 mutation carriers aged 30–49. *Eur J Health Econ* 2007;**8**(2):137–44.
79. Kuhl CK, Schrading S, Strobel K, Schild HH, Hilgers RD, Bieling HB. Abbreviated breast magnetic resonance imaging (MRI): first postcontrast subtracted images and maximum-intensity projection-a novel approach to breast cancer screening with MRI. *J Clin Oncol* 2014;**32**:2304–10.
80. Berg WA, Blume JD, Cormack JB, Mendelson EB, Lehrer D, Bohm-Velez M, et al. Combined screening with ultrasound and mammography vs mammography alone in women at elevated risk of breast cancer. *J Am Med Assoc* 2008;**299**:2151–63.
81. Brem RF, Tabar L, Duffy SW, Inciardi MF, Guingrich JA, Hashimoto BE, et al. Assessing improvement in detection of breast cancer with three-dimensional automated breast US in women with dense breast tissue: the somoinsight study. *Radiology* 2015;**274**:663–73.
82. Sprague BL, Stout NK, Schechter C, van Ravesteyn NT, Cevik M, Alagoz O, et al. Benefits, harms, and cost-effectiveness of supplemental ultrasonography screening for women with dense breasts. *Ann Intern Med* 2015;**162**:157.
83. American College of Radiology. BI-RADS Committee. Breast imaging reporting and data system. Edited by American College of Radiology. American College of Radiology, 1998.
84. Nicholson BT, LoRusso AP, Smolkin M, Bovbjerg VE, Petroni GR, Harvey JA. Accuracy of assigned BI-RADS breast density category definitions. *Acad Radiol* 2006;**13**(9):1143–9.
85. Byng JW, Boyd NF, Fishell E, Jong RA. The quantitative analysis of mammographic densities. *Phys Med Biol* 1994;**39**(10):1629.
86. Boyd NF, Martin L, Yaffe MJ, Minkin S. Mammographic density and breast cancer risk: current understanding and future prospects. *Breast Cancer Res* 2011;**13**(6):223.
87. Highnam R, Brady M, Yaffe MJ, Karssemeijer N, Harvey J. Robust breast composition measurement-VolparaTM. *Digital mammography, lecture notes in computer science*, **vol. 6136**. Springer Berlin Heidelberg; 2010.342–9.
88. Donovan EO, Sergeant J, Harkness E, Morris J, Wilson M, Lim Y, et al. Use of Volumetric breast density measures for the prediction of weight and body mass index *Digital mammography, lecture notes in computer science*, **vol. 8539**. Springer-Verlag Berlin Heidelberg; 2014.282–9.
89. Van Engeland S, Snoeren PR, Huisman H, Boetes C, Karssemeijer N. Volumetric breast density estimation from full-field digital mammograms. *IEEE Trans Med Imaging* 2006;**25**(3):273–82.
90. Moschidis E, Chen X, Taylor C, Astley SM. Texture-based breast cancer prediction in full-field digital mammograms using the dual-tree complex wavelet transform and random forest classification *Breast imaging*. Springer International Publishing; 2014.

91. Nielsen M, Karemore G, Loog M, Raundahl J, Karssemeijer N, Otten JD, et al. A novel and automatic mammographic texture resemblance marker is an independent risk factor for breast cancer. *Cancer Epidemiol* 2011;**35**(4):381–7.
92. Brentnall AR, Harkness EF, Astley SM, Donnelly LS, Stavrinos P, Sampson S, et al. Mammographic density adds accuracy to both the Tyrer-Cuzick and Gail breast cancer risk models in a prospective UK screening cohort. *Breast Cancer Res* 2015;**17**(1):147.
93. Easton DF, Pharoah PD, Antoniou AC, Tischkowitz M, Tavtigian SV, Nathanson KL, et al. Gene-panel sequencing and the prediction of breast-cancer risk. *N Engl J Med* 2015;**372**(23):2243–57.
94. Mealiffe ME, Stokowski RP, Rhees BK, Prentice RL, Pettinger M, Hinds DA. Assessment of clinical validity of a breast cancer risk model combining genetic and clinical information. *J Natl Cancer Inst* 2010;**102**(21):1618–27.
95. Evans DG, Warwick J, Astley SM, Stavrinos P, Sahin S, Ingham S, et al. Assessing individual breast cancer risk within the UK National Health Service Breast Screening Programme: a new paradigm for cancer prevention. *Cancer Prev Res (Phila)* 2012;**5**(7):943–51.
96. Evans DG, Brentnall AR, Harvie M, Dawe S, Sergeant J, Stavrinos P, et al. Breast cancer risk in young women in the National Breast Screening Programme: implications for applying NICE guidelines for additional screening and chemoprevention. Cancer Prevention. *Research* 2014;**7**(10):993–1001.
97. Skarping I, Brand JS, Hall P, Borgquist S. Effects of statin use on volumetric mammographic density: results from the KARMA study. *BMC Cancer* 2015;**15**:435.

CHAPTER

8

BREAST CANCER SCREENING IN THE OLDER WOMAN

Mara A. Schonberg

Division of General Medicine and Primary Care, Beth Israel Deaconess Medical Center, Harvard Medical School, Boston, MA, United States

CHAPTER OUTLINE

Breast Cancer Screening. DOI: http://dx.doi.org/10.1016/B978-0-12-802209-2.00008-5

PLAIN LANGUAGE SUMMARY

It is not certain if mammograms benefit women aged 70 or older. While the chance of breast cancer increases with age, breast cancers tend to grow more slowly among older women. Experts think that a small breast cancer found on an older woman's mammogram would not have caused problems for 5 to 10 years and some of the breast cancers found would never have caused problems. Meanwhile, the average women aged 75 lives 13 more years; those in poor health live less long. Experts recommend that clinicians think about how long an older woman may have to live before recommending mammography screening. Guidelines recommend against screening women who are unlikely to live 10 years and experts encourage women ≥70 years in good health to make an informed decision about whether or not to be screened. The pros to getting a screening mammogram are that mammograms are more likely to find breast cancers when they are small, improving an older woman's chances of only needing minor surgery. In addition, although doctors are unsure that getting a mammogram will lower an older woman's chances of dying from breast cancer, some studies suggest that 2 out of 1000 women aged 70 in good health that continue getting mammograms for 10 years may avoid breast cancer death. However, approximately 100–300 of these women will experience a "false alarm." These women experience an abnormal mammogram but additional tests do not show breast cancer. It is estimated that 20–50 of 1000 women that continue to be screened will experience a benign breast biopsy as a result of having been screened and the majority of older women find their experience with breast biopsies stressful. In addition, around 13 of 1000 women screened will be diagnosed with a breast cancer that would never otherwise have shown up or caused problems in an older woman's lifetime. Since it is difficult to predict which breast cancers will progress and which will not, nearly all older women undergo treatment for breast cancer. Breast cancer treatment for older women usually involves removing the lump of breast cancer from the breast and taking hormonal pills for approximately 5 years. Some older women are also treated with radiation therapy and a few older women in excellent health are treated with chemotherapy. While most older women do well after surgery, many experience side effects from the hormonal pills and from treatment with radiation and/or chemotherapy. To decide whether or not to get a mammogram, older women must consider their health, their risk of breast cancer, and how strongly they feel about the possibility of reducing their risk of death from breast cancer in 10 years with the greater chance of experiencing a false alarm or being diagnosed and treated for a breast cancer that otherwise may not have caused problems. There are educational tools available to help older women weigh these trade-offs and clarify their values and preferences about whether or not to be screened with mammography.

INTRODUCTION

Women ≥70 years are the fastest growing segment of the United States (US) population and breast cancer incidence increases with age peaking between ages 75–79 years (Table 8.1).[1] However, few women ≥70 years were included in the randomized controlled trials evaluating mammography screening and whether or not to screen these women for breast cancer is controversial.[5] National and international guidelines and policies regarding mammography screening for older women vary (Table 8.2). Most US guidelines recommend that clinicians consider an older woman's health and/or life expectancy before recommending screening and some guidelines specifically recommend not screening women with less

Table 8.1 Breast Cancer Incidence Among Women in the US by Race/ethnicity and in the UK, Sweden, Canada, and Australia

Age	White[a]	Black[a]	Hispanic[b]	Chinese[c]	Japanese[c]	Hawaiian/ Filipino[c]	Pacific Islanders[c]	United Kingdom[d]	Sweden[e]	Canada[2]	Australia[3]
55–59	273.8	275.2	185.7	197.1	322.2	537.3	236.6	266.2	248.9	220	264.5
60–64	359.2	328.5	215.1	167.5	400.7	523.8	284.4	318.7	324.8	320	334.9
65–69	430.7	382.4	251.2	182.2	352.2	558.2	292.1	378.5	363.4	320	378.3
70–74	445.4	396.7	284.6	183.4	359.3	567.8	233.0	296.4	336.9	310	301.0
75–79	462.3	405.4	275.7	192.0	358.9	651.3	203.6	331.9	274.3	310	307.9
80–84	436.3	395.8	252.3	223.3	353.9	389.0	148.3	369.7	307.6	270	296.3
85+	365.0	371.9	203.9	224.7	205.2	294.9	101.2	—	—	270	306.9

*Average breast cancer incidence per year per 100,000 women.

[a]*Data from NCI's Surveillance, Epidemiology, and End Results (SEER) Program from 2006–2010.*

[b]*Data from NCI's Surveillance, Epidemiology, and End Results (SEER) Program from 1990–1996 (most recent available for Hispanics).*

[c]*Data from NCI's Surveillance, Epidemiology, and End Results (SEER) Program from 1998–2002 (most recent available for Asian Ethnicities).*

[d]*Data from Thames Registry first breast cancer rates 2005–2009.*[4]

[e]*Data from Statistics Sweden first breast cancer rates 2006–2010.*[4]

Table 8.2 Guidelines for Screening Mammography Among Women 75 Years or Older[a]

Organization	Year Guideline Issued	Mammography Screening Recommendations
United States		
American Board of Internal Medicine Choosing Wisely Campaign	2013[6]	Do not recommend cancer screening in adults with life expectancy of less than 10 years.
American Cancer Society	2015[7]	Women should continue screening mammography as long as their overall health is good and they have a life expectancy of 10 years or longer. If performed, recommend screening every 2 years.
American College of Obstetricians and Gynecologists	2011[8]	Women aged 75 or older should, in consultation with their physicians, decide whether or not to continue mammographic screening. Medical comorbidity and life expectancy should be considered. If performed, recommend screening every year.
American College of Radiology	2008[9]	Screening should stop when life expectancy is < 5 to 7 years or when abnormal results would not be acted on due to age or comorbidities. If performed, recommend screening every year.
National Comprehensive Cancer Network	2013[10]	In older women, mammography screening should be individualized, weighing its potential benefits/risks in the context of the patient's overall health and estimated longevity. If a patient has severe comorbid conditions limiting her life expectancy and no intervention would occur based on the screening findings, then the patient should not undergo screening. If performed, recommend screening every year.
US Preventive Services Task Force	2015[11]	Evidence is insufficient to assess the additional benefits and harms of screening mammography in women 75 years or older. No recommendation (I statement—If the service is offered, patients should understand the uncertainty about the balance of benefits and harms). If performed, recommend screening every 2 years.
Other Countries		
Canadian Task Force on Preventive Health Care	2011[12]	A tailored approach to mammography screening is warranted in women aged 70 years or older. If a woman desires to continue screening mammography, it is justified if her life expectancy exceeds 5–10 years (weak recommendation; low quality evidence). If performed, recommend screening every 2–3 years.
National Health Service, United Kingdom	2010[13]	Women aged 74 or older can request continued mammography screening but do not receive routine invitations. If performed, recommend screening every 3 years.
Netherlands National Institute for Public Health and the Environment	1998[14]	Women up to age 74 are invited to be screened with mammography every 2 years. Women aged 75 or older can request to be screened but do not receive routine invitations.

(*Continued*)

Table 8.2 Guidelines for Screening Mammography Among Women 75 Years or Older (Continued)

Organization	Year Guideline Issued	Mammography Screening Recommendations
The Royal Australian College of General Practitioners	2014[15,16]	Women aged 75 or older (changed from age 70 in 2015) can request continued mammography screening, but they are not targeted to be screened by BreastScreen Australia. Women in this age group should balance the potential benefits and downsides of screening, considering their general health and whether they have other diseases or conditions. If performed, recommend screening every 2 years.
Other Countries Combined		
China[17]	2009	Women up to age 59 are invited to be screened with mammography every 3 years in China.
Finland, Greece, Hungary, Saudi Arabia, Singapore[13,17–19]		Women up to age 64 are invited to be screened with mammography every 2 years in these countries. (In Hungary, women are invited to be screened every year).
Ireland[18]	2000	Women up to age 65 are invited to be screened with mammography every 2 years in Ireland.
Belgium, Denmark, Germany, Iceland, Italy, Luxembourg, Norway, New Zealand, Poland, Portugal, Spain, Switzerland, Uruguay[13,17–19]		Women up to age 69 are invited to be screened with mammography every 2 years in these countries. (In Uruguay, women are invited to be screened every year).
France, Israel, Sweden		Women up to age 74 are invited to be screened with mammography every 2 years in these countries.
Japan, Korea[13,18]		Women up to age 75 are invited to be screened with mammography every 2 years in these countries.

[a]*Recommendations are based on each organization's literature review, consensus process and expert opinion.*

than 10-year life expectancy.[20] The United States Preventive Services Task Force (USPSTF) recommends biennial mammography for women ages 50–74 years and states that there is insufficient evidence to recommend screening to women aged 75 and older.[11] Instead, the USPSTF recommends that if mammography screening is offered to women $\geq$75 years, these women should understand the uncertainty about the balance of benefits and harms before being screened. Despite these recommendations, Medicare has covered biennial screening mammograms for all women aged 65 or older regardless of their age or health since 1991 and has covered annual screening mammograms for women aged 65 and older since 1998. The Affordable Care Act also includes coverage of annual screening mammograms for all women regardless of their age or life expectancy.

In the US, screening is opportunistic. Women initiate screening for themselves or are encouraged to get screened by their physicians. In Canada, Australia, and most European countries screening is implemented through a national screening program where women receive mailed invitations to be screened at regular intervals based on their age. Within these countries, determining the appropriate age to stop inviting older women to be screened is controversial. In Canada, women cease to be invited for mammography screening by age 70.[12] In the UK, the Netherlands, and Australia women stop receiving invitations to be screened by age 74 or age 75 (Table 8.2).[14–16,21] Older women may continue to request to be screened even after they stop receiving screening invitations; however, data from the UK suggest that the majority of older women (82%) stop being screened once they stop receiving screening invitations.[22] In the US, however, approximately 50% of women ≥75 years continue to be screened,[23] including 36% of older women with ≤5 year life expectancy.[24] In the setting of limited data from clinical trials and disparate policies, experts recommend that decision-making around mammography screening for older women consider their *risk of breast cancer*, their *life expectancy*, and their *values and preferences* based on a reasonable and realistic understanding of the benefits and risks of screening. This chapter will review what is known about each of these components of high quality mammography screening decisions for older women.

LATE-LIFE BREAST CANCER RISK

While it is well known that the risk of breast cancer increases with age (Table 8.1), there are few tools available to help inform older women of their individualized risk of breast cancer beyond their age-based risk. The Breast Cancer Risk Assessment Tool (BCRAT), also known as the Gail model, is the most commonly used breast cancer prediction model in primary care settings.[25,26] The model gives older women that are in good health and that are regularly screened a reasonable estimate of their probability of breast cancer within 5 years.[27] For example, based on the model a 75 year old white woman at average risk has 2.2% probability of breast cancer in 5 years.[28] However, the model does not discriminate well which women are more or less likely to develop breast cancer.[6,27] This means that many women categorized at high risk by the model will not get breast cancer while a number of women categorized at low risk will still get breast cancer.

To determine a woman's 5-year probability for developing breast cancer, the BCRAT considers a woman's baseline risk of breast cancer based on her age and race using age and race/ethnic specific population breast cancer incidence rates from NCI's Surveillance, Epidemiology, and End Results (SEER) program (Table 8.1 presents recent incident rates available through SEER as well as breast cancer incidence rates in Canada, Australia, UK, and Sweden).[28] The model then adjusts a woman's probability of breast cancer by considering whether or not a woman has several risk factors for breast cancer including younger age at menarche, older age at her first live birth, a history of first degree relative (mother, sister, daughter) with breast cancer, a history of breast biopsy, and a history of atypical hyperplasia on a breast biopsy.[26] However, some of the risk factors included in the BCRAT, for example, age at menarche and age at first birth, may become less predictive of breast cancer as women age due to the number of years that have passed since these factors influenced older women's estrogen levels.[29–31] In addition, factors that may be more indicative of recent exposure to endogenous estrogens such as obesity,[30] high bone mass,[32] high breast density,[6] postmenopausal hormone therapy,[33] may be more predictive of late-life breast cancer but are not included in the BCRAT. Also, although the model considers a woman's risk of death in 5-years from nonbreast cancer causes, the model assumes that the age-specific hazard of dying from nonbreast cancer causes is the same for all individuals in an age group. However, there is known to be significant variations in older women's health and life expectancy with age.[29]

The model may also overestimate the influence of some risk factors on an older woman's probability of breast cancer. Some of the risk factors included in the model, such as family history of breast cancer and a history of benign breast biopsy, are associated with increased mammography use. Meanwhile, mammography may find some breast cancers before symptoms develop and may even find some cancers that would never have caused problems. Therefore, mammography use may lead to an increased estimated risk of breast cancer among older women who are screened.[34] As a result, some of the increased risk of breast cancer associated with family history and history of breast cancer may be confounded by increased use of mammography among older women with these risk factors. Similarly, whether race is an independent risk factor for late-life breast cancer is uncertain. White women aged 75–84 have a higher incidence of breast cancer than African American women in this age range (Table 8.1), but this difference may also be a result of differential use of mammography by these women.

Due to these limitations, new breast cancer risk models that consider factors associated with late-life breast cancer risk (eg, obesity, higher bone mass) and an older women's individualized competing risk of nonbreast cancer death are needed to better inform decision-making around breast cancer screening for older women.[27] In the meantime, to estimate their risk, older women should consider their age-based risk (see Table 8.1) and slightly increase or decrease their probability of breast cancer based on their family history of breast cancer, their history of benign breast disease, body-mass index, breast density, competing mortality risks, and use of mammography.

UNDERSTANDING THE BENEFITS AND RISKS OF MAMMOGRAPHY SCREENING AMONG OLDER WOMEN

POTENTIAL BENEFITS OF MAMMOGRAPHY SCREENING AMONG OLDER WOMEN

The benefit of mammography screening is finding breast cancer at an early, asymptomatic stage when treatment is expected to be more effective in reducing breast cancer mortality than if treatment were begun later when the cancer presented symptomatically. While mammography screening has been shown to reduce breast cancer mortality by 15% among women in their 40s and by 32% among women in their 60s,[35] whether mammography screening reduces breast cancer mortality for women ≥70 years is not certain. Of the randomized controlled trials of mammography screening, only the Swedish Two-County trial included women ≥70 years and this study only included women up to age 74. A subgroup analysis of women 70–74 years in this trial did not find a significant reduction in breast cancer mortality among women 70–74 years screened every 24–33 months compared to women not offered screening (relative risk: 1.12 95% CI (073–1.72)).[36] To better understand the effectiveness of mammography screening among women 70–73 years, beginning in 2009, the UK's National Health Service Breast Screening Program has randomized the roll-out of extending the age at which women are invited for mammography screening from age 69 to age 73 in a large 10-year cluster randomized controlled trial.[21] It will be several years before the results of this study will be available. In the meantime, investigators have attempted to estimate the effectiveness of mammography screening among women ≥70 years through retrospective cohort studies, simulation models, and by extrapolating data from the randomized controlled trials of mammography screening that included younger women.

Even in the absence of clinical trial data, there are reasons to hypothesize that mammography screening may be beneficial to women ≥70 years. First, breast cancer incidence increases with age and screening tests tend to be more beneficial in a population where the condition is prevalent. Second, the performance (sensitivity, specificity) of mammography screening may improve with age. In the US, the sensitivity of digital mammography screening among women in their 70s has been reported to be around 86–88% with a specificity of 93%, while the sensitivity of mammography screening among women in their 50s is reported to be around 81% with a specificity of 91%.[37,38] In addition, improvements in breast cancer survival seen since 1980 have lagged behind for older women and lower rates of mammography use among women ≥75 years may partially explain this finding. Between 1980 to 1997 the adjusted risk of breast cancer death in newly diagnosed women decreased by 3.6% per year for women <75 years; however, the adjusted risk of breast cancer death decreased only by 1.3% per year for women ≥75 years.[39] This is despite the fact that older women tend to have more favorable tumor characteristics (more estrogen receptor positive (ER+) tumors, lower proliferative rates, and normal p53).[40] Reassurance about one's health may be another potential benefit of mammography for older women; however, there may be more cost-effective ways for physicians to reassure older women about their health.

Retrospective studies evaluating mammography screening among older women

Several retrospective studies have compared breast cancer survival among older women who are screened regularly compared to older women who are not screened or are not screened regularly to better understand mammography's impact on older women's survival.[41–43] Using these methods, McCarthy et al. found that 5-year breast cancer mortality was lower among women 67–84 years (but not for women ≥85 years) that had undergone mammography screening within 2 years of diagnosis compared to women who had not been screened, even after adjusting for comorbidity.[42] McPherson et al. found that among women 65–101 years diagnosed with breast cancer that all-cause mortality was lower among women whose breast cancers were detected through screening compared to women whose breast cancers were detected nonmammographically, except for women with severe or multiple comorbidities.[43] Badgwell et al. found that among women ≥80 years diagnosed with breast cancer, 5-year breast cancer survival was 94% among women who received ≥3 mammograms during the 5 years before breast cancer diagnosis, 88% among women who received 1–2 mammograms in the 5 years before diagnosis, and 82% among women that were not screened.[41] Combined, these studies suggest a survival benefit for mammography screening among older women, especially for older women in good health.

It is important to note, however, that these studies were limited by lead-time, length time, and selection biases inherent in observational data that may explain the positive results.[44] Lead-time bias occurs when screening results in identification of disease earlier than it would have otherwise been detected, thus lengthening survival time between diagnosis and death, without actually altering when death occurs. A retrospective study examining differences in survival following a breast cancer diagnosis among women that were screened compared to women that were not screened that does not adequately account for lead-time bias will overestimate the benefits of mammography screening since a woman whose disease is diagnosed earlier through screening will live longer following diagnosis simply due to earlier detection. Length bias occurs because screening increases the number of slowly progressive or nonprogressive cancers that are identified. These tumors may never become a symptomatic problem (overdiagnosis) but are treated because they are detected. Comparing survival after diagnosis of such tumors to tumors detected nonmammographically will overestimate the benefits of mammography. Selection bias occurs because older women in good health are more likely to choose to be screened and adjusting for comorbidity may not completely account for baseline differences in mortality risk between these women. In fact, the Badgwell et al. study found similar improvements in nonbreast cancer survival among women ≥80 years that were regularly screened compared to women ≥80 years that were not screened suggesting that selection bias may explain the breast cancer survival benefits found to be associated with mammography in this study.[41]

Simulation models

Due to the limitations of retrospective studies, investigators have also attempted to estimate the benefits of mammography screening in older women through microsimulation models. These models make assumptions about the natural history of breast cancer and the efficacy of screening mammography among older women and consider the relationships between breast cancer incidence and mortality, competing causes of death, mammography test characteristics, and breast cancer treatment effects. To understand the effects of continuing biennial and/or annual screening beyond age 69 to age 79 years, Mandelblatt et al. compared results from six different well-established simulation models that use US data. On average, they found that approximately two additional breast cancer deaths are averted and 24 life years gained (LYG) per 1000 older women that continue to be screened.[45] Van Ravesten et al. used three of these microsimulation models to examine the effects of continuing mammography screening from age 74 up to age 96 years. They found that the benefits of screening outweigh the risks up until age 90. At age 74 years, screening results in 7.8 to 11.4 LYG per 1000 women screened which decreases to 4.8 to 7.8 LYG at age 80 years per 1000 women screened and to 1.4 to 2.4 LYG at age 90 per 1000 women screened.[46] By age 90, the life years gained by mammography screening are counterbalanced by the loss of quality of life associated with false positive tests and overdiagnosis. Barratt et al. used a Markov simulation model and national data from Australia on use of mammography, follow-up testing after screening, and on breast cancer and overall mortality to compare women aged 70 who choose to continue biennial screening for 10 years with women who choose to stop being screened at age 69. Similar to Mandelblatt et al., they found that compared to women who stop screening, 2 of 1000 women who choose to continue biennial screening may avoid breast cancer death (6 vs 8 breast cancer deaths per 1000 women who choose to continue screening).[47]

Other studies using simulation models have found that the benefits of mammography screening for older women may be limited to older women with risk factors for breast cancer. Kerlikowske et al. using a Markov simulation model estimated the effects of mammography screening among older women based on their bone density. They found that one of 1064 older women with high bone density that chooses to continue being screened routinely from ages 69 to 79 will avoid breast cancer death. However, they also found that 7143 women with low bone density need to be screened routinely from ages 69 to 79 to prevent one breast cancer death, suggesting that screening is not as effective among older women with low bone density.[48] Schousboe et al. used a Markov microsimulation model to examine the effect of screening women 70–79 years every 3 to 4 years compared to no screening and found that 1–3 fewer women 70–79 years per 1000 die of breast cancer that are screened. However, the benefits of screening were mostly limited to older women with high breast density, a history of breast biopsy, and/or a family history of breast cancer.[49] In addition, in a cost-effective analysis using simulation modeling, Mandelblatt et al. found that screening women to age 79 or to a life expectancy of 9.5 years is cost-effective, especially for older women at higher risk of breast cancer.[50]

Combined, the data from modeling studies suggest that approximately 2 women ≥70 years that choose to continue to be screened with mammography annually or biennially for 10 years may avoid breast cancer death and that the benefits of screening may be greater for older women at higher risk of breast cancer. It is important to note; however, that these modeling studies must make several assumptions about the natural history of breast cancer and the efficacy of mammography screening among older women due to the lack of available data on these outcomes for older women.[45] Therefore, there is more uncertainty when using these models to estimate the effects of mammography screening among older women than for younger women. When breast cancer is assumed to be slower growing and higher rates of overdiagnosis of breast cancer as a result of mammography screening are used in the models, simulation models find that mammography screening is less effective among women ≥70 years.[51]

Other methods for estimating the efficacy of mammography screening among older women

Investigators have also examined incidence rates of advance stage breast cancers before and after implementation of screening within a population to better understand the benefits of screening older women. If mammography screening is effective then advanced stage cancers should decrease in a population while early stage cancers increase after screening is implemented.[52] Using this approach, investigators in the Netherlands examined the incidence of early and advanced stage breast cancer before and after the implementation of mass screening among women aged 70–75 years which occurred in 1998 in the Netherlands. They found that after screening was implemented the incidence of early stage cancers increased by 1.46% while the incidence of advanced stage cancers decreased only by 0.88%. For each "prevented" advanced stage tumor there were 19.7 overdiagnosed breast cancers or breast cancers that would not otherwise have caused problems or symptoms during an older woman's lifetime.[53] Critics of this method of assessing the benefits of screening argue that it overestimates overdiagnosis because it does not adequately account for lead-time bias.

To understand the time-lag to benefitting from mammography screening among older women, Lee et al. examined pooled data from five of the randomized controlled trials evaluating mammography screening.[54] They excluded trials that were considered biased in a Cochrane review of randomized controlled trials of mammography screening and they excluded trials that did not include women >50 years. They found that on average 10.7 years passed before one death was prevented for 1000 women ≥50 years screened with mammography. Therefore, they concluded that mammography screening is most appropriate for older women with >10 year life expectancy.

Summary

Based on the available existing data, approximately 2 women out of 1000 age ≥70 years with life expectancy greater than 10 years may avoid death from breast cancer that chooses to continue being screened with mammography biennially for 10 years. These benefits may be more likely for older women at high risk of breast cancer such as older women with a family history of breast cancer or a history of benign breast biopsy.

RISKS OF MAMMOGRAPHY SCREENING AMONG OLDER WOMEN

Potential harms of mammography screening include anxiety resulting from false positive tests, false reassurance from an erroneously negative test, diagnosis of tumors that otherwise would not have shown up in an older woman's lifetime (overdiagnosis), and complications from work-up and/or treatment of cancer.[29] Among women ≥75 years who undergo biennial screening the cumulative probability of a false-positive mammogram over 10 years ranges from 12–27%[37,47,55–57] and the risk nearly doubles if women are screened annually (48% of women 75 to 89 years screened annually will experience a false positive mammogram).[55] False positive recalls tend to be lower outside the US.[47] While follow-up tests such as diagnostic mammograms and breast ultrasounds are generally low-risk procedures, approximately 10–20% of older women that experience a false positive mammogram will undergo a benign breast biopsy[47,56,57] and this procedure can cause distress, scarring and infection.[58] Among 94 US women ≥65 years that experienced a benign breast biopsy, 76% (71/94) reported a negative psychological consequence (eg, lack of sleep) from screening at the time of breast biopsy[59] and 39% (37/94) reported that they were still experiencing a negative psychological consequence of screening six months after their breast biopsy. A stereotactic breast biopsy may be particularly burdensome to older women, due to the amount of time and positioning required to be on the biopsy table, especially for older women with osteoarthritis.[59] Also, older women who rely on family for transportation may feel that they are burdening family for travel to the breast biopsy. Furthermore, experience with a false positive mammogram has been shown conversely to increase older women's enthusiasm for screening[60] and to increase health care utilization in general.[61]

Overdiagnosis

Overdiagnosis is the major harm of cancer screening for older women since it leads to diagnosis and treatment of tumors that otherwise would never have caused problems in an older woman's lifetime. A breast cancer diagnosis may be particularly burdensome to an older woman due to increasing comorbidity,[62] frailty,[63] declining social networks,[64] less access to medical information,[65] decreased use of counseling,[66] more experience with loss,[66] and lower socioeconomic status.[67] Older women are also more likely to experience adverse effects from breast cancer treatments. Despite this, few studies have attempted to estimate the proportion of screen-detected tumors among women ≥70 years that are likely overdiagnosed.[68] Quantifying overdiagnosis regardless of a woman's age remains a challenge. Estimates of overdiagnosis vary from 0 to 50% of screen-detected breast cancers but all estimates are subject to bias and there is debate about the best methodology.[68,69]

An easy to conceptualize method for estimating overdiagnosis is examining the persistent excess incidence of breast cancer over long-term follow-up among women that were randomized to be screened with mammography compared to women that were not randomized to be screened in the screening trials. Using this methodology, Welch and Black estimated that 24% (95% CI 20–28%) of screen-detected cancers were cases of overdiagnosis based on 15 years of follow-up after the 10 year trial period of the Malmo mammography trial.[70] A randomized controlled trial of mammography screening in Canada of women 40–59 years reported an overdiagnosis rate of 22% for all screen-detected invasive breast cancers after 25 years follow-up.[71] The US rate of overdiagnosis has been estimated to be 22–31% of all breast cancers diagnosed when comparing breast cancer incidence before and after screening was implemented.[72] Combined, these data suggest that around one-fourth of screen-detected breast cancers are overdiagnosed. However, since older women tend to have less aggressive tumors with more favorable biologic characteristics (eg, greater percent of estrogen (ER) positive tumors) and more competing mortality risks, overdiagnosis is thought to increase with age.[45] Furthermore, detection of ductal carcinoma in situ (DCIS), a noninvasive form of breast cancer, which accounts for approximately 16% of all screen-detected breast cancers among women 70–84 years,[73] likely represents overdiagnosis. This is because only about a third of cases of DCIS are thought to develop into invasive cancer after 10–15 years follow-up[74,75] and less than 5% of women diagnosed with DCIS will die of breast cancer within

30 years after diagnosis.[76] Meanwhile, the average life expectancy for women aged 75 is 12.9 years, 9.7 years for women aged 80, and 6.9 years for women aged 85.[77]

Using simulation models, van Ravensteyn et al. estimated changes in the rate of overdiagnosis for screen-detected tumors by age. They found that the models estimated 5 to 32% of women 50–74 years that undergo biennial screening are overdiagnosed, compared to 14–36% of women at age 80, and 28 to 41% of women at age 90 years.[46] Barratt et al. also used simulation modeling to estimate overdiagnosis among older women. They found that 41 out of 1000 women aged 70 that continue to be screened biennially for 10 years will be diagnosed with breast cancer (including DCIS) compared to 24 women who choose to stop being screened (37% more breast cancers detected through screening). Excluding DCIS, they found that 35 women that choose to be screened for the next 10 years will be diagnosed with breast cancer (28% more invasive breast cancers detected compared to women who choose to stop being screened).[47]

Summary

Based on available data, it is reasonable to estimate that 10–30% of women ≥70 years who continue biennial screening will experience a false positive test and 10–20% of these women will undergo a benign breast biopsy which is often a stressful experience for older women. In addition, approximately 30% of screen-detected breast cancers among older women are likely overdiagnosed. If we estimate, based on SEER data, that 44 women out of 1000 aged 75 will be diagnosed with breast cancer over 10 years then approximately 13 (30%) of these women will be diagnosed with a breast cancer that otherwise would not have caused problems in their lifetimes (overdiagnosis). However, since it is not possible to know which screen-detected tumors will progress and which will not, nearly all older women undergo treatment for breast cancer.

EFFICACY OF BREAST CANCER TREATMENT AMONG OLDER WOMEN

Mammography screening will only be beneficial if there is effective treatment available early in the natural course of the disease that results in a better prognosis than treatment given after symptoms develop. However, few breast cancer treatment trials included women aged 70 years and older, especially those with multiple comorbidities. Consequently, the benefit to risk ratio of some breast cancer treatments is not known, making decision-making around treatment also challenging for older women, especially those with comorbidity.[78]

In the US, 97% of women ≥67 years with DCIS or early-stage breast cancer are initially treated with surgery, usually lumpectomy.[79] Since mastectomy and lumpectomy have equivalent survival outcomes; mastectomy is generally reserved for older women with large primary tumors, those who have previously undergone breast irradiation, or those who have multicentric disease.[80] However, some older women with small early stage tumors prefer to be treated with mastectomy so as not to have to undergo multiple surgeries (20% of women ≥70 years will need more surgery after lumpectomy[81]) and to avoid having to decide whether or not to be treated with radiotherapy since radiotherapy is generally not recommended to older women after mastectomy. Many (41%) women ≥70 years experience complications after breast cancer surgery (eg, seromas or infection); however, only 6.5% of older women experience serious complications that warrant delays in discharge, readmission to a hospital, or additional procedures.[82] However, the risk of complications after breast surgery increases with age.[83]

In the UK, 40% of women ≥70 years diagnosed with early stage breast cancer choose to be treated with primary endocrine therapy (PET) to avoid surgery.[84] However, PET is associated with increased local recurrence rates and worse survival among women with ≥5year life expectancy. Therefore, experts recommend limiting the use of PET to women with less than 2 year life expectancy.[85–87]

In addition to surgical treatment, older women diagnosed with early-stage estrogen receptor positive (ER+) breast cancers treated with radiotherapy combined with endocrine therapy (eg, tamoxifen or aromatase inhibitors (AIs)) experience lower risk of local-regional recurrence at 10 years (from 10% to 2%) but no differences in survival compared to women treated with endocrine therapy alone after surgery.[88] Therefore, experts recommend that women ≥70 years with early stage ER+ breast cancers be offered the choice to forgo radiotherapy (RT) after lumpectomy. Despite this, many women ≥70 years with early stage, ER+, breast cancers still receive radiation therapy (70% of women 70–74, 65% of women 75–79, 50% of women 80–84, and 25% of women ≥85 receive radiation therapy after lumpectomy).[89] Meanwhile, radiation therapy can cause fatigue, breast pain, and edema and increases the risk of ischemic heart disease among older women.[90] Also, traveling to a medical center for daily radiation treatments can be burdensome to older women who may be dependent on family for transportation.

Increasingly, older women are offered alternatives to conventional radiotherapy including hypofractionated radiotherapy or accelerated partial breast irradiation (APBI).[91,92] Hypofractionated radiotherapy consists of fewer but higher-dose fractions of radiation generally delivered over 3 weeks rather than the 5 weeks required for conventional radiotherapy. APBI includes techniques that deliver radiotherapy locally to breast tissue with external beam radiation, intraoperative radiotherapy, brachytherapy using multiple interstitial catheters, or intra-cavitary brachytherapy using a balloon catheter. APBI reduces the volume of breast tissue irradiated; it is still considered investigational.[93]

Endocrine therapy for at least 5 years is universally recommended for women ≥70 years with ER+ breast cancers because it reduces breast cancer recurrence by 30–50% at 10 years and improves survival.[94] However, around 20% of older women never initiate endocrine therapy.[95,96] Of those that initiate endocrine therapy, around 75% receive AIs and around 25% receive tamoxifen[95,96]; however, 50% discontinue endocrine therapy before 5 years,[96,97] usually due to side effects.[98,99] Tamoxifen can cause hot flashes and can increase an older woman's risk of endometrial cancer and thromboembolism.[100] Aromatase inhibitors can cause joint pain, myalgias, heart disease, and fractures and may be associated with temporary cognitive decline.[100,101]

Chemotherapy improves survival for healthy, older women with lymph node-positive or hormone receptor-negative invasive cancers.[102] There are limited data to make chemotherapy recommendations for women ≥70 years with early stage breast cancer; however, chemotherapy may be offered to older women in excellent health.[103] Toxicity and mortality from chemotherapy increase with age[104] and short-term cognitive decline may also occur in older women following chemotherapy.[105]

While many older women respond well to breast cancer treatment, it is important to consider the harms of treatment when deciding whether or not to screen these women with mammography since many screen-detected cancers among older women are cases of overdiagnosis.

ESTIMATING REMAINING LIFE EXPECTANCY FOR OLDER WOMEN

Due to the approximate 10-year lag time before an older woman that is screened may avoid breast cancer death as a result of being screened, the American Geriatrics Society and the Society of General Internal Medicine Choosing Wisely campaigns recommend not screening older women for breast cancer who have <10 year life expectancy.[20] The rationale is that while screening may reduce cancer deaths, the mortality benefit occurs years after the test is performed. Meanwhile, older women are at risk of experiencing harms from breast cancer screening immediately and the chance of harm increases as women age and become more frail.[16] Women with <10 year life expectancy are unlikely to live long enough to derive the distant benefit from screening and the balance of potential benefits and harms does not favor recommending screening to these patients.[20]

Since consideration of patient life expectancy is key to high quality screening decisions, several tools are now available to help primary care physicians (PCPs) estimate patient life expectancy when deciding on cancer screening. The Lee-Schonberg index (available at www.ePrognosis.org) considers a patient's age, sex, body mass index, function, mobility, history of cancer, diabetes, emphysema, heart failure and smoking, number of hospitalizations in the past year, and perceived health.[106–109] Adults with >50% risk of mortality within 10 years based on their health score on this index are considered to have an estimated life expectancy <10 years.[108] In addition, Walter and Covinsky using data from 1997 US life tables calculated the upper, middle, and lower quartiles of life expectancy for US adults ≥70 year stratified by sex and age [110] (these tables were recently updated using data from 2008 US Life Tables – Fig. 8.1).[29] They recommend that clinicians estimate whether a patient is in the top, middle, or lower quartile of health for his/her age group and then refer to these stratified life tables to obtain an estimate of patient life expectancy. For example, for a 75 year old woman in poor health, her PCP would use the life expectancy information from the life tables for a 75 year old women in the lowest quartile of life expectancy or 7.4 years and would not recommend screening to this women.[29]

Cho et al. adjusted US life table survival probabilities for adults aged 66 and older without a history of cancer based on the presence or absence of comorbidities.[111] Based on a patient's age, sex, and whether or not they have low, medium, or high comorbidity a clinician may refer to the tables created by Cho et al. to estimate their patients' life expectancy. For example, they found that a 75 year old woman with diabetes has a life expectancy of 11.4 years, while a 75-year old woman with COPD has a life expectancy of 10.2 years, and a 75-year old woman with congestive heart failure (CHF) has a life expectancy of 7.0 years. Based on these data a clinician may choose to recommend screening to a 75-year old woman with diabetes since she has greater than 10 year life expectancy but not to a 75-year old women with CHF since she has less than 10 life expectancy. Similarly, Landsdorp-Vogelaar et al. examined the age at which women should stop being screened for cancer based on the presence or absence of comorbidity to experience the same balance of benefits and risks from screening a woman aged 74 in average health.[112] They found that women with severe comorbidity (eg, those with COPD, chronic renal disease, dementia, CHF, or multiple comorbidities) should stop being screened at age 66 while women with moderate comorbidity (cardiovascular disease, diabetes, or combinations of diabetes with MI, ulcer, or rheumatologic disease) should stop being screened at age 72. They found that women with mild comorbidity (history of MI, ulcer, rheumatologic disease) should stop being screened at age 74 and women with no comorbidity should stop being screened at age 76 to experience the same benefits and risks as screening the average 74-year old US woman.

Using any of these tools or guides combined with clinical judgement may help a clinician estimate whether or not their patient has <10 year life expectancy. Based on patient life expectancy, a clinician may then decide whether or not to recommend mammography screening to an older woman.

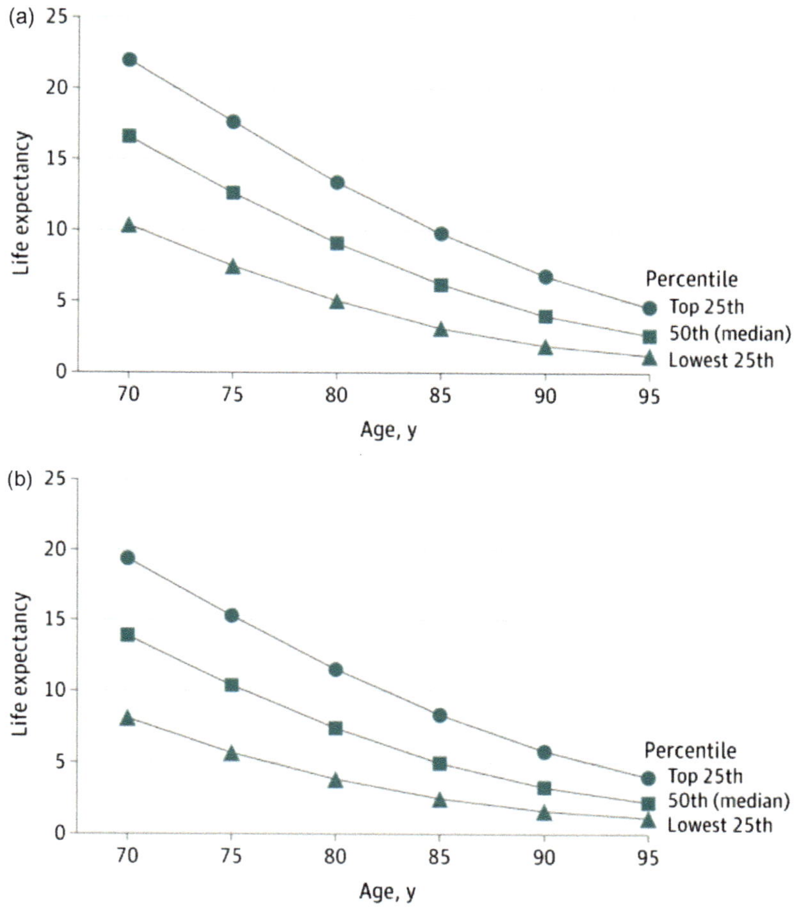

FIGURE 8.1

Upper, middle, and lower quartiles of life expectancy for women and men at selected ages. (a) Women. (b) Men.

*Data are from the 2008 Life Tables of the United States. Reprinted with Permission from J Am Med Assoc 2014;***311***(13):1336–47. doi:10.1001/jama.2014.2834.*

SCREENING AND COGNITIVE IMPAIRMENT

In general, mammography screening should not be recommended to older women with dementia.[113] On average women live 3 to 12 years after being diagnosed with dementia; therefore, the majority of women diagnosed with dementia do not have adequate life expectancy to benefit from screening.[114] Also, the harms of screening may be greater for these women since they may be more frightened by procedures that they cannot understand and may have more difficulty complying with treatment. Despite these concerns, one study found that 18% of older women with severe cognitive impairment underwent mammography screening even though their median life expectancy was 3.3 years.[115] In some cases, a family member or surrogate will ask about mammography for an older woman with dementia. In these cases, it is important for clinicians to thoughtfully discuss the very unlikely chance of benefit with the much greater chance of harm for these women.

SCREENING INTERVALS FOR OLDER WOMEN

While it is not certain that screening women ≥70 year for breast cancer with mammography results in a mortality benefit, data increasingly suggest that if an older women continues to be screened than she should be screened less frequently than annually. With age the biology of tumors shifts to lower risk lesions that grow more slowly and screening tends to preferentially identify lower risk lesions, making 2-year screening intervals for mammography more reasonable than annual.[52] In studies of older women, irrespective of comorbidity, biennial screening is associated with similar reductions in breast cancer mortality as annual screening but lower incidence of false positive tests, breast biopsies, and overdiagnosis.[45,55] The appropriate frequency of screening older women with mammography may also depend on an older woman's breast density, family history of breast cancer, and history of breast biopsy. Among women aged 70–79, with low breast density and no additional breast cancer risk factors, mammography every 3 to 4 years rather than every 2 years was found to be cost-effective.[49] If an older woman chooses to continue to be screened it is important to let her know that screening every other year is associated with the same benefits as being screened every year but with fewer harms.

OTHER SCREENING MODALITIES

CLINICAL BREAST EXAM

There are no data to inform clinicians whether they should stop performing clinical breast exams (CBEs) when they stop recommending mammography screening to older women. Since breast density decreases with age, a CBE is likely to have greater sensitivity and specificity among older women than younger women. Also, CBE is likely associated with less overdiagnosis than mammography screening since a tumor has to be large enough to be palpable for detection. Clinical trials are needed to determine whether CBE leads to reduced breast cancer mortality among older women who choose to stop being screened with mammography. In the meantime, the USPSTF states that there is insufficient evidence to recommend for or against CBEs. The American Geriatrics Society recommends that CBEs be performed periodically.

DIGITAL MAMMOGRAPHY AND COMPUTER-AIDED DETECTION (CAD)

In 2001, the US Congress extended Medicare coverage to digital mammography and computer-aided detection (CAD) even though the benefits of digital mammography compared to film were only noted among premenopausal women, women with dense breasts, and women <50 years.[116] Furthermore, among women 67 to 89 years CAD is associated with increased DCIS detection but not increased detection of invasive disease.[117] CAD is also associated with increased diagnostic testing.[117] Despite these limitations, digital mammography screening increased from 2.0% in 2001–2002 to 29.8% in 2008–2009 among Medicare beneficiaries and CAD increased from 3.2% to 33.1%.[118] During the same time period breast ultrasound use only increased from 4.0 to 4.9% and MRI use only increased from 0.03 to 0.3%, likely due to the fact that these screening modalities are not covered by Medicare. Overall, there was a 47% increase in per-capita costs associated with breast cancer screening among Medicare beneficiaries from 2001 to 2009 without a statistically or clinically significant difference in the incidence of early-stage breast cancer.[118] The additional cost of screening without benefits to screening efficacy leads to mammography screening being less cost-effective for older women.

DIGITAL BREAST TOMOSYNTHESIS

While digital breast tomosynthesis is being rapidly diffused into clinical care, it is not clear if the benefits of tomosynthesis are the same for women of all ages. One study that examined the effect of breast tomosynthesis by age found significant reductions in recall after mammography screening for women aged 40–69 but not for women aged 70 and older.[119] Meanwhile, digital breast tomosynthesis increases the radiation dose that older women are exposed to and the costs of screening.

It is important that the effects of new technologies used to screen for breast cancer at the population level be considered before wide dissemination in order to maximize benefits and minimize harm for older women.

FACTORS INFLUENCING OLDER WOMEN'S SCREENING DECISIONS

Although guidelines recommend that older women be informed of the benefits and risks of mammography screening before being screened, few (21%) women ≥75 year report having discussed the risks of mammography with their clinicians.[120] Physicians report feeling ill-prepared to discuss the benefits and risks of mammography screening with older women due to the lack of clinical trial data on outcomes of screening older women and because these conversations can be challenging and time consuming.[121,122] As a result 70 to 86% of primary care physicians report that they recommend mammography screening to healthy women aged 80 years old.[123]

Patient brochures and public health messages about mammography screening also tend to be uniformly positive, since the dominant approach has been to promote the uptake of screening. In this environment, it is not surprising that many older women overestimate the benefits of mammography screening, are unaware of the lag-time to benefit, and underestimate the harms.[124,125] In fact, 70% of adults report that they plan to continue cancer screening as long as they live.[125] Older women view continuation of cancer screening as something that is done automatically and that is morally obligatory.[124]

While a physician's recommendation is the strongest driver of screening among older women,[24] older women are also influenced by their perceived risk of breast cancer, their access to mammography screening, a family member/friend's experience with breast cancer, and/or a family member/friend's (especially daughter's) recommendation to be screened. Older women with a family history of breast cancer and/or a history of benign breast biopsy are more likely to choose to be screened.[24] Few older women report that they consider their health or life expectancy in deciding whether or not to be screened.[122] For many older women undergoing mammography is not perceived to be a decision, they simply receive a reminder card that it is time to come for their annual mammogram. Others are automatically scheduled for an annual mammogram at the time of their last appointment.

Primary care physicians (PCPs), more so than patients, tend to consider patient age, health, function, and life expectancy when deciding whether or not to screen older women.[122,124,126] Clinicians also consider a patient's living situation, family support, personality (patients with higher anxiety tend to be more likely to be screened),[127] expectations to be screened,[127] previous screening behavior, proximity to cancer treatment sites, and availability of treatment for breast cancer. Some clinicians note that since endocrine therapy is a treatment option for frail patients that they offer screening to older women since there is treatment available if a breast cancer is diagnosed.[122] Screening rates also tend to be higher among older women who see their PCPs frequently[128]; likely because more time with a physician gives physicians more opportunity to discuss screening with older adults and physicians tend to highlight the benefits of screening. Geography also affects screening rates among older women. Higher numbers of PCPs, mammographic facilities, and radiologists per 100,000 residents in an area are associated with higher mammography screening rates for women with limited life expectancy.[128] In addition, physician specialty is associated with different screening recommendations for older women. Obstetricians/gynecologists have 1.69 times the odds the odds of overrecommending screening to older women with terminal illness compared to general practitioners.[123]

Physicians are also influenced by the doctor–patient relationship. Physicians avoid talking about stopping screening with some older women because they fear that such discussions may result in loss of patient trust and negatively impact the doctor–patient relationship.[124] Physicians may also recommend screening to older women due to concerns about litigation if a cancer diagnosis is missed. However, medical-legal experts recommend against reflexively ordering cancer screening to avoid liability risks.[129] Instead, these experts recommend that physicians clearly communicate and document the rationale for the recommended screening strategy and which guideline they are following.[129]

DISCUSSING THE BENEFITS AND RISK OF SCREENING WITH OLDER WOMEN

RECOMMENDATIONS FOR DISCUSSING STOPPING MAMMOGRAPHY SCREENING WITH OLDER WOMEN

To improve the quality of discussions about stopping cancer screening, experts recommend that physicians: (1) initiate and reinitiate discussions about stopping screening with older women; (2) inform older women of the benefits and risks of screening; (3) estimate patient life expectancy and how it affects the ratio of benefits to harms of screening; (4) clarify patients' values around the likely outcomes of being screened or not screened; and (5) focus on health promotion measures that benefit older women within their estimated life expectancy.[29,130]

Physicians may need to initiate discussions about stopping cancer screening more than once and a few years before they actually plan to recommend stopping screening to prepare patients and to set up the expectation that there will be a point when the harms of screening outweigh the potential benefits. While there are few data available for primary care physicians (PCPs) on how to approach talking about prognosis and/or life expectancy with older adults, PCPs may use the calculators on www.eprognosis.org or the Walter et al. stratified life tables (Fig. 8.1) in conjunction with their clinical judgment to

Table 8.3 Pros and Cons of Screening Mammography Among Older Women

Pros	Cons
A mammogram is more likely to find breast cancer when it is small, improving an older woman's chances of only needing a minor surgery.	A mammogram may find a breast cancer that would never have caused problems or symptoms in a woman's lifetime.
Getting a mammogram may lower an older woman's chances of dying from breast cancer.	Getting a mammogram may result in older women getting additional tests (for example, additional mammograms, ultrasounds, and breast biopsies) or treatments. Some of these tests or treatments may cause harm.
Getting a mammogram may help an older woman feel good about her health.	Getting a mammogram may be uncomfortable or cause anxiety.

*Reprinted with Permission from J Am Med Assoc 2014;***311***(13):1336–47. doi:10.1001/jama.2014.2834.*

estimate a patient's risk of mortality in 10 years. Once a PCP has estimated a patient's life expectancy, the PCP can better frame the ratio of benefits to risks of mammography for a patient. Framing cancer screening conversations in terms of increasing harms in relation to decreasing benefits has been found to be most acceptable to older patients and may maintain or promote trust more than citing national guideline recommendations to stop screening based on age cutoffs.[29,124]

Time during a clinic visit should also be used to help patients understand that a decision to stop cancer screening does not mean abandoning health promotion, but rather refocusing health promotion on interventions most likely to benefit patients over a shorter time frame. For example, few older women regularly exercise, yet exercise has been shown to have many late-life benefits including maintaining functional independence. As life expectancy declines, a woman's health may be helped more by focusing on health promotion measures such as exercise, select immunizations, and medication reconciliation rather than mammography screening.

In summary, women ≥70 years should be reminded that there is a choice that needs to be made about whether or not to continue being screened with mammography. For those with <10 year life expectancy, recommendations to stop mammography screening should be framed around how a woman's health problems increase the harms of screening (eg, overdiagnosis) and the need to shift the focus to interventions likely to be beneficial over a shorter time frame (eg, falls prevention, depression screening). For women with ≥10 year life expectancy, screening discussions should elicit from women their values around the outcomes of screening and whether the woman feels the benefits outweigh the risks. Table 8.3 presents a summary of the benefits and risks of mammography screening for older women that can be used when counseling older women.

DECISION AIDS ON MAMMOGRAPHY SCREENING FOR OLDER WOMEN (TABLE 8.4)

Fortunately, decision aids are now available to help inform older women of the benefits and risks of mammography screening and to clarify their values about whether or not to be screened. Decision aids are educational tools that provide detailed and personalized focus on options and outcomes of a decision.[134] To improve older women's decision-making, Schonberg et al. developed and evaluated a

Table 8.4 Tools to Help Patients and Providers With Decision Making Around Mammography Screening for Older Women

Decision Aid	Description	Evaluation	Available at:
A Mammography Decision Aid for Women ≥ 75 years[131]	Includes information on breast cancer risk, likely outcomes if screened or not screened over 5 years, the impact of health/life expectancy on outcomes, and a description of breast cancer treatment options. It also includes a values clarification exercise.	Tested in a pretest-posttest trial of 45 women seen at a Boston academic practice. Found to increase older women's knowledge of the benefits and risks of screening and led to fewer intending to be screened, especially those with short life expectancy.	As supplementary material of referenced publication[131] or by emailing the author at: mschonbe@bidmc.harvard.edu A decision aid based on this tool was developed for older women in New Zealand and is available at: http://nzbcf.org.nz/BREASTCANCER/BreastAwareness/Women70-plus/Screen70plus.aspx
A Mammography Decision Aid for Women Aged 70 Years[132]	This decision aid was designed to help women at age 70 years decide whether or not to continue mammography screening. Includes information on likely outcomes if screened or not screened over 10 years, information on breast cancer risk, and a description of how health may affect outcomes	A large randomized controlled trial of 734 Australian women found that women who used the decision aid were more informed and better able to make an informed choice about whether or not to continue mammography screening.	http://www.psych.usyd.edu.au/cemped/docs/Mammogram_DecisionAid.pdf
ePrognosis Cancer Screening App for iphones and ipads and ePrognosis Cancer Screening Webpage	This decision aid uses prognostic information about older adults to help clinicians and older adults decide if cancer screening is likely to be more beneficial or harmful. The app assesses patient age, gender, body mass index, symptoms, and functional impairment to calculate a mortality risk to help determine if a patient is likely to live >5–10 years.	The app/web page has not been tested in a clinical trial. However, the mortality indices used to estimate life expectancy have been validated.[106,108]	The app is available for free downloading at: https://itunes.apple.com/us/app/eprognosis-cancer-screening/id714539993?mt=8 The web page is available at: http://cancerscreening.eprognosis.org/
Comorbidity-Adjusted Life Expectancy	Presents life expectancy of Women aged 66 and Older stratified by race and the presence or absence of comorbidity (none, low/medium, high) including specific comorbidities (Diabetes, COPD, Congestive Heart Failure).	Effect on screening decisions has not been evaluated.	Table 8.3 in the manuscript shows life expectancy by gender, race, and comorbidity.[111]
Decision Aid for Providers in Making Recommendations About Screening in Older Women[133]	Includes the Walter et al. life tables. Asks physicians to estimate patient life expectancy and if patient has >5 year life expectancy and wants to be screened than encourages physicians to recommend screening.	Providers evaluated the Decision Aid and felt that it would have helped them make recommendations in hypothetical scenarios	The decision aid is available in the manuscript.[133]

decision aid on mammography screening for women ≥75 years.[131] The decision aid includes information on an older woman's breast cancer risk, life expectancy, likely outcomes if screened or not screened for breast cancer, competing mortality risks, breast cancer treatments usually offered to older women, and a values clarification exercise.[131] In a pretest–postest trial of 45 women ≥75 years who received primary care at an academic medical center in Boston, the decision aid was found to increase older women's knowledge of the benefits and risks of mammography, help clarify their values, and led to fewer women intending to be screened, especially those with <10 year life expectancy. In addition to this decision aid, Table 8.4 presents a list of currently available tools to help older women with decision-making around mammography screening.

QUALITY METRICS

Currently, US quality measures for breast cancer screening encourage screening women up to age 75. A physician who appropriately discourages screening in a 74 year old with limited life expectancy could be penalized in this system that uses an age-based "one-size-fits-all" quality measure.[135] The current system discourages a personalized approach to cancer screening. Therefore, US quality measures for cancer screening need to change their focus to encourage informed discussions rather than tallying the proportion of adults that have received a screening test during a specified time period. A more appropriate quality measures would be quantifying the proportion of women that have been informed of the benefits and burdens of mammography screening.[135] In European countries, Canada, and Australia, primary care physicians are encouraged to provide objective, balanced, and easily accessible information on breast cancer screening to their patients to allow them to make the best possible decisions.[136]

SIMILARITIES TO OTHER CANCER SCREENING TESTS

Much of the discussion in this chapter around whether or not to screen older women for breast cancer is also true for considering whether or not to screen older adults for other cancers (eg, colon cancer) or for other diseases. When deciding whether or not to screen an older adult for cancer it is important to consider the individual's risk of disease, life expectancy, and their values and preferences based on an informed understanding of the likely outcomes if screened or not screened. In the case of screening for colon cancer, similar to mammography screening, it is estimated that 1000 older adults need to be screened for colon cancer for one to avoid colon cancer death in 10 years.[54] Therefore, guidelines recommend that older adults with less than 10 year life expectancy not be screened for colon cancer and that decisions around whether or not to screen older adults with >10 year life expectancy for colon cancer be individualized. In addition, there are decision aids available to help older adults decide whether or not to undergo colon cancer screening.[137]

QUESTIONS/FUTURE WORK

Decision making around mammography screening for older women is challenging. To better inform these decisions, new breast cancer prediction models are needed to help older women understand their risk of breast cancer beyond their risk based on age alone. Also, while there are tools available to estimate older women's life expectancy, few of these tools have been validated in a clinical setting. In addition, there is limited data to guide primary care physicians on how to talk to older women about their prognosis in the context of making decisions around mammography screening. While, new technologies are continuously emerging to screen women for breast cancer, these technologies are often incorporated into clinical practice without knowledge of how they will impact the benefits and risks of screening older women. As a result, implementation of these technologies often results in reducing the cost-effectiveness of screening older women. Therefore, it is important to study the effect of new screening technologies among older women before implementation. While decision aids have been developed to help older women with decision-making around screening, whether these tools impact older women's screening decisions is still uncertain and there are few data on how to successfully implement these tools in practice. In addition, since overdiagnosis is the major harm of screening older women, future studies should aim to obtain better estimates of overdiagnosis from screening older women. Data are also needed to better understand the impact of overdiagnosis on older women's quality of life to better inform simulation models estimating the benefits and harms of mammography screening among older women.

CONCLUSIONS

There are few data from clinical trials on the efficacy of mammography screening for women aged 70 years and older. Data from simulation models and retrospective observational studies suggest that screening may benefit women ≥70 years with >10 year life expectancy. However, many women ≥70 years experience harms from being screened including being diagnosed and treated for a breast cancer that would not otherwise have shown up in their lifetime. Risk of overdiagnosis increases as women age and life expectancy decreases. To make informed decisions around mammography screening, older women need to be informed of the lag-time to benefitting from mammography screening and the chance of experiencing immediate harm from being screened. Decision aids are now available to help older women understand the trade-offs that must be weighed when deciding whether or not to be screened. This process of individualized decision-making should be a measure of quality of care rather than whether or not a woman of a certain age receives a screening mammogram.

LIST OF ACRONYMS AND ABBREVIATIONS

CAD	Computer Aided Detection
CBE	Clinical Breast Exam
CHF	Congestive Heart Failure
COPD	Chronic Obstructive Pulmonary Disease
ER+	Estrogen Receptor Positive
LYG	Life years gained
PCP	Primary Care Physician
US	Unites States
USPSTF	United States Preventive Services Task Force

REFERENCES

1. *Data on seer (surveillance, epidemiology and end results) cancer statistics* [cited 09.07.15]. SEER data 1973–2012. Available from: <http://seer.cancer.gov>.
2. Canadian Cancer Statistics. *Table 1.1. Lifetime probability of developing cancer overall and by age group, Canada 2009*. Available at: <http://www.cancer.ca/~/media/cancer.ca/CW/cancer%20information/cancer%20 101/Canadian%20cancer%20statistics/Canadian-Cancer-Statistics-2014-EN.pdf>; 2014 [accessed 11.08.15].
3. Breast Cancer in Australia an Overview. *Table D2.1 Incidence of breast cancer, by age at diagnosis, females, Australia*. Available at <http://www.aihw.gov.au/WorkArea/DownloadAsset.aspx?id=10737423006>; 2008. [accessed 11.08.15].
4. IBIS Breast Cancer Risk Evaluation Tool. *Table 1. Breast cancer rates (per year, 100K) used in the models*. Available at: <http://www.ems-trials.org/riskevaluator>; 2015 [accessed 11.08.15].
5. Gotzsche PC, Nielsen M. Screening for breast cancer with mammography. *Cochrane Databse Syst Rev* 2009;**4** CD001877.
6. Vacek PM, Skelly JM, Geller BM. Breast cancer risk assessment in women aged 70 and older. *Breast Cancer Res Treat* 2011;**130**(1):291–9.
7. Oeffinger KC, Fontham ETH, Etzioni R, Herzig A, Michaelson JS, Shin YT, et al. Breast cancer screening for women at average risk: 2015 Guideline update from the american cancer society. *JAMA* 2015;**314**(15): 1599–614.
8. Bulletin ACoOaGP Breast Cancer Screening. Clinical management guidelines for obstetrician-gynecologists. *Obstet Gynecol* 2011;**118**(2):372–82.
9. Radiology ACo. *ACR practice guideline for the performance of screening and diagnostic mammography*.
10. Network. NCC. *Breast cancer screening and diagnosis. Version 2*. [cited 23.06.15]. Available from: <http://www.nccn.org/professionals/physician_gls/pdf/breast-screening.pdf>; 2013.
11. Force USPST. *Draft recommendation statement. breast cancer: screening*. [cited 23.06.15]. Available from: <http://www.uspreventiveservicestaskforce.org/Page/Document/RecommendationStatementDraft/breast-cancer-screening1>; 2015.
12. Warner E, Heisey R, Carroll JC. Applying the 2011 Canadian guidelines for breast cancer screening in practice. *Can Med Assoc J* 2012;**184**(16):1803–7.
13. System. NH. *NHS breast screening programme: extending the screening age range*. [cited 23.06.15]. Available from: <http://www.cancerscreening.nhs.uk/breastscreen/over-70.html>; 2015.
14. National Institute for Public Health and the Environment. *Ministry of Health WaS. Screening for breast cancer*. [cited 23.06.15]. Available from: <http://www.rivm.nl/en/Documents_and_publications/Common_and_Present/Brochures/Disease_Prevention_and_Healthcare/Breast_cancer_screening_programme>; 2015.
15. Practitioners TRACoG. 9.3 Breast Cancer. *Guidelines for preventive activities in general practice* [cited 23.06.15]; 8th. Available from: <http://www.racgp.org.au/your-practice/guidelines/redbook/early-detection-of-cancers/breast-cancer/>; 2015.
16. Health AGDo. *Expansion of BreastScreen Australia*. [cited 23.06.14]. Available from: <http://www.cancer-screening.gov.au/internet/screening/publishing.nsf/Content/expansion-of-breastscreen-Australia>; 2014.
17. International Cancer Screening Network. *Breast cancer screening program in 26 ICSN countries, 2012: organization, policies, and program reach*. Available at: <http://www.healthcaredelivery.cancer.gov>. [accessed 09.10.15].
18. Dowling EC, Klabunde C, Patnick J, Ballard-Barbash R. Breast and cervical cancer screening programme implementation in 16 countries. *J Med Screen* 2010;**17**:139–46.
19. *Use of breast cancer screening [Internet]. Lyon, France: international agency for research on cancer* [cited 13.08.15]. Available from: <http://www.iarc.fr/en/publications/pdfs-online/prev/handbook7/Handbook7_Breast-3.pdf>; 2002.

20. *Choosing wisely: an initiative of the ABIM foundation. Promoting conversations between providers and patients* [cited 19.05.15]. Available from: <www.choosingwisely.org>.
21. Programme NBS. *Evaluating the age extension to the NHS Breast Screening Programme.* [cited 29.06.15]. Available from: <www.cancerresearchuk.org/cancer-help/trials/a-study-to-evaluate-an-age-extension-of-the-nhs-breast-screening-programme>; 2012.
22. Collins K, Winslow M, Reed MW, Walters SJ, Robinson T, Madan J, et al. The views of older women towards mammographic screening: a qualitative and quantitative study. *Br J Cancer* 2010;**102**(10):1461–7.
23. Yao N, Bradley CJ, Miranda PY. Mammography use after the 2009 debate. *J Clin Oncol* 2014;**32**(35):4023–4.
24. Schonberg MA, Breslau ES, McCarthy EP. Targeting of mammography screening according to life expectancy in women aged 75 and older. *J Am Geriatr Soc* 2013.
25. Amir E, Freedman OC, Seruga B, Evans DG. Assessing women at high risk of breast cancer: a review of risk assessment models. *J Am Geriatr Soc* 2013;**61**(3):388–95.
26. Gail MH, Brinton LA, Byar DP, Corle DK, Green SB, Schairer C, et al. Projecting individualized probabilities of developing breast cancer for white females who are being examined annually. *J Natl Cancer Inst* 1989;**81**(24):1879–86.
27. Schonberg MA, Li VW, Eliassen H, Davis RB, LaCroix AZ, McCarthy EP, et al. Performance of the breast cancer risk assessment tool among women age 75 years and older. *J Natl Cancer Inst* 2016;**108**(3):djv348.
28. Breast Cancer Risk Assessment SAS Macro (Gail Model). Available at: <http://dceg.cancer.gov/tools/risk-assessment/bcrasasmacro>; 2012. [accessed 11.07.15.].
29. Walter LC, Schonberg MA. Screening mammography in older women: a review. *J Am Med Assoc* 2014;**311**(13):1336–47.
30. Sweeney C, Blair CK, Anderson KE, Lazovich D, Folsom AR. Risk factors for breast cancer in elderly women. *Am J Epidemiol* 2004;**160**(9):868–75.
31. Cummings SR, Lee JS, Lui LY, Stone K, Ljung BM, Cauleys JA. Sex hormones, risk factors, and risk of estrogen receptor-positive breast cancer in older women: a long-term prospective study. *Cancer Epidemiol Biomarkers Prev* 2005;**14**(5):1047–51.
32. Cauley JA, Lucas FL, Kuller LH, Vogt MT, Browner WS, Cummings SR. Bone mineral density and risk of breast cancer in older women: the study of osteoporotic fractures. Study of Osteoporotic Fractures Research Group. *J Am Med Assoc* 1996;**276**(17):1404–8.
33. Chlebowski RT, Hendrix SL, Langer RD, Stefanick ML, Gass M, Lane D, et al. Influence of estrogen plus progestin on breast cancer and mammography in healthy postmenopausal women: the Women's Health Initiative Randomized Trial. *J Am Med Assoc* 2003;**289**(24):3243–53.
34. Cook NR, Rosner BA, Hankinson SE, Colditz GA. Mammographic screening and risk factors for breast cancer. *Am J Epidemiol* 2009;**170**(11):1422–32.
35. Pace LE, Keating NL. A systematic assessment of benefits and risks to guide breast cancer screening decisions. *J Am Med Assoc* 2014;**311**(13):1327–35.
36. Nystrom L, Andersson I, Bjurstam N, Frisell J, Nordenskjold B, Rutqvist LE. Long-term effects of mammography screening: updated overview of the Swedish randomised trials. *Lancet* 2002;**359**(9310):909–19.
37. Henderson LM, O'Meara ES, Braithwaite D, Onega T. Breast cancer surveillance consortium. Performance of digital screening mammography among older women in the United States. *Cancer* 2015;**121**(9):1379–86.
38. Kerlikowske K, Hubbard RA, Miglioretti DL, Geller BM, Yankaskas BC, Lehman CD, et al. Comparative effectiveness of digital versus film-screen mammography in community practice in the United States: a cohort study. *Ann Intern Med* 2011;**155**(8):493–502.
39. Smith BD, Jiang J, McLaughlin SS, Hurria A, Smith GL, Giordano SH, et al. Improvement in breast cancer outcomes over time: are older women missing out? *J Clin Oncol* 2011;**29**(35):4647–53.
40. Diab SG, Elledge RM, Clark GM. Tumor characteristics and clinical outcome of elderly women with breast cancer. *J Natl Cancer Inst* 2000;**92**(7):550–6.

41. Badgwell BD, Giordano SH, Duan ZZ, Fang S, Bedrosian I, Kuerer HM, et al. Mammography before diagnosis among women age 80 years and older with breast cancer. *J Clin Oncol* 2008;**26**(15):2482–8.
42. McCarthy EP, Burns RB, Freund KM, Ash AS, Shwartz M, Marwill SL, et al. Mammography use, breast cancer stage at diagnosis, and survival among older women. *J Am Geriatr Soc* 2000;**48**(10):1226–33.
43. McPherson CP, Swenson KK, Lee MW. The effects of mammographic detection and comorbidity on the survival of older women with breast cancer. *J Am Geriatr Soc* 2002;**50**(6):1061–8.
44. Berry DA. Breast cancer screening: controversy of impact. *Breast* 2013(22 Suppl. 2):S73–6.
45. Mandelblatt JS, Cronin KA, Bailey S, Berry DA, de Koning HJ, Draisma G, et al. Effects of mammography screening under different screening schedules: model estimates of potential benefits and harms. *Ann Intern Med* 2009;**151**(10):738–47.
46. van Ravesteyn NT, Stout NK, Schechter CB, Heijnsdijk EA, Alagoz O, Trentham-Dietz A, et al. Benefits and harms of mammography screening after age 74 years: model estimates of overdiagnosis. *J Natl Cancer Inst* 2015;**107**(7).
47. Barratt A, Howard K, Irwig L, Salkeld G, Houssami N. Model of outcomes of screening mammography: information to support informed choices. *B Med J* 2005;**330**(7497):936.
48. Kerlikowske K, Salzmann P, Phillips KA, Cauley JA, Cummings SR. Continuing screening mammography in women aged 70 to 79 years: impact on life expectancy and cost-effectiveness. *J Am Med Assoc* 1999;**282**(22):2156–63.
49. Schousboe JT, Kerlikowske K, Loh A, Cummings SR. Personalizing mammography by breast density and other risk factors for breast cancer: analysis of health benefits and cost-effectiveness. *Ann Intern Med* 2011;**155**(1):10–20.
50. Mandelblatt JS, Schechter CB, Yabroff KR, Lawrence W, Dignam J, Extermann M, et al. Toward optimal screening strategies for older women. *J Gen Intern Med* 2005;**20**(6):487–96.
51. Kramer BS, Elmore JG. Projecting the benefits and harms of mammography using statistical models: proof or proofiness? *J Natl Cancer Inst* 2015;**107**(7).
52. Esserman LJ, Shieh Y, Rutgers EJ, Knauer M, Retel VP, Mook S, et al. Impact of mammographic screening on the detection of good and poor prognosis breast cancers. *Breast Cancer Res Treat* 2011;**130**(3):725–34.
53. de Glas NA, de Craen AJ, Bastiaannet E, Op't Land EG, Kiderlen M, van de Water W, et al. Effect of implementation of the mass breast cancer screening programme in older women in the Netherlands: population based study. *Br Med J* 2014;**349**:g5410.
54. Lee SJ, Boscardin WJ, Stijacic-Cenzer I, Conell-Price J, O'Brien S, Walter LC. Time lag to benefit after screening for breast and colorectal cancer: meta-analysis of survival data from the United States, Sweden, United Kingdom, and Denmark. *Br Med J* 2013;**346**:e8441.
55. Braithwaite D, Zhu W, Hubbard RA, O'Meara ES, Miglioretti DL, Geller B, et al. Screening outcomes in older US women undergoing multiple mammograms in community practice: does interval, age, or comorbidity score affect tumor characteristics or false positive rates? *J Natl Cancer Inst* 2013;**105**(5):334–41.
56. Schonberg MA, Silliman RA, Marcantonio ER. Weighing the benefits and burdens of mammography screening among women age 80 years or older. *J Clin Oncol* 2009;**27**(11):1774–80.
57. Welch HG, Fisher ES. Diagnostic testing following screening mammography in the elderly. *J Natl Cancer Inst* 1998;**90**(18):1389–92.
58. Bruening W, Fontanarosa J, Tipton K, Treadwell JR, Launders J, Schoelles K. Systematic review: comparative effectiveness of core-needle and open surgical biopsy to diagnose breast lesions. *Ann Intern Med* 2010;**152**(4):238–46.
59. Schonberg MA, Silliman RA, Ngo LH, Birdwell RL, Fein-Zachary V, Donato J, et al. Older women's experience with a benign breast biopsy-a mixed methods study. *J Gen Intern Med* 2014;**29**(12):1631–40.
60. Tosteson AN, Fryback DG, Hammond CS, Hanna LG, Grove MR, Brown M, et al. Consequences of false-positive screening mammograms. *JAMA Intern Med* 2014;**174**(6):954–61.

61. Barton MB, Moore S, Polk S, Shtatland E, Elmore JG, Fletcher SW. Increased patient concern after false-positive mammograms: clinician documentation and subsequent ambulatory visits. *J Gen Intern Med* 2001;**16**(3): 150–6.
62. Di Maio M, Perrone F. Quality of life in elderly patients with cancer. *Health Qual Life Outcomes* 2003;**1**:44.
63. Ganz PA, Guadagnoli E, Landrum MB, Lash TL, Rakowski W, Silliman RA. Breast cancer in older women: quality of life and psychosocial adjustment in the 15 months after diagnosis. *J Clin Oncol* 2003;**21**(21): 4027–33.
64. Sammarco A. Quality of life of breast cancer survivors: a comparative study of age cohorts. *Cancer Nurs* 2009;**32**(5):347–56. quiz 57-8.
65. Silliman RA, Balducci L, Goodwin JS, Holmes FF, Leventhal EA. Breast cancer care in old age: what we know, don't know, and do. *J Natl Cancer Inst* 1993;**85**(3):190–9.
66. Mor V, Allen S, Malin M. The psychosocial impact of cancer on older versus younger patients and their families. *Cancer* 1994;**74**(7 Suppl.):2118–27.
67. Ballantyne PJ. Social context and outcomes for the ageing breast cancer patient: considerations for clinical practitioners. *J Clin Nurs* 2004;**13**(3a):11–21.
68. Puliti D, Duffy SW, Miccinesi G, de Koning H, Lynge E, Zappa M, et al. Overdiagnosis in mammographic screening for breast cancer in Europe: a literature review. *J Med Screen* 2012(19 Suppl. 1):42–56.
69. Etzioni R, Gulati R, Mallinger L, Mandelblatt J. Influence of study features and methods on overdiagnosis estimates in breast and prostate cancer screening. *Ann Intern Med* 2013;**158**(11):831–8.
70. Welch HG, Black WC. Overdiagnosis in cancer. *J Natl Cancer Inst* 2010;**102**(9):605–13.
71. Miller AB, Wall C, Baines CJ, Sun P, To T, Narod SA. Twenty five year follow-up for breast cancer incidence and mortality of the Canadian National Breast Screening Study: randomised screening trial. *B Med J* 2014;**348**:g366.
72. Bleyer A, Welch HG. Effect of three decades of screening mammography on breast-cancer incidence. *N Engl J Med* 2012;**367**(21):1998–2005.
73. Ernster VL, Ballard-Barbash R, Barlow WE, Zheng Y, Weaver DL, Cutter G, et al. Detection of ductal carcinoma in situ in women undergoing screening mammography. *J Natl Cancer Inst* 2002;**94**(20):1546–54.
74. Betsill Jr. WL, Rosen PP, Lieberman PH, Robbins GF. Intraductal carcinoma. Long-term follow-up after treatment by biopsy alone. *J Am Med Assoc* 1978;**239**(18):1863–7.
75. Page DL, Dupont WD, Rogers LW, Jensen RA, Schuyler PA. Continued local recurrence of carcinoma 15-25 years after a diagnosis of low grade ductal carcinoma in situ of the breast treated only by biopsy. *Cancer* 1995;**76**(7):1197–200.
76. Schairer C, Mink PJ, Carroll L, Devesa SS. Probabilities of death from breast cancer and other causes among female breast cancer patients. *J Natl Cancer Inst* 2004;**96**(17):1311–21.
77. *E. A. United States Life Tables, 2010; Vol. 63, Number 7. National vital statistics reports 2014* [cited 11.07.15]. Available from: <http://www.cdc.gov/nchs/data/nvsr/nvsr63/nvsr63_07.pdf>.
78. Schonberg MA, Birdwell RL, Bychkovsky BL, Hintz L, Fein-Zachary V, Wertheimer MD, et al. Older women's experience with breast cancer treatment decisions. *Breast Cancer Res Treat* 2014;**145**(1):211–23.
79. Schonberg MA, Marcantonio ER, Li D, Silliman RA, Ngo L, McCarthy EP. Breast cancer among the oldest old: tumor characteristics, treatment choices, and survival. *J Clin Oncol* 2010;**28**(12):2038–45.
80. Morrow M, Jagsi R, Alderman AK, Griggs JJ, Hawley ST, Hamilton AS, et al. Surgeon recommendations and receipt of mastectomy for treatment of breast cancer. *J Am Med Assoc* 2009;**302**(14):1551–6.
81. Wilke LG, Czechura T, Wang C, Lapin B, Liederbach E, Winchester DP, et al. Repeat surgery after breast conservation for the treatment of stage 0 to II breast carcinoma: a report from the National Cancer Data Base, 2004–2010. *JAMA Surg* 2014;**149**(12):1296–305.
82. Lavelle K, Sowerbutts AM, Bundred N, Pilling M, Todd C. Pretreatment health measures and complications after surgical management of elderly women with breast cancer. *Br J Surg* 2015;**102**(6):653–67.

83. de Glas NA, Kiderlen M, Bastiaannet E, de Craen AJ, van de Water W, van de Velde CJ, et al. Postoperative complications and survival of elderly breast cancer patients: a FOCUS study analysis. *Breast Cancer Res Treat* 2013;**138**(2):561–9.
84. Wyld L, Garg DK, Kumar ID, Brown H, Reed MW. Stage and treatment variation with age in postmenopausal women with breast cancer: compliance with guidelines. *Br J Cancer* 2004;**90**(8):1486–91.
85. Biganzoli L, Wildiers H, Oakman C, Marotti L, Loibl S, Kunkler I, et al. Management of elderly patients with breast cancer: updated recommendations of the International Society of Geriatric Oncology (SIOG) and European Society of Breast Cancer Specialists (EUSOMA). *Lancet Oncol* 2012;**13**(4):e148–60.
86. Chakrabarti J, Kenny FS, Syed BM, Robertson JF, Blamey RW, Cheung KL. A randomised trial of mastectomy only versus tamoxifen for treating elderly patients with operable primary breast cancer-final results at 20-year follow-up. *Crit Rev Oncol Hematol* 2011;**78**(3):260–4.
87. Morgan JL, Reed MW, Wyld L. Primary endocrine therapy as a treatment for older women with operable breast cancer – a comparison of randomised controlled trial and cohort study findings. *Eur J Surg Oncol* 2014;**40**(6):676–84.
88. Hughes KS, Schnaper LA, Bellon JR, Cirrincione CT, Berry DA, McCormick B, et al. Lumpectomy plus tamoxifen with or without irradiation in women age 70 years or older with early breast cancer: long-term follow-up of CALGB 9343. *J Clin Oncol* 2013;**31**(19):2382–7.
89. Palta M, Palta P, Bhavsar NA, Horton JK, Blitzblau RC. The use of adjuvant radiotherapy in elderly patients with early-stage breast cancer: changes in practice patterns after publication of Cancer and Leukemia Group B 9343. *Cancer* 2015;**121**(2):188–93.
90. Buchholz TA. Radiation therapy for early-stage breast cancer after breast-conserving surgery. *N Engl J Med* 2009;**360**(1):63–70.
91. Smith GL, Xu Y, Buchholz TA, Giordano SH, Jiang J, Shih YC, et al. Association between treatment with brachytherapy vs whole-breast irradiation and subsequent mastectomy, complications, and survival among older women with invasive breast cancer. *J Am Med Assoc* 2012;**307**(17):1827–37.
92. Bekelman JE, Sylwestrzak G, Barron J, Liu J, Epstein AJ, Freedman G, et al. Uptake and costs of hypofractionated vs conventional whole breast irradiation after breast conserving surgery in the united states, 2008–2013. *J Am Med Assoc* 2014;**312**(23):2542–50.
93. Hattangadi JA, Taback N, Neville BA, Harris JR, Punglia RS. Accelerated partial breast irradiation using brachytherapy for breast cancer: patterns in utilization and guideline concordance. *J Natl Cancer Inst* 2012;**104**(1):29–41.
94. Davies C, Godwin J, Gray R, Clarke M, Cutter D, Darby S, et al. Relevance of breast cancer hormone receptors and other factors to the efficacy of adjuvant tamoxifen: patient-level meta-analysis of randomised trials. *Lancet* 2011;**378**(9793):771–84.
95. Riley GF, Warren JL, Harlan LC, Blackwell SA. Endocrine therapy use among elderly hormone receptor-positive breast cancer patients enrolled in Medicare Part D. *Medicare Medicaid Res Rev* 2011;**1**(4).
96. Sheppard VB, Faul LA, Luta G, Clapp JD, Yung RL, Wang JH, et al. Frailty and adherence to adjuvant hormonal therapy in older women with breast cancer: CALGB protocol 369901. *J Clin Oncol* 2014;**32**(22):2318–27.
97. Nekhlyudov L, Li L, Ross-Degnan D, Wagner AK. Five-year patterns of adjuvant hormonal therapy use, persistence, and adherence among insured women with early-stage breast cancer. *Breast Cancer Res Treat* 2011;**130**(2):681–9.
98. Hershman DL, Kushi LH, Shao T, Buono D, Kershenbaum A, Tsai WY, et al. Early discontinuation and non-adherence to adjuvant hormonal therapy in a cohort of 8,769 early-stage breast cancer patients. *J Clin Oncol* 2010;**28**(27):4120–8.
99. Owusu C, Buist DS, Field TS, Lash TL, Thwin SS, Geiger AM, et al. Predictors of tamoxifen discontinuation among older women with estrogen receptor-positive breast cancer. *J Clin Oncol* 2008;**26**(4):549–55.

100. Burstein HJ, Griggs JJ, Prestrud AA, Temin S. American society of clinical oncology clinical practice guideline update on adjuvant endocrine therapy for women with hormone receptor-positive breast cancer. *J Oncol Pract* 2010;**6**(5):243–6.
101. Agrawal K, Onami S, Mortimer JE, Pal SK. Cognitive changes associated with endocrine therapy for breast cancer. *Maturitas* 2010;**67**(3):209–14.
102. Muss HB, Berry DA, Cirrincione CT, Theodoulou M, Mauer AM, Kornblith AB, et al. Adjuvant chemotherapy in older women with early-stage breast cancer. *N Engl J Med* 2009;**360**(20):2055–65.
103. NCCN. *NCCN guidlelines for treatment of breast cancer. Version 3.* [cited 01.03.15]. Available from: <www.nccn.org>; 2014.
104. Muss HB, Woolf S, Berry D, Cirrincione C, Weiss RB, Budman D, et al. Adjuvant chemotherapy in older and younger women with lymph node-positive breast cancer. *J Am Med Assoc* 2005;**293**(9):1073–81.
105. Hurria A, Rosen C, Hudis C, Zuckerman E, Panageas KS, Lachs MS, et al. Cognitive function of older patients receiving adjuvant chemotherapy for breast cancer: a pilot prospective longitudinal study. *J Am Geriatr Soc* 2006;**54**(6):925–31.
106. Lee SJ, Lindquist K, Segal MR, Covinsky KE. Development and validation of a prognostic index for 4-year mortality in older adults. *J Am Med Assoc* 2006;**295**(7):801–8.
107. Yourman LC, Lee SJ, Schonberg MA, Widera EW, Smith AK. Prognostic indices for older adults: a systematic review. *J Am Med Assoc* 2012;**307**(2):182–92.
108. Schonberg MA, Davis RB, McCarthy EP, Marcantonio ER. External validation of an index to predict up to 9-year mortality of community-dwelling adults aged 65 and older. *J Am Geriatr Soc* 2011;**59**(8):1444–51.
109. Schonberg MA, Davis RB, McCarthy EP, Marcantonio ER. Index to predict 5-year mortality of community-dwelling adults aged 65 and older using data from the National Health Interview Survey. *J Gen Intern Med* 2009;**24**(10):1115–22.
110. Walter LC, Covinsky KE. Cancer screening in elderly patients: a framework for individualized decision making. *J Am Med Assoc* 2001;**285**(21):2750–6.
111. Cho H, Klabunde CN, Yabroff KR, Wang Z, Meekins A, Lansdorp-Vogelaar I, et al. Comorbidity-adjusted life expectancy: a new tool to inform recommendations for optimal screening strategies. *Ann Intern Med* 2013;**159**(10):667–76.
112. Lansdorp-Vogelaar I, Gulati R, Mariotto AB, Schechter CB, de Carvalho TM, Knudsen AB, et al. Personalizing age of cancer screening cessation based on comorbid conditions: model estimates of harms and benefits. *Ann Intern Med* 2014;**161**(2):104–12.
113. Raik BL, Miller FG, Fins JJ. Screening and cognitive impairment: ethics of forgoing mammography in older women. *J Am Geriatr Soc* 2004;**52**(3):440–4.
114. Kua EH, Ho E, Tan HH, Tsoi C, Thng C, Mahendran R. The natural history of dementia. *Psychogeriatrics* 2014;**14**(3):196–201.
115. Mehta KM, Fung KZ, Kistler CE, Chang A, Walter LC. Impact of cognitive impairment on screening mammography use in older US women. *Am J Public Health* 2010;**100**(10):1917–23.
116. Pisano ED, Gatsonis C, Hendrick E, Yaffe M, Baum JK, Acharyya S, et al. Diagnostic performance of digital versus film mammography for breast-cancer screening. *N Engl J Med* 2005;**353**(17):1773–83.
117. Fenton JJ, Xing G, Elmore JG, Bang H, Chen SL, Lindfors KK, et al. Short-term outcomes of screening mammography using computer-aided detection: a population-based study of medicare enrollees. *Ann Intern Med* 2013;**158**(8):580–7.
118. Killelea BK, Long JB, Chagpar AB, Ma X, Wang R, Ross JS, et al. Evolution of breast cancer screening in the Medicare population: clinical and economic implications. *J Natl Cancer Inst* 2014;**106**(8).
119. Haas BM, Kalra V, Geisel J, Raghu M, Durand M, Philpotts LE. Comparison of tomosynthesis plus digital mammography and digital mammography alone for breast cancer screening. *Radiology* 2013;**269**(3):694–700.
120. Fox J, Zikmund-Fisher BJ, Gross CP. Older patient experiences in the mammography decision-making process. *Arch Intern Med* 2012;**172**(1):62–4. Discussion 4.

121. Lewis CL, Griffith J, Pignone MP, Golin C. Physicians' decisions about continuing or stopping colon cancer screening in the elderly: a qualitative study. *J Gen Intern Med* 2009;**24**(7):816–21.
122. Schonberg MA, Ramanan RA, McCarthy EP, Marcantonio ER. Decision making and counseling around mammography screening for women aged 80 or older. *J Gen Intern Med* 2006;**21**(9):979–85.
123. Leach CR, Klabunde CN, Alfano CM, Smith JL, Rowland JH. Physician over-recommendation of mammography for terminally ill women. *Cancer* 2012;**118**(1):27–37.
124. Torke AM, Schwartz PH, Holtz LR, Montz K, Sachs GA. Older adults and forgoing cancer screening: "I Think It Would Be Strange". *JAMA Intern Med* 2013:1–7.
125. Schwartz LM, Woloshin S, Fowler Jr. FJ, Welch HG. Enthusiasm for cancer screening in the United States. *J Am Med Assoc* 2004;**291**(1):71–8.
126. Lewis CL, Esserman D, Deleon C, Pignone MP, Pathman DE, Golin C. Physician decision making for colorectal cancer screening in the elderly. *J Gen Intern Med* 2013.
127. Haggerty J, Tudiver F, Brown JB, Herbert C, Ciampi A, Guibert R. Patients' anxiety and expectations: how they influence family physicians' decisions to order cancer screening tests. *Can Fam Physician* 2005;**51**:1658–9.
128. Tan A, Kuo YF, Goodwin JS. Potential overuse of screening mammography and its association with access to primary care. *Med Care* 2014;**52**(6):490–5.
129. Kachalia A, Mello MM. Breast cancer screening: conflicting guidelines and medicolegal risk. *J Am Med Assoc* 2013;**309**(24):2555–6.
130. Schonberg MA, Walter LC. Talking about stopping cancer screening-not so easy. *JAMA Intern Med* 2013;**173**(7):532–3.
131. Schonberg MA, Hamel MB, Davis RB, Griggs MC, Wee CC, Fagerlin A, et al. Development and evaluation of a decision aid on mammography screening for women 75 years and older. *JAMA Intern Med* 2014;**174**(3):417–24.
132. Mathieu E, Barratt A, Davey HM, McGeechan K, Howard K, Houssami N. Informed choice in mammography screening: a randomized trial of a decision aid for 70-year-old women. *Arch Intern Med* 2007;**167**(19):2039–46.
133. Tisnado DM, Moore AA, Levin JR, Rosen S. Developing and testing a decision aid for use by providers in making recommendations: about mammography screening in older women. *J Appl Gerontol* 2015;**34**(3):343–58.
134. O'Connor AM, Stacey D, Entwistle V, Llewellyn-Thomas H, Rovner D, Holmes-Rovner M, et al. Decision aids for people facing health treatment or screening decisions. *Cochrane Database Syst Rev* 2003(2) CD001431.
135. Onega T, Beaber EF, Sprague BL, Barlow WE, Haas JS, Tosteson AN, et al. Breast cancer screening in an era of personalized regimens: a conceptual model and National Cancer Institute initiative for risk-based and preference-based approaches at a population level. *Cancer* 2014;**120**(19):2955–64.
136. Schopper D, de Wolf C. *Breast cancer screening by mammography: International evidence and the situation in Switzerland [Internet]*. Bern, Switzerland: Swiss Cancer League; 2007. June [cited 13.08.15]. Available from: <http://assets.krebsliga.ch/downloads/short_mammo_report_final_el_.pdf>.
137. *Making a decision about colon cancer screening*. [cited 29.06.15]. Available from: <http://shareddecisionmaking.org/Site/Female%20Age%2080.pdf>; 2010.

CHAPTER

SCREENING WOMEN IN THEIR 40S

9

Heidi D. Nelson[1,2]

[1]Pacific Northwest Evidence-Based Practice Center and Departments of Medical Informatics and Clinical Epidemiology and Medicine, Oregon Health & Science University, Portland, OR, United States, [2]Providence Cancer Center, Providence Health & Services, Portland, OR, United States

CHAPTER OUTLINE

PLAIN LANGUAGE SUMMARY

Women in their 40s face conflicting breast cancer screening guidelines that are based on different interpretations of research and considerations of the benefits and harms of screening.

How well mammography screening reduces death from breast cancer was evaluated in eight randomized controlled trials (RCTs) of women in their 40s. Neither the individual trials, nor an estimate that combined results of all of the trials, showed reduced deaths with screening. Deaths were reduced by 26% to 44% in two studies comparing women in community screening programs with those not screened. However, these studies provided less reliable results than the trials because women were

Breast Cancer Screening. DOI: http://dx.doi.org/10.1016/B978-0-12-802209-2.00009-7

not randomized to screening and control groups. Screening trials also showed that cases of advanced breast cancer as well as deaths from all causes were not reduced with screening.

A false-positive mammography result occurs when the initial report describes an area of suspicion that is later found to be normal after obtaining additional tests and sometimes biopsies. False-positive results are considered harms of screening because a healthy person is subjected to tests and procedures without direct benefit. A false-negative result occurs when a mammogram is interpreted as normal when a tumor actually exists. In this case, patients are harmed when diagnosis and treatment are delayed.

In a large US study, breast cancer rates were lowest among women in their 40s and increased with age, while rates of false-positive results were highest among women in their 40s and decreased with age. Higher false-positive rates were associated with risk factors for breast cancer. Over 50% of women in their 40s had false-positive results over a 10-year period. Rates of false-negative results and recommendations for biopsy did not differ by age. Rates of false-positives, false-negatives, and recommendations for biopsy did not differ by time since previous screening.

Studies suggest potential reductions in false-positive results with combined use of tomosynthesis and mammography compared to mammography alone, while effects on rates of false-negative results and biopsies and how rates vary by patient factors including age are presently unclear. Results of a single trial indicated increased false-positive and biopsy rates with combined mammography and ultrasonography compared with mammography alone.

Additional potential harms of screening include overdiagnosis and overtreatment; radiation exposure; and anxiety, distress, and pain during procedures. Overdiagnosis refers to diagnosing breast cancer for cases that will not cause symptoms. However, current methods of defining, measuring, and estimating the effects of these harms are inadequate, and how to determine their importance for individual women is unclear.

As a result of the current state of evidence and the dilemma of differing guidelines for women in their 40s, shared decision-making has become an important part of the screening process. In shared decision-making, each woman takes an active role in determining the appropriate screening services for her. Screening decisions could be improved by additional research on the effectiveness of screening women in their 40s who have specific risk factors, methods to reduce harms of screening, and approaches that improve communication and further involve women in the screening process.

INTRODUCTION

Breast cancer screening guidelines are the most debated and least congruent for average-risk women in their 40s, and for this reason, it is particularly important for women, clinicians, researchers, and policy makers to understand the evidence behind them. While some guidelines recommend routine screening beginning at age 40,[1,2] most others recommend beginning at age 50[3–5] or at ages in between.[6] Recommendations also differ regarding annual versus biennial mammography and the role of clinical and self-breast examinations. The context of recommendations ranges from providing explicit directions for screening to relying on shared decision-making in which women take a major role in making the screening decision.[7] For many women, their screening choices are primarily driven by their health insurance plan's coverage and by their access to health care services.

Screening guidelines are an important influence on screening practices, even when guidelines are dissimilar. A study of changes in screening practices in a large US health system indicated a significant decline in mammography screening among women in their 40s after release of the U.S. Preventive Services Task Force (USPSTF) recommendations in 2009 despite insurance coverage.[8] During the same time period, screening increased among women age 50 to 74, the age group targeted by the USPSTF recommendations, but not until the Affordable Care Act was implemented soon thereafter providing increased coverage of screening services. These relationships differ throughout health systems worldwide, whether private or public, and are important to understand in order to deliver optimal, yet appropriate, breast cancer screening.

In contrast to the conflicting guidelines regarding screening women at average risk, guideline groups generally agree that high-risk women in their 40s may benefit from initiating more frequent screening at younger ages. Clinically significant risk factors associated with high risk for breast cancer include breast cancer susceptibility gene (BRCA) mutations, mutation status unknown but having a first-degree relative with a BRCA mutation, and other hereditary genetic syndromes associated with more than a 15% lifetime risk, including Li-Fraumeni syndrome, Cowden syndrome, or hereditary diffuse gastric cancer.[9] The degree of risk associated with family history of breast cancer varies according to familial patterns of disease. Estimates of lifetime risk of breast cancer determined by kindred analysis of over 15% or 20% are considered high.

Previous diagnosis of invasive breast cancer, ductal carcinoma in situ (DCIS), or high-risk lesions including lobular carcinoma in situ, atypical ductal hyperplasia, atypical lobular hyperplasia, flat epithelial atypia, papillary atypia, and apocrine atypia significantly increase risk for breast cancer to various levels.[10–12] Also, women with histories of high-dose radiation therapy to the chest between the ages of 10 to 30 years, such as for treatment of Hodgkin lymphoma, are considered at high risk.[13]

Additional factors increase risk for breast cancer to lower levels than for high-risk women, and women in their 40s with these characteristics generally fall within routine screening guidelines. A modeling study indicated that benefits and harms of screening for a hypothetical woman in her 40s is similar to an average-risk woman in her 50s when risk exceeds 2 to 4 times greater than average.[14] However, this screening strategy has not been evaluated in clinical settings.

An important first step in considering risk factors in making screening choices is to identify those that are specific to women in their 40s and determine their impact. Results of a systematic review and analysis of data from a large screening population narrowed the possible potential risk factors to a concise list (Fig. 9.1).[15] These include family history of breast cancer that is less extensive than for high-risk women; prior benign breast biopsy; current use of oral contraceptives; no previous pregnancies; and higher breast density, a radiographic measure of breast tissue that is associated with increased risk for breast cancer and reduced mammography sensitivity. Increased breast density is more common among younger women.[16]

Empiric models that incorporate several of these risk factors have been developed to predict breast cancer risk for individual women.[17] All of the models include age and first-degree family history of breast cancer into their calculations, but vary by other components. However, studies of their diagnostic accuracy indicate that the models are poor predictors of an individual's risk,[17] and it remains unclear how to apply these models to selecting women for screening. Therefore, despite extensive research, screening decisions for women in their 40s remain complex, individualized decisions based on personal consideration of benefits and harms.

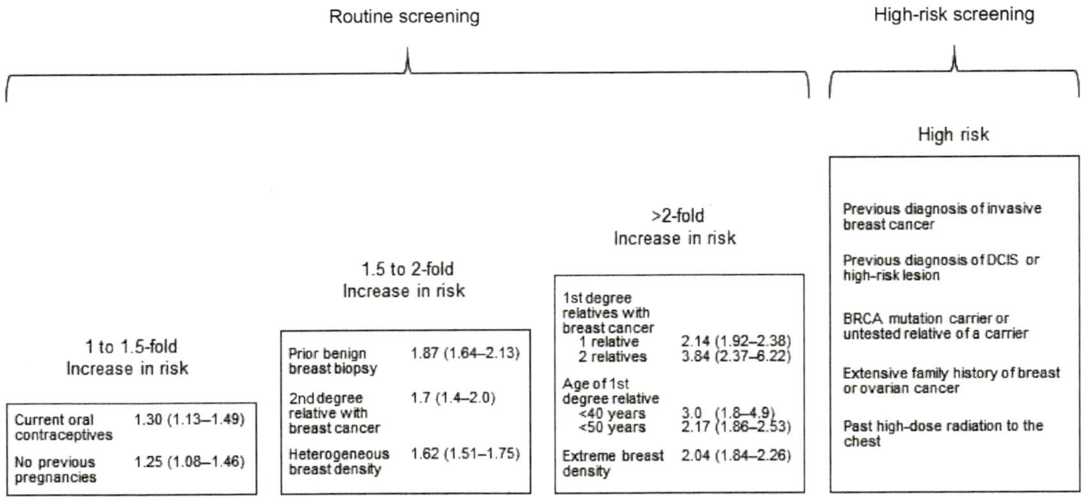

FIGURE 9.1

Risk factors for breast cancer for women in their 40s. Family history of breast cancer, increased breast density, prior benign breast biopsy, current use of oral contraceptives, and no previous pregnancies modestly increase risk for breast cancer in epidemiologic studies of women in their 40s (RR with 95% CI). Additional factors identify women at high risk.

SCREENING BENEFITS

BREAST CANCER MORTALITY

Breast cancer screening trials

Eight main RCTs of breast cancer screening enrolled women in their 40s and reported breast cancer mortality results specifically for them. These include the UK Age trial,[18,19] Canadian National Breast Screening Study 1 (CNBSS-1),[20,21] Health Insurance Plan of Greater New York (HIP) trial,[22] Stockholm trial,[23] Malmö Mammographic Screening Trial (referred to separately as MMST I and MMST II),[24] Swedish Two-County Study (referred to separately as Östergötland and Kopparberg),[25] and Gothenburg trial.[26] The descriptions of trials and meta-analyses in this chapter are based on a systematic review of the most recent trial results.[27,28] In these analyses, the number of trials was counted as the number of discrete data sources contributing to the summary estimate.

All trials were designed as RCTs, although they varied in their recruitment of participants and controls, sizes, methods of randomization, and screening protocols. Additional details of the trials, their screening protocols, and limitations are described in chapter: "Estimates of Screening Benefit: The Randomized Trials of Breast Cancer Screening." Two trials enrolled only women in their 40s (CNBSS-1 and Age),[18,20] while others enrolled various broader age ranges that included women in their 40s.[22–26] The Canadian trials recruited volunteers, the Age trial identified women from general practice lists, and the HIP trial recruited women enrolled in a health insurance plan. The other trials enrolled participants based on their residence in communities.

Age trial

The UK Age trial is particularly relevant to determining screening effectiveness in women in their 40s because it is the only trial designed to specifically evaluate this question.[18,19] The Age trial is also the largest trial, randomizing a total of 160,921 women age 39 to 41 to screening with seven rounds of annual mammography until age 48, or usual care which did not involve routine screening. Women were individually randomized and stratified by group practice, and were offered routine screening at age 50 to 52 in accordance with practice standards at the time. The Age trial is the most recent trial, beginning in 1991, and provides 17.5 years of follow-up results. Adherence was relatively high, 68% of women in the trial attended the prevalent screen, and overall, 81% of women attended at least one screen. The mean number of screens in the trial was 4.5. Follow-up conducted through the National Health Service central register was complete, and the analysis included deaths from breast cancer during the trial and during follow-up.

Limitations of the Age trial include use of standard two-view mammography only at the baseline screen and one-view mammography at subsequent screens. The majority of screens used film mammography, rather than digital. These technical differences make the trial less clinically relevant to current practice where two-view digital mammography is the usual standard. Also, it is unclear how many women in the usual care group received mammography during the trial. The Age investigators have reported concerns about the trial's lack of power to detect statistically significant differences between screening and usual care groups because the trial did not attain recruitment goals, and their initial assumptions regarding population estimates of breast cancer mortality were not accurate because there was an unanticipated decline in mortality rates during the years of the trial.

The initial results of the Age trial, based on a median of 10.7 years of follow-up, indicated a reduction in breast cancer mortality that was not statistically significant [relative risk (RR): 0.83; 95% confidence interval (CI), 0.66 to 1.04].[18] Results of long-term follow-up in the Age trial, as well as the other screening trials, are based on two methods of accrual of breast cancer cases and deaths (further described in chapter: "Estimates of Screening Benefit: The Randomized Trials of Breast Cancer Screening").[27,28] The short case accrual method includes only deaths occurring among cases of breast cancer diagnosed during the screening intervention period, and in some trials, within an additional defined case accrual period. The long case accrual method counts all of the breast cancer cases contributing to breast cancer deaths diagnosed during the screening intervention period plus the follow-up period. In the Age trial, follow-up after a median of 17 years indicated a RR of breast cancer mortality with screening of 0.88 (95% CI, 0.74 to 1.04) for cases diagnosed during the intervention phase; and 0.93 (95% CI, 0.80 to 1.09) for cases diagnosed during the intervention and follow-up phases.[19] While long-term follow-up may have improved the power of the trial to detect differences between comparison groups, these results indicate an even weaker relationship between screening and breast cancer mortality.

Meta-analysis of screening trials

Five of the screening trials reported results using the long case accrual method (Swedish Two-County [Kopparberg and Östergötland],[25] Age,[19] Gothenburg,[26] and CNBSS-1[29]), while four used only the short case accrual method (HIP,[30] Malmö I,[31] Malmö II,[31] and Stockholm[31]). Using the longest case accrual available across all trials, mean durations of screening were 3.5 to 18.8 years, case accrual 7.0 to 21.9 years, and follow-up 11.2 to 21.9 years.

Age-specific summary estimates of breast cancer mortality reduction were derived from meta-analyses that combined results from the trials.[27,28] For women age 40 to 49, neither the individual trials nor the combined estimate indicated statistically significant differences between screening and

Trial	Age at entry, years	Mean follow-up, years	Relative risk (95% CI)
Malmö II	43–49	11.2	0.64 (0.39 to 1.06)
Kopparberg	40–49	12.5	0.73 (0.37 to 1.41)
Östergötland	40–49	12.5	1.02 (0.52 to 1.99)
Age	39–41	17.5	0.93 (0.80 to 1.09)
Gothenburg	39–49	13.8	0.69 (0.45 to 1.05)
HIP	40–49	14.0	0.75 (0.53 to 1.05)
Stockholm	40–49	14.3	1.52 (0.80 to 2.88)
Malmö I	43–49	18.2	0.74 (0.42 to 1.29)
CNBSS-1	40–49	21.9	1.04 (0.87 to 1.24)
Overall (*I^2*=24.0%, *p*=0.230)			**0.92 (0.75 to 1.02)**

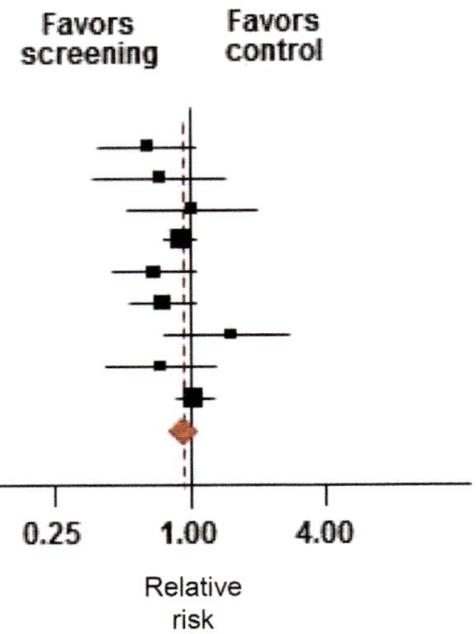

FIGURE 9.2

Effects of screening on breast cancer mortality among women in their 40s. Results of a meta-analysis of trials with estimates based on the longest case accrual methods available indicate no statistically significant differences between screening and nonscreening groups.

Adapted from Ref. 27.

control groups (RR: 0.92; 95% CI, 0.75 to 1.02; nine trials)[19,25–32] (Fig. 9.2). The meta-analysis was repeated using estimates from trials with short case accrual methods to examine differences related to how outcomes were captured. Results indicated a RR of 0.87 (95% CI, 0.72 to 1.00), consistent with a borderline statistically significant difference, although power was reduced in this estimate because fewer cases were included.

Absolute rates of breast cancer mortality reduction were derived from results of meta-analyses of RCTs. Results indicated that three deaths could be reduced (prevented) per 10,000 women screened for 10 years for both the long and short case accrual methods, assuming that differences between screening and control groups were actually statistically significant.

Observational studies

Observational studies of mammography screening provide additional information about screening effectiveness in contemporary populations and settings. However, observational studies are subject to biases that may limit their use in determining effectiveness. Most importantly, they lack comparability of comparison groups that is only attainable through randomization.

Recent comprehensive systematic reviews of observational studies summarize most of the relevant research,[33–36] including reviews conducted by the EUROSCREEN Working Group to assess the effectiveness of population-based mammography screening on breast cancer mortality.[33–35] In general, observational studies of screening indicate more favorable reductions in breast cancer mortality than results of the screening trials. However, most studies included women age 50 and older and their relevance to women in their 40s is uncertain.

Only two observational studies comparing outcomes of participants in screening programs versus nonparticipants reported results specifically for women in their 40s. A large prospective cohort study of the Mammography Screening of Young Women Cohort in Sweden indicated reduced risk for breast cancer deaths for women age 40 to 49 years invited to screening compared with women not invited (RR: 0.74; 95% CI, 0.66 to 0.83).[37] Although the study included over 600,000 women, it is unclear whether comparable groups were maintained over time due to attrition, crossover, adherence, and contamination.

An incidence-based mortality study of over 2 million women age 40 to 79 in Canada compared screening program participants versus nonparticipants.[38] Results were expressed as standardized mortality ratios (SMR), the ratio of the observed breast cancer mortality of screening participants to province-specific breast cancer mortality based on nonparticipant incidence and survival rates. Breast cancer mortality was reduced for women age 40 to 49 years (SMR: 0.56; 95% CI, 0.45 to 0.67). Although the analysis considered the influence of self-selection bias using historical trend data for women age 35 to 39, the validity of this approach is unclear. In the Canadian randomized trials, screening participants were more educated, had fewer pregnancies, and had overall higher risks for breast cancer[20,39] suggesting that women who participate in mammography differ from those who do not. These differences introduce bias and influence results of comparisons between screening and nonscreening groups.

Effects of screening intervals and imaging modalities

No trials directly compared the effect of different screening intervals on breast cancer mortality. A registry-based study in Finland indicated no breast cancer mortality differences between annual and triennial screening among women age 40 to 49 years.[40] No trials or observational studies of screening using digital mammography, tomosynthesis, ultrasound, or magnetic resonance imaging (MRI) provide mortality outcomes for women in their 40s.

ALL-CAUSE MORTALITY

All-cause mortality outcomes were reported for women age 40 to 49 in seven trials [Age,[19] CNBSS-1,[20,21] Stockholm,[23] Malmö II,[24] Swedish Two-County Study (separately reported for Östergötland and Kopparberg),[25] and Gothenburg[26]]. A meta-analysis of results indicated no all-cause mortality differences between screening and control groups (RR: 0.99; 95% CI, 0.95 to 1.05)[27,28] (details in chapter: "Estimates of Screening Benefit: The Randomized Trials of Breast Cancer Screening").

INCIDENCE OF ADVANCED BREAST CANCER

The incidence of advanced breast cancer is another clinically important outcome in determining the effectiveness of screening. The most commonly used measures in studies include clinical stage (0 to IV), number of involved lymph nodes (0, 1 to 3, 4+), and tumor size (mm). However, these measures vary across studies and do not capture important prognostic indicators, such as hormone receptor status. Also, most comparisons using these categories provide differences between screening and comparison groups that represent relatively early stages of disease, rather than advanced stages.

An analysis of the screening trials defined advanced breast cancer based on the most severe disease categories reported by the trials.[27,28] These included stage III and IV disease (ie, regional and metastatic), size 50 mm or greater, or having four or more positive lymph nodes. Trials reporting results specifically for women in their 40s are listed in Table 9.1. Combining estimates based on these definitions of advanced cancer in a meta-analysis indicated no difference with screening for women age 40 to 49 years (RR: 0.98; 95% CI, 0.74 to 1.37; four trials).[21,25,41,42]

The relationship of mammography screening and advanced breast cancer outcomes was also evaluated in analyses of data from the Breast Cancer Surveillance Consortium (BCSC), a collaborative network of mammography registries across the United States, supported by the National Cancer Institute (NCI).[43,44] Registries were linked to pathology databases and tumor registries and included demographic and medical history information from questionnaires.

Since all of the women included in the BCSC database have had previous mammography, studies compared 1-year versus 2-year screening intervals and their relationships with cancer stage at diagnosis (Table 9.2).[45–48] These intervals represent the time between the two most recent screening mammograms prior to diagnosis. Information regarding influences related to selection of specific screening intervals is not available.

In one study, the adjusted proportion of stage III + IV disease among women age 40 to 49 years was lower for women screened 1-year compared to 2-years previously (10.1% vs 14.0%; adjusted difference 4.8%; 95% CI, 1.3% to 8.4%).[47] In a separate analysis, women age 40 to 49 years with extremely dense breasts had increased risks for stage IIB or higher disease (odds ratio, OR: 2.39; 95% CI, 1.06 to 3.39) and tumors >20 mm (OR: 2.39; 95% CI, 1.37 to 4.18) with 2-year compared with 1-year intervals.[46] Differences were not significant for positive lymph nodes, other density categories, other age groups, or when compared with 3-year screening intervals.

In another BCSC study comparing 1-year versus 2-year intervals based on narrower definitions of intervals, there were no significant differences for stage IIB or higher disease, tumor size >15 mm, or positive lymph nodes for women age 40 to 49.[48] When evaluated by menopausal status, premenopausal women diagnosed with invasive breast cancer after a 2-year screening interval were more likely to have stage IIB or higher disease and tumor size >15 mm than those diagnosed after a 1-year interval.

Table 9.1 Screening Trials With Advanced Breast Cancer Outcomes for Women in Their 40s

Trial	Stage	+Lymph Nodes, n[a]	Size, mm[b]	Definition of Advanced Cancer[c]	RR for Advanced Cancer (95% CI)[d]
Age	NR	0, 1–3, 4+	1–9, 10–14, 15–19, 20–29, 30–49, ≥ 50	Size ≥ 50 mm 4+ lymph nodes	0.85 (0.57 to 1.23) 0.77 (0.53 to 1.13)
HIP	I, II, III, IV	NR	NR	Stage III– IV	0.87 (0.48 to 1.58)
CNBSS-1	NR	0, 1–3, 4+	1–9, 10–14, 15–19, 20–39, ≥ 40	Size ≥ 40 mm 4+ lymph nodes	1.18 (0.67 to 2.03) 2.00 (1.20 to 3.34)
Swedish Two-County	I, II, III–IV	0, 1+	1–9, 10–14, 15–19, 20–29, 30–49, ≥ 50	Size ≥ 50 mm	1.57 (0.63 to 3.94)

Adapted from Ref. 27.
Abbreviations: CI, confidence interval; CNBSS, Canadian National Breast Screening Study; HIP, Health Insurance Plan of Greater New York; mm, millimeter; n, number; NR, not reported; RR, relative risk.
[a]*Lymph nodes with micrometastases are classified as Stage IB, otherwise ≥ 1 positive lymph node is classified as Stage IIA or higher.*
[b]*Size ≥ 20 mm is classified as Stage IIA or higher; size ≥ 50 mm is classified as Stage IIB or higher.*
[c]*Represents the highest category of disease reported by the trials.*
[d]*Screening versus control.*

Table 9.2 Observational Studies of Advanced Breast Cancer Outcomes That Included Women in Their 40s

Author, Year	Study Design	Population; Age, Years; Participants, *n*	Study Years; Comparison	Outcome Measures	Results
Buseman et al., 2003[49]	Case series	US, Kaiser Permanente; 42–49 years; 247	1994 to 2000; screened vs unscreened	Stage II–IV; III–IV	• Stage II–IV: 39% (41/105) vs 52% (74/142), $p = 0.06$ • Stage III–IV: 4% vs 9%, $p =$ NR
Goel et al., 2007[45]	Case series	US, Vermont Breast Cancer Surveillance System; > 40 years; 1944	1994 to 2002; 1-year vs 2-year screening intervals	Either Stage IIB+; size > 20 mm; > 1 positive node	21% vs 24%, $p = 0.262$ No statistically significant differences by age
Hubbard et al., 2011[47]	Case series	US, BCSC data, multisite; 40–59 years; 4492	1996 to 2006; 1-year vs 2-year screening intervals	Stage IIB+	Adjusted proportion of cancer stage for 2-year vs 1-year intervals • Stage III or IV for 40–49 years: 4.8 (95% CI, 1.3 to 8.4) • No statistically significant differences for other stages
Kerlikowske et al., 2013[46]	Case series	US, BCSC data, multisite; 40–74 years; 11,474	1996 to 2008; 1-year vs 2-year vs 3-year screening intervals	Stage IIB–IV	Adjusted OR (95% CI) for 2-year vs 1-year intervals • Stages IIB– IV in age 40–49 + extreme breast density: 1.89 (1.06 to 3.39) • Tumor size > 20 mm in age 40–49 + extreme breast density: 2.39 (1.37 to 4.18) • No statistically significant differences for 40–49 years without extreme density, or for any comparisons between 3-year vs 2-year intervals
Miglioretti et al., 2015[48]	Case series	US, BCSC data, multisite; 40–49 years; 15,440	1996 to 2012; 1-year vs 2-year screening intervals	Stage IIB – IV; size > 15 mm; > 1 positive node	Adjusted OR (95% CI) for 2-year vs 1-year intervals, age 40 to 49 • Stages IIB – IV: 1.17 (0.93 to 1.46) • Tumor size > 15 mm: 1.10 (0.98 to 1.21) • Lymph node positive: 1.90 (0.92 to 1.29) • Composite outcome: 1.04 (0.94 to 1.14) Premenopausal • Stages IIB– IV: 1.28 (1.01 to 1.63) • Tumor size > 15 mm: 1.21 (1.07 to 1.37) • Lymph node positive: 1.15 (0.96 to 1.38) • Composite outcome: 1.11 (1.00 to 1.22)

Adapted from Ref. 27.
Abbreviations: BCSC, Breast Cancer Surveillance Consortium; CI, confidence interval; NR, not reported; US, United States; vs, versus.

A smaller BCSC study indicated no differences in outcomes between 1-year versus 2-year intervals,[45] and a non-BCSC study based on health system data also showed no differences between screened and unscreened women.[49]

While the BCSC studies included large numbers of women across the United States, their findings represent the opportunistic screening experiences of a fluctuating population of women. Findings may not be applicable to women not captured by the BCSC. Additional limitations include restrictions of registry data in addressing research questions, such as reliance on predefined data elements and inherent biases of observational data, particularly regarding the comparability of nonrandomized groups. In addition, the screening intervals were based on the time between the last two screening mammograms, not on consistent screening regimens, and the definitions of advanced breast cancer represented relatively early rather than advanced stages of disease.

SCREENING HARMS

FALSE-POSITIVE AND FALSE-NEGATIVE MAMMOGRAPHY RESULTS AND BIOPSIES

A false-positive mammography result occurs when the initial interpretation of a mammogram indicates an area of suspicion that is ultimately determined to be normal after obtaining additional imaging tests and sometimes biopsies. False-positive results are considered harms of screening because a healthy person is subjected to tests and procedures without direct benefit. A false-negative result occurs when a mammogram is interpreted as normal when a tumor actually exists. In this case, patients are harmed when diagnosis and treatment are delayed.

Determining the impact of false-positive and false-negative mammography results and biopsies on women undergoing screening is complex. Rates are dependent on patient factors, imaging technology, and practice variation. Under most conditions, younger women experience higher rates of false-positive mammograms relative to older women, which in turn result in subsequent recommendations for additional imaging and biopsies.

Population-based rates

A recent analysis of BCSC data in the United States estimated rates of false-positive and false-negative mammography results and recommendations for biopsy after a single round of digital mammography screening.[50] Of the 405,191 women aged 40 to 89 screened from 2003 to 2011 (including 113,770 women in their 40s), 2963 were diagnosed with invasive cancer or DCIS within 12 months of screening.

Rates of invasive breast cancer (2.2/1000) and DCIS (1.6/1000) were lowest among women in their 40s and increased across subsequent age categories (Fig. 9.3). Women aged 70 to 79 had the highest rates of invasive cancer (7.2/1000) and DCIS (2.3/1000). In this analysis, DCIS constituted a higher proportion of diagnoses for women in their 40s (35%) compared with older women (22% for age 70 to 79).

While rates of invasive cancer and DCIS were lowest among women in their 40s and increased with age, rates of false-positive mammography results were highest among women in their 40s (121.2/1000) and decreased with age (Fig. 9.4). Rates of false-negative mammography results were generally low for all age groups, ranging from 1.0/1000 to 1.5/1000, and did not differ by age ($p = 0.32$). Rates of recommendations for biopsy after a positive mammography result also did not differ by age (15.6/1000 to 17.5/1000; $p = 0.12$).

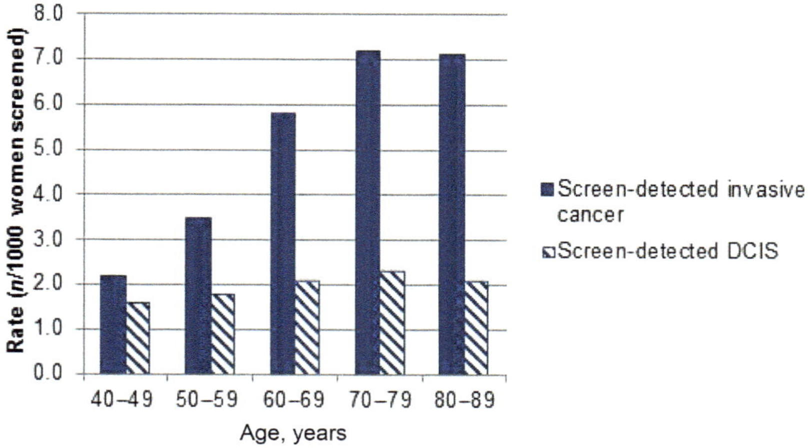

FIGURE 9.3

Age-specific rates of screen-detected invasive cancer and DCIS from a single screening round. Rates are lowest among women in their 40s and increase across subsequent age categories for invasive breast cancer (2.2/1000 women; $p < 0.001$) and DCIS (1.6/1000 women; $p = 0.055$).

Results from Ref. 27.

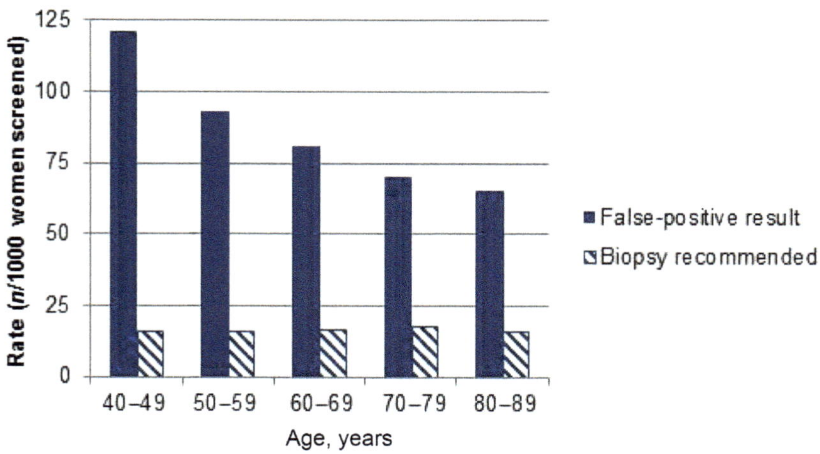

FIGURE 9.4

Age-specific rates of false-positive mammography results and recommendations for biopsy after a positive mammography from a single screening round. Rates of false-positive mammography results are highest among women in their 40s and decrease across subsequent age categories (121.2/1000; $p < 0.001$), while rates of recommendations for biopsy do not differ by age (16.4/1000; $p = 0.12$).

Results from Ref. 27.

These results indicate that mammography screening has a lower yield for younger women, because more women need to be screened in order to diagnose a case of breast cancer. Conversely, screening in older women has a higher yield because fewer women need to be screened in order to diagnose a case. For example, using the BCSC data, for every case of invasive breast cancer detected by mammography screening in women aged 40 to 49 years, 464 women had mammography, 58 were recommended for additional imaging, and 10 were recommended for biopsies.[27,50] In comparison, for women aged 70 to 79, for every case of invasive breast cancer detected by screening, 139 women had mammography, 11 were recommended for additional imaging, and 3 were recommended for biopsies.

Relationships of rates with risk factors and screening intervals

Patient factors related to these outcomes include the presence of known common risk factors for breast cancer specific to women in their 40s.[15] Significantly higher rates were estimated for women with first-degree relatives with breast cancer versus none; heterogeneous or extremely dense breast density versus entirely fat and scattered fibroglandular density; previous benign breast biopsies versus none; and for those who were premenopausal versus perimenopausal or postmenopausal; not currently using oral contraceptives versus users; and had a body mass index less than 30 kg/m^2 (Table 9.3).

When evaluating the effect of time since last mammography, rates of false-positives, false-negatives, and recommendations for biopsy did not differ by interval durations that estimated 1 versus 2-year screening cycles (9 to 18 vs 19 to 30 months; 11 to 14 vs 23 to 26 months).

Cumulative probability rates

While the BCSC analysis provided estimates based on one round of screening, additional observational studies estimated the cumulative probability of false-positive results for women in their 40s after 10 years of screening.[46,47,51] In a study of patients in a US health maintenance organization, the cumulative risk of at least one false-positive mammography result after 10 screening examinations using film mammography was estimated as 56%.[51] Results were similar in a study of film and digital

Table 9.3 Risk Factors Associated With Higher Rates of False-Positive and False-Negative Results and Recommendations for Biopsies

Risk Factor	False-Positive Results	False-Negative Results	Recommendation for Biopsy
One or more first-degree relatives with breast cancer	×	×	×
Breast density[a]			
Heterogeneous	×	×	×
Extreme		×	×
Previous benign biopsy	×		×
Premenopausal[b]	×		
No current use of oral contraceptives	×		×
Body mass index < 30	×		× (<25)

Results from Ref. 27.
[a]*Compared with entirely fat and scattered fibroglandular density.*
[b]*Compared with perimenopausal and postmenopausal.*

mammography based on BCSC data that estimated the 10-year rate as 61% with annual, and 42% with biennial screening.[47] In this study, the cumulative probability of receiving a false-positive biopsy recommendation after 10 years of screening was 7% with annual versus 5% with biennial screening. In a separate analysis of BCSC data, rates of false-positive mammography results and biopsies were highest among women in their 40s receiving annual mammography who had heterogeneously or extremely dense breasts (66% to 69% for mammography; 12% for biopsy).[46]

Rates with different screening modalities

The introduction of newer screening modalities, including digital breast tomosynthesis, MRI, and supplemental ultrasonography, provides opportunities to improve screening outcomes. Although most of the studies of these technologies indicate increased detection of noninvasive and early stage invasive cancer,[52–57] no studies have been done that demonstrate superiority over mammography alone in reducing breast cancer mortality.

In evaluations of screening tomosynthesis, recall rates were generally lower for women screened by combined tomosynthesis and mammography compared with mammography alone,[52–56] although results specifically for women in their 40s were not provided. While one US study reported a reduction of 16 recalls per 1000 women with combined tomosynthesis and mammography, it was accompanied by an increase of 1.3 biopsies per 1000 women.[52] Another US study demonstrated reduced recall rates with combined tomosynthesis and mammography versus mammography alone after controlling for age, breast density, and breast cancer risk (adjusted OR 0.62, 95% CI, 0.55 to 0.70; $p < 0.0001$),[53] although no differences were found in another smaller US study.[55] Lower recall rates were also reported in two European studies (1% vs 2%, $p < 0.0001$[56]; and 53/1000 vs 61/1000; $p = 0.001$[54]). While these studies suggest potential reductions in false-positive results with combined tomosynthesis and mammography, effects on rates of false-negative results and biopsies and how rates vary by patient factors including age are presently unclear.

A recent trial of women age 40 to 49 years in Japan indicated increased recall and biopsy rates with combined mammography and ultrasonography compared with mammography alone (12.6% vs 8.8% recall; 4.5% vs 1.8% biopsy).[57] Use of combined modalities also increased detection of noninvasive and early stage invasive cancer, but not stage II or worse disease.

OVERDIAGNOSIS AND OVERTREATMENT

Overdiagnosis in breast cancer screening refers to assigning a diagnosis of noninvasive or invasive breast cancer to abnormal lesions that are unlikely to become clinically evident in the absence of screening. Overdiagnosed women may be harmed by receiving unnecessary procedures and treatments, also referred to as overtreatment; as well as by the burden of having a cancer diagnosis (see also chapter: "Challenges in Understanding and Quantifying Overdiagnosis and Overtreatment"). For women in their 40s, overdiagnosis is particularly relevant to the diagnosis of DCIS which accounts for a large proportion of screen-detected breast cancer cases. Currently, DCIS is generally treated aggressively despite growing concerns that this approach may be unnecessary.[58,59]

Various methods have been used to estimate overdiagnosis and at least seven different measures of overdiagnosis have been reported,[60] yet there is no consensus defining a standard[61] (see also chapter: "Challenges in Understanding and Quantifying Overdiagnosis and Overtreatment"). Few estimates of overdiagnosis specifically for women in their 40s have been reported. In the Canadian screening trials, estimates for women age 40 to 49 were higher (12.4% to 22.7%) than for age 50 to 59 (9.7%

and 16.0%).[21,62] Unadjusted estimates from 13 observational studies of screening programs included in a systematic review indicated rates ranging from 0% to 54% across all ages; while six studies that adjusted for breast cancer risk and lead-time indicated rates ranging from 1% to 10%.[63] Estimates from other observational studies fall within this broad range. However, since most of the observational studies are based on European service screening programs that do not include women in their 40s, their relevance to this age group is uncertain.

Most of the studies of overdiagnosis are observational and are based on populations that were defined either geographically, or by the times in which exposures and outcomes occurred. Estimates of overdiagnosis describe a population phenomenon, not an individual assessment. Estimates represent averages across populations and are subject to confounders that may not be controlled, and assumptions that may be inaccurate. It is currently not possible to determine a woman's individual risk for overdiagnosis without knowing whether a particular lesion will progress to invasive cancer, how quickly a woman's cancer will advance, and her expected lifetime.

RADIATION EXPOSURE

Although two-view digital mammography and screen-film mammography are considered low dose, low energy radiation, cumulative radiation exposure is highest when screening is initiated at earlier ages and when screening is more frequent. In addition, high rates of additional imaging and subsequent biopsies among women in their 40s subject many women to variable additional levels of radiation exposure. No studies have directly measured the association between radiation exposure from mammography screening and the incidence of radiation-induced cancer and death. A recently published model estimated the number of deaths due to radiation-induced cancer from digital mammography screening as 7.6 per 100,000 in women screened annually between ages 40 to 49.[64] However, this estimate may not be clinically applicable when determining radiation risks for individual woman.

ANXIETY, DISTRESS, AND PAIN DURING PROCEDURES

Anxiety, distress, and pain during procedures are individual experiences that vary widely among women undergoing mammography screening. These experiences are difficult to quantify and evaluate, and their impact specifically on women in their 40s is unclear. Although a large number of descriptive studies reporting these outcomes have been published, results vary.[27,65] In general, studies indicate that women who receive clear communication of their negative mammography results have minimal anxiety with screening, while women recalled for further testing have more anxiety, breast cancer worry, and distress.[66–71] Some women have persistent anxiety, despite eventual negative results,[70,72–75] whereas others have only transient anxiety.[68,76–82] Although studies indicate that many women experience pain with screening procedures, few consider it a deterrent from future screening.[83,84] These responses to mammography screening can adversely affect the quality of life for some women, while others are not impacted.

SHARED DECISION-MAKING

Shared decision-making is a process that involves the patient and clinician in understanding the benefits, harms, and effectiveness of health care tests and treatments; determining personal priorities and values; and mutually agreeing upon a course of action. The goal of shared decision-making is to help align medical care with patients' preferences and values. It is especially useful when the tradeoff between benefits and harms is close, unclear, or unknown, as is the case with mammography screening for women in their 40s. Recent practice guidelines for women in their 40s specifically state that shared decision-making should be part of their screening decision[3,6,7] (see also chapter: "Informed and Shared Decision-Making in Breast Screening").

Patient decision aids are evidence-based tools that involve patients in shared decision-making by providing information about options and outcomes and clarifying personal values. Trials indicate that decision aids for various health conditions are more effective than usual care in providing patients with knowledge and reducing decisional conflict.[85] Despite the potential for decision aids to assist women in their 40s in making informed screening decisions, few resources are currently available.

A patient decision aid developed in the wake of the 2009 USPSTF recommendation that specifically called upon shared decision-making for this age group was recently evaluated for feasibility and effectiveness.[86,87] The aid was based on age-specific evidence of breast cancer risk factors for women in their 40s[15] and benefits and harms of screening,[27] and was developed using the International Patient Decision Aids Standards (IPDAS).[88] Components include a risk tool to identify women with increased breast cancer risk; information about screening and breast cancer; a priority setting activity (Fig. 9.5); and a customized report for the shared decision-making encounter. This report can be emailed to a clinician or electronic chart, or printed for the woman to bring to her clinic appointment.

Results of the study indicated that women using the decision aid in community-based clinics in the United States reported less conflict about their decisions for mammography screening, and felt more confident to make decisions after its use. In addition, clinics were able to integrate use of the aid into usual processes, and the aid enhanced their identification of women at increased risk for breast cancer. Adoption of these types of decision aids into clinical practice may lead to more informed patient choices and more appropriate use of screening services for women in their 40s.

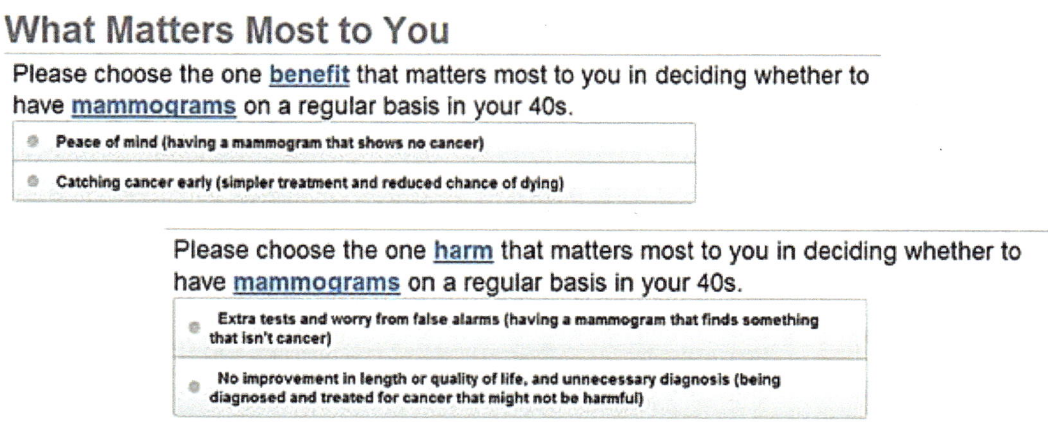

FIGURE 9.5

Patient aids guide shared decision-making for screening women in their 40s. Decision aids provide information about options and outcomes and clarify personal values about benefits and harms. Screenshots provided by the author.

CONCLUSIONS

Women in their 40s face conflicting breast cancer screening guidelines that are based on different interpretations of research and considerations of benefits and harms. While guideline groups generally agree that high-risk women in their 40s may benefit from initiating more frequent screening at younger ages, it remains unclear how to incorporate lower level risk factors in screening decisions.

The effectiveness of mammography screening in reducing breast cancer specific mortality was evaluated in eight RCTs including the UK Age trial that was specifically designed for women in their 40s. Neither the individual trials, nor the combined estimate indicated statistically significant differences between screening and control groups, although some results were borderline. Only two observational studies of women in Sweden and Canada compared outcomes of women in screening programs versus those not and reported results specifically for women in their 40s. Results indicated 26% to 44% reduced risk for breast cancer death, consistent with observational studies of women age 50 and older. However, observational studies are subject to biases that limit their use in determining effectiveness, particularly, they lack comparability of comparison groups that is only attainable through randomization. Results of RCTs and observational studies are consistent in showing no reductions in all-cause death with screening.

The incidence of advanced breast cancer was not reduced in an analysis of screening trials based on the most severe disease categories reported. Most observational studies of screening populations evaluated cancer stage based on time between screens. Results generally indicated earlier stage, smaller size, and fewer positive lymph nodes for 1 versus 2 year intervals. However, in these studies, screening was opportunistic and the definitions of advanced breast cancer represented relatively early rather than advanced stages of disease.

In a large US population, rates of invasive cancer and DCIS were lowest among women in their 40s and increased with age, while rates of false positive results were highest among women in their 40s and decreased with age. Over 50% of women in their 40s had false-positive results over a 10-year period. Rates of false-negative results and recommendations for biopsy after a positive mammography result did not differ by age. Higher false-positive rates were associated with personal risk factors for breast cancer. Rates of false-positives, false-negatives, and recommendations for biopsy did not differ by time since previous screening when comparing 1 versus 2-year intervals.

Observational studies suggest potential reductions in false-positive results with combined tomosynthesis and mammography compared to mammography alone, while effects on rates of false-negative results and biopsies and how rates vary by patient factors including age are presently unclear. Results of a trial in Japan indicated increased recall and biopsy rates with combined mammography and ultrasonography compared with mammography alone.

Additional potential harms of screening include overdiagnosis and overtreatment; radiation exposure; and anxiety, distress, and pain during procedures. However, current methods of defining, measuring, and quantifying their effects are inadequate, and determining their clinical relevance for individual women is unclear.

As a result of the current state of evidence and the dilemma of conflicting guidelines for women in their 40s, shared decision-making has become an important part of the screening process. In shared decision-making, each woman takes an active role in determining the appropriate screening services for her. Screening decisions could be improved by additional research on the effectiveness of screening women in their 40s who have specific risk factors, methods to reduce harms of screening, and approaches that improve communication and further involve women in the screening process.

ACKNOWLEDGMENTS

Spencer Dandy assisted with preparation of this chapter.

GLOSSARY

All-cause mortality deaths due to any cause.

Breast-cancer mortality deaths due to breast cancer.

Breast density a radiographic measure of breast tissue that is associated with increased risk for breast cancer and reduced mammography sensitivity.

Clinical relevance (applicability) how well the research findings from a study translate to other patient populations, settings, and circumstances.

False-negative mammography result a mammogram is interpreted as normal when a tumor actually exists; patients are harmed when diagnosis and treatment are delayed.

False-positive mammography result the initial interpretation of a mammogram indicates an area of suspicion that is ultimately determined to be normal after obtaining additional imaging tests and sometimes biopsies; patients are harmed when they are subjected to tests and procedures without direct benefits.

Long case accrual method counts all of the breast cancer cases contributing to breast cancer deaths diagnosed during the screening intervention period plus the follow-up period. This method has been referred to as the "follow-up" method of analysis by some investigators.

Meta-analysis statistical methods to combine results from two or more studies to provide summary estimates.

Overdiagnosis and overtreatment assigning a diagnosis of breast cancer to abnormal lesions that are unlikely to become clinically evident in the absence of screening. Overdiagnosed women may be harmed by receiving unnecessary procedures and treatments, also referred to as overtreatment; as well as by the burden of having a cancer diagnosis.

Randomization the assignment of screening or control groups is not predictable by the participant, researchers, and others and important confounders are equally distributed among comparison groups, including confounders that are unrecognized or not measured.

Randomized controlled trial (RCT) provides direct comparisons between screened and control groups; are regarded as the strongest study design to determine effectiveness, because a well-designed RCT is less susceptible to bias than other study designs.

Relative risk (RR) expresses risk for disease in terms of one group of individuals compared to another (eg, women randomized to the screening group vs control group).

Shared decision-making a process that involves the patient and clinician in understanding the benefits, harms, and effectiveness of health care tests and treatments; determining personal priorities and values; and mutually agreeing upon a course of action.

Short case accrual method includes only deaths occurring among cases of breast cancer diagnosed during the screening intervention period, and in some trials, within an additional defined case accrual period. This has been referred to as the "evaluation method" of analysis by some investigators.

LIST OF ACRONYMS AND ABBREVIATIONS

BCSC Breast Cancer Surveillance Consortium
BRCA Breast cancer susceptibility gene
CI Confidence interval

CNBSS-1	Canadian National Breast Screening Study 1
DCIS	Ductal carcinoma in situ
HIP	Health Insurance Plan of Greater New York
MMST	Malmö Mammographic Screening Trial
MRI	Magnetic resonance imaging
NCI	National Cancer Institute
RCT	Randomized controlled trial
RR	Relative risk
SMR	Standardized mortality ratio
USPSTF	U.S. Preventive Services Task Force

REFERENCES

1. American College of Obstetrics and Gynecology Practice bulletin no. 122: breast cancer screening. *Obstet Gynecol* 2011;**118**:372–82.
2. Lee CH, Dershaw DD, Kopans D, Evans P, Monsees B, Monticciolo D, et al. Breast cancer screening with imaging: recommendations from the Society of Breast Imaging and the ACR on the use of mammography, breast MRI, breast ultrasound, and other technologies for the detection of clinically occult breast cancer. *J Am Coll Radiol* 2010;**7**:18–27.
3. U.S. Preventive Services Task Force. Screening for breast cancer: U.S. Preventive Services Task Force recommendation statement. *Ann Intern Med*; published online Jan. 12, 2016.
4. Canadian Task Force on Preventive Health Care, Tonelli M, Connor Gorber S, et al. Recommendations on screening for breast cancer in average-risk women aged 40–74 years [Erratum appears in CMAJ. 2011 Dec 13;183(18):2147]. *CMAJ* 2011;**183**:1991–2001.
5. Giordano L, von Karsa L, Tomatis M, Majek O, de Wolf C, Lancucki L, et al. Mammographic screening programmes in Europe: organization, coverage and participation. *J Med Screen* 2012;**19**:72–82.
6. Oeffinger KC, Fontham EH, Etzioni R, Herzig A, Michaelson JS, Shih YCT, et al. Breast cancer screening for women at average risk: 2015 guideline update from the American Cancer Society. *JAMA* 2015;**314**: 1599–614.
7. Qaseem A, Snow V, Sherif K, Aronson M, Weiss KB, Owens DK, et al. Screening mammography for women 40 to 49 years of age: a clinical practice guideline from the American College of Physicians [Summary for patients in Ann Intern Med. 2007 Apr 3;146(7):I20; PMID: 17404347]. *Ann Intern Med* 2007; **146**:511–5.
8. Nelson HD, Weerasinghe R, Wang L, Grunkemeier G. Mammography screening in a large health system following the U.S. Preventive Services Task Force recommendations and the Affordable Care Act. *PLoS One* 2015;**10**:e0131903.
9. Nelson HD, Pappas M, Zakher B, Mitchell JP, Okinaka-Hu L, Fu R. Risk assessment, genetic counseling, and genetic testing for BRCA-related cancer in women: a systematic review to update the U.S. Preventive Services Task Force recommendation. *Ann Intern Med* 2014;**160**:255–66.
10. Coopey S, Mazzola E, Buckley J, Sharko J, Belli AK, Kim EM, et al. The role of chemoprevention in modifying the risk of breast cancer in women with atypical breast lesions. *Breast Cancer Res Treat* 2012;**136**:627–33.
11. Tice JA, O'Meara ES, Weaver DL, Vachon C, Ballard-Barbash R, Kerlikowske K. Benign breast disease, mammographic breast density, and the risk of breast cancer. *J Natl Cancer Inst* 2013;**105**:1043–9.
12. Tice JA, Miglioretti DL, Li CS, Vachon CM, Gard CC, Kerlikowske K. Breast density and benign breast disease: risk assessment to identify women at high risk of breast cancer. *J Clin Oncol* 2015;**33**:3137–43.
13. Moskowitz CS, Chou JF, Wolden SL, Bernstein JL, Malhotra J, Novetsky D, et al. Breast cancer after chest radiation therapy for childhood cancer. *J Clin Oncol* 2014;**32**:2217–23.

14. van Ravesteyn NT, Miglioretti DL, Stout NK, Lee SJ, Schechter CB, Buist DSM, et al. What level of risk tips the balance of benefits and harms to favor screening mammography starting at age 40? *Ann Intern Med* 2012;**156**:609–17.
15. Nelson HD, Zakher B, Cantor A, Fu R, Griffin J, O'Meara ES, et al. Risk factors for breast cancer for women aged 40 to 49 years: a systematic review and meta-analysis. *Ann Intern Med* 2012;**156**:635–48.
16. Sprague BL, Gangnon RE, Burt V, Trentham-Dietz A, Hampton JM, Wellman RD, et al. Prevalence of mammographically dense breasts in the United States. *J Natl Cancer Inst* 2014;**106**(10). Available from: http://dx.doi.org/10.1093/jnci/dju255.
17. Nelson HD, Smith ME, Griffin JC, Fu R. Use of medications to reduce risk for primary breast cancer: a systematic review for the U.S. Preventive Services Task Force. *Ann Intern Med* 2013;**158**:604–14.
18. Moss SM, Cuckle H, Evans A, Johns L, Waller M, Bobrow L, et al. Effect of mammographic screening from age 40 years on breast cancer mortality at 10 years' follow-up: a randomised controlled trial. *Lancet* 2006;**368**:2053–60.
19. Moss SM, Wale C, Smith R, Evans A, Cuckle H, Duffy SW. Effect of mammographic screening from age 40 years on breast cancer mortality in the UK Age trial at 17 years' follow-up: a randomised controlled trial. *Lancet Oncol* 2015;**16**:1123–32.
20. Miller AB, Baines CJ, To T, Wall C. Canadian National Breast Screening Study-1: breast cancer detection and death rates among women aged 40 to 49 years. *CMAJ* 1992;**147**:1459–76.
21. Miller AB, To T, Baines CJ, Wall C. The Canadian National Breast Screening Study-1: breast cancer mortality after 11 to 16 years of follow-up. A randomized screening trial of mammography in women age 40 to 49 years. *Ann Intern Med* 2002;**137**:305–12.
22. Shapiro S, Venet W, Strax P, Venet L, Roeser R. Ten- to fourteen-year effect of screening on breast cancer mortality. *J Natl Cancer Inst* 1982;**69**:349–55.
23. Frisell J, Lidbrink E, Hellstrom L, Rutgvist LE. Followup after 11 years—update of mortality results in the Stockholm mammographic screening trial. *Breast Cancer Res Treat* 1997;**45**:263–70.
24. Andersson I, Aspegren K, Janzon L, Landberg T, Lindholm K, Linell F, et al. Mammographic screening and mortality from breast cancer: the Malmö mammographic screening trial. *BMJ* 1988;**297**:943–8.
25. Tabár L, Fagerberg G, Chen HH, Duffy SW, Smart CR, Gad A, et al. Efficacy of breast cancer screening by age. New results from the Swedish Two-County Trial. *Cancer* 1995;**75**:2507–17.
26. Bjurstam N, Bjorneld L, Warwick J, Sala E, Duffy SW, Nystrom L, et al. The Gothenburg breast screening trial. *Cancer* 2003;**97**:2387–96.
27. Nelson HD, Cantor A, Humphrey L, Fu R, Pappas M, Daeges M, Griffin J. *Screening for breast cancer: a systematic review to update the 2009 U.S. Preventive Services Task Force Recommendation.* Evidence Synthesis No. 124. AHRQ Publication No. 14-05201-EF-1. Rockville, MD: Agency for Healthcare Research and Quality; 2016.
28. Nelson HD, Fu R, Cantor A, Pappas M, Daeges M, Humphrey L. Effectiveness of breast cancer screening: systematic review and meta-analysis to update the 2009 U.S. Preventive Services Task Force Recommendation. *Ann Intern Med*; published online Jan. 12, 2016.
29. Miller AB, Wall C, Baines CJ, Sun P, To T, Narod SA. Twenty five year follow-up for breast cancer incidence and mortality of the Canadian National Breast Screening Study: randomised screening trial. *Br Med J* 2014;**348**:g366.
30. Habbema JD, van Oortmarssen GJ, van Putten DJ, Lubbe JT, van der Maas PJ. Age-specific reduction in breast cancer mortality by screening: an analysis of the results of the Health Insurance Plan of Greater New York study. *J Natl Cancer Inst* 1986;**77**:317–20.
31. Nyström L, Andersson I, Bjurstam N, Frisell J, Nordenskjöld B, Rutgvist LE. Long-term effects of mammography screening: updated overview of the Swedish randomised trials. *Lancet* 2002;**359**:909–19.
32. Moss S, Johns L, Cuckle H, Bobrow L, Evans A, Kutt L, et al. *Randomised controlled trial of mammographic screening in young women: updated results on incidence and mortality.* <http://conference.ncri.org.uk/abstracts/2009/abstracts/B35.htm>; 2009 [accessed 18.09.14].

33. Broeders M, Moss S, Nyström L, Njor S, Jonsson H, Paap E, et al. The impact of mammographic screening on breast cancer mortality in Europe: a review of observational studies. *J Med Screen* 2012;**19**(Suppl. 1): 14–25.
34. Moss SM, Nyström L, Jonsson H, Paci E, Lynge E, Njor S, et al. The impact of mammographic screening on breast cancer mortality in Europe: a review of trend studies. *J Med Screen* 2012;**19**(Suppl. 1):26–32.
35. Njor S, Nyström L, Moss S, Paci E, Broeders M, Segnan N, et al. Breast cancer mortality in mammographic screening in Europe: a review of incidence-based mortality studies. *J Med Screen* 2012;**19**(Suppl. 1):33–41.
36. Harris R, Yeatts J, Kinsinger L. Breast cancer screening for women ages 50 to 69 years a systematic review of observational evidence. *Prev Med* 2011;**53**:108–14.
37. Hellquist BN, Duffy SW, Abdsaleh S, Björneld L, Bordas P, Tabar L, et al. Effectiveness of population-based service screening with mammography for women ages 40 to 49 years: evaluation of the Swedish Mammography Screening in Young Women (SCRY) cohort. *Cancer* 2011;**117**:714–22.
38. Coldman A, Phillips N, Wilson C, Decker K, Chiarelli AM, Brisson J, et al. Pan-Canadian study of mammography screening and mortality from breast cancer. *J Natl Cancer Inst* 2014:106. Available from: http://dx.doi.org/10.1095/jnci/dju261.
39. Miller AB, Baines CJ, To T, Wall C. Canadian National Breast Screening Study-2: breast cancer detection and death rates among women aged 50 to 59 years. *CMAJ* 1992;**147**:1477–88.
40. Parvinen I, Chiu S, Pylkkänen L, Klemi P, Immonen-Räihä P, Kauhava L, et al. Effects of annual vs triennial mammography interval on breast cancer incidence and mortality in ages 40–49 in Finland. *Br J Cancer* 2011;**105**:1388–91.
41. Chu KC, Smart CR, Tarone RE. Analysis of breast cancer mortality and stage distribution by age for the Health Insurance Plan clinical trial. *J Natl Cancer Inst* 1988;**80**:1125–32.
42. Moss S, Thomas I, Evans A, Thomas B, Johns L, Trial Management Group. Randomised controlled trial of mammographic screening in women from age 40: results of screening in the first 10 years. *Br J Cancer* 2005;**92**:949–54.
43. Ballard-Barbash R, Taplin SH, Yankaskas BC, Ernster VL, Rosenberg RD, Carney PA, et al. Breast Cancer Surveillance Consortium: a national mammography screening and outcomes database. *Am J Roentgenol* 1997;**169**:1001–8.
44. National Cancer Institute. *Breast Cancer Surveillance Consortium: Evaluating Screening Performance in Practice. NIH Publication No. 04-5490*. Bethesda, MD: National Cancer Institute, National Institutes of Health, U.S. Department of Health and Human Services. <http://breastscreening.cancer.gov/espp.pdf>; 2004 [accessed 19.09.14].
45. Goel A, Littenberg B, Burack RC. The association between the pre-diagnosis mammography screening interval and advanced breast cancer. *Breast Cancer Res Treat* 2007;**102**:339–45.
46. Kerlikowske K, Zhu W, Hubbard RA, Geller B, Dittus K, Braithwaite D, et al. Outcomes of screening mammography by frequency, breast density, and postmenopausal hormone therapy. *JAMA Intern Med* 2013;**173**:807–16.
47. Hubbard RA, Kerlikowske K, Flowers CI, Yankaskas BC, Zhu W, Miglioretti DL. Cumulative probability of false-positive recall or biopsy recommendation after 10 years of screening mammography: a cohort study [Summary for patients in Ann Intern Med. 2011 Oct 18;155(8):I14; PMID: 22007059]. *Ann Intern Med* 2011;**155**:481–92.
48. Miglioretti DL, Zhu W, Kerlikowske K, Sprauge BL, Onega T, Buist DS, et al. Breast tumor prognostic characteristics and biennial vs annual mammography, age, and menopausal status. *JAMA Oncol* 2015;**1**(8):1069–77.
49. Buseman S, Mouchawar J, Calonge N, Byers T. Mammography screening matters for young women with breast carcinoma: evidence of downstaging among 42–49-year-old women with a history of previous mammography screening. *Cancer* 2003;**97**:352–8.

50. Nelson HD, O'Meara ES, Kerlikowske K, Balch S, Miglioretti D. Factors associated with rates of false-positive and false-negative results from digital mammography screening: an analysis of registry data. *Ann Intern Med*; published online Jan. 12, 2016.
51. Elmore JG, Barton MB, Moceri VM, Polk S, Arena PJ, Fletcher SW. Ten-year risk of false positive screening mammograms and clinical breast examinations [see comment]. *N Engl J Med* 1998;**338**:1089–96.
52. Friedewald SM, Rafferty EA, Rose SL, Durand MA, Plecha DM, Greenberg JS, et al. Breast cancer screening using tomosynthesis in combination with digital mammography. *JAMA* 2014;**311**:2499–507.
53. Haas BM, Kalra V, Geisel J, Raghu M, Durand M, Philpotts LE. Comparison of tomosynthesis plus digital mammography and digital mammography alone for breast cancer screening. *Radiology* 2013;**269**:694–700.
54. Skaane P, Bandos AI, Gullien R, Eben EB, Ekseth U, Haakenaasen U, et al. Comparison of digital mammography alone and digital mammography plus tomosynthesis in a population-based screening program. *Radiology* 2013;**267**:47–56.
55. Rose SL, Tidwell AL, Bujnoch LJ, Kushwaha AC, Nordmann AS, Sexton Jr R, et al. Implementation of breast tomosynthesis in a routine screening practice: an observational study. *Am J Roentgenol* 2013;**200**:1401–8.
56. Ciatto S, Houssami N, Bernardi D, Caumo F, Pellegrini M, Brunelli S, et al. Integration of 3D digital mammography with tomosynthesis for population breast-cancer screening (STORM): a prospective comparison study. *Lancet Oncol* 2013;**14**:583–9.
57. Ohuchi N, Suzuki A, Sobue T, Kawai M, Yamamoto S, Zheng YF, et al. Sensitivity and specificity of mammography and adjunctive ultrasonography to screen for breast cancer in the Japan Strategic Anti-cancer Randomized Trial (J-START): a randomised controlled trial. *Lancet* 2015; published online Nov. 4, 2015.
58. Narod SA, Iqbal J, Giannakeas V, Sopik V, Sun P. Breast cancer mortality after a diagnosis of ductal carcinoma in situ. *JAMA Oncol* 2015;**1**:888–96.
59. Esserman L, Yau C. Rethinking the standard for ductal carcinoma in situ treatment. *JAMA Oncol* 2015;**1**:881–3.
60. de Gelder R, Heijnsdijk EAM, van Ravesteyn NT, Fracheboud J, Draisma G, de Koning HJ. Interpreting overdiagnosis estimates in population-based mammography screening. *Epidemiol Rev* 2011;**33**:111–21.
61. Independent UKPoBCS The benefits and harms of breast cancer screening: an independent review. *Lancet* 2012;**380**:1778–86.
62. Miller AB, To T, Baines CJ, Wall C. Canadian National Breast Screening Study-2: 13-year results of a randomized trial in women aged 50–59 years. *J Natl Cancer Inst* 2000;**92**:1490–9.
63. Puliti D, Duffy SW, Miccinesi G, de Koning H, Lynge E, Zappa M, et al. Overdiagnosis in mammographic screening for breast cancer in Europe: a literature review. *J Med Screen* 2012;**19**(Suppl. 1):42–56.
64. Yaffe MJ, Mainprize JG. Risk of radiation-induced breast cancer from mammographic screening [Erratum appears in Radiology. 2012 Jul;264(1):306]. *Radiology* 2011;**258**:98–105.
65. Nelson HD, Pappas M, Cantor A, Griffin J, Daeges M, Humphrey L. Harms of breast cancer screening: systematic review to update the 2009 U.S. Preventive Services Task Force recommendation. *Ann Intern Med*; published online Jan. 12, 2016.
66. Brett J, Bankhead C, Henderson B, Watson E, Austoker J. The psychological impact of mammographic screening. A systematic review. *Psychooncology* 2005;**14**:917–38.
67. Hafslund B, Nortvedt MW. Mammography screening from the perspective of quality of life: a review of the literature. *Scand J Caring Sci* 2009;**23**:539–48.
68. Lowe JB, Balanda KP, Del Mar C, Hawes E. Psychologic distress in women with abnormal findings in mass mammography screening. *Cancer* 1999;**85**:1114–8.
69. Hislop TG, Harris SR, Jackson J, Thorne SE, Rousseau EJ, Coldman AJ, et al. Satisfaction and anxiety for women during investigation of an abnormal screening mammogram. *Breast Cancer Res Treat* 2002;**76**:245–54.
70. Brett J, Austoker J. Women who are recalled for further investigation for breast screening: psychological consequences 3 years after recall and factors affecting re-attendance. *J Public Health Med* 2001;**23**:292–300.

71. Ong G, Austoker J, Brett J. Breast screening: adverse psychological consequences one month after placing women on early recall because of a diagnostic uncertainty. A multicentre study. *J Med Screen* 1997;**4**:158–68.
72. Aro AR, Pilvikki Absetz S, Van Elderen TM, van der Ploeg E, van der Kamp LJ. False-positive findings in mammography screening induces short-term distress—breast cancer-specific concern prevails longer. *Eur J Cancer* 2000;**36**:1089–97.
73. Brett J, Austoker J, Ong G. Do women who undergo further investigation for breast screening suffer adverse psychological consequences? A multi-centre follow-up study comparing different breast screening result groups five months after their last breast screening appointment. *J Public Health Med* 1998;**20**:396–403.
74. Lerman C, Trock B, Rimer BK, Boyce A, Jepson C, Engstrom PF. Psychological and behavioral implications of abnormal mammograms. *Ann Intern Med* 1991;**114**:657–61.
75. Lampic C, Thurfjell E, Sjödén PO. The influence of a false-positive mammogram on a woman's subsequent behaviour for detecting breast cancer. *Eur J Cancer* 2003;**39**:1730–7.
76. Cockburn J, Staples M, Hurley SF, De Luise T. Psychological consequences of screening mammography. *J Med Screen* 1994;**1**:7–12.
77. Ekeberg Ø, Skjauff H, Kåresen R. Screening for breast cancer is associated with a low degree of psychological distress. *Breast* 2001;**10**:20–4.
78. Gilbert FJ, Cordiner CM, Affleck IR, Hood DB, Mathieson D, et al. Breast screening: the psychological sequelae of false-positive recall in women with and without a family history of breast cancer. *Eur J Cancer* 1998;**34**:2010–4.
79. Gram IT, Lund E, Slenker SE. Quality of life following a false positive mammogram. *Br J Cancer* 1990;**62**:1018–22.
80. Lampic C, Thurfjell E, Bergh J, Sjöden PO. Short- and long-term anxiety and depression in women recalled after breast cancer screening. *Eur J Cancer* 2001;**37**:463–9.
81. Lidbrink E, Levi L, Pettersson I, Rosendahl I, Rutgvist LE, de la Torre B, et al. Single-view screening mammography: psychological, endocrine and immunological effects of recalling for a complete three-view examination. *Eur J Cancer* 1995;**31**:932–3.
82. Sandin B, Chorot P, Valiente RM, Lostao L, Santed MA. Adverse psychological effects in women attending a second-stage breast cancer screening. *J Psychosom Res* 2002;**52**:303–9.
83. Armstrong K, Moye E, Williams S, Berlin JA, Reynolds EE. Screening mammography in women 40 to 49 years of age: a systematic review for the American College of Physicians. *Ann Intern Med* 2007;**146**:516–26.
84. Whelehan P, Evans A, Wells M, Macgillivray S. The effect of mammography pain on repeat participation in breast cancer screening: a systematic review. *Breast* 2013;**22**:389–94.
85. Stacey D, Legare F, Col NF, Bennett CL, Barry MJ, Eden KB, et al. Decision aids for people facing health treatment or screening decisions. *Cochrane Database Syst Rev* 2014;**1**:CD001431.
86. Eden KB, Scariati P, Klein K, Watson L, Remiker M, Hribar M, et al. Mammography decision aid reduces decisional conflict for women in their forties considering screening. *J Womens Health (Larchmt)* 2015;**24**(12):1013–20.
87. Scariati P, Nelson L, Watson L, Bedrick S, Eden KB. Impact of a decision aid on reducing uncertainty: pilot study of women in their 40s and screening mammography. *BMC Med Inform Decis Mak* 2015;**15**:89.
88. Collaboration IPDAS. IPDAS 2005: criteria for judging the quality of patient decision aids; 2014. Disponibile a: www ipdas ohri ca/IPDAS_checklist pdf Ultimo accesso. 18.

CHAPTER

SCREENING FOR BREAST CANCER IN WOMEN WITH DENSE BREASTS

10

Jeffrey A. Tice[1] and Karla Kerlikowske[2]

[1]Division of General Internal Medicine, Department of Medicine, University of California, San Francisco, CA, United States, [2]General Internal Medicine Section, Department of Veteran Affairs, San Francisco, CA, and Departments of Medicine and Epidemiology and Biostatistics, University of California, San Francisco, CA, United States

CHAPTER OUTLINE

Breast Cancer Screening. DOI: http://dx.doi.org/10.1016/B978-0-12-802209-2.00010-3

PLAIN LANGUAGE SUMMARY

Mammography is the only screening test that reduces death from breast cancer in randomized trials. However, it does not detect all cancers that are present. One of the reasons that mammography misses cancers is that dense areas on the image can obscure cancers. Both breast cancers and breast density show up as white on mammograms so it is more difficult to identify cancer in an area of density. Digital mammography improves the detection of breast cancers in dense breasts, but cancers are still missed. This raises the question about the potential benefits of additional screening with different technology.

Four approaches have been advocated to identify cancers in women with dense breasts and normal screening mammograms: hand-held ultrasound, automated breast ultrasound, breast magnetic resonance imaging (MRI), and digital breast tomosynthesis. All four of these technologies generate multiple images representing slices of the breast that allow the radiologist to visualize the breast with less overlapping tissue. This is particularly useful in dense breasts because overlapping dense tissue may hide breast cancer.

No clinical trials demonstrate that supplemental screening reduces death from breast cancer. Studies do show that all four techniques identify additional cancers in women with normal mammograms. Hand-held ultrasound is the best studied: it identifies an additional two cancers per 1000 women screened, but is time-consuming, dependent on the skill of the operator, and requires more biopsies to find one cancer than other techniques. Automated breast ultrasound was developed to remove the operator dependency, shorten the time of image acquisition, and improve the efficiency of ultrasound, but suffers from the same high number of biopsies performed to find one cancer. MRI finds the most additional cancers, but is very expensive, time-intensive, and requires intravenous contrast. It is only practical for women at the highest risk for breast cancer, such as carriers of mutations in the BRCA genes. Tomosynthesis, on the other hand, finds an additional two cancers per 1000 women screened and requires a similar number of biopsies to find one cancer as traditional digital screening mammography; however, as currently practiced it doubles the radiation dose. It is the most promising technology.

Not all women with dense breasts require additional imaging. Breast density information can be combined with a woman's risk for breast cancer to target those women at highest risk for missed cancers. Using a risk-based strategy, only about one in four women with dense breasts would be recommended for supplemental screening.

INTRODUCTION

This chapter summarizes the evidence on the comparative clinical effectiveness of standard screening mammography and supplemental imaging to screen women with mammographically dense breasts following a negative mammogram. As of 2015, 24 states in the United States have passed legislation requiring mammography facilities to notify women with dense breasts about their density. For example, on April 1, 2013 a law[1] went into effect in California requiring mammography facilities to inform women with dense breasts about the potential for "masking" and the increased risk of breast cancer associated with dense breast tissue. Masking occurs when breast cancers are hidden by dense breast tissue on a mammogram, which, like cancer, appears white. The law requires the following language be included in reports sent to women who have dense breast tissue:

> Your mammogram shows that your breast tissue is dense. Dense breast tissue is common and is not abnormal. However, dense breast tissue can make it harder to evaluate the results of your mammogram and may also be associated with an increased risk of breast cancer. This information about the results of your mammogram is given to you to raise your awareness and to inform your conversations with your doctor. Together, you can decide which screening options are right for you. A report of your results was sent to your physician.[1]

The primary motivation for the law is to alert women to the masking effect of dense breast tissue on their mammograms. However, dense breast tissue may also play an important role by identifying women at high enough risk for breast cancer to warrant additional imaging with a different technology. A number of new technologies and new applications of existing technologies have been promoted to enhance screening in women with dense breasts. These include hand-held and automated breast ultrasound, magnetic resonance imaging (MRI), and digital breast tomosynthesis (DBT).

This chapter will summarize the evidence about film and digital screening mammography in women with dense breasts and the harms and benefits of supplemental screening after a normal screening mammography examination. We will also assess ways to estimate the overall risk of breast cancer for women with dense breasts and a negative mammogram to guide the decision about which women are more likely, and which less, to benefit from supplemental screening.

BACKGROUND

BREAST CANCER

Breast cancer is the most common cancer in women worldwide. There were approximately 1.7 million new cases of breast cancer and 552,000 deaths from breast cancer in 2012.[2] In the United States, mortality from breast cancer has declined by about 2.2% per year since 1990, a 28% overall decline.[3] The median values from a series of models estimated that a little more than half of the decline was due to improvements in therapy for breast cancer and that a little less than half (46%) was due to early diagnosis from mammography while a more recent study in Norway found only 33% of the reduction in breast cancer mortality was due to screening.[4,5] An analysis of 30 years of data from the United States Surveillance, Epidemiology, and End Results (SEER) data also called into question the contributions of screening mammography to decreasing breast cancer mortality.[6] Bleyer and Welch estimated that 31% of breast cancer diagnosed with mammography represents "overdiagnosis" (ie, identification of cancers unlikely to cause significant morbidity or mortality) and concluded that screening mammography has had, at best, only a small effect on breast cancer mortality.[6]

SCREENING FOR BREAST CANCER

The primary method worldwide used to screen for breast cancer is mammography. Nine large clinical trials established the efficacy of screening mammography by randomizing over 600,000 women and following them for 10–20 years.[7–25] The results have been summarized in many systematic reviews and meta-analyses.[26–41] There is general consensus that, for women between the ages of 50 and 69 years, screening mammography reduces breast cancer mortality by approximately 20% to 25% after 15 years of follow-up.[36] For average-risk women between the ages of 40 and 49 years, there remains controversy about whether the benefits of routine mammography outweigh the harms, such that most countries that offer mammography do not offer routine screening to women aged 40–49 years and some recommend a discussion of the benefits and harms of mammography allowing women to decide on screening based on their personal preference.[42–45]

DIGITAL MAMMOGRAPHY

Mammography was traditionally performed with film. It was one of the last radiographic procedures to transition from film to digital imaging because mammography requires extremely high resolution to be effective. Digital image acquisition improves the signal to noise ratio of X-ray detection over a wider contrast range than film.[46–48] Digital enhancement of the images at computer workstations may also improve the accuracy of mammographic interpretation.[47] In particular, increased contrast resolution improves the detection of low contrast lesions in radiographically dense breasts. Digital mammography has become the standard across the United States. As of October 1, 2015, 97.5% (14,769/15,153) of all US mammography machines accredited by the Food and Drug Administration (FDA) are full-field digital.[49]

MAMMOGRAPHIC BREAST DENSITY

Mammographic density refers to areas within the breast that absorb significant amounts of X-ray energy and show up as relatively white areas on the mammogram. These correspond to regions in the breast that are rich in epithelial and stromal tissue while the nondense (darker gray areas) correspond to regions that are predominantly fat.

In the United States, the Breast Imaging Reporting and Data System (BI-RADS) of the American College of Radiology[50] classifies density in the following four breast composition categories:

a. The breasts are almost entirely fatty.
b. There are scattered areas of fibroglandular density.
c. The breasts are heterogeneously dense, which may obscure small masses.
d. The breasts are extremely dense, which lowers the sensitivity of mammography.

The prevalence of high breast density (BD; heterogeneous or extremely dense tissue) is 43% in women 40–74 years old, which represents almost 28 million women in the United States.[51] The prevalence varies by age declining from 57% for women between the ages of 40 and 44 years to 28% for women ages 85 years and older. High BD using the BI-RADS categories is also more common in Asian women.[52]

It has been known for years that the sensitivity of film mammography is lower in women with dense breasts than in women with fatty breasts.[53] There is a masking effect due to mammographic density. In the Breast Cancer Surveillance Consortium (BCSC), a US collaboration of breast imaging registries, the sensitivity of film mammography decreased markedly with increasing density (see Table 10.1).[54] This

Table 10.1 Sensitivity of Film and Digital Mammography by Breast Density

Study	Type	BI-RADS Density Category			
		Almost Entirely Fatty (a)	Scattered Fibroglandular Densities (b)	Heterogeneously Dense (c)	Extremely Dense (d)
BCSC (Carney 2003)[54]	Film	88.2	82.1	68.9	62.2
DMIST (Pisano 2005)[55]	Film			55[a]	
	Digital			70[a]	
BCSC (Kerlikowske 2011)[57]	Film	85.7	85.1	79.3	68.1
	Digital	78.3	86.6	82.1	83.6

[a]*The DMIST study reported results for the combined high-density categories only.*

study evaluated the results from 463,372 screening film mammograms performed between 1996 and 1998. Among women in the low density categories, the sensitivity of mammography was 88% and 82% for density categories a and b, respectively, but this decreased to 69% for women with heterogeneously dense breasts and to 62% for women with extremely dense breasts.[54]

BD AND DIGITAL MAMMOGRAPHY

As described above, the increased contrast resolution of digital mammography improves the detection of low contrast lesions in radiographically dense breasts. Thus digital mammography should improve the sensitivity of mammography in women with dense breast tissue compared to film.

The Digital Mammography Imaging Screening Trial (DMIST) study is the largest trial directly comparing digital mammography to plain film mammography ($n = 42{,}760$).[55] All women were screened with both film and digital mammography on the same visit. Mammograms were read independently by radiologists blinded to the results of the other mammogram. In DMIST, digital mammography had the same recall and biopsy rates as film mammography. Digital mammography was more sensitive than film for younger women with denser breasts (59.1% vs 27.3%, $p = 0.\ 0013$).[56] Among women of all ages with either heterogeneously dense or extremely dense breasts, digital mammography was also more sensitive than film mammography (70% vs 55%, $p = 0.02$, Table 10.2). Similarly, in women with dense breast tissue there was a trend towards greater specificity with digital mammography (91% vs 90%, $p = 0.09$) and the overall accuracy of digital mammography, as measured by the area under the receiver operator curve, was greater than that of film mammography (0.78 vs 0.68, $p = 0.003$).[55]

The BCSC has reported on the accuracy of screening mammography based on a comparison of 231,034 digital mammograms and 638,252 film mammograms performed between January 1, 2000 and December 31, 2006.[57] Similar to the prior study, the sensitivity of film mammography decreased from 86% to 68% across the four BD categories (see Table 10.2). However, for digital mammography, the sensitivity of digital mammography remained greater than 80% for the highest density categories and did *not* appear to decrease with increasing density (see Table 10.2). As in the DMIST trial, digital mammography was significantly more sensitive than film mammography in women with dense breasts, but had lower specificity.

Table 10.2 Cancer Detection, Sensitivity, and Specificity of Digital Mammography by Breast Density

Study	Type	BI-RADS Density Category			
		Almost Entirely Fatty (a)	Scattered Fibroglandular Densities (b)	Heterogeneously Dense (c)	Extremely Dense (d)
BCSC (Kerlikowske 2011)[57]	Rate[a]	1.8	3.3	4.8	5.1
	Sens	78	87	82	84
	Spec	95	91	87	89

[a]Rate = breast cancer detection rate per 1000 women screened.

Table 10.3 Recall Rates and Cancer Detection Using Film and Digital Mammography in Large Studies of Screening Irrespective of Density

Study	Type	Mammograms, *n*	Recall Rate per 1000	Biopsy Rate per 1000	Cancer Detection per 1000	PPV3
DMIST (Pisano 2005)[55]	Film	42,555	86	16.0	4.1	24.4
	Digital	42,555	86	15.9	4.4	26.0
Vestfold (Vigeland 2008)[58]	Film	324,763	42	NR	6.5	15.1
	Digital	18,239	41	NR	7.7	18.5
BCSC (Kerlikowske 2011)[57]	Film	638,252	93	10.6	3.8	24.7
	Digital	231,034	100	11.0	3.8	25.3

Note: PPV3, the positive predictive value for biopsies performed.

Table 10.2 shows the cancer detection rate and specificity in addition to the sensitivity of digital mammography by BI-RADS density category in the BCSC study. Despite concerns about the test performance of mammography in dense breasts, more breast cancers are found per 1000 digital screening mammograms in the dense breast categories than in the nondense categories. This highlights the general principle that the yield of screening tests is greater as the underlying risk of the population screened goes up. Women with dense breasts are at higher risk, so the cancer detection rate is higher. These data also suggest that the masking effect of BD is reduced when digital mammography is used.

Table 10.3 summarizes important outcomes with film and digital mammograms in the three largest studies that report data on both digital and film mammography.[55,57,58] These are useful benchmarks to use when evaluating the potential yield of additional imaging compared to no additional imaging. The biopsy rate and cancer detection rate did not differ between women screened with digital or film mammography in any of these studies, although the recall rate for digital was higher in the BCSC (100 vs 93 per 1000, $p < 0.001$). When cancer detection was stratified by BD in the BCSC, no statistical differences were found between digital and film mammography. However, there was a nominal trend toward higher cancer detection in women with extremely dense breasts (5.1 vs 3.8 per 1000, $p = 0.17$); the authors concluded that this was primarily due to better detection in women aged 40–49 with extremely dense breasts.

It is worth noting in Table 10.3 that in Europe, the recall rate for mammography is generally about half that observed in the United States.[59–61] Thus, one of the harms of mammography, recalls for false-positive imaging results, is less common in Europe. It is important to keep this in mind when evaluating how to apply the results from studies of supplemental screening performed in Europe versus the United States to different countries performing mammography.

In summary, the findings from both the DMIST and BCSC studies, along with the results from other high-quality studies, highlight a critical difference between digital and film mammography in women with dense breasts. The studies find that digital mammography is more sensitive than film mammography in women with dense breasts. Therefore, the masking effect of BD observed with film mammography is reduced, but not eliminated with digital mammography.

SUPPLEMENTAL SCREENING MODALITIES FOR BREAST CANCER SCREENING

There are many imaging approaches to screen for breast cancer in addition to mammography. Breast MRI has been increasing since the American Cancer Society recommended the use of MRI to screen women at highest risk for breast cancer in 2007, based primarily on genetic susceptibility.[62] Hand-held ultrasound has been used as a diagnostic tool to evaluate women with breast masses and has been promoted by some as a screening tool.[63] The FDA has approved automated whole breast ultrasound, which scans and records ultrasound images of the entire breast, for breast cancer screening.[64,65] Finally, DBT, a three-dimensional (3D) extension of digital mammography, has been viewed as holding significant promise in breast cancer screening.[66–68] Other imaging modalities, such as contrast-enhanced mammography, thermography, diffuse optical tomography, sestamibi, positron emission mammography, dedicated breast computed tomography, electrical impedance scanning, MRI spectroscopy, and breast-specific gamma imaging are still in early investigational phases[69,70] and will not be considered further.

All four of the advanced imaging technologies considered in this chapter produce multiple 2D images of the breast. This is particularly relevant in mammographically dense breasts because breast cancers may be obscured by superimposed dense tissue.

HAND-HELD ULTRASOUND OF THE BREAST

Hand-held ultrasound (HHUS) is widely used at breast imaging centers to evaluate breast masses and to guide both cyst aspiration and percutaneous breast biopsy procedures. It is particularly useful to differentiate fluid filled cysts from solid masses (cysts are rarely cancerous). Over time, HHUS has evolved to use higher frequency sound waves to generate images of the breast with improved resolution. In addition, earlier generations of HHUS were not able to penetrate deeply into breast tissue and had a limited field of view. Advantages of ultrasound include its widespread availability and the ability to evaluate tissue that is dense on mammography without additional ionizing radiation, which can potentially increase the risk for future cancers. It is also perceived to be more comfortable than mammography because it does not require compression of the breasts.

Ultrasound also has limitations. The primary concern with HHUS is the high number of false-positive findings, which often lead to unnecessary biopsies. There are also concerns about the operator dependency and reproducibility of the examinations. Like MRI, HHUS takes time. The average length of time for breast HHUS imaging in a recent study was 19 minutes.[71] In that study and many others, a breast radiologist performed the ultrasound, but technologists are also performing screening ultrasounds. At a minimum, the breast radiologist needs to be available to review static images saved by the performing technologist in real time so that additional images can be acquired if necessary.

AUTOMATED WHOLE BREAST ULTRASOUND

Automated whole breast ultrasound (ABUS) uses computer driven ultrasound transducers to scan the entire breast under the guidance of a technician. A technician compresses the woman's breasts to her chest wall and applies ultrasound gel. A breast-shaped transducer is placed on the compressed breast and automatically scans the entire breast. The entire procedure, including patient preparation, takes about 15 minutes to complete.[64,65] ABUS reduces the need for radiologists to perform the scan and decreases the length of time of the exam, thus addressing two of the shortcomings of HHUS. It also produces a scan that should have less operator dependence. The radiologist can review the scan independently using software that displays the images individually or sequentially in a movie mode. The primary drawbacks to ABUS are the high number of false-positive examinations, inability to image very large breasts, the storage requirements for the data acquired during the scan, and the time required to read the images.[64,65]

BREAST MRI

MRI uses strong magnetic fields to image the breast, rather than ionizing radiation. The system uses computational algorithms to generate detailed cross-sectional views of the breast. Mammography requires repositioning of the breast for each desired view. In contrast, the MRI examination is typically performed with the woman in the prone position lying on a platform placed in the MR chamber that allows the breast to extend dependently from the woman and does not require repositioning. A contrast agent, gadolinium, is injected through an intravenous catheter (IV) to improve the images of the breast.

In studies of high-risk women, MRI approximately doubles the number of breast cancers that are detected compared to film mammography or breast ultrasound.[72–79] However, several factors limit the widespread use of MRI for screening. These include an increase in false-positive test results, the need for placement of an intravenous catheter to infuse contrast, the length of time required for the examination, the cost of the examination, limited availability of breast MRI facilities (with special breast-specific magnetic coils and biopsy capability), and contraindications to the use of MRI due to claustrophobia, pacemakers, and other metallic implants. In addition, mammography has been found to be more sensitive than MRI for the detection of ductal carcinoma in situ, a noninvasive cell abnormality in the milk ducts, and some invasive breast cancers, so the two are typically used together.[43,62,80]

DIGITAL BREAST TOMOSYNTHESIS

DBT uses a conventional X-ray source that sweeps along an arc around the breast to acquire multiple 2D digital images.[66,68,81] Breast compression is performed using the same device and technique as conventional digital mammography. The procedure to obtain each digital view is complete in less than 20s.

One of the advantages of DBT is that the images can be acquired immediately following the digital mammogram. Like MRI, computational algorithms synthesize the resulting 2D digital images to create tomograms (ie, slices) allowing for a 3D reconstruction of the breast. The tomograms can be displayed individually (similar to enhanced conventional mammograms) or in a dynamic movie mode.

There are several drawbacks to DBT. The dose of ionizing radiation for DBT is about the same as or a little higher than that used for a conventional digital mammography. Currently, a standard digital image is also acquired, so the total dose is at least twice that of digital mammography alone.[66,67] The technology and algorithms used for DBT are still in evolution.[66,68,81] One of the crucial areas is the development of techniques to biopsy lesions that are only seen on DBT.[82] DBT can also be used to generate a virtual 2D digital mammogram (referred to as synthetic 2D mammogram), which could eliminate the need for performing digital mammography and thus eliminate the excess ionizing radiation. This technology has been developed and approved by the FDA for clinical use, has not been used in studies cited in this chapter (see chapter "Evolution of Mammography Screening: From Film Screen to Digital Breast Tomosynthesis" in this book for evidence on DBT with synthetic 2D mammography). Finally, the reading time for DBT is about twice that required for digital mammography.[66,67]

SCREENING HAND-HELD BREAST ULTRASOUND (HHUS) STUDIES IN WOMEN WITH DENSE BREASTS

HHUS is the most studied supplemental screening technology for women with dense breasts ($n > 80{,}000$).[83–100] In general, women in these studies underwent mammography first and those with negative mammogram results were subsequently screened by HHUS.

JAPAN STRATEGIC ANTICANCER RANDOMIZED TRIAL

In Japan, investigators in the Japan Strategic Anticancer Randomized Trial (J-START) trial[101] randomized 72,998 asymptomatic woman women ages 40–49 years to mammography plus HHUS or mammography alone twice over a 2-year period. All women also underwent clinical breast examination. In the first round of screening, the cancer detection rate with the combination of mammography and HHUS was higher than that of mammography alone (5.0 per 1000 vs 3.3 per 1000, $p = 0.003$). As expected, the sensitivity was higher in the group receiving both tests (91.1% vs 77.0%, $p = 0.004$) and the specificity was lower (87.7% vs 91.4%, $p < 0.0001$). Fewer interval cancers were detected in the dual screened arm of the study (0.05% vs 0.10, $p = 0.034$). The recall rate of the HHUS group was higher than that of the mammography group (12.6% vs 8.8%) as was the biopsy rate (4.5% vs 1.8%). The study does not directly address the question of the added value of HHUS in women with dense breasts because the study screened all women ages 40–49 years. However young Asian women have a very high prevalence of dense breasts, so the results are a reasonable approximation.

AMERICAN COLLEGE OF RADIOLOGY IMAGING NETWORK 6666 TRIAL

The American College of Radiology Imaging Network (ACRIN) 6666 trial[71,102] is the only US prospective clinical trial of HHUS with follow-up for multiple screening rounds. The population studied was higher risk than that of a typical screening population, so the biopsy rate, cancer detection rate, and positive predictive values will be higher than those of a screening population. For instance, in the first round the biopsy rate based on mammography was 14.4 per 1000 examinations, the cancer detection rate was 7.5 per 1000 examinations, and the PPV3, which represents the percentage of biopsies that are positive for cancer, was 31%, all of which are higher than expected for mammography in a screening population (10 per 1000, 5 per 1000, 25%, respectively).

The ACRIN 6666 trial recruited 2809 high-risk women to receive both mammography (film or digital) and ultrasound in a randomized order.[71] High-risk was defined by at least one of the following: a personal history of breast cancer; positive for BRCA1 or BRCA2 mutation; a lifetime risk ≥25%, a 5-year risk ≥2.5% or ≥1.7% with extremely dense breast tissue; prior biopsy with atypical ductal hyperplasia, atypical lobular hyperplasia, lobular carcinoma in situ or atypical papilloma; or prior mantle radiation. The study also required that the women have at least one quadrant of one breast with heterogeneously dense or extremely dense tissue on a prior mammogram.

In the first screening round, mammography detected 20 cancers (cancer detection rate 7.6 per 1000 examinations) and ultrasound detected an additional 14 cancers (5.9 per 1000 examinations).[102] There were two interval cancers so the sensitivity of mammography was 55.6% (20/36) and the sensitivity of ultrasound in women with negative mammograms was 87.5% (14/16). The number of recalls increased from 306 with mammography alone to 707 with mammography plus ultrasound, a 2.3-fold increase in the recall rate (from 115.1 per 1000 examinations to 265.9 per 1000). The number of breast biopsies increased from 65 to 272, a 4.2-fold increase (from 24.4 per 1000 examinations to 102.3 per 1000). The PPV3 for ultrasound in women with negative mammograms was only 6.8%.

In round 3, women were offered MRI in addition to HHUS and mammography.[102] The 612 women in the MRI substudy had higher risk for breast cancer and were younger than those who declined participation.[103] In this group of participants, mammography alone detected five cancers, ultrasound detected an additional two cancers (sensitivity for the combination 43.8%, cancer detection rate 11.4 per 1000 examinations) and MRI detected nine additional cancers (sensitivity 100%, incremental cancer detection rate 14.7 per 1000 examinations and combined cancer detection rate 26.1 per 1000 examinations). The nine cancers detected by MRI only were small (median 8.5 mm) and all were lymph node negative. Both cancers seen only with HHUS (not mammography) were also diagnosed with MRI. The high cancer detection rate in the women in the MRI group reflects the high underlying risk for cancer in the women who agreed to participate in the substudy. The recall rate was 85.0 per 1000 examinations for mammography alone, 163.4 per 1000 for the combination of mammography plus HHUS, and 260.0 per 1000 for MRI. The biopsy rate was 62.1 per 1000 examinations for the combination of mammography plus HHUS and 132.3 per 1000 for the combination with MRI. The PPV3 for MRI in women with a negative mammogram was 22.4%, which is much higher than that of ultrasound.

In this high-risk population, supplemental screening with HHUS produced a relatively high yield of cancers the first round of screening, approximately doubling the cancer detection rate, but this decreased with subsequent rounds. In order to find the additional cancers, the recall rate more than doubled so that one in four women (26.6%) were recalled in the first round. The number of biopsies performed increased by a factor of 4. In the first round, the combination of ultrasound plus mammography led to almost as many biopsies (10.2% of women) as women recalled with mammography alone (11.5% of women). The addition of MRI more than doubled the cancer detection rate of mammography plus ultrasound, but was associated with an even higher recall rate and a doubling of the biopsy rate. The PPV3 for ultrasound in women with negative mammograms was very low (6.8% round 1, 7.1% rounds 2 and 3) compared to mammography alone (29.1% round 1, 38.1% rounds 2 and 3). The PPV3 for MRI in women with negative mammograms was 22.4%.

OBSERVATIONAL STUDIES

We reviewed 15 observational studies on HHUS.[83–99,101] The participants in these studies had a mean age usually in the 50s with a broad range (25–91 years). Most included asymptomatic women presenting for screening mammography who were found to have dense breasts, although the definition of high BD varied somewhat. The majority of the studies were done outside of the United States. Four retrospective cohorts[95,97,99,100] described the findings in Connecticut, the first state in the United States requiring mandatory BD notification. These studies represent the best evidence in the US population for the incremental cancer detection rate with HHUS in average-risk women with dense breasts, although they do not have data on interval cancer rate. Two other studies in the United States[86,87] reported results from imaging performed in the year 2000 and earlier. A radiologist performed the HHUS in the majority of the studies. Nine of the studies reported no follow-up of participants. This means that the sensitivity, specificity, and negative predictive value reported from those studies will overestimate the true values.

The biopsy rate for women having HHUS after normal mammography ranged from 12–114 per 1000 examinations with a median of 46, which is threefold higher than with mammography. There was also a wide range of estimates across the studies for the recall rate (2.0% to 11.7%, median 6.5%) and the PPV3 (3.2% to 18.4%, median 7.1%). The heterogeneity of these results was likely due to a combination of factors. These include the study design (prospective, retrospective), the use of film or digital mammography, differences in the assessment of mammography across countries, whether a radiologist or a technician performed the HHUS, the level of experience and training of the person performing the HHUS, and differences in the populations studied (age distribution, breast cancer risk factors, time since last mammogram).

Most of the cancers detected by HHUS after negative mammography are small, node negative, early stage cancers. These are the cancers that are potentially curable by early detection before they potentially develop into cancers with a poorer prognosis. Cancers at an early stage also require less aggressive therapy: the patient may be eligible for lumpectomy rather than mastectomy and may not require systemic chemotherapy. Thus early detection may improve both quality and quantity of life. On the other hand, many of these early stage cancers may not have progressed before the next routine screening examination with mammography. Thus, they may ultimately have been detected and cured with mammographic screening alone. In addition, some proportion of these cancers may represent overdiagnosis: the identification of a cancer that would not have ever progressed to cause symptoms prior to the death of that individual woman (see chapter "Challenges in Understanding and Quantifying Over-Diagnosis and Over-Treatment" for more information on overdiagnosis). The identification of such cancers would lead to unnecessary labeling of the woman as someone who has cancer as well as unnecessary surgery and chemotherapy (ie, overtreatment). The only way to test which of these two competing hypotheses is true would be to perform a randomized trial comparing the two approaches to breast cancer screening.

SUMMARY: SCREENING HHUS OF THE BREAST

There are no studies evaluating the impact of adding HHUS to mammographic screening among women with dense breast tissue that address the key patient-centered outcomes of breast cancer mortality and disease-free survival. The available body of evidence, focusing largely on shorter-term outcomes of recall, biopsy, cancer detection, and false-positive rates, is limited by multiple factors. There were a

Table 10.4 Key Findings From Selected Studies of HHUS

Study	Recall Rate Per 1000	Biopsy Rate Per 1000	PPV3 (%)	Cancer Detection Rate Per 1000
J-START, Japan[101]	126	45	11.1	5.0
Corsetti (2011), Italy[94]	59.3	13	7.5	4.4
Hooley (2012), United States[95]	56.7	56.7	5.7	3.2
Weigert (2012), United States[97]	49.6	48.3	6.7	3.2
Parris (2013), United States[99]	33.5	32.8	5.5	1.8
Weigert (2015), United States[100]	42.3	42.3	3.0	1.3
ACRIN 6666, United States[102]	185.7	88.0	6.8	5.9

Table 10.5 Estimated Incremental Yield of HHUS After Negative Digital Mammography in Women With Dense Breast Tissue

Statistic	Digital Mammography	Incremental Yield With HHUS	Uncertainty
Recall rate per 1000	128	98	High
Biopsy rate per 1000	17.8	49	Low-moderate
CDR per 1000	4.2	2–3	Low
PPV3	24%	7%	Low

large number of studies, but the heterogeneity of the study designs, populations, and results preclude the use of meta-analytic techniques to combine the results. The majority of the studies had a negative film-screen mammography examination followed by supplemental screening ultrasound, were retrospective, did not fully report the recall rate, and were not able to calculate sensitivity because women with negative mammograms were not followed for interval cancer. The best estimates for sensitivity and specificity in the United States come from the ACRIN 6666 trial (87.5% and 81.9%, respectively) because it was a well-conducted prospective trial.[102] The incremental cancer detection rate from the four studies on the Connecticut experience was approximately 2 additional cancers per 1000. The results from Connecticut are more likely to be representative of routine clinical practice in the United States and to represent average-risk women with dense breasts. Table 10.4 summarizes the key statistics from the six with direct evidence and the ACRIN 666 study (high quality indirect evidence).

Estimates of incremental yield based on these data are shown in Table 10.5. There is a low level of uncertainty around the PPV3 because it was fairly consistent in the literature. The cancer detection rate comes primarily from the three studies describing the experience in Connecticut. There is high uncertainty about the recall rate because of the lack of direct evidence from studies of HHUS in women with dense breast tissue and because of the heterogeneity of the findings in the studies. In all of the prospective studies the recall rate was greater than 100 per 1000 examinations.

These estimates suggest that HHUS would find an additional 2–3 cancers more than those found by digital mammography with a PPV3 of 7%. There would be approximately 98 additional recalls and 49 additional biopsies in order to identify these cancers.

Table 10.6 Estimated Incremental Yield of ABUS After Negative Digital Mammography in Women With Dense Breast Tissue

Statistic	Digital Mammography	Incremental Yield With ABUS	Uncertainty
Recall rate per 1000	128	98	High
Biopsy rate per 1000	17.8	49	High
CDR per 1000	4.2	2–3	High
PPV3	24%	7%	High

AUTOMATED WHOLE BREAST ULTRASOUND (ABUS) STUDIES IN WOMEN WITH DENSE BREASTS

There are four studies[64,104–106] of ABUS evaluating approximately 9000 participants. The study of Kelly and colleagues offers the only reasonable estimates (sensitivity 67.6%, specificity 92.9%, recall rate 74.8 per 1000, biopsy rate 12.1 per 1000, cancer detection rate 3.7 per 1000), but the validity and relevance of these data are limited by concerns about spectrum bias and the use of film rather than digital mammography, which would decrease the cancer detection rate of mammography in the population of women with dense breasts. In addition, in an unreported proportion of the women, ABUS was performed between 5 and 8 months after mammography and likely found some cancers that it would not have identified at the time of mammography. Across the four studies, the recall rate varied from 5 to 207 per 1000 examinations, the biopsy rate was not reported or up to 15 per 1000 examinations, the PPV3 from not reported to 31% and the cancer detection rate ranged from 0 to 7.6 per 1000 examinations. Overall, the paucity of studies, the lack of high-quality studies, and the wide range of estimates across the three studies mean that there is considerable uncertainty surrounding all of the estimates for the diagnostic test statistics for ABUS.

Because of the uncertainty described above, we felt that the most reliable estimates for the test characteristics for ABUS come from the HHUS literature, but with high uncertainty. Estimates based on these data are shown in Table 10.6 and are identical to those for HHUS.

SCREENING BREAST MRI STUDIES

There are no studies of breast MRI to screen women with dense breasts. There is one study in progress in the Netherlands designed to address this question.[107] MRI has been studied for breast cancer screening in women deemed to be at high risk either by personal history, family history, or because they were known carriers of either a BRCA1 or BRCA2 mutation.[72–79,108–119] These women have a lifetime risk greater than 20%, rather than the 10%–20% lifetime risk for most women with high BD. No studies have demonstrated that MRI reduces the risk of death from breast cancer: there are no studies comparing women screened with MRI to other women screened with mammography alone and none of the studies of the test characteristics of MRI are of sufficient duration or size to evaluate patient-oriented outcomes such as the breast cancer recurrence or death from breast cancer.

The sensitivity of MRI for breast cancer ranged from 77% to 100%. The sensitivity of mammography (25–59%) and ultrasound (13–65%) in these studies was about half that of MRI. In the largest three studies,[74–76] which included 52% of the cancers in all 14 studies, the sensitivity of MRI ranged from 71% to 91% while the sensitivity of mammography ranged from 32% to 40%. However, the specificity of MRI is consistently lower than mammography. In the same three studies, the specificity of MRI ranged from 81% to 97% compared to 93% to 99% for mammography, and in each individual study the specificity of MRI was lower than that of mammography. Because breast cancer is relatively uncommon, even in these very high-risk populations, the lower specificity of MRI translates into a much higher number of false-positive results. One study suggested that the high false-positive rate decreases after the initial MRI.[108] In that study the rate of false-positive results declined from 14% initially to 8.2% on subsequent MRI's, but was still substantially higher than the 4.6% false-positive rate for mammography.[108]

It is worth noting that the sensitivity of mammography and ultrasound were similar to each other in each of the five studies that report the sensitivity of all three screening technologies. The sensitivity of mammography and ultrasound in these studies is much lower than the sensitivity usually reported for these tests. The low sensitivity is due to the large number of cancers that are found by MRI alone—more than typically appear as interval cancers in the year following a screening examination. This suggests that many of the cancers detected by MRI would not have been diagnosed without MRI for more than 1 year after the examination. Early detection of cancers that would have become clinically apparent at a later date should translate into a higher cure rate and the need for less aggressive therapies, but some proportion of the cancers detected by MRI are likely to represent overdiagnosis—cancers that never would have become symptomatic in a woman's life.

SUMMARY: SCREENING MRI OF THE BREAST

There are no data evaluating MRI in a general screening population with dense breasts, nor in populations at intermediate risk (15% to 20% lifetime risk). There is one ongoing study.[107] The data from high-risk populations suggests that the addition of MRI would more than double the cancer detection rate (best estimate 2.4-fold increase) with a fourfold increase in the recall rate (best estimate 4.3-fold increase). Estimates based on these data are shown in Table 10.7. There is a high level of uncertainty around these values because of the lack of direct evidence from studies of MRI in women with dense breast tissue and because of the heterogeneity of the findings in the studies of high-risk women summarized in Table 10.6.

Table 10.7 Estimated Incremental Yield of MRI After Negative Digital Mammography in Women With Dense Breast Tissue Based on Performance of MRI in Mutation Carriers

Statistic	Digital Mammography	Incremental Yield With MRI	Uncertainty
Recall rate per 1000	128	100	High
Biopsy rate per 1000	17.8	17–36	High
CDR per 1000	4.2	8	High
PPV3	24%	22–48%	High

These estimate suggest that MRI would find an additional eight cancers more than those found by digital mammography with a PPV3 between 22% and 48%. There would be approximately 100 additional recalls and between 17 and 36 additional biopsies in order to identify these cancers.

The studies comparing mammography, ultrasound, and MRI in very high-risk women described in the section on MRI help with the comparative effectiveness of the three technologies. In the six studies evaluating all three technologies,[75,77,79,102,111,120] mammography detected 48 cancers, ultrasound detected 53, and MRI detected 116. Ultrasound detected 19 cancers that were not detected by mammography, which represents 40% (19/48) more cancers detected. Four cancers (3%) were detected only on ultrasound. These studies suggest that the addition of HHUS would increase the cancer detection rate by about 40% (best estimate 1.4-fold increase) more than mammography alone, but that HHUS does not increase the cancer detection rate when added to mammography plus MRI.

DBT STUDIES IN WOMEN WITH DENSE BREASTS

Nine studies[67,121–128] evaluated the use of DBT in more than 600,000 women presenting for routine screening for breast cancer found that DBT increased the cancer detection rate relative to mammography while decreasing the recall rate and the biopsy rate. The results were consistent despite the different methods for interpretation used in the three different countries (Norway, Italy, United States). The same increase in cancer detection and decrease in recall rate was seen in women with both low- and high-density mammograms.

There are several limitations to these results, when considering DBT for supplemental screening following a normal mammogram with dense breast tissue. First, DBT has been studied primarily in combination with digital mammography in all women coming in for breast cancer screening, not as supplemental screening for women with dense breasts. In addition, the data from the two US studies[122,123] have significant uncertainty because they studied the results in two different populations that may not be directly comparable.

Estimates based on these data are shown in Table 10.8. These estimates are artificial because they reflect the use of DBT as supplemental screening rather that as the primary screening modality. As discussed elsewhere, the evidence is consistent that DBT for primary screening decreases recall rates

Table 10.8 Estimated Incremental Yield of DBT After Negative Digital Mammography in Women With Dense Breast Tissue

Statistic	Digital Mammography	Incremental Yield With DBT	Uncertainty
Recall rate per 1000	128	20*	Moderate
Biopsy rate per 1000	17.8	5	Low
CDR per 1000	4.2	1–3	Low
PPV3	24%	25%	Low

**This represents the estimate for recalls for women with negative mammograms and dense breasts who are screened a second time with DBT and not the results for DBT as a primary screening modality.*

compared with digital mammography, while increasing the cancer detection rate by 1–2 cancers per 1000 screens while maintaining a PPV of about 25%.

These estimate suggest that DBT used as supplemental screening in women with dense breasts would find an additional 1–3 cancers more than those found by digital mammography with a PPV3 of 25%. There would be approximately 20 additional recalls and 5 additional biopsies in order to identify these cancers.

SUMMARY

Table 10.9 summarizes the estimates for each of the four technology based on the clinical data published through mid-2015. Many of the estimates have a high degree of uncertainty and will likely change as more high-quality data become available. However, they provide reasonable estimates of the clinical benefits and harms relative to each other.

Table 10.9 highlights the low PPV3 of ultrasound compared to the other technologies, which translates into a large number of unnecessary biopsies for every cancer detected by ultrasound. The table also clearly illustrates that DBT has a much lower recall rate than the other technologies and that MRI detects the greatest number of additional breast cancers.

Thus, we know with a high degree of certainty that all forms of supplemental screening find additional breast cancers. Most of the cancers are small, lymph node negative, and thus are potentially curable. MRI finds the most cancers and DBT has the fewest false-positives. HHUS results in the largest number of false-positive biopsies. If DBT is used for primary screening, it decreases overall recall rates while increasing cancer detection rates. There are no studies addressing whether supplemental screening would be beneficial in women with dense breasts who were screened with DBT.

Finally, use of a woman's risk for subsequent breast cancer can identify a subset of women most likely to benefit from supplemental screening. Limiting supplemental screening to those at highest risk would reduce the number of women recommended for additional tests by approximately 75%.

The major unanswered question is whether the identification of additional cancers through supplemental screening improves outcomes for women. Some advocates of supplemental screening will argue that the majority of the cancers identified through supplemental screening are early stage cancers with an excellent prognosis following treatment. These represent the spectrum of cancers identified with mammography that led to the reduction in mortality seen with the randomized trials of screening

Table 10.9 Summary of the Key Statistics for Four Supplemental Screening Technologies in Women With Dense Breasts

Statistic	Digital Mammography	Incremental Yield		
		MRI	HHUS/ABUS	DBT
Recall rate per 1000	128	100	98	20
Biopsy rate per 1000	17.8	17–36	49	5
CDR per 1000	4.2	8	2–3	1–3
PPV3	24%	22–48%	7%	25%

mammography. In their view, there can be no question that patient outcomes will be improved with supplemental screening. Others will argue that many of these supplemental screen-detected cancers would have been cured when detected on physical exam or subsequent screening mammograms and that some of these cancers represent overdiagnosis, which leads to net harm for the patient. They will highlight the growing evidence for significant overdiagnosis with mammography alone. These individuals will suggest that much of the incremental cancer detection rate with HHUS (2–6 or more per 1000 examinations), which is much higher than the expected interval cancer rate (1 per 1000 examinations), can only represent overdiagnosis. Only large randomized trials can definitively answer this question.

WHO SHOULD RECEIVE SUPPLEMENTAL SCREENING?

One of the goals of supplemental screening is to detect cancers that are not seen on screening mammography that will present as interval cancers prior to the next screening. A study of more than 350,000 women between the ages of 40 and 74 years screened as part of the US BCSC suggested that both risk and BD were important to consider when making the decision to perform additional screening tests.[129] Investigators at the BCSC developed a model that uses BI-RADS density in combination with a woman's age, race/ethnicity, family history, and history of breast biopsies to estimate her 5-year risk for breast cancer.[52] A web-based calculator using the BCSC model is available for women and their physicians (https://tools.bcsc-scc.org/BC5yearRisk/calculator.htm) as well as an application for iPhones and iPads (https://itunes.apple.com/us/app/bcsc-risk-calculator/id919034661?ls=1&mt=8). Using this tool, the study found that half of women with heterogeneously or extremely dense breasts did not have a high risk of interval cancer. High interval cancer rates were observed for women with extremely dense breasts with a 5-year risk ≥1.67% or higher and women with heterogeneously dense breasts and a 5-year risk ≥2.5%, combined these groups represent 24% of women with dense breasts. Supplemental ultrasound, DBT, and MRI needed to be examined in these high-risk groups to determine whether these imaging modalities can identify interval cancers missed on digital mammography.

LIST OF ACRONYMS AND ABBREVIATIONS

2D	Two-Dimensional
3D	Three-Dimensional
ABUS	Automated Whole Breast Ultrasound
ACRIN	American College of Radiology Imaging Network
BD	Breast Density
BI-RADS	Breast Imaging Reporting and Data System
BRCA	BReast CAncer susceptibility gene
CDR	Cancer Detection Rate
DBT	Digital Breast Tomosynthesis
DMIST	Digital Mammography Imaging System Trial
FDA	Food and Drug Administration
HHUS	Hand Held Ultrasound
IV	Intravenous
J-START	Japan Strategic Anticancer Randomized Trial

MRI Magnetic Resonance Imaging
PPV3 Positive Predictive Value 3: Percentage of breast biopsies that are cancer
SEER Surveillance, Epidemiology, and End Results

REFERENCES

1. An act to add and repeal Section 123222.3 of the Health and Safety Code, relating to mammograms. In: Legislature CS, ed. *SB1538*.
2. Ferlay J, Soerjomataram I, Dikshit R, et al. Cancer incidence and mortality worldwide: sources, methods and major patterns in GLOBOCAN 2012. *Int J Cancer* 2015;**136**(5):E359–86.
3. Ries LAG, Melbert D, Krapcho M, editors. *SEER cancer statistics review, 1975– 2005*. Bethesda, MD: National Cancer Institute; 2008.
4. Berry DA, Cronin KA, Plevritis SK, et al. Effect of screening and adjuvant therapy on mortality from breast cancer. *N Engl J Med* 2005;**353**(17):1784–92.
5. Kalager M, Zelen M, Langmark F, Adami HO. Effect of screening mammography on breast-cancer mortality in Norway. *N Engl J Med* 2010;**363**(13):1203–10.
6. Bleyer A, Welch HG. Effect of three decades of screening mammography on breast-cancer incidence. *N Engl J Med* 2012;**367**(21):1998–2005.
7. Alexander FE. The Edinburgh randomized trial of breast cancer screening. *J Natl Cancer Inst Monogr* 1997(22):31–5.
8. Andersson I, Aspegren K, Janzon L, et al. Mammographic screening and mortality from breast cancer: the malmo mammographic screening trial. *BMJ* 1988;**297**(6654):943–8.
9. Andersson I, Janzon L. Reduced breast cancer mortality in women under age 50: updated results from the malmo mammographic screening program. *J Natl Cancer Inst Monogr* 1997(22):63–7.
10. Bjurstam N, Bjorneld L, Duffy SW, et al. The Gothenburg Breast Cancer Screening Trial: preliminary results on breast cancer mortality for women aged 39–49. *J Natl Cancer Inst Monogr* 1997(22):53–5.
11. Bjurstam N, Bjorneld L, Duffy SW, et al. The Gothenburg breast screening trial: first results on mortality, incidence, and mode of detection for women ages 39–49 years at randomization. *Cancer* 1997;**80**(11):2091–9.
12. Frisell J, Lidbrink E. The Stockholm mammographic screening trial: risks and benefits in age group 40–49 years. *J Natl Cancer Inst Monogr* 1997(22):49–51.
13. Frisell J, Lidbrink E, Hellstrom L, Rutqvist LE. Followup after 11 years-update of mortality results in the Stockholm mammographic screening trial. *Breast Cancer Res Treat* 1997;**45**(3):263–70.
14. Miller AB, Baines CJ, To T, Wall C. Canadian National Breast Screening Study: 2. Breast cancer detection and death rates among women aged 50 to 59 years. *CMAJ* 1992;**147**(10):1477–88.
15. Miller AB, Baines CJ, To T, Wall C. Canadian National Breast Screening Study: 1. Breast cancer detection and death rates among women aged 40 to 49 years. *CMAJ* 1992;**147**(10):1459–76.
16. Miller AB, To T, Baines CJ, Wall C. The Canadian National Breast Screening Study: update on breast cancer mortality. *J Natl Cancer Inst Monogr* 1997(22):37–41.
17. Miller AB, To T, Baines CJ, Wall C. Canadian National Breast Screening Study-2: 13-year results of a randomized trial in women aged 50–59 years. *J Natl Cancer Inst* 2000;**92**(18):1490–9.
18. Miller AB, To T, Baines CJ, Wall C. The Canadian National Breast Screening Study-1: breast cancer mortality after 11 to 16 years of follow-up. A randomized screening trial of mammography in women age 40 to 49 years. *Ann Intern Med* 2002;**137**(5 Part 1):305–12.
19. Nystrom L, Andersson I, Bjurstam N, Frisell J, Nordenskjold B, Rutqvist LE. Long-term effects of mammography screening: updated overview of the Swedish randomised trials. *Lancet* 2002;**359**(9310):909–19.
20. Shapiro S. Periodic screening for breast cancer: the HIP Randomized Controlled Trial. Health Insurance Plan. *J Natl Cancer Inst Monogr* 1997(22):27–30.

21. Shapiro S, Venet W, Strax P, Venet L. Current results of the breast cancer screening randomized trial: the health insurance plan (HIP) of greater New York study. In: Day N, Miller A, editors. *Screening for Breast Cancer*. Toronto Lewiston, NY: Huber; 1988. p. 3–15.
22. Tabar L, Fagerberg G, Chen HH, et al. Efficacy of breast cancer screening by age. New results from the Swedish Two-County Trial. *Cancer* 1995;**75**(10):2507–17.
23. Tabar L, Fagerberg G, Duffy SW, Day NE. The Swedish two county trial of mammographic screening for breast cancer: recent results and calculation of benefit. *J Epidemiol Commun Health* 1989;**43**(2):107–14.
24. Tabar L, Vitak B, Chen HH, et al. The Swedish Two-County Trial twenty years later. Updated mortality results and new insights from long-term follow-up. *Radiol Clin North Am* 2000;**38**(4):625–51.
25. Moss SM, Cuckle H, Evans A, Johns L, Waller M, Bobrow L. Effect of mammographic screening from age 40 years on breast cancer mortality at 10 years' follow-up: a randomised controlled trial. *Lancet* 2006;**368**(9552):2053–60.
26. Breast-cancer screening with mammography in women aged 40–49 years. Swedish Cancer Society and the Swedish National Board of Health and Welfare. *Int J Cancer*. 1996;**68**(6):693–9. (PMID 8980168).
27. Armstrong K, Moye E, Williams S, Berlin JA, Reynolds EE. Screening mammography in women 40 to 49 years of age: a systematic review for the American College of Physicians. *Ann Intern Med* 2007;**146**(7):516–26.
28. Cox B. Variation in the effectiveness of breast screening by year of follow-up. *J Natl Cancer Inst Monogr* 1997(22):69–72.
29. Elwood JM, Cox B, Richardson AK. The effectiveness of breast cancer screening by mammography in younger women. *Online J Curr Clin Trials* 1993 [Doc No 32:23,227 words; 195 paragraphs].
30. Glasziou PP. Meta-analysis adjusting for compliance: the example of screening for breast cancer. *J Clin Epidemiol* 1992;**45**(11):1251–6.
31. Glasziou PP, Woodward AJ, Mahon CM. Mammographic screening trials for women aged under 50. A quality assessment and meta-analysis. *Med J Aust* 1995;**162**(12):625–9.
32. Gotzsche PC, Nielsen M. Screening for breast cancer with mammography. *Cochrane Database Syst Rev* 2006(4):CD001877.
33. Gotzsche PC, Olsen O. Is screening for breast cancer with mammography justifiable? *Lancet* 2000; **355**(9198):129–34.
34. Hendrick RE, Smith RA, Rutledge III JH, Smart CR. Benefit of screening mammography in women aged 40–49: a new meta-analysis of randomized controlled trials. *J Natl Cancer Inst Monogr* 1997(22): 87–92.
35. Humphrey LL, Helfand M, Chan BK, Woolf SH. Breast cancer screening: a summary of the evidence for the U.S. Preventive Services Task Force. *Ann Intern Med* 2002;**137**(5 Part 1):347–60.
36. Kerlikowske K. Efficacy of screening mammography among women aged 40 to 49 years and 50 to 69 years: comparison of relative and absolute benefit. *J Natl Cancer Inst Monogr* 1997(22):79–86.
37. Kerlikowske K, Grady D, Rubin SM, Sandrock C, Ernster VL. Efficacy of screening mammography. A meta-analysis. *JAMA* 1995;**273**(2):149–54.
38. Nystrom L, Rutqvist LE, Wall S, et al. Breast cancer screening with mammography: overview of Swedish randomised trials. *Lancet* 1993;**341**(8851):973–8.
39. Ringash J. Preventive health care, 2001 update: screening mammography among women aged 40–49 years at average risk of breast cancer. *CMAJ* 2001;**164**(4):469–76.
40. Smart CR, Hendrick RE, Rutledge III JH, Smith RA. Benefit of mammography screening in women ages 40 to 49 years. Current evidence from randomized controlled trials. *Cancer* 1995;**75**(7):1619–26.
41. Myers ER, Moorman P, Gierisch JM, et al. Benefits and harms of breast cancer screening: a systematic review. *JAMA* 2015;**314**(15):1615–34.
42. Screening for breast cancer: U.S. Preventive Services Task Force recommendation statement. *Ann Intern Med*. 2009;**151**(10):716–26, [W-236]. (PMID 19920272).
43. Bevers TB, Anderson BO, Bonaccio E, et al. NCCN clinical practice guidelines in oncology: breast cancer screening and diagnosis. *J Natl Compr Canc Netw* 2009;**7**(10):1060–96.

44. Lee CH, Dershaw DD, Kopans D, et al. Breast cancer screening with imaging: recommendations from the Society of Breast Imaging and the ACR on the use of mammography, breast MRI, breast ultrasound, and other technologies for the detection of clinically occult breast cancer. *J Am Coll Radiol* 2010;**7**(1):18–27.
45. Smith RA, Brooks D, Cokkinides V, Saslow D, Brawley OW. Cancer screening in the United States, 2013: a review of current American Cancer Society guidelines, current issues in cancer screening, and new guidance on cervical cancer screening and lung cancer screening. *CA Cancer J Clin* 2013;**63**(2):88–105.
46. Feig SA, Yaffe MJ. Digital mammography. *Radiographics* 1998;**18**(4):893–901.
47. Pisano ED, Cole EB, Hemminger BM, et al. Image processing algorithms for digital mammography: a pictorial essay. *Radiographics* 2000;**20**(5):1479–91.
48. Pisano ED, Zong S, Hemminger BM, et al. Contrast limited adaptive histogram equalization image processing to improve the detection of simulated speculations in dense mammograms. *J Digit Imaging* 1998;**11**(4):193–200.
49. United States Food and Drug Administration. *Mammography quality standards act and program*. <http://www.fda.gov/Radiation-EmittingProducts/MammographyQualityStandardsActandProgram/FacilityScorecard/ucm113858.htm/>; 2015 [accessed 15.10.13].
50. Sickles E, D'Orsi C, Bassett L, Mendelson E, Morris E. ACR BI-RADS Atlas® mammography *ACR BI-RADS Atlas®, breast imaging reporting and data system*. Reston, VA: American College of Radiology; 2013.
51. Sprague BL, Gangnon RE, Burt V, et al. Prevalence of mammographically dense breasts in the United States. *J Natl Cancer Inst* 2014;**106**(10). (The PMID is 25217577; full text available at PMCID PMC4200066).
52. Tice JA, Cummings SR, Smith-Bindman R, Ichikawa L, Barlow WE, Kerlikowske K. Using clinical factors and mammographic breast density to estimate breast cancer risk: development and validation of a new predictive model. *Ann Intern Med* 2008;**148**(5):337–47.
53. Kerlikowske K, Grady D, Barclay J, Sickles EA, Ernster V. Effect of age, breast density, and family history on the sensitivity of first screening mammography. *JAMA* 1996;**276**(1):33–8.
54. Carney PA, Miglioretti DL, Yankaskas BC, et al. Individual and combined effects of age, breast density, and hormone replacement therapy use on the accuracy of screening mammography. *Ann Intern Med* 2003;**138**(3):168–75.
55. Pisano ED, Gatsonis C, Hendrick E, et al. Diagnostic performance of digital versus film mammography for breast-cancer screening. *N Engl J Med* 2005;**353**(17):1773–83.
56. Pisano ED, Hendrick RE, Yaffe MJ, et al. Diagnostic accuracy of digital versus film mammography: exploratory analysis of selected population subgroups in DMIST. *Radiology* 2008;**246**(2):376–83.
57. Kerlikowske K, Hubbard RA, Miglioretti DL, et al. Comparative effectiveness of digital versus film-screen mammography in community practice in the United States: a cohort study. *Ann Intern Med* 2011;**155**(8):493–502.
58. Vigeland E, Klaasen H, Klingen TA, Hofvind S, Skaane P. Full-field digital mammography compared to screen film mammography in the prevalent round of a population-based screening programme: the Vestfold County Study. *Eur Radiol* 2008;**18**(1):183–91.
59. Hofvind S, Vacek PM, Skelly J, Weaver DL, Geller BM. Comparing screening mammography for early breast cancer detection in Vermont and Norway. *J Natl Cancer Inst* 2008;**100**(15):1082–91.
60. Jensen A, Geller BM, Gard CC, et al. Performance of diagnostic mammography differs in the United States and Denmark. *Int J Cancer* 2010;**127**(8):1905–12.
61. Smith-Bindman R, Chu PW, Miglioretti DL, et al. Comparison of screening mammography in the United States and the United kingdom. *JAMA* 2003;**290**(16):2129–37.
62. Saslow D, Boetes C, Burke W, et al. American cancer society guidelines for breast screening with MRI as an adjunct to mammography. *CA Cancer J Clin* 2007;**57**(2):75–89.
63. Mahoney MC, Newell MS, Screening MR. Imaging versus screening ultrasound. Pros and Cons. *Magn Reson Imaging Clin N Am* 2013;**21**(3):495–508.
64. Giuliano V, Giuliano C. Using automated breast sonography as part of a multimodality approach to dense breast screening. *J Diag Med Sonogra* 2012;**28**(4):159–65.
65. Kelly KM, Richwald GA. Automated whole-breast ultrasound: advancing the performance of breast cancer screening. *Semin Ultrasound, CT MRI* 2011;**32**(4):273–80.

66. Houssami N, Skaane P. Overview of the evidence on digital breast tomosynthesis in breast cancer detection. *Breast* 2013;**22**(2):101–8.
67. Skaane P, Bandos AI, Gullien R, et al. Comparison of digital mammography alone and digital mammography plus tomosynthesis in a population-based screening program. *Radiology* 2013;**267**(1):47–56.
68. Kopans DB, Skaane P. Digital breast tomosynthesis: a better mammogram. *Radiology* 2013;**267**(3):968–9.
69. Drukteinis JS, Mooney BP, Flowers CI, Gatenby RA. Beyond mammography: new frontiers in breast cancer screening. *Am J Med* 2013;**126**(6):472–9.
70. Yang WT. Emerging techniques and molecular imaging in breast cancer. *Semin Ultrasound CT MRI* 2011;**32**(4):288–99.
71. Berg WA, Blume JD, Cormack JB, et al. Combined screening with ultrasound and mammography vs mammography alone in women at elevated risk of breast cancer. *JAMA* 2008;**299**(18):2151–63.
72. Berg WA, Gutierrez L, NessAiver MS, et al. Diagnostic accuracy of mammography, clinical examination, US, and MR imaging in preoperative assessment of breast cancer. *Radiology* 2004;**233**(3):830–49.
73. Hagen AI, Kvistad KA, Maehle L, et al. Sensitivity of MRI versus conventional screening in the diagnosis of BRCA-associated breast cancer in a national prospective series. *Breast* 2007;**16**(4):367–74.
74. Kriege M, Brekelmans CT, Boetes C, et al. Efficacy of MRI and mammography for breast-cancer screening in women with a familial or genetic predisposition. *N Engl J Med* 2004;**351**(5):427–37.
75. Kuhl CK, Schrading S, Leutner CC, et al. Mammography, breast ultrasound, and magnetic resonance imaging for surveillance of women at high familial risk for breast cancer. *J Clin Oncol* 2005;**23**(33):8469–76.
76. Leach MO, Boggis CR, Dixon AK, et al. Screening with magnetic resonance imaging and mammography of a UK population at high familial risk of breast cancer: a prospective multicentre cohort study (MARIBS). *Lancet* 2005;**365**(9473):1769–78.
77. Sardanelli F, Podo F, D'Agnolo G, et al. Multicenter comparative multimodality surveillance of women at genetic-familial high risk for breast cancer (HIBCRIT study): interim results. *Radiology* 2007;**242**(3):698–715.
78. Tilanus-Linthorst MM, Obdeijn IM, Bartels KC, de Koning HJ, Oudkerk M. First experiences in screening women at high risk for breast cancer with MR imaging. *Breast Cancer Res Treat* 2000;**63**(1):53–60.
79. Warner E, Plewes DB, Hill KA, et al. Surveillance of BRCA1 and BRCA2 mutation carriers with magnetic resonance imaging, ultrasound, mammography, and clinical breast examination. *JAMA* 2004;**292**(11): 1317–25.
80. Mann RM, Kuhl CK, Kinkel K, Boetes C, Breast MRI. Guidelines from the European Society of Breast Imaging. *Eur Radiol* 2008;**18**(7):1307–18.
81. Sechopoulos I. A review of breast tomosynthesis. Part I. The image acquisition process. *Med Phys* 2013;**40**(1):014301.
82. Viala J, Gignier P, Perret B, et al. Stereotactic vacuum-assisted biopsies on a digital breast 3D-tomosynthesis system. *Breast J* 2013;**19**(1):4–9.
83. Kolb TM, Lichy J, Newhouse JH. Occult cancer in women with dense breasts: detection with screening US—diagnostic yield and tumor characteristics. *Radiology* 1998;**207**(1):191–9.
84. Maestro C, Cazenave F, Marcy PY, Bruneton JN, Chauvel C, Bleuse A. Systematic ultrasonography in asymptomatic dense breasts. *Eur J Radiol* 1998;**26**(3):254–6.
85. Buchberger W, Niehoff A, Obrist P, DeKoekkoek-Doll P, Dunser M. Clinically and mammographically occult breast lesions: detection and classification with high-resolution sonography. *Semin Ultrasound CT MR* 2000;**21**(4):325–36.
86. Kaplan SS. Clinical utility of bilateral whole-breast US in the evaluation of women with dense breast tissue. *Radiology* 2001;**221**(3):641–9.
87. Kolb TM, Lichy J, Newhouse JH. Comparison of the performance of screening mammography, physical examination, and breast US and evaluation of factors that influence them: an analysis of 27,825 patient evaluations. *Radiology* 2002;**225**(1):165–75.
88. Crystal P, Strano SD, Shcharynski S, Koretz MJ. Using sonography to screen women with mammographically dense breasts. *Am J Roentgenol* 2003;**181**(1):177–82.

89. Leconte I, Feger C, Galant C, et al. Mammography and subsequent whole-breast sonography of nonpalpable breast cancers: the importance of radiologic breast density. *Am J Roentgenol* 2003;**180**(6):1675–9.
90. Corsetti V, Ferrari A, Ghirardi M, et al. Role of ultrasonography in detecting mammographically occult breast carcinoma in women with dense breasts. *Radiol Med* 2006;**111**(3):440–8.
91. Brancato B, Bonardi R, Catarzi S, et al. Negligible advantages and excess costs of routine addition of breast ultrasonography to mammography in dense breasts. *Tumori* 2007;**93**(6):562–6.
92. De Felice C, Savelli S, Angeletti M, et al. Diagnostic utility of combined ultrasonography and mammography in the evaluation of women with mammographically dense breasts. *J Ultrasound* 2007;**10**(3):143–51.
93. Corsetti V, Houssami N, Ferrari A, et al. Breast screening with ultrasound in women with mammography-negative dense breasts: evidence on incremental cancer detection and false positives, and associated cost. *Eur J Cancer* 2008;**44**(4):539–44.
94. Corsetti V, Houssami N, Ghirardi M, et al. Evidence of the effect of adjunct ultrasound screening in women with mammography-negative dense breasts: interval breast cancers at 1 year follow-up. *Eur J Cancer* 2011;**47**(7):1021–6.
95. Hooley RJ, Greenberg KL, Stackhouse RM, Geisel JL, Butler RS, Philpotts LE. Screening US in patients with mammographically dense breasts: initial experience with Connecticut Public Act 09–41. *Radiology* 2012;**265**(1):59–69.
96. Leong LC, Gogna A, Pant R, Ng FC, Sim LS. Supplementary breast ultrasound screening in Asian women with negative but dense mammograms-a pilot study. *Ann Acad Med Singapore* 2012;**41**(10):432–9.
97. Weigert J, Steenbergen S. The Connecticut experiment: the role of ultrasound in the screening of women with dense breasts. *Breast J* 2012;**18**(6):517–22.
98. Girardi V, Tonegutti M, Ciatto S, Bonetti F. Breast ultrasound in 22,131 asymptomatic women with negative mammography. *Breast* 2013;**22**(5):806–809.
99. Parris T, Wakefield D, Frimmer H. Real world performance of screening breast ultrasound following enactment of Connecticut Bill 458. *Breast J* 2013;**19**(1):64–70.
100. Weigert J, Steenbergen S. The Connecticut experiments second year: ultrasound in the screening of women with dense breasts. *Breast J* 2015;**21**(2):175–80.
101. Ohuchi N, Suzuki A, Sobue T, et al. Sensitivity and specificity of mammography and adjunctive ultrasonography to screen for breast cancer in the Japan Strategic Anti-cancer Randomized Trial (J-START): a randomised controlled trial. *Lancet* 2015. [Epub ahead of print].
102. Berg WA, Zhang Z, Lehrer D, et al. Detection of breast cancer with addition of annual screening ultrasound or a single screening MRI to mammography in women with elevated breast cancer risk. *JAMA* 2012;**307**(13):1394–404.
103. Berg WA, Blume JD, Adams AM, et al. Reasons women at elevated risk of breast cancer refuse breast MR imaging screening: ACRIN 6666. *Radiology* 2010;**254**(1):79–87.
104. Kelly KM, Dean J, Lee SJ, Comulada WS. Breast cancer detection: radiologists' performance using mammography with and without automated whole-breast ultrasound. *Eur Radiol* 2010;**20**(11):2557–64.
105. Stoblen F, Landt S, Stelkens-Gebhardt R, Sehouli J, Rezai M, Kummel S. First evaluation of the diagnostic accuracy of an automated 3D ultrasound system in a breast screening setting. *Anticancer Res* 2011;**31**(8):2569–74.
106. Arleo EK, Saleh M, Ionescu D, Drotman M, Min RJ, Hentel K. Recall rate of screening ultrasound with automated breast volumetric scanning (ABVS) in women with dense breasts: a first quarter experience. *Clin Imaging* 2014;**38**(4):439–44.
107. Emaus MJ, Bakker MF, Peeters PH, et al. MR imaging as an additional screening modality for the detection of breast cancer in women aged 50– 75 years with extremely dense breasts: the DENSE Trial Study Design. *Radiology* 2015;**277**(2):527–37.
108. Kriege M, Brekelmans CT, Boetes C, et al. Differences between first and subsequent rounds of the MRISC breast cancer screening program for women with a familial or genetic predisposition. *Cancer* 2006;**106**(11):2318–26.

109. Kuhl CK, Schmutzler RK, Leutner CC, et al. Breast MR imaging screening in 192 women proved or suspected to be carriers of a breast cancer susceptibility gene: preliminary results. *Radiology* 2000;**215**(1):267–79.
110. Lehman CD, Blume JD, Weatherall P, et al. Screening women at high risk for breast cancer with mammography and magnetic resonance imaging. *Cancer* 2005;**103**(9):1898–905.
111. Lehman CD, Isaacs C, Schnall MD, et al. Cancer yield of mammography, MR, and US in high-risk women: prospective multi-institution breast cancer screening study. *Radiology* 2007;**244**(2):381–8.
112. Podo F, Sardanelli F, Canese R, et al. The Italian multi-centre project on evaluation of MRI and other imaging modalities in early detection of breast cancer in subjects at high genetic risk. *J Exp Clin Cancer Res* 2002;**21**(3 Suppl):115–24.
113. Morris EA, Liberman L, Ballon DJ, et al. MRI of occult breast carcinoma in a high-risk population. *Am J Roentgenol* 2003;**181**(3):619–26.
114. Port ER, Park A, Borgen PI, Morris E, Montgomery LL. Results of MRI screening for breast cancer in high-risk patients with LCIS and atypical hyperplasia. *Ann Surg Oncol* 2007;**14**(3):1051–7.
115. Stoutjesdijk MJ, Boetes C, Jager GJ, et al. Magnetic resonance imaging and mammography in women with a hereditary risk of breast cancer. *J Natl Cancer Inst* 2001;**93**(14):1095–102.
116. Yu J, Park A, Morris E, Liberman L, Borgen PI, King TA. MRI screening in a clinic population with a family history of breast cancer. *Ann Surg Oncol* 2008;**15**(2):452–61.
117. Warner E, Plewes DB, Shumak RS, et al. Comparison of breast magnetic resonance imaging, mammography, and ultrasound for surveillance of women at high risk for hereditary breast cancer. *J Clin Oncol* 2001;**19**(15):3524–31.
118. Trecate G, Vergnaghi D, Manoukian S, et al. MRI in the early detection of breast cancer in women with high genetic risk. *Tumori* 2006;**92**(6):517–23.
119. Hartman AR, Daniel BL, Kurian AW, et al. Breast magnetic resonance image screening and ductal lavage in women at high genetic risk for breast carcinoma. *Cancer* 2004;**100**(3):479–89.
120. Kuhl C, Weigel S, Schrading S, et al. Prospective multicenter cohort study to refine management recommendations for women at elevated familial risk of breast cancer: the EVA trial. *J Clin Oncol* 2010;**28**(9):1450–7.
121. Ciatto S, Houssami N, Bernardi D, et al. Integration of 3D digital mammography with tomosynthesis for population breast-cancer screening (STORM): a prospective comparison study. *Lancet Oncol* 2013;**14**(7):583–9.
122. Haas BM, Kalra V, Geisel J, Raghu M, Durand M, Philpotts LE. Comparison of tomosynthesis plus digital mammography and digital mammography alone for breast cancer screening. *Radiology* 2013;**269**(3):694–700.
123. Rose SL, Tidwell AL, Bujnoch LJ, Kushwaha AC, Nordmann AS, Sexton Jr R. Implementation of breast tomosynthesis in a routine screening practice: an observational study. *Am J Roentgenol* 2013;**200**(6):1401–8.
124. Skaane P, Bandos AI, Gullien R, et al. Prospective trial comparing full-field digital mammography (FFDM) versus combined FFDM and tomosynthesis in a population-based screening programme using independent double reading with arbitration. *Eur Radiol* 2013;**23**(8):2061–2071.
125. McCarthy AM, Kontos D, Synnestvedt M, et al. Screening outcomes following implementation of digital breast tomosynthesis in a general-population screening program. *J Natl Cancer Inst* 2014;**106**(11). (PMID 25313245/PMCID PMC4271033).
126. Durand MA, Haas BM, Yao X, et al. Early clinical experience with digital breast tomosynthesis for screening mammography. *Radiology* 2015;**274**(1):85–92.
127. Friedewald SM, Rafferty EA, Rose SL, et al. Breast cancer screening using tomosynthesis in combination with digital mammography. *JAMA* 2014;**311**(24):2499–507.
128. Greenberg JS, Javitt MC, Katzen J, Michael S, Holland AE. Clinical performance metrics of 3D digital breast tomosynthesis compared with 2D digital mammography for breast cancer screening in community practice. *Am J Roentgenol* 2014;**203**(3):687–93.
129. Kerlikowske K, Zhu W, Tosteson AN, et al. Identifying women with dense breasts at high risk for interval cancer: a cohort study. *Ann Intern Med* 2015;**162**(10):673–81.

CHAPTER

SCREENING WOMEN WITH KNOWN OR SUSPECTED CANCER GENE MUTATIONS

11

Xuan-Anh Phi[1], Anna M. Chiarelli[2,3] and Geertruida H. de Bock[1]

[1]Department of Epidemiology, University Medical Center Groningen, University of Groningen, Groningen, The Netherlands, [2]Prevention and Cancer Control, Cancer Care Ontario, Toronto, ON, Canada, [3]Dalla Lana School of Public Health, University of Toronto, Toronto, ON, Canada

CHAPTER OUTLINE

PLAIN LANGUAGE SUMMARY

Women with certain genetic mutations (eg, *BRCA1* and *BRCA2*) or with familial risk (without a known gene mutation but with a strong family history of breast or ovarian cancer) are at an elevated risk of developing breast cancer; from 57% to 65% in women with a *BRCA1* mutation and from 45% to 49% in women with a *BRCA2* mutation. The risk of developing breast cancer for women with familial risk depends on number, closeness and age of relatives with breast and ovarian cancer and is between the population risk (11%) and of women with known gene mutations. In some countries, these women at elevated (high) breast cancer risk are offered screening with annual magnetic resonance imaging (MRI) and mammography starting at age 30 or earlier, with the goal of detecting breast cancers at an early stage. This chapter reviews evidence on the benefits and the harms of breast cancer screening strategies in these women. Large-scale studies in women with a *BRCA* gene mutation have been conducted, whereas

Breast Cancer Screening. DOI: http://dx.doi.org/10.1016/B978-0-12-802209-2.00011-5

evidence for women at familial risk is limited. Recent evidence supports screening women at high risk with both MRI and mammography annually because this strategy detects most (84–94%) breast cancers and a large proportion are detected at an early stage. However, this strategy results in more false-positive results (ie, additional imaging and biopsies in women without cancer) compared to screening with a single modality, and some breast cancers are still missed by screening. Further, young women at elevated risk who undergo mammography before age 30 may be at an increased risk of radiation-induced breast cancer. In addition, using MRI is more expensive than mammography, and is more invasive as it requires intravenous contrast. The evidence on whether screening with both MRI and mammography saves lives is based on few, limited studies. Simulation models suggest that yearly screening with both MRI and mammography from age 30 is the most cost-effective strategy for women at elevated risk.

GENERAL INTRODUCTION AND STRUCTURE OF THE CHAPTER

As women with known or suspected gene mutations have an increased lifetime breast cancer risk with an earlier age of onset, there has been much attention focused on effective breast screening of this high-risk population. In this chapter, the evidence regarding breast cancer screening in these women is reviewed. Evidence is based on studies considering different aspects of breast cancer screening including screening accuracy, mortality reduction, potential harms, and cost-effectiveness.

GENETIC PREDISPOSITION TO BREAST CANCER

In the past two decades several major genes have been identified that are associated with an increased lifetime risk of breast cancer, such as *BRCA1*, *BRCA2*, *TP53, CDH1*, *STK11*, and *PTEN*.[1,2] The two most common high-risk cancer-predisposing genes are *BRCA1* and *BRCA2*, and their association with breast cancer as well as ovarian cancer has been extensively studied. Other genes, such as *TP53, STK11*, and *PTEN*, are rarer and associated with broader tumor syndromes. Guidelines on breast cancer prevention and management in *BRCA* families are based on very large series; however, large studies are not possible for the rarer tumor syndromes. Genes like *PALB2, NF1, MEN1, RECQL*, and *CHEK2* mutations, especially the *CHEK2*1100delC* mutation, are known to be associated with a moderately increased risk of breast cancer and breast cancer recurrence; in general breast cancer risk management in these carriers has not been studied as extensively as in *BRCA* carriers. The largest group however, are the women with an increased risk due to a substantial family history, but without any detectable genetic mutation. In this section we will examine the breast cancer risk related to women with *BRCA1/2* gene mutations and to women with a substantial family history of breast cancer without a proven gene mutation.

BRCA1 and BRCA2 gene mutations and their penetrance

The *BRCA1* and *BRCA2* gene mutations are related to the Hereditary Breast Ovarian Cancer Syndrome.[1] The *BRCA* genes are tumor suppressor genes and belong to a family of genes involved in DNA repair or for eliminating DNA that cannot be repaired. Pathogenic mutations in either of these genes impair this process. The wild-type allele *BRCA* gene mutations are dominantly inherited which means any child of a *BRCA* mutation carrier has a 50% chance of carrying the mutation.

BRCA1 and *BRCA2* are the two most common high-risk cancer-predisposing genes. Although the estimated prevalence in the general population is low (0.11% and 0.12%, respectively),[3,4] carriers have an increased lifetime risk of breast cancer and associated earlier age at onset. From two metaanalyses based on retrospective studies, the estimated cumulative risk of breast cancer by the age of 70 vary from 57% (95% confidence interval (CI) 47–66) to 65% (95% CI 44–78) in women with a *BRCA1* mutation and from 45% (95% CI 31–56) to 49% (95% CI 40–57) in women with a *BRCA2* mutation.[5,6] These estimated breast cancer risks were confirmed in a prospective study,[7] and vary by type and location of *BRCA1/2* mutations,[8] as well as by methods of risk estimation.[9]

Women with high familial risk

Women with a suspected genetic predisposition include women who have a strong family history of breast cancer or with a family history of ovarian cancer without a proven mutation. These women are at increased risk of breast cancer and are referred to as women at familial risk for breast cancer. Though there is no single definition of strong family history of breast cancer, generally accepted criteria include: (1) at least three breast and/or ovarian cancer cases from the same side in a family (first or second degree relatives); or (2) two breast cancer cases diagnosed before the age of 40; or (3) a family member with both breast and ovarian cancer; (4) two breast cancer cases in first degree relatives, with at least one case diagnosed before age 50; (5) any male relative with breast cancer; and (6) Ashkenazi Jewish ancestry with a family member with breast cancer, particularly triple-negative breast cancer diagnosed before age 60.[10–12]

Risk assessment tools are designed to identify women at risk of carrying a mutation in a high-risk gene or to identify the risk of developing breast cancer during their lifetime with or without such a mutation.[13] A recent study concluded that for current clinical practice, the IBIS (or Tyrer-Cuzick) model based on the International Breast Intervention Study and the Breast and Ovarian Analysis of Disease Incidence and Carrier Estimation Algorithm (BOADICEA) models are the most accurate for assessing the risk of breast cancer.[14] BOADICEA is used to compute *BRCA1/2* mutation carrier probabilities and age-specific risks of breast and ovarian cancer.[15] However, there is much variation between countries in the use of these risk assessment tools as well as in the applied thresholds for recommending testing or screening.[16]

CHARACTERISTICS OF *BRCA*-ASSOCIATED BREAST CANCERS RELATED TO SCREENING

Several studies observed differences in the pathology of *BRCA1/2* associated breast tumors as compared to non-*BRCA*-associated breast tumors. In general, *BRCA1/2* associated breast tumors more frequently are estrogen and progesterone receptor positive, where *BRCA2*-related tumors are more likely to have a lobular morphology and *BRCA1*-related tumors a medullary carcinoma morphology.[7] In general, women with a *BRCA1/2* mutation have a significantly faster growth rate of their tumors than women with sporadic breast cancer.[17] It is likely that this faster tumor growth rate in *BRCA* mutation carriers is due to a combined effect of having a *BRCA* mutation and the relatively young age at cancer diagnosis, where this effect is more pronounced in *BRCA1* than in *BRCA2*.[18] In addition, the mean preclinical duration in *BRCA1* mutation carriers is supposed to be shorter than in *BRCA2* mutation carriers.[19]

SCREENING WOMEN WITH KNOWN OR SUSPECTED GENE MUTATION

Because screening mammography has been shown to be effective in reducing breast cancer mortality, screening for breast cancer is applied widely in many countries either through a national screening program or through clinical guidelines for average risk women, usually starting between the ages of 40 and 50 with intervals of 1–3 years. Women with known or suspected gene mutations have an increased lifetime breast cancer risk with an earlier age of onset, therefore, much attention has been focused on effective screening of this high-risk population. Although mammography screening is effective in the early detection of breast cancer in average risk women, its sensitivity to detect breast cancer in this high-risk group is much lower. Therefore, most studies have examined the sensitivity of the addition of screening tests to mammography for screening of younger women with known or suspected gene mutation using a nonrandomized design. Recent evidence from prospective cohort studies suggest that women at high risk for breast cancer benefit from screening, which includes breast MRI in addition to mammography, at an earlier age and shorter intervals than usually recommended for population screening. Although MRI with mammography is more sensitive than mammography alone, its specificity is lower, leading to false-positives and unnecessary tests. Further, repeated screening of young women with mammography annually before the age of 40 may increase the risk of breast cancer due to radiation exposure.[20] To minimize the risk of radiation-induced cancer in young women, some guidelines recommend starting screening with MRI alone at the age of 25, while delaying screening with mammography until the age of 30.[21,22] The decision on what age to start screening with mammography, therefore, should consider both the benefit of early detection and the potential harm of false-positives and increased risk of radiation-induced cancer.

EFFECTIVENESS OF SCREENING WOMEN WITH A KNOWN OR SUSPECTED GENE MUTATION

International collaborative groups have published guidelines for the managing and surveillance of women at high risk for breast cancer, often based on experts' opinion.[23–28] Preventive options for these women include risk-reducing mastectomy, salpingo-oophorectomy or use of tamoxifen. Although prophylactic mastectomy offers the greatest reduction in breast cancer risk, an international comparison of the uptake of this preventive option found that the minority of women opt for this.[29] Therefore, it is important to identify in addition an acceptable and effective screening strategy. Many prospective cohort studies have been conducted examining the effectiveness of breast cancer screening in this high-risk population that includes MRI of the breast in addition to mammography. This section summarizes the evidence on the effectiveness of screening with MRI as an adjunct to mammography as compared to mammography-only in women with *BRCA* gene mutations and women at familial risk for breast cancer. The effectiveness of screening strategies is summarized in terms of expected benefits, such as improved cancer detection, the potential reduction in breast cancer mortality, cost-effectiveness of screening strategies, and the potential harms such as false-positives and false-negatives and radiation-induced tumor risk.

The literature was searched for studies reporting on screening for breast cancer in high-risk women from 1990 to 2015, to identify and summarize relevant evidence on this issue. Women were considered to have a high-risk of developing breast cancer if they had a *BRCA1* or a *BRCA2* mutation, or had a high familial risk without a known gene mutation. In a study setting, MRI and mammography had to be performed prospectively and simultaneously and these two tests had to be read independently of each other. In a real-world screening setting, MRI and mammography are not interpreted independently of each other. Prospective and model-based studies included are those that reported the screening sensitivity and specificity of MRI and mammography or related data from which sensitivity and specificity could be derived; those that examined survival or mortality rate; and those that compared cost-effectiveness of screening strategies.

INCREASED SENSITIVITY OF SCREENING MRI AS AN ADJUNCT TO MAMMOGRAPHY

Evidence from prospective studies and metaanalyses

Fourteen prospective cohort studies including seven single center and seven multicenter studies were published through 2015[30–43] (see Table 11.1). These studies report sensitivity, specificity, and cancer yield (how many additional cancers detected by each screening modality) of screening modalities in a high-risk population.

Based on these studies, three metaanalyses have been performed[44,45,46] (Table 11.1). Two of the metaanalyses included screening studies in which women at high risk for breast cancer due to gene mutation or strong family history were included.[44,45] The most recently published metaanalysis, consisting of individual patient data (IPD) from six large studies, reported data only on women with *BRCA* genes and it used a common categorization of screening test results.[46]

Evidence in women with a *BRCA1* or *BRCA2* mutation

Overall, in women with a *BRCA1* or a *BRCA2* mutation, studies found low mammography sensitivity (the sensitivity ranged from 0% to 53%) and a much higher sensitivity of MRI (range 50–100%) in particular for MRI and mammography (range 70–100%) (Table 11.1). The incremental sensitivity of MRI compared to mammography alone ranged from 40% to 100%.[32–35,38–41] Sensitivity of mammography was higher in women with a *BRCA2* mutation than in women with a *BRCA1* mutation, possibly because of the higher proportion of Ductal Carcinoma in Situ (DCIS) in women with a *BRCA2* mutation.[32,34] Related to this, the incremental sensitivity of MRI was observed to be higher in women with a *BRCA1* mutation than in women with a *BRCA2* mutation, as MRI is less sensitive for DCIS.

The Lord et al. systematic review[44] included five prospective studies with a total of 2059 women with a *BRCA1/2* mutation or at high familial risk, reporting screening accuracy of the combination of MRI and mammography with or without breast ultrasound and clinical breast examination (CBE). A metaanalysis of the three studies that compared MRI and mammography versus mammography alone estimated a sensitivity of the combination of MRI and mammography of 94% (95% CI 86–98) and an incremental sensitivity of MRI as an adjunct to mammography of 58% (95% CI 47–70).[44] The incremental sensitivity of MRI decreased when it was compared as an adjunct to mammography plus ultrasound or to the combination of mammography, ultrasound plus CBE.[44] The main limitations of this review were that data for estimates of sensitivity and specificity of screening modalities were not reported, and that the pooled estimate was based on two different definitions of a positive screening test, which might result in biased estimates (one study used BI-RADS 0,3–5 as positive test and others used BI-RADS 4,5 as positive test).[44]

The Warner et al. systematic review[45] included 11 prospective studies with a total of 4983 women with a *BRCA1/2* mutation or at high familial risk, reporting screening accuracy of MRI alone, mammography alone, and the combination if available. In this review, data were pooled for varying definitions of a positive test, and this showed that the sensitivity of screening modalities slightly decreased when the definition of a positive screening test was less strict.[45] Using the stricter definition of BI-RADs scores of 4 and 5 considered to be positive, the sensitivity for mammography-only was 32% (95% CI 23–41) (based on seven studies, 4084 women), and the sensitivity for the combination of MRI and mammography was 84% (95% CI 70–97) (based on five studies, 1897 women), resulting in an incremental sensitivity for MRI of 52% (95% CI 42–62). The increase in sensitivity was traded off by a decrease in specificity from 98.5% of mammography-only, to 95.2% of the combination of MRI and mammography.[45]

Table 11.1 Overview of Studies Reporting Screening Accuracy of Magnetic Resonance Imaging (MRI) and Mammography Screening in Women With a Known or Suspected Gene Mutation

Author, Year, Study/Time Frame	Study Design/ Reading Policy	Positive Test	Follow-Up and Intermediate Tests	Risk Category	Total (*n*)	Breast Cancers (*n*)	MRI Sens–Spec (%)	Mammography Sens–Spec (%)	Ultrasound Sens–Spec (%)	MRI+ Mammography Sens–Spec (%)
Prospective Studies Including Annual MRI and Mammography Simultaneously										
Passaperuma et al. (2012) Toronto-Canada[30] 11/1997–6/2009	Single center study/Single reading	BI-RADS 0,3,4,5	Positive test: Biopsy. If MRI is positive but no other tests are, MRI is repeated within 1 month Intermediate test: (BI-RADS 3) 6,12,24-month follow-up	Total	496	57	86–90	19–97	NA	NA
				BRCA1	267	31	90–NA	19–NA	NA	NA
				BRCA2	229	26	80–NA	20–NA	NA	NA
				Familial risk	0	0	NA	NA	NA	NA
Sardanelli et al. (2011) Italy[31] HIBCRIT 1 Study 6/2000–1/2007	Multicenter study/Single reading	BI-RADS 4,5	Positive test: Biopsy Negative test: 12-month follow-up Intermediate test: (BI-RADS 3) 4-month follow-up	Total	501	52	91.3–96.7	50–99	52–98.4	NA
				BRCA1	184	21	NA	NA	NA	NA
				BRCA2	146	10	NA	NA	NA	NA
				Familial risk	171	21	NA	NA	NA	NA
Leach et al. (2005) UK[32] MARIBS 8/1997–5/2004	Multicenter study/ Double reading	BI-RADS 0,3,4,5	Positive test: Biopsy Negative test: 12-month follow-up No intermediate test	Total	649	35	77–81	40–93	NA	94–77
				BRCA1	82	13	92–79	23–92	NA	92–74
				BRCA2	43	12	58–82	50–94	NA	92–78
				Familial risk	524	10	NA	NA	NA	NA
Riedl et al. (2015) Austria[33] 1/1999–7/2006	Single center study/Single reading	BI-RADS 4,5	Positive test: Biopsy Negative test: Follow-up till the last round Intermediate test: (BI-RADS 3) 6-month follow-up	Total	559	40	85.7–92.3	37.5–97.1	37.5–96.9	95–88.2
				BRCA1/2	156	16	81.3–94.3	43.8–98.9	37.5–99.1	87.5–NA
				Familial risk	297	24	95.8–NA	33.3–NA	37.5–NA	100–NA

Rijnsburger (2010) The Netherlands[34] MRISC 11/1999–3/2006	Multicenter study/Single reading	BI-RADS 0,3,4,5	Positive test: Biopsy Negative test: If imaging test was negative and CBE was suspect, additional test was required Intermediate test: (BI-RADS 0,3) US w/wo fine needle aspiration or imaging test	Total	2157	97	70.7–89.7	41.3	NA	
				BRCA1	422	35	66.7–91	25–94.6	NA	70.8–NA
				BRCA2	172	18	69.2–91	61.5–93.8	NA	92.3–NA
				Familial risk	1563	44	73–89.2	46–94.6	NA	89.2–NA
Trop et al. (2010) Montreal-Canada [35] 8/2003–5/2007	Single center study/Single reading	BI-RADS 4,5	Positive test: Biopsy Negative test: Follow-up till the last round Intermediate test: (BI-RADS 3) 6-month follow-up	Total	184	12	83–93.6	58–95.4	42–93.8	100–NA
				BRCA1	75	6	83.3–NA	50–NA	50–NA	NA
				BRCA2	68	5	80–NA	60–NA	20–NA	NA
				Familial risk	41	1	100–NA	100–NA	100–NA	NA
Lehman et al. (2005) USA [36] 7/1999–1/2002	Multicenter study/Single reading	BI-RADS 4,5	Positive test: Biopsy	Total	390	4	100–NA	25–NA	NA	NA
Lehman et al. (2007) USA [37] 11/2002–4/2003	Multicenter study/Single reading	BI-RADS 3,4,5	Positive test: Biopsy	Total	190	6	100–NA	66.7–NA	16.7–NA	NA
				BRCA1	41	2	100–NA	0	0	NA
				BRCA2	39	1	100–NA	0	0	NA
				Familial risk	110	3	100–NA	66.7–NA	33.4–NA	NA
Kuhl et al. (2005) Germany [38] 3/1996–2/2002	Single center study/ Double reading	BI-RADS 4,5	Positive test: Biopsy Negative test: Follow-up	Total	529	43	90.7–NA	32.6–NA	39.5–NA	93–NA
				BRCA1/2	43	8	100–NA	37.5–NA	25–NA	100–NA
				Familial risk	486	35	88.6–NA	NA	NA	NA
Kuhl et al. (2010) Germany [39] 10/2002–12/2005	Multicenter study/Single reading	BI-RADS 4,5	Positive test: Biopsy Negative test: Follow-up	Total	687	27	92.6–98.4	33.3–99.1	37–98	100–97.5
				BRCA1	53	NA	NA	NA	NA	NA
				BRCA2	12	NA	NA	NA	NA	NA
				Familial risk	622	NA	NA	NA	NA	NA

(*Continued*)

Table 11.1 Overview of Studies Reporting Screening Accuracy of Magnetic Resonance Imaging (MRI) and Mammography Screening in Women With a Known or Suspected Gene Mutation (Continued)

Author, Year, Study/Time Frame	Study Design/ Reading Policy	Positive Test	Follow-Up and Intermediate Tests	Risk Category	Total (*n*)	Breast Cancers (*n*)	MRI Sens–Spec (%)	Mammography Sens–Spec (%)	Ultrasound Sens–Spec (%)	MRI+ Mammography Sens–Spec (%)
Hagen et al. (2007) Norway [40] 2002–01/2006	Multicenter study/Single reading	BI-RADS 3,4,5	Positive test: Biopsy Negative test: Follow-up till the last round Intermediate test: (BI-RADS 3) short term follow-up	Total	491	21	86–NA	48–NA	NA	95.2–NA
				BRCA1	445	19	84–NA	53–NA	NA	94.7–NA
				BRCA2	46	2	100–NA	0–NA	NA	100–NA
Weinstein et al. (2009) USA[41] 5/2002–7/2007	Single center study/Single reading	BI-RADS 0,3,4,5	Final conclusion made by consensus combining all results from different modalities. If all the tests gave suspicious finding, biopsy was performed	Total	609	0.18	71–NA	33 (FSM) 39 (DM)	17–88	95–NA
				BRCA1	27	2	50–NA	50 (FSM) 50 (DM)	0	100–NA
				BRCA2	17	2	0	100 (DM)	0	100–NA
				Familial risk	565	14	78.6–NA	35.7 (DM) 35.7 (FSM)	21–NA	93–NA
Cortesi et al. (2006) Modena study, Italy[42] 1/1994–9/2000	Single center study/Single reading	Not specified		Total	1325	36	100–NA	78–NA	50–NA	NA
				BRCA1/2	48	4	100–NA	50–NA	75–NA	NA
				High risk	647	21	NA	90–NA	52–NA	NA
				Intermediate risk	257	8	NA	50–NA	50–NA	NA
				Slightly increased	346	3	NA	100–NA	0	NA

Warner et al. (2004) Toronto, Canada[43] 11/1997–3/2003	Single center study/Single reading	BI-RADS 4,5	Positive test: Biopsy If MRI is positive but no other tests are, MRI is repeated within 1 month Intermediate test: (BI-RADS 3) 6,12,24-month follow-up	*BRCA1/2*	236	22	77–NA	36–NA	33–NA	NA
Prospective Study on Additional Value of Ultrasound/Clinical Breast Examination to Screening										
Bosse et al. (2014) 1/1997–10/2008[48]	Single-center study/Single reading	BI-RADS 4,5	Positive test: Biopsy	Total	221	27	100–55.5	27–82.3	81–84.2	NA
Tilanus-Linthorst et al. (2000) 1/1994–4/1998[49]	Single-center study/Single reading	Not reported	Not reported	Women at high risk (>15%)	678	50	8–NA* (only in subgroup of high risk over 25% risk underwent MRI)	68–NA	62–NA	NA
Metaanalysis of High-Risk Screening Studies										
	Included study		**Study population**	**Test threshold**	**MRI+ Mammography Sens–Spec (%) (95% CI)**			**Mammography Sens–Spec (%) (95% CI)**	**MRI Sens–Spec (%) (95% CI)**	
Lord et al. (2007)[46]	Kuhl et al. (2005)[38] MARIBS study (2005)[32] Lehman et al.[36] HIBCRIT study 2006 (interim results)[82] Warner et al. (2004)[43]		Women with *BRCA1/2* mutation and women at familial risk		94 (86–98)–NA Incremental sensitivity: 58% (95% CI 47–70)			NA	NA	

(*Continued*)

Table 11.1 Overview of Studies Reporting Screening Accuracy of Magnetic Resonance Imaging (MRI) and Mammography Screening in Women With a Known or Suspected Gene Mutation (Continued)

Author, Year, Study/Time Frame	Study Design/ Reading Policy	Positive Test	Follow-Up and Intermediate Tests	Risk Category	Total (*n*)	Breast Cancers (*n*)	MRI Sens–Spec (%)	Mammography Sens–Spec (%)	Ultrasound Sens–Spec (%)	MRI+ Mammography Sens–Spec (%)
Warner et al. (2008)[47]	Kuhl et al. (2005)[38] MRISC study (2004)[55] Warner et al. (2001)[83] Warner et al. (2004)[43] Trecate et al. (2006)[84] Hartman et al. (2004)[85] Lehman et al. (2005)[36] Lehman et al. (2007)[37] Hagen et al. (2007)[40] MARIBS study (2005)[32]		Women with *BRCA1/2* mutation and women at familial risk	BI-RADS 3,4,5 as positive	94 (90–97)–77.2 (74.7–79.7)			39 (37–41)–94.7 (93–96.5)	77 (70–84)–86.3 (80.9–91.7)	
				BI-RADS 4,5 as positive	84 (70–797)–95.2 (93.7–96.6)			32 (23–41)-98.5 (97.8–99.2)	75 (62–88)–96.1 (94.8–97.4)	
Phi et al. (2015)[53]	Montreal Canada study 2010[35] MARIBS study 2005[32] HIBCRIT study 2011[31] Austria study 2015 [33] MRISC study 2010[34] Toronto Canada study 2012[30]		Women with *BRCA1/2* mutation	BI-RADS 0,3,4,5 as positive	93.4 (79.7–98.1)–80.3 (72.5–86.3)			39.4 (30–49.7)–93.7 (88.8–96.5)	85.3 (69.3–93.7)–84.7 (79–89.1)	
Roeke et al. (2014)[50]	Tilanus-Linthorst (2000)[45] Warner et al. (2001)[83] Warner et al. (2004)[43] MRISC study (2010)[34] Kuhl CK et al. (2010)[39] Montreal Canada study (2010)[35] HIBCRIT study (2011)[31]		Women with *BRCA1/2* mutation and women at familial risk	NA	Cancer yield by clinical breast examination: 0–4%			NA	NA	

The Phi et al. metaanalysis[46] consisting of IPD from six large prospective studies, and reported data on 1951 women with *BRCA* genes using a common categorization of screening test results. Considering a BI-RADS 3,4, or 5 as a positive test, the IPD estimated sensitivity of the combination of MRI and mammography was 93.4% (95% CI 80.2–98) and the incremental sensitivity of MRI was 53.8%, which is similar to the Warner et al. metaanalysis in 2008 (incremental sensitivity of 55%) when using the same cutoff point.[46] In the general population, the sensitivity of mammography increases with increasing age and decreasing breast density. However, the IPD metaanalysis showed that mammography sensitivity was lower in women with a genetic mutation regardless of age (for women aged <50: 40% (95% CI 30.5–50.3) and for women older than 50: 38.1% (95% CI 22.4–56.7)),[46] suggesting that screening with mammography alone would not be sufficient for these high-risk women over the age of 50. The evidence suggests that MRI continues to contribute to a high sensitivity in women with a *BRCA1* or *BRCA2* mutation older than 50 years old.[46]

Evidence for women at high familial risk

The sensitivity and specificity of screening modalities were reported separately for women at high familial risk in a few studies.[33–35,37,38,41,42] Women without a gene mutation, but at high familial risk for breast cancer, comprised varying proportions of the total study population in the studies (22.3–92.8%), as these women have a lower expected incidence of breast cancer, which is reflected by the small number of observed breast cancers (Table 11.1). The reported sensitivity and specificity estimates are comparable to those for women with *BRCA1/2* mutation in the few studies that had more than five breast cancer cases.[33,34,41] However, as the observed incidence of breast cancer is lower in these women without a gene mutation, but at high familial risk for breast cancer, the positive predictive values of the screening will be lower and the negative predictive values will be higher than observed in the mutation carriers. Therefore, based on the trade-off of the lower positive and higher negative predictive values, the decision to add MRI to mammography in breast cancer screening may be different for this population. Further research is needed to strengthen the current evidence for this population on the added value of MRI to mammography in breast cancer screening.

Heterogeneity across studies

Due to the heterogeneity of methodology used, there are limitations when comparing results amongst the prospective studies evaluating the screening accuracy of MRI and mammography in high-risk women. First, these studies were conducted over different time periods, ranging from 1994 until 2011, during which the sensitivity and specificity of MRI may have improved. Second, the definition for a positive screening result was not consistent though all studies used BI-RADS assessments to classify the outcomes of screening. In some studies a positive screening test was defined as a BI-RADS 0,3,4,5,[30,32,34,37,40,41] whereas in others a positive screening test was defined as BI-RADS 4, 5.[31,33,35,36,38,39,43] Usually a BI-RADS 4 or 5 is followed by a biopsy. However, a BI-RADS 3 was either followed by additional imaging,[34] within 4 months,[31] or within 6 months.[30,35,38] In one study, BI-RADS 0 also lead to additional testing.[34] Third, the time between screening tests varied with screening modalities performed on the same day,[30,32,40–42] within 1 month of each other,[33,35] or 6 weeks to 3 months of each other.[35–39] Fourth, some studies only included women with a *BRCA1/2* mutation[30,40,43] and others included women with *BRCA* mutations and with strong family history equivalent to a lifetime risk of breast cancer higher than 20%.[31–39,41,42] This lifetime risk of breast cancer was defined and assessed by different risk assessment tools such as lifetime risk of being a carrier by *BRCA*PRO,[35,37,39] or lifetime risk of developing breast cancer by the Gail or Claus model,[31,33,34,36,38] or a study-specific risk model.[32] Finally, inclusion criteria such as whether women with a personal history of breast cancer were excluded,[32,34] or the age of recruitment differed between studies (age 35[32]; age 25[30,31,33,34,36–39,41,43]; or no specific age[40,42]).

Evidence from effectiveness studies evaluating screening program for high-risk women

Most of the prospective studies comparing MRI and mammography screening are efficacy studies in which annual MRI and mammography are performed simultaneously, and in which the results are blinded to ensure the comparison. There has been only one study of a real-world setting within a tailored screening program. A study from Ontario, Canada, reported first year results for the Ontario Breast Screening High Risk Program that offers annual MRI and mammography to women aged 30–69 years simultaneously but the results of both tests were not blinded.[47] This study showed that no breast cancers were additionally detected by mammography and all the cancers were detected by MRI.[47] The highest cancer detection (30.8/1000) was reported among women who were known gene mutation carriers.

Conclusions for cancer detection in women at high risk

Given the above evidence (summarized in Table 11.1), breast MRI screening as an adjunct to mammography improves the sensitivity of breast cancer detection in women with *BRCA1/2* mutations, both in younger women and in women over the age of 50 years. For women without a *BRCA* mutation, the combination of MRI and mammography was also shown to be the most sensitive. However as the observed incidence of breast cancer is lower in these women without a gene mutation, the positive predictive values of the screening will be lower and the negative predictive values will be higher than observed in the mutation carriers. The evidence for women at familial risk is limited and does not consider different risk levels, and further research is needed to give more robust evidence in this particular population considering different risk levels. The prospective studies were heterogeneous in terms of methodology and study population and the aggregated metaanalyses were based on those studies. The most robust evidence comes from the IPD metaanalysis where the heterogeneity was minimized by using individual data from six studies, using common categorization of screening test results and women with similar risk profile.

THE ROLE OF OTHER SCREENING MODALITIES

Breast ultrasound

In addition to MRI and mammography, some studies included ultrasound (US) in their screening protocol.[31,33,35,37,39,41,42] When US was performed annually with MRI and mammography, US alone had low sensitivity similar to mammography alone in women with or without *BRCA* mutation, ranging from 0% to 52% [31,33,37,39,41] (Table 11.1). No breast cancers were detected by US only. In other settings, where US was offered semiannually,[35,38,42,48] the sensitivity was 39.5–77%,[35,38,42,48,49] and in one study three of 25 cancers were detected by US only,[48] suggesting US as a screening modality every 6 months might help to detect more breast cancers. However, the cancer detection benefit should be balanced with the harm of screening, such as false-negative, and balanced with the cost per additional cancer detected.

Clinical breast examination

The contribution of CBE in screening women with or without *BRCA* mutation, was reviewed in a recent publication.[50] The sensitivity of CBE ranged from 3% to 50% and the cancer yield of CBE was from 0% to 3% or 4% of the total breast cancers.[50] The two studies reporting the contribution of CBE to be about 3–4% of the breast cancers [34,45] had less screened detected breast cancers compared to other studies in which no additional breast cancers were detected by only CBE. Further, these two studies performed CBE semiannually compared to annually in the other studies. Another study which was not included in the review reported that biannual CBE detected four intervals cancers.[42] Therefore, the contribution of annual CBE in screening women at high risk for breast cancer did not improve breast cancer detection. However, semi-annual CBE was shown to have a small contribution to breast cancer detection, though the evidence is very limited. It is important to balance the benefit with the harm of screening, as the price for detecting more breast cancer should be acceptable.

POTENTIAL MORTALITY BENEFITS OF SCREENING WITH MRI

Early stage breast cancers are expected to have a better prognosis and to have an improved survival rate. The main goal of breast cancer screening is therefore to increase the rate of early stage tumor detection and to reduce mortality. To evaluate the mortality benefit of screening, there is a need for data derived from prospective studies including a control group with a long-term follow-up and for model-based studies, estimating survival rate due to screening with MRI and mammography as compared to no screening or mammography-only screening. In this section, results are reported from prospective studies that include a control group and from a model-based study using populations from prospective studies which estimated survival rates due to screening with MRI and mammography[19,51,52,53] (Table 11.2). The prospective studies either performed MRI and mammography in a study setting where the results of two tests were blinded (the MRISC study)[52] or in a daily practice setting where the results of the test were not blinded (the Norway and UK study).[51,53]

Evidence for women with BRCA1/2 mutations

The MRISC study compared metastasis-free-survival of patients with breast cancer and with *BRCA1/2* mutations or with familial risk undergoing intensive screening consisting of biannual CBE, annual MRI and mammography between the ages of 25 and 70 years, to matched controls, that were unscreened if less than 50 or screened with mammography if 50 years or older by risk group, year of diagnosis, and age at diagnosis.[52] The 10-year metastasis-free-survival rate was significantly higher in the screened compared to control group (90% vs 77%, $p = 0.008$; HR = 0.36, 95% CI 0.16–0.8). However, this did not result in a statistically significant improvement in overall survival in the intensively screened group (88%) compared to the control group (78%, $p = 0.064$; HR = 0.51, 95% CI 0.24–1.06). For women with a *BRCA1* mutation, the metastasis-free-survival rate was just above the significance level (88% in screening group vs 72% in control group, $p = 0.055$; HR = 0.3, 95% CI 0.08–1.13). While for women with a *BRCA2* mutation, the metastasis-free-survival rate was not significantly different (88% in screened group vs 83% in unscreened group, $p = 0.739$; HR = 0.21, 95% CI 0.12–4.45).

A study from Norway examined survival rates of patients with a *BRCA1*-associated breast cancer aged 25–74 years who underwent annual MRI and mammography screening as part of a national MRI-based surveillance program.[53] The overall 5- and 10-year survival rates for women with a *BRCA1*-related breast cancer were 75% (95% CI 56–86) and 69% (95% CI 48–83), respectively.[53] The survival rates were higher for women diagnosed with breast cancer at age 50 and above and for women diagnosed with small cancers (size below 1.0 cm). For stage 1 breast cancer, women with a *BRCA1* mutation had a 5-year survival of 82%, which is lower than that for the general Norway population which is 98% ($p < 0.05$). As survival for *BRCA1* patients was less than expected, this study did not recommend offering MRI-based screening as an alternative to preventive mastectomy in these women.

Table 11.2 Overview of Studies Reported Survival Rate of Screening with Magnetic Resonance Imaging (MRI) and Mammography in Women with a Known or Suspected Gene Mutation

No	Authors/Year of Publication	Design/Population/Analysis/Endpoint	Outcomes		Comparison	Hazard Ratio
1	Evans et al. (2014)[51] MARIBS	Design: Prospective study Population: Women with *BRCA1/2* or TP53 mutation and women at equivalent risk (40% lifetime risk), age 35–55 MRI group: Screened annually with MRI and mammography (simultaneously and later every 6 months) Mammography group: Screened annually with mammography Unscreened group: Women with *BRCA1/2* mutation with breast cancer aged <55, no intensive screening Analysis: Kaplan–Meier survival curves, log rank test, cox regression adjusted for age at diagnosis Endpoint: Censored or death	10-year survival MRI group	95.30%	MRI vs Unscreened	HR=0.13 (0.032–0.05), p=0.004
			10-year survival Unscreened group	73.70%	MRI vs Mammography	HR=NR, p=0.075
			10-year survival Mammography group	87.70%	Mammography vs Unscreened	HR=0.52 (0.24–1.11), p=0.09
					MRI vs Unscreened for *BRCA1* carriers	HR=0.21 (0.051–0.89), p=0.03
					Screened vs Unscreened for *BRCA2* carriers	HR=0.21 (0.066–0.67), p=0.008
2	Saadatmand et al. (2015)[52] MRISC	Design: Prospective study Population: Women with *BRCA1/2* mutation and women at familial risk (15–50% risk), age 25–70 Cases: Women screened with annual MRI and mammography, semi-annual CBE Controls: Matched with cases in risk, year of diagnosis, age at diagnosis. only screened after age 50 in National population screening (mutation identified after diagnosis) Analysis: Kaplan–Meier curves, unadjusted cox proportional hazard model, model adjusted for lead time bias and survival bias Endpoint: Censored, death, distant metastases	10-year metastasis-free-survival (MFS) of screened group	90%	MFS Screened vs Unscreened	HR=0.36 (0.16–0.8), p=0.008
			10-year MFS of unscreened group	77%	MFS Screened vs Unscreened for *BRCA1* carriers	HR=0.3 (0.08–1.13), p=0.055
			10-year MFS of screened group for *BRCA1* carriers	88%	MFS Screened vs Unscreened for *BRCA2* carriers	HR=0.74 (0.12–4.45), p=0.739
			10-year MFS of unscreened group for *BRCA1* carriers	72%		
			10-year MFS of screened group for *BRCA2* carriers	88%		
			10-year MFS of unscreened group for *BRCA2* carriers	83%		

3	Moller et al. (2013)[53]	Design: Prospective study Population: Case: women with *BRCA1* mutation screened with mammography and MRI annually, age 25–75 Comparison group: General population from National cancer registry Analysis: Kaplan–Meier curves Endpoint: Breast cancer diagnosis or prophylactic mastectomy	10-year survival for stage 1 BC	82%	$p<0.05$ compared to screened cohort	
			10-year survival for stage 1 BC from general population	98%		
4	Heijnsdijk et al. (2012)[19] MRISC, MARIBS, Canadian	Design: Simulation model Population: Women with *BRCA1/2* mutations from three prospective studies: MRISC, MARIBS, Canadian Screened with mammography and/or MRI Analysis: Simulation with MISCAN Outcome: Mortality reduction compared to no screening	Mortality reduction mammography (age 25–60), *BRCA1* carriers	41.90%		
			Mortality reduction mammography (age 25–60), *BRCA2* carriers	46.80%		
			Mortality reduction Mammography and MRI study protocol, *BRCA1* carriers	50.10%		
			Mortality reduction Mammography and MRI study protocol, *BRCA2* carriers	61.60%		

In the UK study, data from two prospective cohorts (the MARIBS cohort and surveillance program) were used to compare survival in women aged 35–55 years at high risk due to known or suspected genes.[51] The MRI group was screened with annual MRI and mammography as in the MARIBS study, or with MRI and mammography alternating every 6 months in the surveillance program. The mammogram group included women who were *BRCA1/2* mutation carriers and/or at equivalent risk who had received mammography screening only, and the unscreened group were women with *BRCA1/2* who had not undergone surveillance. They reported a 10-year survival of 95% in the MRI group, which was higher than the mammogram only group (87.7%) and statistically significantly higher than that of the unscreened group (74%, $p = 0.002$). Among the *BRCA1* carriers screened with MRI, there was a less pronounced but still statistically significant survival advantage (91.6%) compared to unscreened women (78%) ($p = 0.03$; HR = 0.21, 95% CI 0.051–0.89). There were no deaths among women with a *BRCA2* mutation undergoing MRI screening and 10-year survival of those being screened (with MRI or mammography) (94%) was better than that in the unscreened population (76%) ($p = 0.008$, HR = 0.21, 95% CI 0.07–0.67). This study showed a survival benefit from screening with MRI with mammography, particularly in *BRCA2* carriers.

A model-based study, using data from three prospective studies for *BRCA* carriers,[19] predicted and compared mortality reduction among screening protocols which included mammography alone or the combination of MRI and mammography at different ages. The study population included women from the United Kingdom,[32] the Netherlands,[34,54] and Canada.[43,54] The model predicted breast cancer mortality reduction of the combination of MRI and mammography to be 48–62% higher than that of mammography alone, which ranged from 42% to 47%. Screening with only MRI led to an estimated 49–61% mortality reduction. The study also showed that the expected mortality reduction is higher for women with a *BRCA2* mutation than for women with a *BRCA1* mutation. This was explained by the different tumor growth rates that are associated with each of the gene mutations. However, the authors do note several limitations of their study. The models are based on an overall small number of cancers and there was only a small proportion of women older than 50 years of age included. In addition, prior prophylactic mastectomy and screening history of the participating women could not be taken into account and survival estimates were based on the age- and stage-specific survival rates for noncarriers. Also, a substantial proportion of the women were screened with mammography before entering the study. Finally, the breast cancer incidence without screening is unknown, and as women treated for breast cancer before entering the study were mostly excluded, these cancers were missing from the model.

Evidence for women at high familial risk

Women at high familial risk for breast cancer were included in the UK study and the MRISC study mentioned above, however, only the MRISC study reported survival rate for this particular group.[52] In the high familial risk group, screening with MRI and mammography was shown to improve survival significantly: 95% for the screening group vs 78% for the control group ($p = 0.024$; HR = 0.21, 95% CI 0.04–0.95). This estimate was comparable to that estimated for women with a *BRCA1/2* mutation in the same study (90%) and in the UK study (95%).[51]

Heterogeneity across studies and biases

The results from the three prospective studies are not comparable due to the heterogeneity in methodology. Firstly, the studies differ regarding the included study populations. The MRISC and the UK study included women with *BRCA1/2* mutations or with familial risk, however, they used different risk criteria to identify familial risk and age at recruitment.[51,52] The Norway cohort only included women with a

BRCA1 mutation[53] which would lead to a higher breast cancer incidence and thus reflect more of a benefit in mortality for these mutation carriers. Secondly, the control groups in these studies were selected differently. The Dutch study selected a control group that was matched for breast cancer risk, year, and age at diagnosis, and included women without intensive screening. The UK study selected two unmatched control groups, including women at high risk for breast cancer who received only mammography or no screening. The Norway study compared their finding to what can be expected from the general population. Thirdly, the studies used different analysis methods. The women's baseline characteristics were adjusted by matching in the MRISC study[52] and by analysis in the UK and Norway study.[51,53]

Comparing survival between the screening and unscreened group in a nonrandomized design introduces several biases such as lead time bias, survival bias, and selection bias. Lead time bias occurs when the tumor is detected by screening at an earlier stage than that at which it becomes clinically diagnosed. The apparent benefit from screening might be due to the fact that tumors were diagnosed earlier in time, which may appear to increase the survival time (even in the absence of screening benefit) as the women live longer. It is uncertain whether the survival rate is improved due to the actual benefit of screening or due to lead time bias in the UK study. Selection bias may have occurred in the Norway study as the screening group was at higher risk than the general population control group. In the UK study, it was not described why women with *BRCA* mutations in the no screening group had not undergone intensive surveillance, although a subset of women aged 50–55 years were screened by mammography. Survival bias may have occurred in the MRISC study as they selected a control group of women with *BRCA1/2* mutations who were tested after being diagnosed with breast cancer, meaning they had to survive long enough to be tested. However, in the MRISC study, the analysis was adjusted for lead time and survival bias.

Conclusion from survival perspective

In conclusion, there have been a few prospective studies and one model-based study investigating the effect of MRI as an adjunct to mammography on survival in women with or without *BRCA1/2* mutation, and limited data have been reported for women with familial risk. Although, the studies found improved survival from MRI screening in women with a *BRCA1/2* mutation compared to no screening, the results compared to mammography screening are variable. Results from the Norway cohort suggest that the improvement of survival was not completely explained by detecting early stage tumors. The survival effect is different for women with a *BRCA1* or *BRCA2* mutation, where it seems that *BRCA2* mutation carriers might benefit more from screening than *BRCA1* mutation carriers. As these prospective studies have several limitations due to their nonrandomized design and the model-based study included various assumptions and exclusions, the results should be interpreted with caution.

POTENTIAL HARMS OF SCREENING WITH MRI AND MAMMOGRAPHY

The purpose of breast cancer screening is to detect early stage tumors so that they will have a better prognosis. A perfect screening test would correctly identify any breast abnormality in a very early stage as breast cancer or as a precancer lesion, which means that this test will have a 100% sensitivity. However, every screening test has its limitations and in general, an improvement in sensitivity usually comes with a decrease in specificity. Sensitivity and specificity are measures of the diagnostic accuracy of a test. Sensitivity measures how accurately a screening test captures true cases of a disease in a population. If the sensitivity is low, the test will miss many cancers, resulting in a high rate of false-negative results or interval cancers. A high specificity is also desirable as it reflects the ability of a test to accurately identify cases that are not cancer, therefore reducing the number of false-positive cases. Another issue to be considered in breast cancer screening in young women, is the potential harm by induced radiation risk for breast cancer, due to mammographic screening. This section discusses the potential harms of screening with annual MRI and mammography in women at high risk for breast cancer: high false-negative rate or low sensitivity, high false-positive rate or low specificity, and radiation-induced tumor risk.

High false-negative rate or low sensitivity

False-negative cases are breast cancer cases diagnosed between screening rounds and referred to as interval cancers. Due to a low sensitivity of mammography in screening high-risk women, MRI is added. Although the sensitivity of screening is improved due to the addition of MRI, the sensitivity is still not optimized to 100%. Among the prospective studies, the interval cancer rate ranged from 0% to 17%.[30–43] Interval cancers are a heterogeneous group comprised of those in which recognizable signs of tumor existed at the time of screening but were "missed" for technical or interpretive reasons and those that were not detectable at screening. A study from Austria found that an interval tumor (G3, pT1c, negative nodal status medullary carcinoma) was not visible in review.[33] The interval cancer rate is higher for women with a *BRCA1* mutation compared to women with a *BRCA2* mutation, supporting the faster tumor growth rate of *BRCA1*-associated breast cancers.[34] Interval cancers are not only early stage tumors or DCIS. In addition, invasive breast cancer, high grade tumor, and even triple-negative tumor were not detected by screening.[30] Improvement in standards, technique, and radiologist experience are needed to improve the sensitivity of the screening and to reduce false-negative cases.

High false-positive rate or low specificity

Although combining MRI and mammography in breast cancer screening will increase the sensitivity, it will also reduce the specificity compared to a single modality, as the disagreement of the two test results regarding which cases are positive for the presence of breast cancer, will yield per definition more false-positive cases. A high false-positive rate is reflected by a low specificity which was also observed in the prospective high-risk screening studies[31–33,38,39] and the two metaanalyses.[45,46,53] The specificity of the combination of MRI and mammography ranged from 77% to 97.7% for women with or without a *BCA1/2* mutation, which was in all studies lower than the mammography specificity. The IPD metaanalysis estimates the specificity of MRI and mammography at about 80.3% (95% CI 72.5–86.2) which is substantially lower than the specificity of mammography alone (93.6%, 95% CI 88.8–96.5) and also of MRI alone (84.7, 95% CI 79–89.1).[46] The Warner et al. metaanalysis gave similar estimates.[45]

Radiation-induced tumor risk

Exposure to chest radiation at a young age increases the risk of breast cancer.[20,56–58] Therefore, annual screening with mammography starting at a young age may increase risk of breast cancer. In addition, women with a *BRCA1/2* mutation are more sensitive to radiation at all ages, partially due to the impairment of proper repair of DNA double-strand breaks.[59] The following section discusses the studies reporting radiation risk in women with a *BRCA1/2* mutation and in women with high familial risk.

Evidence for women with a *BRCA1/2* gene mutation

Three studies, with partly overlapping study populations, support the association between radiation exposure (chest X-ray or mammogram) and breast cancer risk among women with a *BRCA1/2* mutation.[60–62] (Table 11.3) The overall odds ratios ranged from 1.06 (95% CI 0.66–1.71) to 4.29

Table 11.3 Overview of Evidence on Radiation-Induced Breast Cancer Risk in Women With a Known or Suspected Gene Mutation

No	Authors/Year of Publication	Design/population/Analysis	Exposure/Groups	Population vs Control	Results (OR or HR (95% CI), *p* Value)
1	Giannakeas et al. (2014)[66]	Design: Prospective study Population: *BRCA1/2* carriers without history of breast cancer at baseline, age 30–70 Analysis: Hazard ratio was adjusted for reproductive factors, family history, oophorectomy and family country of residence	Exposure: Mammography screening Cases: *BRCA* carriers exposed Controls: *BRCA* carriers not exposed	*BRCA1* carriers exposed vs nonexposed *BRCA2* carriers exposed vs nonexposed	HR=0.79 (0.53–1.19), p=0.26 HR=0.9 (0.35–2.34), p=0.83
2	John et al. (2013)[63]	Design: Case–control study Population: *BRCA1/2* carriers, aged <50 Data from three cancer registries: United States, Canada, and Australia/New Zealand Analysis: OR adjusted for age, study site, family history, and number of full terms of pregnancies	Exposure: Diagnostic X-ray (not mammography) Cases: *BRCA1/2* carriers with breast cancer Controls: *BRCA1/2* carriers with no history of breast cancer	*BRCA1* carriers exposed vs nonexposed any chest X-ray *BRCA2* carriers exposed vs nonexposed any chest X-ray	OR=1.21 (0.75–2.3) OR=1.13 (0.59–2.18)
3	Lecarpentier et al. (2012) (GENEPSO)[61]	Design: Retrospective study Population: *BRCA1/2* carriers, age >18, median age 40 Analysis: Weighted cox regression model	Exposure: Chest X-ray (not mammography) Cases: *BRCA1/2* carriers exposed Controls *BRCA1/2* carriers not exposed	*BRCA1/2* carriers exposed vs nonexposed *BRCA1/2* carriers exposed vs nonexposed age <20 *BRCA1/2* carriers exposed vs nonexposed age >20	HR=4.29 (2.09–8.81), p<0.0001 HR=4.16 (2.03–8.56), p<0.0001 HR=6.45 (2.86–14.6), p<0.0002
4	Andrieu et al. (2006)[62]	Design: Retrospective study Population: *BRCA1/2* carriers from GENEPSO, GEO-HEBON, EMBRACE, IBCCS collaboration group, age >18, mean age 41.5 Analysis: Weighted cox regression model on incident cohort; women with censored or diagnosis within 5 years before the interview, follow-up only within this 5 years	Exposure: Chest X-ray (not mammography) Cases: *BRCA1/2* carriers exposed Controls: *BRCA1/2* carriers not exposed	*BRCA1/2* carriers exposed vs nonexposed *BRCA1/2* carriers exposed vs nonexposed age ≤40 *BRCA1/2* carriers exposed vs nonexposed age >40 *BRCA1* carriers exposed vs nonexposed *BRCA2* carriers exposed vs nonexposed *BRCA1/2* carriers exposed vs nonexposed age <20	HR=1.75 (1.1–2.8), p<0.05 HR=2.75 (1.4–5.3), p<0.01 HR=1.35 (0.7–2.6) HR=1.91 (1.1–3.3), p<0.05 HR=1.71 (0.4–8.2) HR=5.21 (1.6–17.5)

(Continued)

Table 11.3 Overview of Evidence on Radiation-Induced Breast Cancer Risk in Women With a Known or Suspected Gene Mutation (Continued)

No	Authors/Year of Publication	Design/population/Analysis	Exposure/Groups	Population vs Control	Results (OR or HR (95% CI), *p* Value)
5	Pijpe et al. (2012)[60]	Design: Retrospective study Population: *BRCA1/2* carriers from GENEPSO (France), EMBRACE (UK), HEBON (Netherlands), age >18 Analysis: Weighted cox regression model on incident cohort; women with censored or diagnosis within 5 years before the interview, follow-up only within this 5 years	Exposure: Diagnostic radiation (including mammography) Cases: *BRCA1/2* carriers exposed Controls: *BRCA1/2* carriers not exposed	*BRCA1/2* carriers exposed vs nonexposed before age 20	HR=1.62 (1.02–2.58)
				BRCA1/2 carriers exposed vs nonexposed age 20–29	HR=1.43 (0.93–2.21)
				BRCA1/2 carriers exposed vs nonexposed before age 30	HR=1.90 (1.2–3.0)
				BRCA1/2 carriers exposed vs nonexposed age 30–39	HR=1.06 (0.66–1.71)
				BRCA1/2 carriers exposed vs nonexposed before age 40	HR=1.91 (1.12–3.26)
6	Goldfrank et al. (2006)[64]	Design: Retrospective study Population: *BRCA1/2* carriers, age >19 Analysis: Logistic regression	Exposure: Mammography Cases: *BRCA1/2* carriers with breast cancer Controls: *BRCA1/2* carriers without breast cancer	*BRCA1/2* carriers with BC vs unaffected *BRCA1/2* carriers	OR=0.94 (0.88=1.0), p=0.06
				BRCA1 carriers with BC vs unaffected *BRCA1* carriers	OR=0.99 (0.90–1.1), p=0.84
				BRCA2 carriers with BC vs unaffected *BRCA2* carriers	OR=0.91 (0.83–1.0), p=0.06
7	Gronwald et al. (2008)[67]	Design: Retrospective study Population: *BRCA1* carriers and noncarriers with breast cancer between age 30 and 50 years Analysis: Logistic regression	Exposure: Chest X-ray Cases: *BRCA1* carriers with breast cancer Controls: Noncarriers with breast cancer	*BRCA1* carriers with BC vs control, chest X-ray before age 20	OR=1.7 (0.9–3.0), p=0.08
				BRCA1 carriers with BC vs control, chest X-ray age 20–30	OR=1.6 (1.0–2.5), p=0.06
				BRCA1 carriers with BC vs control, chest X-ray before age 30	OR=1.8 (1.2–2.9), p=0.01

8	Narod et al. (2006)[65]	Design: Retrospective study Population: *BRCA* carriers with and without breast cancer, matched for age, mutation and country of residency, mean age 47 Analysis: Logistic regression	Exposure: Screening mammography Cases: *BRCA* carriers with breast cancer Controls: *BRCA* carriers without breast cancers	*BRCA* carriers with BC vs unaffected *BRCA* carriers	OR=1.03 (0.85–1.25), p=0.78
				BRCA carriers with BC vs unaffected *BRCA* carriers, first mammogram ≤30	OR=1.0 (0.78–1.29), p=0.99
				BRCA carriers with BC vs unaffected *BRCA* carriers, first mammogram 31–40	OR=1.11 (0.82–1.4), p=0.4
				BRCA carriers with BC vs *BRCA* carriers without BC, first mammogram ≥40	OR=0.92 (0.66–1.29), p=0.63
9	Ma et al. (2008)[69]	Design: Retrospective study Population: Women with family history between age 20–49 Analysis: Multivariate unconditional logistic regression model adjusted for potential confounders	Exposure: Chest X-ray (including mammogram) Cases: With breast cancer Controls: Without breast cancer	Cases with family history vs control with family history, 1–4 chest X-ray	OR=1.24 (0.83–1.84)
				Cases with family history vs control with family history, ≥5 chest X-ray	OR=2.14 (1.14–4.04)
10	John et al. (2007)[68]	Design: Retrospective study Population: Women with breast cancer, 55% between age 40 and 54 years Analysis: Unconditional logistic regression	Exposure: Therapeutic and diagnostic chest radiation (excluding Mammography) for tuberculosis and pneumonia Cases: Women with breast cancer with family history indicating increased genetic risk Controls: sisters of cases who were not diagnosed with breast cancer and unrelated population without breast cancer	Cases with family history vs all controls age at exposure <20	OR=2.61 (1.51–4.51)
				Cases with family history vs all controls age at exposure 20–39	OR=2.64 (1.35–5.17)
				Cases with family history vs all controls age at exposure >40	OR=1.84 (0.39–8.72)

(95% CI 2.09–8.81).[60–62] The results from these three studies were contradictory to other studies,[63–67] showing no significant association between radiation exposure and breast cancer risk in women with a *BRCA* mutation at all ages (OR <1[65,67] and OR >1[63,64,66]) (Table 11.3). These conflicting results may be due to age, as much younger women from the age of 18 were included in the three studies that support the overall association between radiation exposure and breast cancer risk, whereas other studies included older women.

The radiation-induced risk of breast cancer increases with decreasing age at exposure. In women with a *BRCA* mutation exposed to radiation before the age of 20, the evidence shows a strong positive association with breast cancer risk with an OR or HR ranging from 1.62 (95% CI 1.02–2.58)[60] to 4.16 (95% CI 2.03–8.56) compared to nonexposed carriers.[61] Another international study reported an HR of 1.76 (95% CI 0.9–34) for all women with breast cancer and a HR of 5.21 (95% CI 1.6–17.5) for the incidence cohort,[62] considering only women who were diagnosed with breast cancer within 5 years of the interview which means the survival bias was minimized.

Two studies reported results for women with a *BRCA1/2* mutation exposed to radiation before age 30. The GENE-RAD-RISK study reported breast cancer risk to be highest before the age of 30 (OR 1.90 (95% CI 1.2–3)) and similar to the risk before the age of 40 between carriers exposed and nonexposed to radiation including mammography.[60] The Gronwald et al. study[67] compared the breast cancer risk between women with *BRCA1* mutation-associated breast cancers and women with sporadic breast cancers who had been exposed to radiation from chest X-rays before age 30 and developed breast cancer at age 50 or younger. The results show a significant increase in risk of breast cancer in women with a *BRCA1* mutation compared to noncarriers exposed to radiation younger than 30 years old (OR 1.8 (95% CI 1.2–2.9)).[67] When stratifying by age group at exposure (younger than 20 and between 20 and 30) the OR estimates were similar but were no longer statistically significantly different due to the small number of cases and controls.

Three studies reported a significant association between radiation and breast cancer risk in mutation carriers who were exposed to radiation before the age of 40.[60,62,65] The estimated odds ratios were 1.56 (95% CI 1.07–2.27) for women diagnosed with breast cancer before age 40,[65] 1.91 (95% CI 1.12–3.26),[60] and 2.75 (95% CI 1.4–5.3).[62] However, when analyzing separately for women exposed to radiation between the ages of 30–40, the association was no longer significant for women before the age of 40 (Narod et al.: OR: 1.11 (95% CI 0.82–14)[65]; GENE-RAD-RISK study: 1.06 (95% CI 0.63–1.71)[60]) while the association for women younger than 30 remained significant. The significant effect for those aged under 40 could be primarily due to the significant effect in women younger than 30. Contradictorily, the only prospective study did not support the association between radiation and breast cancer risk in women with a *BRCA1/2* mutation.[66]

Evidence for women at familial risk without a *BRCA* mutation

A multiple center case–control study from the Breast Cancer Family Registry in Ontario, Canada and in Melbourne and Sydney in Australia,[68] found a significant increase in risk of breast cancer in women who were exposed to diagnostic chest X-rays for pneumonia or tuberculosis at an age younger than 40. The ORs were 3.09 (95% CI 1.46–6.54) for women exposed to X-rays at younger than 20 years of age, and 2.68 (95% CI 1.2–5.98) for women exposed to X-rays more than 5 times between ages 20 and 39 for breast cancer cases compared to controls (sisters or unrelated population without breast cancers).[69] Another study focusing on women with breast cancer between ages 20 and 49, found that radiation exposure increased breast cancer risk significantly with OR of 1.34 (95% CI 1.04–1.74) compared to women without breast cancer.[69]

Limitations of radiation exposure studies

The main limitation of the studies examining the association of radiation exposure and breast cancer risk is the use of self-reported data on exposure, which can show recall bias. Therefore, results stratifying by type of diagnostic test, dose of X-ray, and age at exposure need to be interpreted with caution. Another potential bias was survival bias, which means that women needed to survive long enough to complete the questionnaire or interview. Some of the studies tried to minimize this bias by only considering women with complete information within 1[67] or 5 years after censoring or events (incident cohort).[63,65] Some studies analyzed data using weighted cox regression models in order to reduce testing bias. Testing bias occurred when affected *BRCA1/2* carriers would have been oversampled due to the fact that they were from high-risk families and qualified for genetic testing.[60–62]

The results were variable between studies, partially due to differences in study population inclusion criteria and exposure definitions. In all studies, exposures included diagnostic chest X-ray, however, among those a few studies[60,64–67,69] included mammograms. It could be that women with breast cancer had suspicious mammograms leading to further diagnostic exposure which increased the X-ray dose. Two studies included only women with *BRCA1/2* mutations younger than 50 years[63,67,69]; one study included only women with *BRCA1* mutations exposed to radiation before age 30 and developed breast cancer afterward at age 50 or younger[67]; while other studies did not have an age limit at recruitment which may have increased the exposure to X-ray due to older age. The three positive studies overlapped in study populations, which could explain their similar results.[60–62]

The minimal induction time for breast cancer risk after radiation exposure is about 10–15 years in the general population.[70] This was not taken into account in most of the studies as there was no clear information about the interval time between exposure and event, or recent radiation exposures, which probably would not have contributed to breast cancer risk, were also included in the analysis.[61–63,67–69] One study adjusted for this induction time in their analysis by using a 5-year time lag in the model under the assumption that women with *BRCA* mutation are more sensitive to radiation than women in the general population.[60] By doing so, they excluded exposure from diagnostic mammography related to the breast cancer diagnosis, which would not contribute to induction of breast cancer. Two studies that excluded mammography reported within 1 year of breast cancer diagnosis[64,65] and the prospective study excluded all the mammograms during their follow-up period of 4.8 years.[66]

Conclusion

In general, exposure to radiation was more likely to increase breast cancer risk primarily for younger women before the age of 30. There was some evidence supporting starting mammography screening from the age of 30 for *BRCA* women as the association between radiation exposure and breast cancer risk in women aged 30–40 has not been clearly proven. The limited studies focusing on women at familial risk without gene mutation supported the association between exposure to radiation at a younger age and an increased breast cancer risk.

COST-EFFECTIVENESS OF SCREENING STRATEGIES INCLUDING MRI AS AN ADJUNCT TO MAMMOGRAPHY

This section discusses the cost-effectiveness of screening strategies in women with a *BRCA*/12 mutation or strong familial risk (Table 11.4). The majority of the studies are model-based, reporting incremental cost-effectiveness for the combination of MRI and mammography compared to mammography alone[73–80]

Table 11.4 Overview of Cost-Effectiveness Analysis of Screening With Magnetic Resonance Imaging (MRI) and Mammography in Women With a Known or Suspected Gene Mutation

No	Authors/Year of Publication	Design/Population/Outcome	Screening Strategies	ICER (95% CI)
1	Tilanus-Linthorst et al. (2000)[71]	Design: Prospective Population: Women 25 and older with an over 25% lifetime risk of breast cancer and >50% density at mammogram Outcome: Additional cost per breast cancer detected compared to mammography alone	Annual MRI+ mammography vs mammography alone	€13,930 per additional breast cancer detected
2	Griebsch et al. (2006)[72]	Design: Prospective Population: Women age 35–49 with >0.9% 1 year risk Outcome: Additional cost per breast cancer detected compared to mammography alone	Annual MRI+ mammography vs mammography alone	£28,284 per additional breast cancer detected
3	Pataky et al. (2013)[73]	Design: Individual simulation study Population: Hypothetical cohort of women, with *BRCA1/2* mutations, being screened from age 25 Outcome: Incremental cost per QALY gained compared to mammography alone	Annual MRI (age 25–64) and mammography (age 30–79), alternating every 6 months, vs mammography alone (age 30–79)	$50,911 per QALY gained
4	Taneja et al. (2009)[74]	Design: Individual simulation study Population: Hypothetical cohort of women, with *BRCA1/2* mutations or lifetime risk >20%, being screened from age 40 Outcome: Incremental cost per QALY gained with MRI and mammography compared to mammography alone	*BRCA1/2* mutation carriers: annual MRI+ mammography vs mammography alone Women with lifetime risk >20%: annual MRI+ mammography vs mammography alone	$24,545 per QALY gained $284,000 per QALY gained
5	de Bock et al. (2013)[75]	Design: Validated individual simulation model (SiMRiSC), including radiation-induced breast cancer risk Population: Hypothetical cohort of women with *BRCA1/2* mutation, being screened at several starting ages Output: Incremental cost per life year gained	Dutch, *BRCA1* carriers (annual MRI (age 25–60) and mammography (age 30–60), followed by biennial mammography until age 75) vs UK, *BRCA1* carriers (Annual MRI (age 30–50) and mammography (age 30–50), followed by mammography every 3 years till age 70) Dutch, *BRCA2* carriers vs UK, *BRCA2* carriers	€2900 per life year gained €5500 per life year gained

6	Cott Chubiz et al. (2013)[76]	Design: Individual simulation study Population: Hypothetical cohort of women with *BRCA1/2* mutation, being screened at several starting ages Output: Incremental cost per QALY gained	*BRCA1* carriers: Digital mammography and MRI alternating at 6-month intervals beginning at age 25 years vs digital mammography alone	$978,500 per QALY gained
			BRCA1 carriers: Digital mammography and MRI alternating at 6-month intervals beginning at age 30 years vs digital mammography alone	$74,200 per QALY gained
			BRCA2 carriers: Digital mammography and MRI alternating at 6-month intervals beginning at age 25 years vs digital mammography alone	Eliminated
			BRCA2 carriers: Digital mammography and MRI alternating at 6-month intervals beginning at age 30 years vs digital mammography alone	$215,700 per QALY
7	Norman et al. (2007)[77]	Design: Individual simulation study Population: Hypothetical cohort of women with *BRCA1* mutation, being screened from ages 30–39 and 40–49 years Output: incremental cost per QALY gained, compared to the previous cost-effective strategy	Cohort aged 40–49: Mammography vs no screening	£2913 per QALY gained
			Cohort aged 40–49: MRI vs mammography screening	£7781 per QALY gained
			Cohort aged 30–39: Mammography vs no screening	£5240 per QALY gained
			Cohort aged 30–39: MRI vs mammography screening	£13,486 per QALY gained
8	Lee et al. (2010)[78]	Design: Individual simulation study Population: Hypothetical cohort of women with *BRCA1* mutation, being screened from age 25 Output: Incremental cost per QALY gained, compared to the previous cost-effective strategy	Annual MRI and mammography vs annual mammography	$69,125 per QALY gained

(*Continued*)

Table 11.4 Overview of Cost-Effectiveness Analysis of Screening With Magnetic Resonance Imaging (MRI) and Mammography in Women With a Known or Suspected Gene Mutation (Continued)

No	Authors/Year of Publication	Design/Population/Outcome	Screening Strategies	ICER (95% CI)
9	Plevritis et al. (2006)[79]	Design: Individual simulation study Population: Hypothetical cohort of women with BRCA1/2 mutation, being screened at several starting ages Output: Incremental cost per QALY gained, compared to annual mammography	*BRCA1*: Annual MRI and mammography vs annual mammography from the ages of 25–69	$88,651 per QALY gained
			BRCA1: Annual MRI from the ages of 35–54 and mammography vs annual mammography from the ages of 25–69	$55.420 per QALY gained
			BRCA2: Annual MRI and mammography vs annual mammography from the ages of 25–69	$188,034 per QALY gained
			BRCA2: Annual mammography age 25–69 and MRI by age 30–69	$130.695 per QALY gained
10	Saadatmand et al. (2013)[80]	Design: Individual simulation model: validated MISCAN model Population: Hypothetical cohort of women aged 25–70 with a *BRCA1/2* mutation or with risk of >15% from MRISC prospective screening study Output: Mortality reduction and costs per life-year gained (LYG), compared to population breast cancer screening (biennial from ages 50–75)	Annual mammography and clinical breast examination from age 35 to 50 years followed by biennial mammography until 75 years vs population breast cancer screening	Mortality reduction: 17% $54,665 per LYG
			Clinical breast examination every 6 months and annual mammography and MRI from age 35 to 50 years followed by biennial mammography until 75 years vs population breast cancer screening	Mortality reduction: 25% $134,932 per LYG

(see Table 11.4). Two prospective studies reported the cost per additional breast cancer detected (Dutch, United Kingdom) of adding MRI to mammography screening.[71,72] Different thresholds have been used to define a more cost-effective program: €20,000 or $100,000 or £20,000 per life year gained (LYG) or quality-adjusted life year gained (QALY).

Evidence for women with a BRCA1/2 mutation

Two prospective studies (Dutch and United Kingdom) reported that screening with an MRI adjunct to mammography resulted in an acceptable cost-effectiveness ratio.[71,72] The Dutch study examined the value of screening with an MRI adjunct to mammography as compared to screening with mammography-only in women aged 25 years and over who were at a high risk for breast cancer. The UK study included the screening of women aged 35–49 years. The Dutch study reported lower additional costs per LYG than the UK study (€13,930 and £28,284, respectively), which was mainly due to the fact that the Dutch study used the official costs related to mammography, MRI, and biopsies, whereas the UK study also included costs of additional work-up, administration, equipment, or other costs related to consumables, contract medium, and capital charges.[72]

Several modeling studies found that adding MRI to mammography screening in women with *BRCA1* or *BRCA2* mutations may be cost-effective compared to mammography alone, mainly depending on the incidence of breast cancer and the MRI costs[73,74,76–80] (see Table 11.4). In addition, it is found that screening for breast cancer in women with a *BRCA1* mutation is more cost-effective than screening for breast cancer in women with a *BRCA2* mutation[75,76,79] (see Table 11.4). The main reason being that the risk of developing breast cancer is higher in *BRCA1* compared to *BRCA2* carriers, leading to more benefit in life-years and quality-adjusted life-years gained in *BRCA1* carriers than in *BRCA2* carriers.

Two model-based studies investigated the cost-effectiveness of alternating MRI and mammography screening every 6 months.[73,76] The first study showed that screening women with *BRCA1/2* mutations with annual MRI from age 25 to 65 years plus screening with mammography every 6 months starting at age 30 until the age of 79 compared to mammography alone has an incremental cost of $50,911 per QALY gained.[73] The other study showed that alternating MRI and mammography screening every 6 months from age 30 compared to annual mammography alone in women with a *BRCA1* mutation is cost-effective with an incremental cost of $74,200 per QALY gained but this screening strategy is not cost-effective for women with *BRCA2* mutation[76] (see Table 11.4).

Evidence for young women with BRCA1/2 mutations

There is conflicting evidence on the cost-effectiveness of screening women with a *BRCA1/2* mutation under the age of 35. One model-based study from the United States reported that screening with MRI and mammography starting from the age of 25 compared to age 35 is not cost-effective, resulting in an increasing cost per QALY from $111,387 to $475,932.[79] This contrasts with the finding from a UK study showing that screening with MRI and mammography in women with a *BRCA1* mutation aged 30–49 years was more cost-effective compared to screening with mammography alone or no screening (ICER per QALY was £3449 for screening between age 30 and 39 and £7785 for screening between age 40 and 49).[77] A possible explanation for this difference is variations in modeling. First, in the US study, women were screened from age 25 to 70 or 35 to 70 years and followed until the end of life,[79] whereas in the UK study, MRI and mammography or mammography-alone screening were compared for women aged 30–39 versus 40–49.[77] In addition, for women with *BRCA1* mutations, screening sensitivity was an output in the US study[79] with a lower value (35% for mammography alone and 85% for mammography plus MRI) than in the UK study where sensitivity was an input of the model[77] and estimated to be higher (40% for mammography alone and 94% for mammography plus MRI).

A modeling study comparing different screening strategies for high-risk women with *BRCA1* or *BRCA2* mutations found the Dutch recommendation (annual MRI at age 25–30 years, mammography and MRI at age 30–60 years, and biennial mammography at age 60–75 years) to be the most cost-effective option.[75] The highly intensive US strategy (annual mammography and MRI from age 25 years to end of life) was only found to be cost-effective in the Netherlands if the Dutch are willing to pay €50,000 per LYG. The UK strategy (MRI and mammography at age 30–50 years, national screening program at age 50–70) saved relatively little in costs and resulted in greater life-years lost.[75]

Evidence for women at high familial risk

Studies on the cost-effectiveness of screening with MRI as an adjunct to mammography in women with suspected gene mutations are very limited. One model-based study shows that in women at a moderate breast cancer lifetime risk (>20%), the incremental cost per QALY was only cost-effective given an assumed prevalence of undiagnosed breast cancer of 3% or 4%.[74] Another study, simulating a high-risk population from a Dutch cohort, included women with familial risk with a cumulative risk of >15%. This study compared different screening schedules including both MRI and mammography and compared these to the population screening program in which women are screened with mammography biennially from age 50 to 75.[80] The results showed that adding annual MRI and mammography with semi-annual CBE from age 35 to 50 compared to the population breast cancer screening program reduced mortality by 25% at a cost per LYG of $134,932, which was not considered cost-effective. However, these results are not presented separately for women at high familial risk versus those with a *BRCA1/2* mutation.

Heterogeneity across study

The model-based and prospective studies are heterogeneous in methodology resulting in different estimates for the cost-effectiveness of screening in women with a *BRCA1/2* mutation or at high familial risk. There were differences in the values for the input parameters, as the input parameters of the models were derived from different literature sources or from a clinical cohort.[71,80,81] Some studies derived data for adherence to screening and survival from the general population,[76,78] while another study determined the survival rate for women with a *BRCA1* mutation aged 30–49 by the assumption that there was an improvement of 15% in 5-year survival of the study population compared to the general population.[77] Only a few studies modeled the induction risk due to radiation exposure.[75–77] Different screening scenarios were modeled. Except for one study,[76] the screening parameters related to mammography were based on film-mammography data, which does not represent the current practice of using digital mammography. The models considered the screened cohort as a fixed cohort instead of a dynamic one. The generalizability of the outcomes of the model-based studies is limited as most are not externally validated.[72] Although the prospective studies reported the costs based on their practice, there were differences in cost components and large differences in cost prices. Some studies included only the costs of screening whereas others considered also the costs of treatment procedures and follow-up. Different threshold values were used to determine cost-effective strategies partially due to different currencies that makes the interpretation of the results difficult to generalize.

Conclusion from economic perspective

Overall, in terms of additional cost per LYG or QALY, screening with MRI as an adjunct to mammography is considered to be cost-effective starting at age 35, if a threshold of €20,000 or $100,000 or £20,000 is applied. Screening for women with a *BRCA1* mutation is more cost-effective than for women with a *BRCA2* mutation. Further cost-effectiveness research on populations with increased familial risk without *BRCA* mutations is needed to further explore the impact in this population and the associated screening regime and benefit. Nevertheless, the results presented here need to be interpreted with caution because of the fact that the studies were conducted in different countries and may overoptimize real practice.

CONCLUSION

This chapter summarizes the evidence regarding the benefits and potential harms of breast cancer screening with MRI as an adjunct to mammography in women with a *BRCA1/2* mutation or at familial risk of breast cancer. The two most common high-risk cancer-predisposing genes are *BRCA1* and *BRCA2*, and their association with breast cancer as well as ovarian cancer has been extensively studied and established. Other gene mutations, which also play a role in the increased risk for breast cancer, are being investigated for clinical relevance. The benefits of screening high-risk women are reflected by the increased cancer detection, potential for mortality reduction, and cost-effectiveness. The potential harms of screening include low specificity, false-negative cases, and radiation-induced cancer risk.

Breast MRI screening as an adjunct to mammography has been shown to improve sensitivity for breast cancer detection by 52% and 53% in women with *BRCA1/2* mutations, respectively, both in younger women and in women over the age of 50.[46] An improvement in survival has also been observed in studies comparing screening with both MRI and mammography to no screening and to screening with mammography alone, however, the association with improved survival was not always significant and these studies had methodological shortcomings. Screening with MRI as an adjunct to mammography starting at age 35 was shown to be cost-effective for women with a *BRCA1* mutation, and probably also for women with a *BRCA2* mutation. However, cost-effectiveness studies relied on uncertain parameters, as all are model-based or prospective in design with specific study protocols and bias in cost computing. There are conflicting results on cost-effectiveness regarding outcomes for women younger than 35 years of age. Combining MRI and mammography lowers screening specificity compared to a single modality. Exposure to radiation from mammography is more likely to increase breast cancer risk primarily for younger women under the age of 30. Over the age of 30, the association between radiation exposure and breast cancer risk is less clear.

For women at high familial risk, there is evidence supporting screening with annual MRI and mammography regarding improved sensitivity for cancer detection. Evidence shows similar survival benefits by screening with MRI and mammography for women at high familial risk as for women with a *BRCA1/2* mutation. There is limited evidence supporting the cost-effectiveness of screening with MRI and mammography in women at high familial risk. There are similar concerns regarding radiation-induced breast cancer risk for women at high familial risk as for young women with a *BRCA1/2* mutation. However, since women at high familial risk have a lower expected breast cancer incidence than those with a *BRCA1/2* mutation, the interpretation of the results may be different from that for women with a *BRCA1/2* mutation. The evidence for women at familial risk is limited and does not consider different risk levels. Further research is needed to give more robust evidence in this particular population considering the different risk levels.

REFERENCES

1. Shiovitz S, Korde LA. Genetics of breast cancer: a topic in evolution. *Ann Oncol* 2015;**26**(7):1291–9.
2. Kurian AW, Hare EE, Mills MA, Kingham KE, McPherson L, Whittemore AS, et al. Clinical evaluation of a multiple-gene sequencing panel for hereditary cancer risk assessment. *J Clin Oncol* 2014;**32**(19):2001–9.
3. Whittemore AS, Gong G, Itnyre J. Prevalence and contribution of BRCA1 mutations in breast cancer and ovarian cancer: results from three U.S. population-based case-control studies of ovarian cancer. *Am J Hum Genet* 1997;**60**(3):496–504.
4. Peto J, Collins N, Barfoot R, Seal S, Warren W, Rahman N, et al. Prevalence of BRCA1 and BRCA2 gene mutations in patients with early-onset breast cancer. *J Natl Cancer Inst* 1999;**91**(11):943–9.
5. Chen S, Parmigiani G. Meta-analysis of BRCA1 and BRCA2 penetrance. *J Clin Oncol* 2007;**25**(11):1329–33.
6. Antoniou A, Pharoah PD, Narod S, Risch HA, Eyfjord JE, Hopper JL, et al. Average risks of breast and ovarian cancer associated with BRCA1 or BRCA2 mutations detected in case series unselected for family history: a combined analysis of 22 studies. *Am J Hum Genet* 2003;**72**(5):1117–30.
7. Mavaddat N, Barrowdale D, Andrulis IL, Domchek SM, Eccles D, Nevanlinna H, et al. Pathology of breast and ovarian cancers among BRCA1 and BRCA2 mutation carriers: results from the Consortium of Investigators of Modifiers of BRCA1/2 (CIMBA). *Cancer Epidemiol Biomarkers Prev* 2012;**21**(1):134–47.
8. Rebbeck TR, Mitra N, Wan F, Sinilnikova OM, Healey S, McGuffog L, et al. Association of type and location of BRCA1 and BRCA2 mutations with risk of breast and ovarian cancer. *JAMA* 2015;**313**(13):1347–61.
9. Vos JR, Hsu L, Brohet RM, Mourits MJ, de Vries J, Malone KE, et al. Bias correction methods explain much of the variation seen in breast cancer risks of BRCA1/2 mutation carriers. *J Clin Oncol* 2015;**33**(23):2553–62.
10. Balmana J, Diez O, Rubio IT, Cardoso F, ESMO Guidelines Working Group. BRCA in breast cancer: ESMO Clinical Practice Guidelines. *Ann Oncol* 2011;**22**(Suppl. 6):vi31–4. September.
11. *CG 164 Familial breast cancer: NICE Guidance [Internet].* <http://guidance.nice.org.uk/CG164/NICEGuidance/pdf/English>; 2013.
12. *NCCN [Internet].* <www.nccn.org>.
13. Amir E, Freedman OC, Seruga B, Evans DG. Assessing women at high risk of breast cancer: a review of risk assessment models. *J Natl Cancer Inst* 2010;**102**(10):680–91.
14. Jacobi CE, de Bock GH, Siegerink B, van Asperen CJ. Differences and similarities in breast cancer risk assessment models in clinical practice: which model to choose? *Breast Cancer Res Treat* 2009;**115**(2):381–90.
15. Lee AJ, Cunningham AP, Kuchenbaecker KB, Mavaddat N, Easton DF, Antoniou AC, et al. BOADICEA breast cancer risk prediction model: updates to cancer incidences, tumour pathology and web interface. *Br J Cancer* 2014;**110**(2):535–45.
16. Gadzicki D, Evans DG, Harris H, Julian-Reynier C, Nippert I, Schmidtke J, et al. Genetic testing for familial/hereditary breast cancer-comparison of guidelines and recommendations from the UK, France, the Netherlands and Germany. *J Community Genet* 2011;**2**(2):53–69.
17. Tilanus-Linthorst MM, Kriege M, Boetes C, Hop WC, Obdeijn IM, Oosterwijk JC, et al. Hereditary breast cancer growth rates and its impact on screening policy. *Eur J Cancer* 2005;**41**(11):1610–7.
18. Tilanus-Linthorst MM, Obdeijn IM, Hop WC, Causer PA, Leach MO, Warner E, et al. BRCA1 mutation and young age predict fast breast cancer growth in the Dutch, United Kingdom, and Canadian magnetic resonance imaging screening trials. *Clin Cancer Res* 2007;**13**(24):7357–62.

19. Heijnsdijk EA, Warner E, Gilbert FJ, Tilanus-Linthorst MM, Evans G, Causer PA, et al. Differences in natural history between breast cancers in BRCA1 and BRCA2 mutation carriers and effects of MRI screening-MRISC, MARIBS, and Canadian studies combined. *Cancer Epidemiol Biomarkers Prev* 2012;**21**(9):1458–68.
20. Jansen-van der Weide MC, Greuter MJ, Jansen L, Oosterwijk JC, Pijnappel RM, de Bock GH. Exposure to low-dose radiation and the risk of breast cancer among women with a familial or genetic predisposition: a meta-analysis. *Eur Radiol* 2010;**20**(11):2547–56.
21. *Richtlijn mammacarcinoom (Breast Cancer National Guideline) [Internet].* <http://www.heelkunde.nl/uploads/_a/Gk/_aGkhzjRsgiYhbhbFWFETQ/Mammacarcinoom2012.pdf>; 2012 [accessed 13.02.12].
22. Singer CF, Tea MK, Pristauz G, Hubalek M, Rappaport C, Riedl C, et al. Guideline for the prevention and early detection of breast and ovarian cancer in high risk patients, particularly in women from HBOC (hereditary breast and ovarian cancer) families. *Wien Klin Wochenschr* 2012;**124**(9–10):334–9.
23. Eccles DM, Evans DG, Mackay J. Guidelines for a genetic risk based approach to advising women with a family history of breast cancer. UK Cancer Family Study Group (UKCFSG). *J Med Genet* 2000;**37**(3):203–9.
24. Vasen HF, Haites NE, Evans DG, Steel CM, Moller P, Hodgson S, et al. Current policies for surveillance and management in women at risk of breast and ovarian cancer: a survey among 16 European family cancer clinics. European Familial Breast Cancer Collaborative Group. *Eur J Cancer* 1998;**34**(12):1922–6.
25. Evans DG, Lalloo F. Risk assessment and management of high risk familial breast cancer. *J Med Genet* 2002;**39**(12):865–71.
26. Eisinger F, Alby N, Bremond A, Dauplat J, Espie M, Janiaud P, et al. Recommendations for medical management of hereditary breast and ovarian cancer: the French National Ad Hoc Committee. *Ann Oncol* 1998;**9**(9):939–50.
27. Moller P, Evans G, Haites N, Vasen H, Reis MM, Anderson E, et al. Guidelines for follow-up of women at high risk for inherited breast cancer: consensus statement from the Biomed 2 Demonstration Programme on Inherited Breast Cancer. *Dis Markers* 1999;**15**(1–3):207–11.
28. Warner E, Heisey RE, Goel V, Carroll JC, McCready DR. Hereditary breast cancer. Risk assessment of patients with a family history of breast cancer. *Can Fam Physician* 1999;**45**:104–12.
29. Metcalfe KA, Birenbaum-Carmeli D, Lubinski J, Gronwald J, Lynch H, Moller P, et al. International variation in rates of uptake of preventive options in BRCA1 and BRCA2 mutation carriers. *Int J Cancer* 2008;**122**(9):2017–22.
30. Passaperuma K, Warner E, Causer PA, Hill KA, Messner S, Wong JW, et al. Long-term results of screening with magnetic resonance imaging in women with BRCA mutations. *Br J Cancer* 2012;**107**(1):24–30.
31. Sardanelli F, Podo F, Santoro F, Manoukian S, Bergonzi S, Trecate G, et al. Multicenter surveillance of women at high genetic breast cancer risk using mammography, ultrasonography, and contrast-enhanced magnetic resonance imaging (the high breast cancer risk Italian 1 study): final results. *Invest Radiol* 2011;**46**(2):94–105.
32. Leach MO, Boggis CR, Dixon AK, Easton DF, Eeles RA, Evans DG, et al. Screening with magnetic resonance imaging and mammography of a UK population at high familial risk of breast cancer: a prospective multicentre cohort study (MARIBS). *Lancet* 2005;**365**(9473):1769–78.
33. Riedl CC, Luft N, Bernhart C, Weber M, Bernathova M, Tea MK, et al. Triple-modality screening trial for familial breast cancer underlines the importance of magnetic resonance imaging and questions the role of mammography and ultrasound regardless of patient mutation status, age, and breast density. *J Clin Oncol* 2015;**33**(10):1128–35. February 23.
34. Rijnsburger AJ, Obdeijn IM, Kaas R, Tilanus-Linthorst MM, Boetes C, Loo CE, et al. BRCA1-associated breast cancers present differently from BRCA2-associated and familial cases: long-term follow-up of the Dutch MRISC Screening Study. *J Clin Oncol* 2010;**28**(36):5265–73.
35. Trop I, Lalonde L, Mayrand MH, David J, Larouche N, Provencher D. Multimodality breast cancer screening in women with a familial or genetic predisposition. *Curr Oncol* 2010;**17**(3):28–36.
36. Lehman CD, Blume JD, Weatherall P, Thickman D, Hylton N, Warner E, et al. Screening women at high risk for breast cancer with mammography and magnetic resonance imaging. *Cancer* 2005;**103**(9):1898–905.

37. Lehman CD, Isaacs C, Schnall MD, Pisano ED, Ascher SM, Weatherall PT, et al. Cancer yield of mammography, MR, and US in high-risk women: prospective multi-institution breast cancer screening study. *Radiology* 2007;**244**(2):381–8.
38. Kuhl CK, Schrading S, Leutner CC, Morakkabati-Spitz N, Wardelmann E, Fimmers R, et al. Mammography, breast ultrasound, and magnetic resonance imaging for surveillance of women at high familial risk for breast cancer. *J Clin Oncol* 2005;**23**(33):8469–76.
39. Kuhl C, Weigel S, Schrading S, Arand B, Bieling H, Konig R, et al. Prospective multicenter cohort study to refine management recommendations for women at elevated familial risk of breast cancer: the EVA trial. *J Clin Oncol* 2010;**28**(9):1450–7.
40. Hagen AI, Kvistad KA, Maehle L, Holmen MM, Aase H, Styr B, et al. Sensitivity of MRI versus conventional screening in the diagnosis of BRCA-associated breast cancer in a national prospective series. *Breast* 2007;**16**(4):367–74.
41. Weinstein SP, Localio AR, Conant EF, Rosen M, Thomas KM, Schnall MD. Multimodality screening of high-risk women: a prospective cohort study. *J Clin Oncol* 2009;**27**(36):6124–8.
42. Cortesi L, Turchetti D, Marchi I, Fracca A, Canossi B, Rachele B, et al. Breast cancer screening in women at increased risk according to different family histories: an update of the Modena Study Group experience. *BMC Cancer* 2006;**6**:210.
43. Warner E, Plewes DB, Hill KA, Causer PA, Zubovits JT, Jong RA, et al. Surveillance of BRCA1 and BRCA2 mutation carriers with magnetic resonance imaging, ultrasound, mammography, and clinical breast examination. *JAMA* 2004;**292**(11):1317–25.
44. Lord SJ, Lei W, Craft P, Cawson JN, Morris I, Walleser S, et al. A systematic review of the effectiveness of magnetic resonance imaging (MRI) as an addition to mammography and ultrasound in screening young women at high risk of breast cancer. *Eur J Cancer* 2007;**43**(13):1905–17.
45. Warner E, Messersmith H, Causer P, Eisen A, Shumak R, Plewes D. Systematic review: using magnetic resonance imaging to screen women at high risk for breast cancer. *Ann Intern Med* 2008;**148**(9):671–9.
46. Phi X, Houssami N, Obdeijn I, Warner E, Sardanelli F, Leach MO, et al. Magnetic resonance imaging improves breast screening sensitivity in BRCA mutation carriers age >/ = 50 years: evidence from an individual patient data meta-analysis. *J Clin Oncol* 2014;**33**(4):349–56. December 22.
47. Chiarelli AM, Prummel MV, Muradali D, Majpruz V, Horgan M, Carroll JC, et al. Effectiveness of screening with annual magnetic resonance imaging and mammography: results of the initial screen from the ontario high risk breast screening program. *J Clin Oncol* 2014;**32**(21):2224–30.
48. Bosse K, Graeser M, Gossmann A, Hackenbroch M, Schmutzler RK, Rhiem K. Supplemental screening ultrasound increases cancer detection yield in BRCA1 and BRCA2 mutation carriers. *Arch Gynecol Obstet* 2014;**289**(3):663–70.
49. Tilanus-Linthorst MM, Bartels CC, Obdeijn AI, Oudkerk M. Earlier detection of breast cancer by surveillance of women at familial risk. *Eur J Cancer* 2000;**36**(4):514–9.
50. Roeke T, van Bommel AC, Gaillard-Hemmink MP, Hartgrink HH, Mesker WE, Tollenaar RA. The additional cancer yield of clinical breast examination in screening of women at hereditary increased risk of breast cancer: a systematic review. *Breast Cancer Res Treat* 2014;**147**(1):15–23.
51. Evans DG, Kesavan N, Lim Y, Gadde S, Hurley E, Massat NJ, et al. MRI breast screening in high-risk women: cancer detection and survival analysis. *Breast Cancer Res Treat* 2014;**145**(3):663–72.
52. Saadatmand S, Obdeijn IM, Rutgers EJ, Oosterwijk JC, Tollenaar RA, Woldringh GH, et al. Survival benefit in women with BRCA1 mutation or familial risk in the MRI screening study (MRISC). *Int J Cancer* 2015;**137**(7):1729–38. March 26.
53. Moller P, Stormorken A, Jonsrud C, Holmen MM, Hagen AI, Clark N, et al. Survival of patients with BRCA1-associated breast cancer diagnosed in an MRI-based surveillance program. *Breast Cancer Res Treat* 2013;**139**(1):155–61.

54. Warner E, Hill K, Causer P, Plewes D, Jong R, Yaffe M, et al. Prospective study of breast cancer incidence in women with a BRCA1 or BRCA2 mutation under surveillance with and without magnetic resonance imaging. *J Clin Oncol* 2011;**29**(13):1664–9.
55. Kriege M, Brekelmans CT, Boetes C, Besnard PE, Zonderland HM, Obdeijn IM, et al. Efficacy of MRI and mammography for breast-cancer screening in women with a familial or genetic predisposition. *N Engl J Med* 2004;**351**(5):427–37.
56. Drooger JC, Hooning MJ, Seynaeve CM, Baaijens MH, Obdeijn IM, Sleijfer S, et al. Diagnostic and therapeutic ionizing radiation and the risk of a first and second primary breast cancer, with special attention for BRCA1 and BRCA2 mutation carriers: a critical review of the literature. *Cancer Treat Rev* 2015;**41**(2):187–96.
57. Berrington de Gonzalez A, Berg CD, Visvanathan K, Robson M. Estimated risk of radiation-induced breast cancer from mammographic screening for young BRCA mutation carriers. *J Natl Cancer Inst* 2009;**101**(3):205–9.
58. Preston DL, Mattsson A, Holmberg E, Shore R, Hildreth NG, Boice Jr. JD. Radiation effects on breast cancer risk: a pooled analysis of eight cohorts. *Radiat Res* 2002;**158**(2):220–35.
59. Powell SN, Kachnic LA. Roles of BRCA1 and BRCA2 in homologous recombination, DNA replication fidelity and the cellular response to ionizing radiation. *Oncogene* 2003;**22**(37):5784–91.
60. Pijpe A, Andrieu N, Easton DF, Kesminiene A, Cardis E, Nogues C, et al. Exposure to diagnostic radiation and risk of breast cancer among carriers of BRCA1/2 mutations: retrospective cohort study (GENE-RAD-RISK). *BMJ* 2012;**345**:e5660.
61. Lecarpentier J, Noguès C, Mouret-Fourme E, Stoppa-Lyonnet D, Lasset C, Caron O, et al. Variation in breast cancer risk with mutation position, smoking, alcohol, and chest X-ray history, in the French National BRCA1/2 carrier cohort (GENEPSO). *Breast Cancer Res Treat* 2011;**130**(3):927–38.
62. Andrieu N, Easton DF, Chang-Claude J, Rookus MA, Brohet R, Cardis E, et al. Effect of chest X-rays on the risk of breast cancer among BRCA1/2 mutation carriers in the international BRCA1/2 carrier cohort study: a report from the EMBRACE, GENEPSO, GEO-HEBON, and IBCCS Collaborators' Group. *J Clin Oncol* 2006;**24**(21):3361–6.
63. John EM, McGuire V, Thomas D, Haile R, Ozcelik H, Milne RL, et al. Diagnostic chest X-rays and breast cancer risk before age 50 years for BRCA1 and BRCA2 mutation carriers. *Cancer Epidemiol Biomarkers Prev* 2013;**22**(9):1547–56.
64. Goldfrank D, Chuai S, Bernstein JL, Ramon Y, Cajal T, Lee JB, et al. Effect of mammography on breast cancer risk in women with mutations in BRCA1 or BRCA2. *Cancer Epidemiol Biomarkers Prev* 2006;**15**(11):2311–3.
65. Narod SA, Lubinski J, Ghadirian P, Lynch HT, Moller P, Foulkes WD, et al. Screening mammography and risk of breast cancer in BRCA1 and BRCA2 mutation carriers: a case-control study. *Lancet Oncol* 2006;**7**(5):402–6.
66. Giannakeas V, Lubinski J, Gronwald J, Moller P, Armel S, Lynch HT, et al. Mammography screening and the risk of breast cancer in BRCA1 and BRCA2 mutation carriers: a prospective study. *Breast Cancer Res Treat* 2014;**147**(1):113–8.
67. Gronwald J, Pijpe A, Byrski T, Huzarski T, Stawicka M, Cybulski C, et al. Early radiation exposures and BRCA1-associated breast cancer in young women from Poland. *Breast Cancer Res Treat* 2008;**112**(3):581–4.
68. John EM, Phipps AI, Knight JA, Milne RL, Dite GS, Hopper JL, et al. Medical radiation exposure and breast cancer risk: findings from the Breast Cancer Family Registry. *Int J Cancer* 2007;**121**(2):386–94.
69. Ma H, Hill CK, Bernstein L, Ursin G. Low-dose medical radiation exposure and breast cancer risk in women under age 50 years overall and by estrogen and progesterone receptor status: results from a case-control and a case-case comparison. *Breast Cancer Res Treat* 2008;**109**(1):77–90.
70. *National Research Council (US) Committee on Health Effects of Exposure to Low Levels of Ionizing Radiations (BEIR VII)*; 1998.
71. Tilanus-Linthorst MM, Obdeijn IM, Bartels KC, de Koning HJ, Oudkerk M. First experiences in screening women at high risk for breast cancer with MR imaging. *Breast Cancer Res Treat* 2000;**63**(1):53–60.

72. Griebsch I, Brown J, Boggis C, Dixon A, Dixon M, Easton D, et al. Cost-effectiveness of screening with contrast enhanced magnetic resonance imaging vs X-ray mammography of women at a high familial risk of breast cancer. *Br J Cancer* 2006;**95**(7):801–10.
73. Pataky R, Armstrong L, Chia S, Coldman AJ, Kim-Sing C, McGillivray B, et al. Cost-effectiveness of MRI for breast cancer screening in BRCA1/2 mutation carriers. *BMC Cancer* 2013;**13** 339,2407-13-339.
74. Taneja C, Edelsberg J, Weycker D, Guo A, Oster G, Weinreb J. Cost effectiveness of breast cancer screening with contrast-enhanced MRI in high-risk women. *J Am Coll Radiol* 2009;**6**(3):171–9.
75. de Bock GH, Vermeulen KM, Jansen L, Oosterwijk JC, Siesling S, Dorrius MD, et al. Which screening strategy should be offered to women with BRCA1 or BRCA2 mutations? A simulation of comparative cost-effectiveness. *Br J Cancer* 2013;**108**(8):1579–86.
76. Cott Chubiz JE, Lee JM, Gilmore ME, Kong CY, Lowry KP, Halpern EF, et al. Cost-effectiveness of alternating magnetic resonance imaging and digital mammography screening in BRCA1 and BRCA2 gene mutation carriers. *Cancer* 2013;**119**(6):1266–76.
77. Norman RP, Evans DG, Easton DF, Young KC. The cost-utility of magnetic resonance imaging for breast cancer in BRCA1 mutation carriers aged 30-49. *Eur J Health Econ* 2007;**8**(2):137–44.
78. Lee JM, McMahon PM, Kong CY, Kopans DB, Ryan PD, Ozanne EM, et al. Cost-effectiveness of breast MR imaging and screen-film mammography for screening BRCA1 gene mutation carriers. *Radiology* 2010;**254**(3):793–800.
79. Plevritis SK, Kurian AW, Sigal BM, Daniel BL, Ikeda DM, Stockdale FE, et al. Cost-effectiveness of screening BRCA1/2 mutation carriers with breast magnetic resonance imaging. *JAMA* 2006;**295**(20):2374–84.
80. Saadatmand S, Tilanus-Linthorst MM, Rutgers EJ, Hoogerbrugge N, Oosterwijk JC, Tollenaar RA, et al. Cost-effectiveness of screening women with familial risk for breast cancer with magnetic resonance imaging. *J Natl Cancer Inst* 2013;**105**(17):1314–21.
81. Koleva-Kolarova RG, Zhan Z, Greuter MJ, Feenstra TL, De Bock GH. Simulation models in population breast cancer screening: a systematic review. *Breast Breast* 2015;**24**(4):354–63.
82. Sardanelli F, Podo F, D'Agnolo G, Verdecchia A, Santaquilani M, Musumeci R, et al. Multicenter comparative multimodality surveillance of women at genetic-familial high risk for breast cancer (HIBCRIT study): interim results. *Radiology* 2007;**242**(3):698–715.
83. Warner E, Plewes DB, Shumak RS, Catzavelos GC, Di Prospero LS, Yaffe MJ, et al. Comparison of breast magnetic resonance imaging, mammography, and ultrasound for surveillance of women at high risk for hereditary breast cancer. *J Clin Oncol* 2001;**19**(15):3524–31.
84. Trecate G, Vergnaghi D, Manoukian S, Bergonzi S, Scaperrotta G, Marchesini M, et al. MRI in the early detection of breast cancer in women with high genetic risk. *Tumori* 2006;**92**(6):517–23.
85. Hartman AR, Daniel BL, Kurian AW, Mills MA, Nowels KW, Dirbas FM, et al. Breast magnetic resonance image screening and ductal lavage in women at high genetic risk for breast carcinoma. *Cancer* 2004;**100**(3):479–89.

CHAPTER

IMAGING SURVEILLANCE OF WOMEN WITH A PERSONAL HISTORY OF BREAST CANCER

12

Janie M. Lee[1] and Nehmat Houssami[2]

[1]Department of Radiology, University of Washington, Seattle, WA, United States,
[2]School of Public Health, Sydney Medical School, University of Sydney, Sydney, NSW, Australia

CHAPTER OUTLINE

Breast Cancer Screening. DOI: http://dx.doi.org/10.1016/B978-0-12-802209-2.00012-7

PLAIN LANGUAGE SUMMARY

Following successful treatment of first breast cancers, women remain at risk of cancer recurrence in the treated breast and also new cancers in the other breast (second breast cancers), which are associated with increased rates of cancer detection in other parts of the body and with death from breast cancer. Imaging surveillance after breast cancer treatment aims to detect second breast cancers before symptoms develop, permitting treatments which may improve survival and maintain quality of life.

This chapter reviews the evidence which supports the use of annual mammography for imaging surveillance in women with a history of breast cancer. Evidence that mammography is underused among breast cancer survivors, especially as time since completing treatment increases, offers an opportunity to improve how mammography can be used to improve survival. In addition, new technologies for detecting breast cancer, such as digital breast tomosynthesis (DBT), breast ultrasound, and breast magnetic resonance imaging (MRI) will be reviewed. DBT, also known as "3D mammography," uses the same X-ray source as digital mammography and moves in an arc around the breast to collect digital information. By presenting images of thin "slices" within the breast, DBT more clearly shows true breast lesions and reduces false-positive findings due to overlapping normal breast tissue. MRI uses strong magnetic fields to image the breast, rather than ionizing radiation. Its ability to detect cancers is very high, and MRI is recommended for breast cancer screening in women with very strong family histories, especially those who are at very high risk of developing breast cancer due to gene mutations such as *BRCA1* and *BRCA2*. The benefit of breast MRI use in breast cancer survivors who do not have these risk factors is still being studied. Breast ultrasound uses high frequency sound waves to examine breast tissue, and a strength of ultrasound is its ability to differentiate cystic from solid breast masses. The main limitation of breast ultrasound when it is used for breast cancer screening or surveillance, is the high number of biopsies which are recommended, most of which have benign (not cancer) results.

We are also improving our understanding of cancer biology, and new information about breast cancer subtypes may help to guide treatment selection and improve survival. Information about how breast cancer subtype is related to detection of first and second cancers is needed to help women decide which imaging tests should be used for imaging surveillance. Other factors, such as quality of life, costs of care, and care that takes into account a woman's individual preferences and values, are also important. It is critical for patients and their doctors to consider these additional factors when making decisions about treatment and imaging surveillance, so that women can lead longer, healthier lives once their treatment is done. This chapter will review the current evidence and highlight critical knowledge gaps where further study is needed to improve clinical care and outcomes.

BACKGROUND

Globally, 28.8 million individuals alive in 2008 were cancer survivors who had been diagnosed within the last 5 years.[1] When identifying survivors by cancer site, female breast cancer is the most prevalent neoplasm worldwide, at approximately one in six cancer survivors. In the United States alone, approximately 232,000 women were diagnosed with invasive breast cancer in 2013.[2] Advances in screening and treatment of primary breast cancer (PBC) have improved survival for many of these women,[2] and the number of breast cancer survivors will continue to increase.[2,3] Women who survive their initial diagnosis of breast cancer remain at risk of subsequent local recurrence (LR) and new primary cancers in the contralateral breast (second breast cancers), which are associated with increased rates of distant metastases and breast cancer mortality.[4,5]

Posttreatment surveillance aims to detect asymptomatic second breast cancers, permitting interventions to potentially improve survival and maintain quality of life.[6] Based on randomized controlled trials (RCTs) demonstrating the effectiveness of screening mammography in reducing breast cancer mortality[7,8] (see also chapter: Estimates of Screening Benefit: The Randomized Trials of Breast Cancer Screening) and on observational studies suggesting effectiveness for posttreatment surveillance,[6,9–11] current guidelines[2,12–19] are consistent in their recommendations supporting the use of mammography in women following treatment for PBC.

With advances in breast imaging technology, additional options beyond mammography are now available for screening and surveillance. These modalities include DBT, as well as breast ultrasound and MRI. In addition, improvements in our understanding of tumor biology, and specifically in the classification of tumors by gene expression profiles or "molecular subtypes," are providing independent prognostic information to guide tailored selection of breast cancer treatment. The provision of clinical care is increasingly focusing on patient centered outcomes beyond survival, such as quality of life, costs of care, and shared decision making based on patient preferences and values.

This chapter will consider these three recent trends influencing imaging surveillance regimen selection.

SELECTING AN APPROPRIATE SURVEILLANCE REGIMEN

Surveillance testing extends beyond application of the test itself. Rather, it is an episode of care that begins with the surveillance test and also includes the subsequent cascade of diagnostic evaluation of positive test results and incidental findings, as well as treatment of the targeted disease. Achieving an overarching balance of benefits and harms with surveillance includes consideration of events within entire episodes of care[20] (Fig. 12.1).

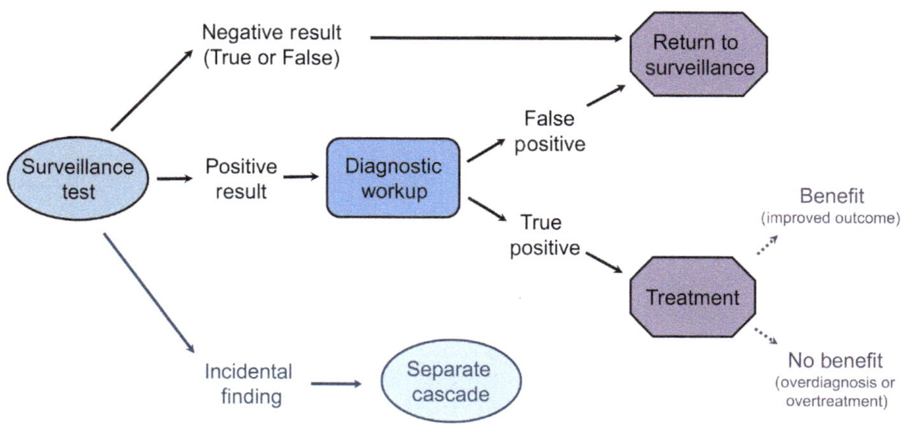

FIGURE 12.1

Cascade of care.

NEGATIVE TEST RESULTS

A highly specific surveillance test, one which correctly excludes patients without the targeted disease, is an essential characteristic of a surveillance test. Ideally, these patients with true negative results will gain reassurance that they do not have disease recurrence. When recurrence is present but the test result is negative (false-negative), the disease will continue to progress until it presents symptomatically, and the patient will not have gained the benefits of earlier detection. A negative surveillance test could potentially provide false reassurance and cause an individual to delay seeking care for a symptom, causing further harm.

POSITIVE TEST RESULTS

Because a population under screening or surveillance has no signs or symptoms of disease, it is important to consider the diagnostic consequences of a positive test result.[21,22] An important potential harm of surveillance is false-positive results. Individuals with false-positive results will incur all the subsequent diagnostic consequences of a positive test—invasive biopsies, increased costs, and anxiety about having a life-threatening recurrence—but gain none of the benefits, as recurrent disease is not present.[20,23–25] The likelihood of having false-positive results increases with an increased surveillance timeframe or with more frequent surveillance intervals, both of which increase the total number of lifetime surveillance episodes, and also with decreasing disease prevalence.[26] Because of these factors, the potential harms of false-positive surveillance results are most likely to accrue in individuals at lower risk of having recurrent disease.

A highly sensitive surveillance test should detect most patients with the targeted disease (a high true-positive proportion), enabling earlier diagnosis of recurrence and access to effective treatments. These patients are the only ones with the potential to benefit from surveillance and to achieve improved long-term outcomes, such as reduced breast cancer mortality and increased overall survival.

Even with a highly sensitive test, an important consequence of screening and surveillance is the potential for harm from overdiagnosis and overtreatment.[24,27–29] *Overdiagnosis* and *overtreatment* occur when surveillance testing detects asymptomatic disease that would not have become clinically apparent over an individual's lifetime, or when detection results in treatment of disease that would not have shortened an individual's life expectancy (see also chapters: Challenges in Understanding and Quantifying Overdiagnosis and Overtreatment; Treatment of Screen-Detected Breast Cancer: Can We Avoid or Minimize Overtreatment?). Both of these scenarios occur more frequently when older populations with higher competing mortality risks undergo surveillance. Due to the invasiveness of treatment and associated morbidity, overdiagnosis and overtreatment may be among the most significant potential harms associated with surveillance.

INCIDENTAL FINDINGS

Incidental findings, discovered during image interpretation that are unrelated to the indication of the study, are a routine part of diagnostic radiology.[30] In examinations with larger fields of view, such as breast MRI, there is potential for the discovery of incidental findings that are unrelated to the targeted disease. For example, Niell et al.[31] reported that of 2324 patients receiving breast MRI examinations performed for any indication, 86 patients (3.7%) had extramammary findings for which additional imaging evaluation was recommended, and nine patients (0.4%) had clinically important findings. Potential harms from incidental findings may result from complications of unnecessary invasive procedures, increased costs, and undue patient anxiety for what is ultimately determined to be a benign lesion.[32] These "incidentalomas" place patients and their providers in a difficult situation, as it may not be possible to predict which will be clinically significant and which will not at the time of examination interpretation.

BALANCING THE BENEFITS AND POTENTIAL HARMS OF SURVEILLANCE

The burden of proof for the effectiveness of screening and surveillance is higher than that for diagnostic tests and treatments. Of all the individuals who will undergo surveillance, only those with true-positive test results who receive effective treatment and are not overdiagnosed/overtreated will obtain its primary benefits, which include decreased morbidity and mortality.[20,21] As we increasingly focus on providing value-based healthcare, with the goal of improving patient outcomes while maintaining or decreasing healthcare costs,[33] the important outcomes to measure extend beyond those of mortality reduction. Outcomes that matter are condition-specific and multidimensional—including overall survival, time without symptoms, quality of life, and the financial consequences of choosing alternative treatments. No single outcome will fully capture the effects of surveillance. Implementation of new imaging-based surveillance tests in clinical practice will increasingly hinge on the successful conduct of research on a scale and with a level of rigor not seen in the past.[34]

The challenge and opportunity for future research studies of imaging-based surveillance are to provide evidence on multiple outcomes to characterize not only its benefits but also its downstream consequences and potential harms. Improved quality of life or reduced disease-specific mortality must be considered in the context of radiation-induced risks, utilization of additional resources to evaluate incidental findings, false-positive test results, and the potential for overdiagnosis and overtreatment. The budget impact and cost-effectiveness of new surveillance regimens are also important factors for which examination prior to adoption and implementation should be considered.

MODALITIES FOR IMAGING SURVEILLANCE

MAMMOGRAPHY—ASSOCIATION WITH SURVIVAL

The primary modality for breast cancer screening is mammography—a fast, noninvasive, relatively inexpensive screening test that has been shown in RCTs to reduce breast cancer mortality in women ages 40–74[7,8] (more detailed discussion in chapter: Estimates of Screening Benefit: The Randomized Trials of Breast Cancer Screening). While the benefit of surveillance mammography to detect asymptomatic second breast cancers in women with a personal history of treated breast cancer is presumed, no RCTs comparing surveillance strategies have been conducted. The evidence support for surveillance mammography is based on the established mortality reduction from screening mammography trials, and also from results of observational studies. A review of the medical literature[35] reported that studies of mammographic surveillance varied in terms of study design, focusing on asymptomatic versus symptomatic detection of second breast cancers, mammographic versus clinical detection, or routine versus nonroutine follow-up. Across varying study designs, their results were consistent in reporting that earlier detection of second breast cancers was associated with reduced mortality.

In three studies evaluating survival from the time of PBC diagnosis, which minimizes lead time bias due to earlier diagnosis of second breast cancers with surveillance, the results were consistent. The largest study[9] of 1044 consecutive women with a second breast cancer, compared asymptomatic detection versus symptomatic detection of second breast cancers. The hazard ratio (HR) for breast cancer mortality after asymptomatic detection of second breast cancer, adjusted for length bias, was 0.53–0.73. In another study of women with contralateral breast cancer (CBC; $n = 656$) and matched controls,[10] the HR for breast cancer mortality after mammographic detection versus other means of detection was 0.31 (95% CI (confidence interval): 0.16–0.63). A study comparing exposure to surveillance mammography to no surveillance reported an HR for breast cancer mortality with mammography exposure to be 0.22–0.37, after adjusting for age, stage, and therapy received.[11]

A metaanalysis[6] of the impact of early detection of second breast cancers on survival reported improved survival for women if a recurrence was found by surveillance mammography compared with clinical detection (HR = 2.44, 95% CI: 1.78–3.35) or if a recurrence was detected in asymptomatic women compared to those with symptoms (HR = 1.56, 95% CI: 1.36–1.79). Based on a pooled HR of 1.68 for earlier detection, the authors further estimated that the absolute breast cancer mortality reduction achievable was 17–28%.

Current clinical guidelines issued since 2010 for imaging surveillance after treatment of PBC are consistent in their recommendation of annual surveillance mammography for at least the first 5 years following treatment (Table 12.1). Organizations supporting surveillance mammography include the American Society of Clinical Oncology (ASCO),[12] the National Comprehensive Cancer Network (United States),[17] the American Cancer Society,[2] the American College of Radiology,[16] the Society of Breast Imaging,[14] the European School of Oncology (ESO),[15] and the National Institute for Health and Care Excellence (NICE, United Kingdom).[18,19] While the organizations based in the United States recommend annual surveillance mammography without specifying a milestone for cessation, the ESO recommends a 1 to 2-year surveillance interval for postmenopausal women, and NICE bases surveillance in posttreatment year 6 and beyond on patient age at diagnosis and "patient risk category."

Additional evidence supports the effectiveness of adherence to clinical guidelines. In a series of cohort studies,[36–38] the most recent being a study of 1846 women with stage I and II PBC who were at least 65 years old receiving care in six integrated health care delivery systems with complete ascertainment of surveillance mammograms,[37] receipt of any surveillance mammography was associated with reduced breast cancer mortality. Further, each additional surveillance mammogram received was associated with a 0.69-fold decrease in the odds of breast cancer mortality (95% CI: 0.52–0.92).

MAMMOGRAPHY PERFORMANCE

A systematic review of surveillance mammography test performance from 1990 to 2006[39] identified two studies[40,41] which reported sensitivities of 64% and 67%, and specificities of 97% and 85% for film mammography performance. Both studies had relatively small sample sizes of 83 and 105 patients, respectively. A more recent study of surveillance mammography accuracy was conducted within the Breast Cancer Surveillance Consortium, where multiple mammography registries across the United States are linked with tumor registries. Examining 58,870 mammograms in 19,078 women with a personal history of breast cancer (American Joint Committee on Cancer[42] stage I or II), Houssami et al.[43] reported more robust and also similar results. While the cancer detection rate was higher in women with a prior history of breast cancer (PHBC) compared to women without this history (6.8 vs 4.4 per

Table 12.1 Evidence-Based Guidelines for Imaging Surveillance After Treatment of Primary Breast Cancer

Organization	Imaging Surveillance Recommendation	
American Society of Clinical Oncology[12]	Women who have undergone breast-conserving surgery	• Posttreatment mammogram 1 year after initial mammogram, and at least 6 months after completion of radiation therapy. • Followed by annual mammography. Not recommended for routine surveillance: • Other imaging (chest X-ray, bone scan, liver ultrasound, CT, PET, MRI). • Tumor marker testing (CA 15-3, CA 27.29, or CEA).
National Comprehensive Cancer Network[17]		• Annual mammography. Not recommended: • Laboratory or imaging studies for metastases screening (v2.2015) if no clinical signs and symptoms suggestive of recurrent disease.
American Cancer Society[2]		• Annual mammography beginning at age 40. • Talk with their doctors about benefits and limitations of adding MRI to yearly mammography.
American College of Radiology/Society of Breast Imaging[14,16]		• Annual mammography from time of diagnosis. • Stage I BC Appropriateness criteria indicate breast MRI may be appropriate in selected patients, depending on risk assessment, in addition to, not as a replacement for mammogram. Not recommended: • Additional imaging with chest X-ray, bone scan, CT, PET/CT, or nonbreast MRI.
European School of Oncology (ESO)[15]	Premenopausal women	• Annual mammography.
	Postmenopausal women	• Every 1–2 year(s). Note: • Breast MRI recommendations not specified. • German Cancer Society (AGO) recommendations are for surveillance mammography q6 months for 2 years, then annually afterward. Breast MRI not recommended.
National Institute for Health and Care Excellence (NICE, United Kingdom)[18,19]		• Annual mammography for first 5 years after treatment, or until National Health Service screening age, then "stratify screening frequency in line with patient risk category." Not recommended: • US or MRI for routine posttreatment surveillance for early invasive BC or DCIS.
International Agency for Research on Cancer (IARC)[13]	Women with personal history of breast cancer	• "Inadequate" evidence that ultrasound increases the cancer detection rate.

1000 screens, respectively) the accuracy of surveillance mammography was significantly lower (all comparisons $p < 0.001$ except as noted). In women with PHBC, sensitivity was 65.4% and specificity was 98.3%. In a matched cohort of women in the same registries without PHBC, sensitivity of screening mammography was 76.5% and specificity was 99.0%. Sensitivity of surveillance mammography was also lower in the initial 5 years (60.2%) than after 5 years from primary cancer treatment (70.8%), and similar for detection of in-breast recurrence (66.3%) and contralateral second cancers (55.1%, $p = 0.96$).

Two subsequent studies,[44,45] also conducted within the Breast Cancer Surveillance Consortium, evaluated risk factors for interval invasive second breast cancer presentation after negative surveillance mammography. Houssami et al.[44] identified age at PBC diagnosis <40 years (OR = 3.41), extremely dense breasts on mammography (OR = 2.55) and treatment with breast conservation without radiation (OR = 2.67) as significant predictors of an interval invasive breast cancer within 1 year of a negative surveillance mammogram. Because approximately 70% of in-breast recurrences occur within 5 years of treatment,[46–48] Lee et al.[45] estimated the 5-year risk of interval invasive second breast cancers. From a cohort of 15,114 women with 47,717 surveillance mammograms diagnosed with American Joint Committee on Cancer stage 0–II unilateral breast cancer from 1996 to 2008, 325 surveillance detected and 138 interval invasive second breast cancers were identified. The cumulative incidence of second breast cancers after 5 years was 54.4 per 1000 women. The 5-year risk of interval invasive second cancer was based on four independent predictors: PBC grade (OR = 1.95), PBC mode of detection (OR = 2.01 for interval PBC presentation), treatment with breast conservation without radiation (OR = 3.27) and heterogeneously dense breasts on mammography (OR = 1.54). The range of risk for women varied substantially, from 0.07% to 6.11%.

These results suggest that aggressive tumor biology in a woman's first breast cancer, as demonstrated by higher grade or clinical presentation after negative screening mammography, may continue to mediate her subsequent surveillance outcomes. Additional factors related to PBC diagnosis and treatment—increased breast density, breast conservation treatment without radiation therapy—contribute to variation in subsequent interval second breast cancer risk.

It is possible that the selective application of adjunctive testing, based on factors known at the time of PBC diagnosis and treatment, to supplement surveillance mammography, either with a more frequent surveillance interval[49] or with another modality, such as breast MRI[50–54] or ultrasound,[55,56] could reduce interval invasive second breast cancers. Further studies are needed to examine the potential contribution of supplemental modalities or alternative regimens to improving surveillance outcomes.

DBT FOR SCREENING

DBT[57] is an innovation upon digital mammography. DBT was designed to eliminate overlapping breast tissue which may obscure breast cancers on standard mammography, when a three-dimensional breast is projected onto a two-dimensional image plane. Using the same X-ray source as digital mammography, a DBT unit moves in an arc around the breast to acquire information from a volume of breast tissue. Computational processing of the digital data reconstructs high-resolution images of thin 0.5–1.0mm "slices" through the breast tissue at doses similar to standard digital mammography. By presenting images of specific planes within the breast, DBT enables clearer visualization of true breast lesions and reduces false-positive findings due to superimposition of adjacent normal breast tissue. DBT images can be obtained in combination with standard digital mammography, or the digital DBT data can be reconstructed to produce a "synthetic" mammographic view along with the thinner slice images, eliminating the need for a standard digital mammogram and reducing exposure to ionizing radiation.

Studies evaluating DBT compared with digital mammography for breast cancer screening are discussed in greater detail in chapter "Evolution of Mammography Screening: From Film Screen to Digital Breast Tomosynthesis." Overall, across varying study designs and locations, the studies of DBT for breast cancer screening support decreased recall rates and stable to increased cancer detection, with increased detection more apparent for studies conducted with biennial screening regimens. The primary benefit at the population level is reduction of false-positive screening results and avoidance of diagnostic evaluations in the subsequent cascade of care. With incomplete follow-up in reports to date, and with early reporting of DBT used primarily in prevalence screening, it remains unclear whether the stable to increased cancer detection with DBT will persist with its use in subsequent incidence screening. In addition, it is not yet clear whether the detection of early cancers with DBT will result in improved patient outcomes such as reduced breast cancer mortality and improved overall survival, or whether some overdiagnosis and overtreatment of breast cancers has occurred. Both scenarios are likely, and additional studies with longer-term follow-up are warranted to confirm the presumed benefit of screening with DBT.

DBT FOR POSTTREATMENT SURVEILLANCE

The early reports of DBT performance have evaluated women presenting for routine breast cancer screening in various settings. While there is consistency of results in demonstrating decreased recall rate from screening and probable increase in cancer detection, these characteristics are associated with the underlying prevalence of breast cancer in the population being screened. Sensitivity and specificity, test performance measures which are independent of disease prevalence, have yet to be reported for most studies, due in part to the need for complete follow-up for identification of interval breast cancers.

The studies to date have not focused on DBT performance within subgroups, based on patient demographics or risk factors, such as family history of breast cancer, personal history of breast cancer, or mammographic density. The Oslo study[58] included women invited to undergo routine biennial screening as part of the Oslo, Norway screening program. The only exclusions reported were disabled women unable to stand and women with breast implants. The STORM trial[59] focused on asymptomatic women at standard population risk for breast cancer in Italy. The sites in the Friedewald et al.[60] study in the United States focused on examinations performed for a screening indication, without further specification of population characteristics. Lourenco et al.'s retrospective single institution analysis[61] similarly studied examinations performed for a screening indication. While none of the studies reported excluding women with a personal history of breast cancer, this specific population of women was not the focus of any of the screening studies reported to date.

It is possible that the improved performance of DBT compared with DM will also be observed in women with a personal history of breast cancer. However, given that the accuracy of mammography in women is decreased in women with prior breast cancer compared to women without this history,[43] it is not yet clear whether and to what extent performance improvements with DBT will offset the known performance limitations of mammography for these women. Further studies are needed to evaluate DBT performance for women at varying risk levels and with varying underlying risk factors, including personal history of breast cancer.

Current guidelines do not discuss DBT separately from mammography (Table 12.1).

BREAST MRI

MRI uses strong magnetic fields to image the breast, rather than ionizing radiation. Because the detection of breast cancer by MRI is based on changes related to cancer neovascularity, intravenous contrast is a required component of the examination. The sensitivity of breast MRI is not limited by mammographic breast density, and studies of breast MRI for supplemental screening women at increased genetic or familial risk of breast cancer have demonstrated high sensitivity, ranging from 68% to 100%. Warner et al.'s metaanalysis[62] of studies reported sensitivity of 75–77% and specificity of 86–93%. Of the eleven studies included for analysis, nine included women with a PHBC in addition to genetic and familial risk factors for breast cancer. Based on these high-risk screening studies, the American Cancer Society and National Comprehensive Cancer Network recommend breast MRI for supplemental screening women with lifetime risk of breast cancer >20%, with use of familial risk assessment models.[17,63]

However, women with sporadic breast cancer were not included in these study populations. While it is likely that surveillance MRI has an improved ability to detect asymptomatic second breast cancer compared with mammography, current evidence is limited, based on relatively small single institution studies. Brennan et al.[50] performed a retrospective review of 144 women with prior breast cancer who received breast MRI for surveillance. Of these women, 44 (31%) underwent biopsy prompted by MRI, and 17 women (12%) were subsequently diagnosed with second breast cancer (cancer detection rate 118 per 1000 examinations). The cancer yield of biopsy (positive predictive value) was 39%.

Schact et al.[52] performed a retrospective review of 208 women with prior breast cancer, of which MRI surveillance detected 6 second breast cancers (cancer detection rate 29 per 1000 examinations). When compared with 345 women receiving screening MRI with family history as the sole risk factor, the cancer detection rate was similar, at 20 per 1000 examinations (7/345).

Gweon et al.[54] studied 932 surveillance breast MRI examinations in 607 women after breast conservation therapy (BCT) in Korea, with MRI performed at the request of clinicians or patients. The median age of women receiving MRI surveillance was 48 years (range 20–72 years). Ten second breast cancers were identified by MRI. The cancer detection rate for prevalence imaging was 18 per 1000 women (95% CI: 16–21 per 1000 women). The cancer yield of biopsy performed (PPV3) was 44% (10/23). Multivariable analysis identified age younger than 50 years at initial diagnosis and greater than 24-month interval between initial surgery and screening MRI as independent predictors of MRI-detection of second breast cancer ($p < 0.02$ for both factors).

Giess et al.[53] evaluated 1194 MRI examinations in 691 women with a personal history of breast cancer, in which 12 second breast cancers were detected by MRI surveillance. The median age of women receiving MRI surveillance was 47 years. The cancer detection rate for MRI was 10 per 1000 examinations (95% CI: 5–18 per 1000), and the average time from PBC diagnosis to second breast cancer detection was 6.2 years (range 1–23 years). Eight of the twelve surveillance detected second breast cancers were in the ipsilateral breast, and four were new primary cancers in the contralateral breast. The cancer yield of biopsy performed (PPV3) was 18% (12/67).

Lehman et al.[51] compared the performance of breast MRI in 915 asymptomatic women with a personal history of breast cancer, and 606 women with a genetic or family history of breast cancer (GFH). The cancer detection rates in both groups were comparable (20 per 1000 examinations in both groups, $p > 0.99$). The cancer yield of biopsy (PPV3) was greater in women with a personal history (25%) compared with women with GFH (15%), but the difference was not significant ($p = 0.19$). Sensitivity was comparable in both groups of women (80% for personal history and 79% for GFH, $p > 0.99$) and specificity was higher in women with a personal history (94%, compared with 86% in women with GFH, $p < 0.001$). The improvement in specificity for women with prior breast cancer was attributable in part to having a prior breast MRI available for comparison, either at the time of first cancer diagnosis to evaluate extent of disease, or a prior surveillance MRI.

While these results suggest that the performance of breast MRI for posttreatment surveillance is comparable to that of MRI for screening women at increased genetic and familial risk of breast cancer, the variation in reported cancer detection rates may be related to relatively small sample sizes for surveillance cohorts, as well as differential selection of women to receive MRI surveillance across studies. Further studies of MRI performance and outcomes in women with a personal history of breast cancer are warranted to guide the appropriate use of breast MRI.

Currently, the American Cancer Society does not recommend for or against breast MRI use for post-treatment surveillance, recommending instead that these women talk with their doctors about the benefits and limitations of adding MRI to the yearly mammogram. The National Comprehensive Cancer Network[17] and European School of Oncology[15] do not specify recommendations regarding breast MRI. ASCO[12] and the NICE (United Kingdom)[18,19] both recommend against breast MRI for routine surveillance, while the American College of Radiology and Society of Breast Imaging[14,16] support MRI use in selected patients based on risk assessment.

BREAST ULTRASOUND

Breast ultrasound employs high frequency sound waves to evaluate specific findings identified by physical examination or mammography. It is widely used primarily in the diagnostic setting, and a strength of ultrasound is its ability to differentiate cystic from solid breast masses. Advantages of ultrasound include the ability to evaluate tissue without ionizing radiation exposure associated with mammography, and the lack of breast compression when hand-held ultrasound (HHUS) transducers are used. Automated whole breast ultrasound (ABUS) is a relatively new technology that standardizes imaging acquisition using an automated transducer, rather than a hand-held one, and allows simultaneous visualization of a volume of breast tissue in multiple planes.[64] Whole breast ultrasound is considered an appropriate supplemental screening test in women who are at high risk for developing breast cancer and cannot receive a breast MRI examination,[65] and has been studied for supplemental screening in women with mammographically dense breasts.[66,67]

The main limitation of breast ultrasound for screening, either HHUS or ABUS, is the high number of false-positive findings,[66,67] which often lead to biopsies ultimately demonstrating benign disease. Image acquisition time, which is longer than that of screening mammography, is a limitation for both HHUS and ABUS, and operator dependency is an additional limitation of HHUS. ABUS requires breast compression while the patient lays supine, and multiple views of each breast are required in a standardized screening examination.

Most studies of breast ultrasound as a supplemental screening modality have focused on women with mammographically dense breasts,[67] with varying additional risk factors, such as family history or personal history of breast cancer. Of 12 screening ultrasound studies conducted since 2000, the American College of Radiology Imaging Network (ACRIN) 6666 study[55,56] was the only prospective study evaluating the combination of mammography plus HHUS compared mammography alone, with

1 year follow-up for multiple screening rounds. In this study, 1426 of 2659 women (53%) had a personal history of breast cancer.

In the first screening round[55,56,68] conducted from 2004 to 2006, the cancer detection rate for mammography alone was 7.6 per 1000 examinations, and mammography/HHUS detected an additional 5.3 cancers per 1000 examinations. However, the number of recalls for additional evaluation increased 2.3-fold, from 115 per 1000 examinations for mammography alone to 266 per 1000 examinations for mammography/HHUS. The number of breast biopsies increased 4.2-fold, from 24 per 1000 examinations with mammography to 102 per 1000 with mammography/HHUS. The cancer yield for biopsies performed (PPV3) for HHUS was 8.6%, indicating that greater than 90% of biopsies performed revealed benign disease.

By the third screening round,[56,68] the mammography examinations had transitioned from film to digital, and mammography alone detected 9.9 cancers per 1000 examinations. Mammography plus ultrasound detected an additional 4.2 cancers per 1000. For women with a personal history of breast cancer, the incremental cancer detection rate for HHUS was the same as in women without this history. The recall rate in the second and third screening rounds remained high, at 94 per 1000 examinations for mammography alone and 168 per 1000 for mammography/HHUS, a 1.8-fold increase. Breast biopsies remained increased with mammography/HHUS screening (3.5-fold increase compared with mammography alone), and the cancer yield following biopsy remained low at 7.1%.

While breast ultrasound may detect additional breast cancers not seen on mammography in women with treated breast cancer, the risk of false-positive biopsies as a diagnostic consequence is far greater. No current guidelines support the use of breast ultrasound, either HHUS or ABUS, for supplemental surveillance in women with treated breast cancer (Table 12.1).

ADHERENCE TO GUIDELINES

The United States Institute of Medicine has identified three categories of health care quality problems: overuse, underuse, and misuse.[69] *Overuse* is the provision of a health care service under circumstances in which its potential for harm exceeds the possible benefit. *Underuse* is the failure to provide a health care service when it would have produced a favorable outcome for the patient. *Misuse* occurs when an appropriate service has been selected but a preventable complication occurs and the patient does not receive the full potential benefit of the service. Efforts to correct problems of overuse, underuse, and misuse aim to increase appropriate use of health care services to improve patient and population outcomes.

EVIDENCE OF OVERUSE

Efforts to promote quality and evidence-based care include the Choosing Wisely initiative of the American Board of Internal Medicine Foundation (ABIMF), which partnered with specialty societies to identify commonly ordered diagnostic tests or treatments that lack evidence of meaningful benefit for patients.[70] The partnership between the ABIMF and the ASCO identified lack of adherence to breast cancer surveillance guidelines as one of its Top Five Choosing Wisely practices in Oncology. In particular, the recommendation is to avoid using advanced imaging or circulating biomarker testing to monitor for recurrence in asymptomatic patients who have been treated for breast cancer with curative intent.[71]

The evidence for this recommendation is based on prior randomized trials. Two such trials conducted in Italy[72–74] found that regularly scheduled chest radiographs, bone scans, and abdominal ultrasounds did not improve survival. A subsequent randomized trial comparing four different follow-up schedules for early-stage breast cancer patients after primary treatment conducted in Finland found that more intensive surveillance increased costs but did not improve patient disease-free or overall survival.[75] Specific testing which the Choosing Wisely initiative recommends against are: positron-emission tomography (PET), PET-CT, and radionuclide bone scanning, as well as the biomarkers CEA (carcinoembryonic antigen), CA (cancer antigen)15-3, and CA27-29.

Despite clinical practice guidelines and the further support of efforts such as the Choosing Wisely initiative, overuse of diagnostic testing in asymptomatic breast cancer survivors has been reported. In a population-based study of 11,219 women treated for early-stage breast cancer conducted in Canada,[76] substantial variation in adherence to guideline recommendations was identified, with both overuse and underuse of surveillance testing observed. Specifically, while approximately two-thirds of women received surveillance mammography in each follow-up year (range 68–73%), over half received additional surveillance imaging (chest X-ray, bone scan, ultrasound, or abdominal/pelvic imaging), consistent with overuse of surveillance imaging. Multivariable analysis indicated that higher comorbidity, receipt of mastectomy for PBC treatment, and seeing both a primary care physician and an oncologist in follow-up increased the odds of having greater than recommended imaging surveillance.

In the United States, Ramsey et al.[77] studied 39,650 early-stage breast cancer survivors aged 65 or older. In this cohort, 16,653 (42%) received at least one tumor marker assessment within 2 years of treatment. When adherence to the Choosing Wisely surveillance recommendation was evaluated among patients enrolled with a regional commercial health insurer,[78] approximately half (53%) of 629 women treated for American Joint Committee on Cancer Stages I or II breast cancer received at least one surveillance imaging or biomarker test that was not recommended. It was noted that additional testing increased with stage of PBC.

When evidence regarding a health intervention is sparse, there may be a pro-intervention, pro-technology bias in clinical decision making.[79] Breast MRI was not among the diagnostic tests included in the Choosing Wisely recommendations for breast cancer surveillance. While guidance on whether and how to apply breast MRI for surveillance is not definitive, its utilization has increased over time. Wernli et al.[80] studied breast MRI use in the United States Breast Cancer Surveillance Consortium and reported that the rate of screening breast MRI increased between 2005 and 2009, from 0.8 to 4.3 per 1000 women. Of women receiving screening breast MRI, 44.9% had a PHBC. Stout et al.[81] studied MRI utilization in a community-based population with commercial health insurance in New England, and reported similar findings. Breast MRI use for posttreatment surveillance increased substantially between 2003 and 2009, from 0.23 to 3.17 per 1000 women, and then stabilized, with the rate in 2011 at 2.81 per 1000 women. While the relative utilization rates have increased substantially, the absolute rate of utilization (less than 1% of women) and the apparent stabilization of utilization in more recent years with available data suggest that overuse of breast MRI is not widespread.

EVIDENCE OF UNDERUSE

Despite evidence of improved survival with asymptomatic mammographic detection of in-breast recurrence and evidence of the effectiveness of adherence to mammographic surveillance recommendations,[36–38] observational studies report underuse of mammographic surveillance among breast cancer survivors. In a study with 10 years of longitudinal follow-up of 3965 women diagnosed with early-stage (I or II) breast cancer during 1990–2008, Wirtz et al.[82] found that 79% of women received surveillance mammography within the first year following completion of PBC treatment. Receipt of surveillance mammography steadily declined through the sixth year of follow up to 68%, and then became relatively stable, ranging from 63% to 66% during the seventh through tenth years of follow-up. In adjusted analyses, factors predicting underuse of surveillance mammography included patient, tumor, treatment, and imaging characteristics. Age was the most significant predictor, with both younger (<40 years) and older women (≥80 years) having lower odds of receiving surveillance mammography. Higher comorbidity and smoking were also associated with underuse of surveillance. Women with PBC stage II and those treated with mastectomy or lumpectomy without radiation therapy were also less likely to receive surveillance mammography after treatment. Women with more outpatient visits (primary care provider, oncologist, or both), and women with screening-detected breast cancers were more likely to have received surveillance mammography.

These findings are consistent with prior studies in different populations across the United States. Keating et al.[83] studied 44,511 women aged 65 and older diagnosed with early-stage (I or II) breast during 1992–99. Similar to Wirtz et al.'s report,[82] 77.6% of women received surveillance mammography within 1 year of completing treatment, and receipt of mammography declined over time, with 56.7% receiving it by the third year of follow-up. Underuse was associated with women who were older, black or Hispanic, unmarried, living in areas with lower median incomes and fewer high school graduates (all $p < 0.001$). Receipt of surveillance mammography also varied significantly across geographic regions ($p < 0.001$). Two additional studies conducted within integrated health systems[84,85] reported similar declines in surveillance mammography use following PBC treatment, with age and comorbidity associated with underuse. As with Wirtz et al.'s study, surgical treatment and outpatient follow-up visits were also significant predictors of surveillance mammography use.

Grunfeld et al.[76] conducted a population-based study of 11,219 women in Canada who were treated for early-stage breast cancer. In this cohort, approximately two-thirds of women received surveillance mammography in each year of follow-up (ranging from 68% to 73%), with no significant decline over time, and this finding was persistent across age groups as well. Underuse of surveillance mammography was associated with older age (>80 years), rural residence and higher comorbidity.

Opportunities exist to reduce ineffective overuse of diagnostic technology, and to reduce underuse of surveillance mammography known to improve patient outcomes. The variety of factors, intrinsic and extrinsic to individual women, predicting both overuse and underuse, indicate that effective interventions will need to be implemented at multiple levels within a health care system. While complex and multidimensional, the goals of protecting patients from harm, increasing use of beneficial tests to improve outcomes, and reducing the financial burden on patients and health care systems must be pursued as we increasingly seek to provide care that brings value to our patients.

BREAST CANCER SUBTYPES

Breast cancer has historically been perceived as a single disease with varying morphologic features and clinical behavior. Over time, immunohistochemistry (IHC) has enabled the classification of breast cancer based on the phenotypic expression of estrogen, progesterone, and human epidermal growth factor receptor 2 (HER2) receptors, which predicts response to treatment with endocrine therapy and trastuzumab, respectively. The identification of hormonal receptors and HER2, along with additional pathologic variables, such as tumor size, histologic grade, and lymph node status, has guided treatment decisions and predicted long-term outcomes for women diagnosed with breast cancer.

More recently, gene expression profile analysis, or "molecular subtyping" using DNA microarrays, has changed our understanding of breast cancer biology.[86–88] Rather than a single heterogeneous disease, breast cancer is increasingly recognized as a complex pathologic condition with multiple pathways which vary in progression rates and outcomes. An emerging approach to understanding breast cancer involves classification by subtype, (also referred to as "intrinsic subtype") each with a distinct "molecular" signature providing independent prognostic information that can be used to refine and guide treatment decisions. In addition to identifying genes which regulate the expression of estrogen receptors (ER), progesterone receptors (PR), and HER2, additional components of a tumor's molecular signature include proliferation-related genes, such as Ki-67, p53, epidermal growth factor receptor (EGFR), genes typical of luminal, myoepithelial, and basal cells (cytokeratins 5/6 or 8/18, and P-cadherin), as well as the degree of expression of these genes.

At least four distinct molecular subtypes of breast cancer have been identified. *Luminal A* breast cancers have high expression of ER and PR, low expression of HER2, low expression of proliferation genes, and have a favorable prognosis. *Luminal B* breast cancers, while also having high expression of ER and PR, have either high expression of HER2 or high expression of proliferation-related genes without over-expression of HER2, and are associated with an intermediate to poor prognosis. There is variable classification of Luminal B breast cancers into *Luminal B (HER2-positive)* and *Luminal B (HER2-negative)* subgroups, related to the different classification criteria and to different treatment regimens for these two subgroups.[89] Breast cancers with high HER2 expression and low ER and PR expression are classified as *HER2 enriched*. While historically having a poor prognosis, the availability of trastuzumab as an effective treatment for HER2-positive breast cancers has significantly improved prognosis for women with this breast cancer subtype. *Basal* subtype breast cancers have low expression of ER and PR, low expression of HER2, high expression of proliferation-related genes and high expression of basal cytokeratins, and are associated with a poor prognosis. Without the additional benefit of endocrine or trastuzumab-based therapy, the primary treatment for basal subtype breast cancers is systemic adjuvant chemotherapy. *Luminal-HER2* has been suggested as an additional subtype to separate breast cancers with both high ER/PR expression and high HER2 expression from those with low ER/PR expression and high HER2 expression.[86] Normal breast-like and Claudin-low profiles have also been suggested as an additional subtypes with intermediate prognosis,[87] and are less widely accepted as distinct subtypes.

Molecular subtypes largely correspond with subtype classification based on immunohistochemical markers, specifically ER, PR, HER2, Ki-67, and grade. While there is substantial overlap, there are also discrepant classifications when using molecular subtyping compared with IHC classification. For example, approximately 75% of "triple negative" breast cancers (ER-negative, PR-negative, HER2-negative by IHC) are "basal" in molecular subtype, with the other 25% comprised of other subtypes.[86] However, due to the more widespread availability of IHC testing, and the expense related to genetic profile analysis, IHC-based subtyping is frequently used in clinical decision-making. While varying definitions for classification of breast cancer subtypes using IHC rather than gene expression data exist, the St. Gallen International Breast Cancer Conference is an annual meeting with participants from over 130 countries worldwide, and its 2011 Expert Panel provided surrogate definitions of molecular subtypes of breast cancer based on IHC characteristics.[89]

There are several commercially available genomic assays for identifying breast cancer subtype using various genes, primarily the Oncotype DX (which is a 21-gene assay) and MammaPrint assays (which evaluates 70 genes).[87,88] The Oncotype DX assay has been endorsed by the American Society of Clinical Oncology and the National Comprehensive Cancer Network to predict the risk of subsequent recurrence, and to guide the selection of low risk ER-positive, node-negative breast cancer patients who many not need adjuvant chemotherapy. Ongoing clinical trials such as the Trial Assigning Individualized Options for Treatment (TAILORx) in the United States using Oncotype DX and the Microarray in Node Negative and 0–3 Positive Lymph Node Disease May Avoid Chemotherapy Trial (MINDACT) in Europe using the MammaPrint will provide prospective randomized comparisons between genomic testing and clinical factors in clinical decision making and treatment selection.

SUBTYPE AND RELAPSE EVENTS

Breast cancer subtype is associated with local and regional relapse. Voduc et al.[90] studied 2985 women with PBC, diagnosed between 1986 and 1992 in British Columbia, Canada. Median age at diagnosis was 59 years, and median follow-up time was 12 years. Six subtypes (*Luminal A, Luminal B, Luminal-HER2, HER2, Basal, and triple-negative nonbasal*) were classified based on tissue microarrays constructed from archival tissue blocks of the PBCs. Factors used in classification included ER, PR, HER2, Ki-67, EGFR, and CK 5/6. Forty-two percent of patients received BCT including radiation therapy, and 58% received mastectomy, with 25% of mastectomy patients also receiving radiation therapy. Fifty-seven percent of patients received adjuvant systemic therapy, either chemotherapy (20%), endocrine therapy (31%), or both (7%). No patients received trastuzumab.

For LR, defined as recurrence within the ipsilateral breast or chest wall (and thus, detectable by surveillance mammography), 10-year event rates varied significantly across subtypes. For women treated with BCT or mastectomy, those with *Luminal A* breast cancers had the lowest LR rate (8% at 10 years). While women with *HER2* subtype cancers had significantly higher 10-year LR rates (21% after BCT and 17% after mastectomy), it is also important to note that treatment guidelines in place during the dates of diagnosis did not include routine use of trastuzumab. Multivariable analysis indicated that younger age at diagnosis (<40 years) and *HER2* subtype independently predicted LR in women treated with BCT. For women treated with mastectomy, multivariable analysis identified *non-luminal A* subtype as an independent predictor of chest wall recurrence and regional nodal recurrence.

Similar results have been reported in the United States. Two studies examined women diagnosed with invasive breast cancer treated with breast conservation and radiation therapy, with Nguyen et al.'s[91] study population being a subset of Arvold et al.'s subsequent study.[92] Of 1434 consecutive patients diagnosed with invasive breast cancer from 1997 to 2006 in an academic comprehensive cancer center, five breast cancer subtypes were approximated from IHC analysis: *Luminal A* (ER- or PR-positive, HER2-negative, grade 1 or 2), *Luminal B* (ER/PR-positive, HER2-negative, grade 3), *Luminal-HER2* (ER/PR-positive, HER2-positive), *HER2* (ER/PR-negative, HER2-positive), and *Triple Negative* (ER, PR, and HER2-negative). While 91% of patients received adjuvant systemic therapy, no patients received trastuzumab.

Five-year LR rates varied significantly by breast cancer subtype, with *Luminal A* subtype having the best prognosis (0.8%) and nonluminal *HER2* and *Triple Negative* subtypes having the highest LR rates (10.8% and 6.7%, respectively). Multivariable analysis confirmed the association of nonluminal subtype with increased LR risk, and identified younger age was an additional independent predictor of LR risk.

Breast cancer subtype is also associated with risk of developing distant metastases. Nguyen et al.[91] reported that *Luminal B* and *Basal* subtypes were associated with increased 5-year rates of distant metastases. Kennecke et al.[93] studied 3726 patients diagnosed from 1986 to 1992 in British Columbia with median follow-up of 14.8 years. Their results indicated that breast cancer subtypes are not only associated with variable rates of developing distant metastases, they are also associated with distinct patterns of metastatic spread and significant differences in survival after relapse. Bone was the most common metastatic site in all subtypes except *Basal* tumors, which had a higher rate of brain, lung, and distant nodal metastases. There were also distinct differences in the timing of distant relapse. Women with nonluminal subtypes experienced distant relapse primarily within the first 5 years after PBC treatment, while women with luminal subtypes, including *Luminal-HER2*, experienced a more constant rate of relapse between 5 and 15 years posttreatment. Of note, *Luminal B* tumors had a distant relapse rate at 15 years which was equivalent to that of basal subtype tumors. Multivariable analysis indicated that even after development of distant metastases, women with *Luminal A* subtype breast cancers had the longest median duration of survival (2.2 years), while women with *Basal* subtype cancers had the shortest median survival (0.5 years, $p < 0.001$).

While there are differences across studies in the definitions of used to classify breast cancer subtypes, the results across studies are consistent in reporting that the *Luminal A* subtype has the most favorable prognosis, and *HER2* and *Basal* subtypes have the least favorable prognosis. The evidence also favors improvement in prognosis over time for women with HER2-enriched breast cancers, due to the increasing use of trastuzumab for treating this subtype.

Less evidence is available regarding the association of breast cancer subtypes and new cancers in the contralateral breast following treatment of PBC. Nichols et al.[94] examined CBC incidence using the United States Surveillance, Epidemiology, and End Results database from 1975 to 2006. Breast cancers were stratified by ER-status, with insufficient data to enable full mapping of molecular subtypes based on IHC markers. The analysis identified a decline in CBC incidence since 1985. This overall decrease was driven by declining CBC rates in women with ER-positive breast cancers, likely related to increasing use of adjuvant endocrine therapy for treating these breast cancers. Further analysis indicated that CBC rates were dependent on age at diagnosis of first breast cancer and ER-status. CBC incidence demonstrated a bimodal pattern related to age at diagnosis, with relative peaks around age 30 and 70. CBC incidence was also higher after ER-negative first cancers compared with ER-positive first cancers (annual incidence ranges for women aged 40–69 years: 0.0045–0.0053 vs 0.0024–0.0036, respectively). CBC rates were not impacted by adjustment for time since diagnosis.

IMAGING OF BREAST CANCER SUBTYPES

The current evidence about how breast cancer subtype mediates imaging detection of breast cancers is sparse. Retrospective comparison of screen-detected and interval cancers in population-based screening programs in Norway,[95] Italy,[96] and Spain[97] suggest that *Triple-negative* or *Basal* subtype cancers are associated with interval presentation after a negative screening mammogram at initial diagnosis. PBC not seen on mammography is also associated with mammographically occult local relapse ($p = 0.036$) and with lower relapse free survival at 10 years ($p < 0.05$).[98] These studies suggest an association between subtype and mode of detection for PBCs and possibly for second breast cancers following completion of treatment. An association between of PBC subtype and surveillance imaging performance and outcomes has yet to be established.

KNOWLEDGE GAPS AND AREAS FOR FURTHER RESEARCH

Further research is needed to guide understanding of current surveillance options and to inform the development and selection of future surveillance regimens. The evidence supports mammography use for detecting second breast cancers earlier, with an association with improved survival. At the same time, the available evidence also suggests that the effectiveness of mammography may be further improved, via interventions to decrease underuse of surveillance mammography, through improvement in diagnostic accuracy as the mainstay of breast imaging screening and surveillance shifts from digital mammography to DBT, and possibly with supplemental imaging modalities such as MRI.

Current critical knowledge gaps include the identification of relevant risk factors and their integration into improved risk prediction tools. Further exploration of molecular subtypes and how they mediate the detection of both primary and second breast cancers is needed. Risk prediction that combines information known at the time of diagnosis and treatment of first breast cancers—patient characteristics, such as age and family history, tumor characteristics, such as subtype and stage, imaging characteristics, such as mammographic breast density, mode of detection of first cancer, and treatment factors, such as the receipt of radiation therapy, and adjuvant endocrine therapy or trastuzumab—may guide the selection of women for surveillance strategies based on second breast cancer risk, or risk of interval breast cancer with surveillance mammography alone.

Improved risk stratification and risk communication may help to identify women who will benefit from surveillance with annual mammography alone, and efforts to achieve adherence with this approach may further improve patient outcomes. For other women who may benefit from supplemental surveillance, evaluation of the performance and comparative effectiveness of multimodality surveillance regimens are needed, as current approaches to measuring imaging performance are based on single-modality assessment.[99] If more intensive surveillance for women at increased risk of second breast cancers can be supported by evidence, application of these new surveillance regimens will be associated with increased costs. The budget impact of more intensive surveillance and its downstream diagnostic consequences should also be measured, so that value of these regimens, defined by the achievable outcomes relative to the cost of obtaining them,[33] may be projected prior to adoption and implementation.

As we increasingly focus on providing patient-centered care, consideration of patient preferences and shared decision making will play a greater role in the optimal selection of imaging surveillance regimens for breast cancer survivors. The trade-offs related to multimodality surveillance in particular, in which additional testing will be associated with an increased false-positive testing results, require communication and exploration. Balancing the potential benefit of earlier detection with anxiety related to diagnostic testing and its subsequent cascade of care will vary according to the values and preferences of individual women.[100,101] Informed and shared decision making is a complex and difficult goal; both patients and providers would benefit from tools to improve this process.

Tremendous progress has been and continues to be made in our understanding of breast cancer development, detection, and treatment. Advances in these areas are enabling women to survive their initial treatment and live longer, healthier lives. Surveillance imaging with current and emerging approaches have the potential to further extend survival and improve outcomes. Closing critical knowledge gaps in technology evaluation, risk assessment, and shared decision making will enable evidence-based selection of tailored imaging surveillance regimens to improve individual and population-level outcomes.

LIST OF ACRONYMS AND ABBREVIATIONS

ABUS	Automated whole breast ultrasound
BCT	Breast conservation therapy
BRCA	Breast cancer susceptibility gene
CA	Cancer antigen
CBC	Contralateral breast cancer
CEA	Carcinoembryonic antigen
DBT	Digital breast tomosynthesis
ER	Estrogen receptors
GFH	Genetic family history
HER	Human epidermal growth factor receptor
HHUS	Hand-held ultrasound
HR	Hazard ratio
HR	Hormone receptors
IHC	Immunohistochemistry
LR	Local recurrence
MRI	Magnetic resonance imaging
PET	Positron-emission tomography
PH	Personal history
PHBC	Prior history of breast cancer
PR	Progesterone receptors
RCTs	Randomized controlled trials

REFERENCES

1. Bray F, Ren JS, Masuyer E, Ferlay J. Global estimates of cancer prevalence for 27 sites in the adult population in 2008. *Int J Cancer* 2013;**132**(5):1133–45.
2. American Cancer Society. *Breast cancer facts & figures 2013–2014*. Atlanta, GA: American Cancer Society, Inc.; 2013.
3. Parry C, Kent EE, Mariotto AB, Alfano CM, Rowland JH. Cancer survivors: a booming population. *Cancer Epidemiol Biomarkers Prev* 2011;**20**:1996–2005.
4. Anderson SJ, Wapnir I, Dignam JJ, Fisher B, Mamounas EP, Jeong JH, et al. Prognosis after ipsilateral breast tumor recurrence and locoregional recurrences in patients treated by breast-conserving therapy in five National Surgical Adjuvant Breast and Bowel Project protocols of node-negative breast cancer. *J Clin Oncol* 2009;**27**(15):2466–73.
5. Komoike Y, Akiyama F, Iino Y, Ikeda T, Akashi-Tanaka S, Ohsumi S, et al. Ipsilateral breast tumor recurrence (IBTR) after breast-conserving treatment for early breast cancer. *Cancer* 2006;**106**(1):35–41.
6. Lu WL, Jansen L, Post WJ, Bonnema J, Van de Velde JC, De Bock GH. Impact on survival of early detection of isolated breast recurrences after the primary treatment for breast cancer: a meta-analysis. *Breast Cancer Res Treat* 2009;**114**(3):403–12.
7. Nelson HD, Tyne K, Naik A, Bougatsos C, Chan BK, Humphrey L, et al. Screening for breast cancer: an update for the U.S. Preventive Services Task Force. *Ann Intern Med* 2009;**151**(10):727–37. W237–42.
8. Tabar L, Vitak B, Chen TH, Yen AM, Cohen A, Tot T, et al. Swedish two-county trial: impact of mammographic screening on breast cancer mortality during 3 decades. *Radiology* 2011;**260**(3):658–63.

9. Houssami N, Ciatto S, Martinelli F, Bonardi R, Duffy SW. Early detection of second breast cancers improves prognosis in breast cancer survivors. *Ann Oncol* 2009;**20**:1505–10.
10. Lu W, Schaapveld M, Jansen L, Bagherzadegan E, Sahinovic MM, Baas PC, et al. The value of surveillance mammography of the contralateral breast in patients with a history of breast cancer. *Eur J Cancer* 2009;**45**:3000–7.
11. Paszat L, Sutradhar R, Grunfeld E, Gainford C, Benk V, Bondy S, et al. Outcomes of surveillance mammography after treatment of primary breast cancer: a population-based case series. *Breast Cancer Res Treat* 2009;**114**:169–78.
12. Khatcheressian JL, Hurley P, Bantug E, Esserman LJ, Grunfeld E, Halberg F, et al. Breast cancer follow-up and management after primary treatment: American Society of Clinical Oncology clinical practice guideline update. *J Clin Oncol* 2013;**31**(7):961–5.
13. Lauby-Secretan B, Scoccianti C, Loomis D, Benbrahim-Tallaa L, Bouvard V, Bianchini F, et al. Breast-cancer screening—viewpoint of the IARC Working Group. *N Engl J Med* 2015;**372**:2353–8.
14. Lee CH, Dershaw DD, Kopans D, Evans P, Monsees B, Monticciolo D, et al. Breast cancer screening with imaging: recommendations from the Society of Breast Imaging and the ACR on the use of mammography, breast MRI, breast ultrasound, and other technologies for the detection of clinically occult breast cancer. *J Am Coll Radiol* 2010;**7**(1):18–27.
15. Lin NU, Thomssen C, Cardoso F, Cameron D, Cufer T, Fallowfield L, et al. International guidelines for management of metastatic breast cancer (MBC) from the European School of Oncology (ESO)-MBC Task Force: Surveillance, staging, and evaluation of patients with early-stage and metastatic breast cancer. *Breast* 2013;**22**(3):203–10.
16. Moy L, Newell MS, Bailey L, Barke LD, Carkaci S, D'Orsi C, et al. ACR Appropriateness Criteria stage I breast cancer: initial workup and surveillance for local recurrence and distant metastases in asymptomatic women. *J Am Coll Radiol* 2014;**11**(12 Pt A):1160–8.
17. National Comprehensive Cancer Network. Breast Cancer, v.2.2015; 2015.
18. National Institute for Health and Care Excellence. *Early and locally advanced breast cancer: diagnosis and treatment (CG80)*. United Kingdom: National Institute for Health and Care Excellence; 2009.
19. National Institute for Health and Care Excellence. Review of Clinical Guideline (CG80)—Breast cancer (early & locally advanced): diagnosis and treatment. In: Practice CfC, editor. United Kingdom: National Institute for Health and Clinical Excellence; 2012.
20. Harris RP, Wilt TJ, Qaseem A. A value framework for cancer screening: advice for high-value care from the American college of physicians. *Ann Intern Med* 2015;**162**:712–7.
21. Black WC, Welch HG. Screening for disease. *AJR Am J Roentgenol* 1997;**168**(1):3–11.
22. Obuchowski NA, Graham RJ, Baker ME, Powell KA. Ten criteria for effective screening: their application to multislice CT screening for pulmonary and colorectal cancers. *AJR Am J Roentgenol* 2001;**176**(6):1357–62.
23. Brewer NT, Salz T, Lillie SE. Systematic review: the long-term effects of false-positive mammograms. *Ann Intern Med* 2007;**146**:502–10.
24. Harris RP, Sheridan SL, Lewis CL, Barclay C, Vu MB, Kistler CE, et al. The harms of screening: a proposed taxonomy and application to lung cancer screening. *JAMA Intern Med* 2014;**174**(2):281–5.
25. Tosteson AN, Fryback DG, Hammond CS, Hanna LG, Grove MR, Brown M, et al. Consequences of false-positive screening mammograms. *JAMA Intern Med* 2014;**174**(6):954–61.
26. Hubbard RA, Kerlikowske K, Flowers CI, Yankaskas BC, Zhu W, Miglioretti DL. Cumulative probability of false-positive recall or biopsy recommendation after 10 years of screening mammography. *Ann Intern Med* 2011;**155**:481–92.
27. Esserman LJ, Shieh Y, Thompson I. Rethinking screening for breast cancer and prostate cancer. *JAMA* 2009;**302**:1685–92.
28. Welch HG, Black WC. Overdiagnosis in cancer. *J Natl Cancer Inst* 2010;**102**(9):605–13.
29. Smith RA. Counterpoint: overdiagnosis in breast cancer screening. *J Am Coll Radiol* 2014;**11**:648–52.

30. Brown SD. Professional norms regarding how radiologists handle incidental findings. *J Am Coll Radiol* 2013;**10**:253–7.
31. Niell BL, Bennett D, Sharma A, Gazelle GS. Extramammary findings on breast MR examinations: frequency, clinical relevance, and patient outcomes. *Radiology* 2015;**276**:56–64.
32. Ding A, Eisenberg JD, Pandharipande PV. The economic burden of incidentally detected findings. *Radiol Clin North Am* 2011;**49**(2):257–65.
33. Porter ME. What is value in health care? *N Engl J Med* 2010;**363**:2477–81.
34. Thrall JH. Building research programs in diagnostic radiology. Part III. Clinical and translational research. *Radiology* 2007;**243**(1):5–9.
35. Houssami N, Ciatto S. Mammographic surveillance in women with a personal history of breast cancer: how accurate? How effective? *Breast* 2010;**19**:439–45.
36. Lash TL, Clough-Gorr K, Silliman RA. Reduced rates of cancer-related worries and mortality associated with guideline surveillance after breast cancer therapy. *Breast Cancer Res Treat* 2005;**89**:61–7.
37. Lash TL, Fox MP, Silliman RA. Reduced mortality rate associated with annual mammograms after breast cancer therapy. *Breast J* 2006;**12**:2–6.
38. Lash TL, Fox MP, Buist DSM, Wei F, Field TS, Frost FJ, et al. Mammography surveillance and mortality in older breast cancer survivors. *J Clin Oncol* 2007;**25**:3001–6.
39. Robertson C, Arcot Ragupathy SK, Boachie C, Dixon JM, Fraser C, Hernandez R, et al. *The clinical effectiveness and cost-effectiveness of different surveillance mammography regimens after the treatment for primary breast cancer: systematic reviews, registry database analyses and economic evaluation*. United Kingdom: Health Technology Assessment; 2011.
40. Bone B, Aspelin P, Isberg B, Perbeck L, Veress B. Contrast-enhanced MR imaging of the breast in patients with breast implants after cancer surgery. *Acta Radiol* 1995;**36**:111–6.
41. Drew PJ, Kerin MJ, Turnbull LW, Imrie M, Carleton PJ, Fox JN, et al. Routine screening for local recurrence following breast-conserving therapy for cancer with dynamic contrast-enhanced magnetic resonance imaging of the breast. *Ann Surg Oncol* 1998;**5**:265–70.
42. American Joint Commission on Cancer. *Manual for staging of cancer*. 6th ed. Philadelphia, PA; 2002.
43. Houssami N, Abraham LA, Miglioretti DL, Sickles EA, Kerlikowske K, Buist DS, et al. Accuracy and outcomes of screening mammography in women with a personal history of early-stage breast cancer. *JAMA* 2011;**305**(8):790–9.
44. Houssami N, Abraham LA, Kerlikowske K, Buist DS, Irwig L, Lee J, et al. Risk model for second screen-detected or interval breast cancers in women with a personal history of breast cancer participating in mammography screening. *Cancer Epidemiol Biomarkers Prev* 2013;**22**:946–61.
45. Lee JM, Buist DSM, Houssami N, Dowling EC, Halpern EF, Gazelle GS, et al. Five-year risk of interval invasive second breast cancer. *J Natl Cancer Inst* 2015;**107**: djv109.
46. Early Breast Cancer Trialists' Collaborative Group. Effects of chemotherapy and hormonal therapy for early breast cancer on recurrence and 15-year survival: an overview of the randomized trials. *Lancet* 2005;**365**:1687–717.
47. Early Breast Cancer Trialists' Collaborative Group. Effects of radiotherapy and of differences in the extent of surgery for early breast cancer on local recurrence and 15-year survival: an overview of the randomised trials. *Lancet* 2005;**366**:2087–106.
48. Early Breast Cancer Trialists' Collaborative Group. Relevance of breast cancer hormone receptors and other factors to the efficacy of adjuvant tamoxifen: patient-level meta-analysis of randomised trials. *Lancet* 2011;**378**:771–84.
49. Arasu VA, Joe BN, Lvoff NM, Leung JWT, Brenner JR, Flowers CI, et al. Benefit of semiannual ipsilateral mammographic surveillance following breast conservation therapy. *Radiology* 2012;**264**:371–7.
50. Brennan S, Liberman L, Dershaw DD, Morris E. Breast M.R.I. screening of women with a personal history of breast cancer. *AJR* 2010;**195**:510–6.

51. Lehman CD, Lee JM, DeMartini WB, Hippe DS, Rendi MH, Kalish G, et al. Screening MRI in women with a personal history of breast cancer. *J Natl Cancer Inst* 2016;**108**(3). pii: djv349. Available from: http://dx.doi.org/10.1093/jnci/djv349. Print 2016 Mar. PubMed PMID: 26744477.
52. Schacht DV, Yamaguchi K, Lai J, Kulkarni K, Sennett CA, Abe H. Importance of a personal history of breast cancer as a risk factor for the development of subsequent breast cancer: results from screening breast MRI. *AJR* 2014;**202**:289–92.
53. Giess CS, Poole PS, Chikarmane SA, Sippo DA, Birdwell RL. Screening breast MRI in patients previously treated for breast cancer: diagnostic yield for cancer and abnormal interpretation rate. *Acad Radiol* 2015;**22**(11):1331–7. Available from: http://dx.doi.org/10.1016/j.acra.2015.05.009. Epub 2015 Jul 2. PubMed PMID: 26142951.
54. Gweon HM, Cho N, Han W, Yi A, Moon HG, Noh DY, et al. Breast MR Imaging Screening in women with a history of breast conservation therapy. *Radiology* 2014;**272**:366–73.
55. Berg WA, Blume JD, Cormack JB, Mendelson EB, Lehrer D, Bohm-Velez M, et al. Combined screening with ultrasound and mammography vs mammography alone in women at elevated risk of breast cancer. *JAMA* 2008;**299**(18):2151–63.
56. Berg WA, Zhang Z, Lehrer D, Jong RA, Pisano ED, Barr RG, et al. Detection of breast cancer with addition of annual screening ultrasound or a single screening MRI to mammography in women with elevated breast cancer risk. *JAMA* 2012;**307**:1394–404.
57. Baker JA, Lo JY. Breast tomosynthesis: state-of-the-art and review of the literature. *Acad Radiol* 2011;**18**:1298–310.
58. Skaane P, Bandos AI, Gullien R, Eben EB, Ekseth U, Haakenaasen U, et al. Comparison of digital mammography alone and digital mammography plus tomosynthesis in a population-based screening program. *Radiology* 2013;**267**:47–56.
59. Ciatto S, Houssami N, Bernardi D, Caumo F, Pellegrini M, Brunelli S, et al. Integration of 3D digital mammography with tomosynthesis for population breast-cancer screening (STORM): a prospective comparison study. *Lancet Oncol* 2013;**14**:583–9.
60. Friedewald SM, Rafferty EA, Rose SL, Durand MA, Plecha DM, Greenberg JS, et al. Breast cancer screening using tomosynthesis in combination with digital mammography. *JAMA* 2014;**311**:2499–507.
61. Lourenco AP, Barry-Brooks M, Baird GL, Tuttle A, Mainiero MB. Changes in recall type and patient treatment following implementation of screening digital breast tomosynthesis. *Radiology* 2015;**274**:337–42.
62. Warner E, Messersmith H, Causer P, Elsen A, Shumak R, Plewes D. Systematic review: using magnetic resonance imaging to screen women at high risk for breast cancer. *Ann Intern Med* 2008;**148**:671–9.
63. Saslow D, Boetes C, Burke W, Harms S, Leach MO, Lehman CD, et al. American cancer society guidelines for breast screening with MRI as an adjunct to mammography. *CA Cancer J Clin* 2007;**57**(2):75–89.
64. Lander MR, Tabar L. Automated 3-D breast ultrasound as a promising adjunctive screening tool for examining dense breast tissue. *Semin Roentgenol* 2011;**46**:302–8.
65. American College of Radiology. *Appropriateness guideline: breast cancer screening*. United States; 2012.
66. Houssami N, Ciatto S. The evolving role of new imaging methods in breast screening. *Prev Med* 2011;**53**(3):123–6.
67. Scheel JR, Lee JM, Sprague BL, Lee CI, Lehman CD. Screening ultrasound as an adjunct to mammography in women with mammographically dense breasts. *Am J Obstet Gynecol* 2015;**212**:9–17.
68. Ollendorf DA, Loos AM, Tice JA, Lee JM, Pearson SD. Institute for Clinical and Economic Review *Appropriate imaging for breast cancer screening in special populations*. Boston, MA: Final appraisal document for the Washington State Health Care authority Health Technology Assessment Committee; 2014.
69. Chassin MR, Galvin RW. Quality NRoHC. The urgent need to improve health care quality. Institute of Medicine National Roundtable on Health Care Quality. *JAMA* 1998;**280**:1000–5.
70. Schnipper LE, Lyman GH, Blayney DW, Hoverman JR, Raghavan D, Wollins DS, et al. American Society of Clinical Oncology 2013 top five list in oncology. *J Clin Oncol* 2013;**31**(34):4362–70.

71. Henry NL, Hayes DF, Ramsey SD, Hortobagyi GN, Barlow WE, Gralow JR. Promoting quality and evidence-based care in early-stage breast cancer follow-up. *J Natl Cancer Inst* 2014;**106**(4): dju034.
72. Del Turco MR, Palli D, Cariddi A, Ciatto S, Pacini P, Distante V. The efficacy of intensive follow-up testing in breast cancer cases. *Ann Oncol* 1995;**6**:S37–9.
73. GIVIO Investigators G Impact of follow-up testing on survival and health-related quality of life in breast cancer patients: a multicenter randomized controlled trial. *JAMA* 1994;**271**(50):1587–92.
74. Palli D, Russo A, Saieva C, Ciatto S, Rosselli Del Turco M, Distante V, et al. Intensive vs clinical follow-up after treatment of primary breast cancer: 10 year update of a randomized trial. *JAMA* 1999;**281**(17):1586.
75. Kokko R, Hakama M, Holli K. Follow-up cost of breast cancer patients with localized disease after primary treatment: a randomized trial. *Breast Cancer Res Treat* 2005;**93**(3):255–60.
76. Grunfeld E, Hodgson DC, Del Giudice ME, Moineddin R. Population-based longitudinal study of follow-up care for breast cancer survivors. *J Oncol Pract* 2010;**6**:174–81.
77. Ramsey SD, Henry NL, Gralow JR, Mirick DK, Barlow W, Etzioni R, et al. Tumor marker usage and medical care costs among older early-stage breast cancer survivors. *J Clin Oncol* 2015;**33**(2):149–55.
78. Ramsey SD, Fedorenko C, Chauhan R, McGee R, Lyman GH, Kreizenbeck K, et al. Baseline estimates of adherence to American Society of Clinical Oncology/American Board of Internal Medicine Choosing Wisely Initiative among patients with cancer enrolled with a large regional commercial health insurer. *J Oncol Pract* 2015;**11**:338–43.
79. Timble JW, Fox DS, Van Busum K, Schneider E. Five reasons that many comparative effectiveness studies fail to change patient care and clinical practice. *Health Aff* 2012;**31**:2168–75.
80. Wernli KJ, DeMartini WB, Ichikawa L, Lehman CD, Onega T, Kerlikowske K, et al. Patterns of breast magnetic resonance imaging use in community practice. *JAMA Intern Med* 2013;**174**:125–32.
81. Stout NK, Nekhlyudov L, Li L, Malin ES, Ross-Degnan D, Buist DS, et al. Rapid increase in breast magnetic resonance imaging use. *JAMA Intern Med* 2013;**174**:114–21.
82. Wirtz HS, Boudreau DM, Gralow JR, Barlow WE, Gray S, Bowles EJ, et al. Factors associated with long-term adherence to annual surveillance mammography among breast cancer survivors. *Breast Cancer Res Treat* 2014;**143**(3):541–50.
83. Keating NL, Landrum MB, Guadagnoli E, Winer EP, Ayanian JZ. Surveillance testing among survivors of early-stage breast cancer. *J Clin Oncol* 2007;**25**:1074–81.
84. Doubeni CA, Field TS, Yood MU, Rolnick SJ, Quessenberry CP, Fouayzi H, et al. Patterns and predictors of mammography utilization among breast cancer survivors. *Cancer* 2006;**106**:2482–8.
85. Field TS, Doubeni CA, Fox MP, Buist DSM, Wei F, Geiger AM, et al. Under utilization of surveillance mammography among older breast cancer survivors. *J Gen Intern Med* 2007;**23**:158–63.
86. Cancer Genome Atlas Network. Comprehensive molecular portraits of human breast tumors. *Nature* 2012;**490**:61–70.
87. Reis-Filho JS, Pusztai L. Gene expression profiling in breast cancer: classification, prognostication, and prediction. *Lancet* 2011;**378**:1812–23.
88. Sotiriou C, Pusztai L. Gene-expression signatures in breast cancer. *N Engl J Med* 2009;**360**(8):790–800.
89. Goldhirsch A, Wood WC, Coates AS, Gelber RD, Thurlimann B, Senn H-J. Strategies for subtypes—dealing with the diversity of breast cancer: highlights of the St. Gallen International Expert Consensus on the Primary Therapy of Early Breast Cancer 2011. *Ann Oncol* 2011;**22**:1736–47.
90. Voduc KD, Cheang MCU, Tyldesley S, Gelmon K, Nielsen TO, Kennecke H. Breast cancer subtypes and the risk of local and regional relapse. *J Clin Oncol* 2010;**28**:1684–91.
91. Nguyen PL, Taghian AG, Katz MS, Niemierko A, Abi Raad RF, Boon WL, et al. Breast cancer subtype approximated by estrogen receptor, progesterone receptor, and HER-2 is associated with local and distant recurrence after breast-conserving therapy. *J Clin Oncol* 2008;**26**(14):2373–8.
92. Arvold ND, Taghian AG, Niemierko A, Abi Raad RF, Sreedhara M, Nguyen PL, et al. Age, breast cancer subtype approximation, and local recurrence after breast-conserving therapy. *J Clin Oncol* 2011;**29**:3885–91.

93. Kennecke H, Yerushalmi R, Woods R, Cheang MC, Voduc D, Speers CH, et al. Metastatic behavior of breast cancer subtypes. *J Clin Oncol* 2010;**28**:3271–7.
94. Nichols HB, Berrington de Gonzalez A, Lacey JVJ, Rosenberg PS, Anderson WF. Declining incidence of contralateral breast cancer in the United States from 1975 to 2006. *J Clin Oncol* 2011;**29**:1564–9.
95. Collett K, Stefansson IM, Eide J, Braaten A, Wang H, Eide GE, et al. A basal epithelial phenotype is more frequent in interval breast cancers compared with screen detected tumors. *Cancer Epidemiol Biomarkers Prev* 2005;**14**:1108–12.
96. Caldarella A, Puliti D, Crocetti E, Bianchi S, Vezzosi V, Apicella P, et al. Biological characteristics of interval cancers: a role for biomarkers in the breast cancer screening. *J Cancer Res Clin Oncol* 2013;**139**:181–5.
97. Domingo L, Salas D, Zubizarreta R, Bare M, Sarriugarte G, Barata T, et al. Tumor phenotype and breast density in distinct categories of interval cancer: results of population-based mammography screening in Spain. *Breast Cancer Res* 2014;**16**(1):R3.
98. Yang T-IJ, Yang Q, Haffty BG, Moran MS. Prognosis for mammographically occult, early-stage breast cancer patients treated with breast-conservation therapy. *Int J Radiat Oncol Biol Phys* 2010;**76**:79–84.
99. American College of Radiology *Breast imaging reporting and data system atlas*, 4th ed. Reston, VA: American College of Radiology; 2003.
100. Hoffmann TC, Del Mar C. Patients' expectations of the benefits and harms of treatments, screening, and tests: a systematic review. *JAMA Intern Med* 2015;**175**(2):274–86.
101. Simard S, Thewes B, Humphris G, Dixon M, Hayden C, Mireskandari S, et al. Fear of cancer recurrence in adult cancer survivors: a systematic review of quantitative studies. *J Cancer Surviv* 2013;**7**(3):300–22.

CHAPTER

13

EVOLUTION OF MAMMOGRAPHY SCREENING: FROM FILM SCREEN TO DIGITAL BREAST TOMOSYNTHESIS

Sophia Zackrisson[1] and Nehmat Houssami[2]

[1]Department of Translational Medicine, Diagnostic Radiology, Lund University, Skåne University Hospital, Malmö, Skåne, Sweden, [2]School of Public Health, Sydney Medical School, University of Sydney, Sydney, NSW, Australia

CHAPTER OUTLINE

PLAIN LANGUAGE SUMMARY

Mammography screening has been adopted in many countries and population health programs because randomized trials showed that it reduces the risk of dying from breast cancer. These randomized trials used screen-film mammography (SFM) which means that the X-ray beams are captured on a film cassette. The films are then developed and reviewed on a light-box by the physician. However, technical developments have witnessed an evolution from screen-film to digital mammography (DM) which

Breast Cancer Screening. DOI: http://dx.doi.org/10.1016/B978-0-12-802209-2.00013-9

means that a specially designed digital so-called "detector" captures the X-rays (replacing the film) and converts the information to a digital image, which is displayed on a high-resolution computer monitor, and transmitted and stored just like computer files. The evidence prompting a change to DM screening came from studies comparing detection for SFM and DM (one of these was a randomized trial) that showed roughly similar or higher cancer detection using DM compared to SFM. There were also some technical efficiencies underlying a general shift to digital imaging in medical practice. In very recent years, a new technology known as digital breast tomosynthesis (DBT, or tomosynthesis), essentially a quasi-three-dimensional mammogram, has become available. So far, tomosynthesis seems capable of detecting more breast cancers then standard DM and it could potentially reduce false-alarms (known as false recalls or false-positive screen) but different studies show mixed findings on this issue. Although some countries have started to use tomosynthesis for screening, and several trials have been or are being done to address evidence gaps around this new technology, there are no recommendations to change to tomosynthesis screening because it is not yet known whether using tomosynthesis adds health benefit above what might be achieved with standard mammography screening.

INTRODUCTION

Since the 1980s mammography screening has been implemented in many countries, including population-based programs, following the results of the randomized controlled trials (RCTs) of mammography screening, as described in chapter "Estimates of Screening Benefit: The Randomized Trials of Breast Cancer Screening." Alongside widespread adoption of mammography screening, there has been a continuous and substantial technical development from SFM to full-field digital mammography (FFDM) and very recently also the introduction of digital breast tomosynthesis (DBT). This technical evolution calls for new evidence regarding the performance of screening using new mammography technologies, and the evidence needed to translate new technologies into screening practice.

This chapter has three main sections, beginning with a brief overview of the technical background and development of the different mammography-based modalities. The second part focuses on the trials and studies that form the basis of the evidence for screening with FFDM versus SFM, and the rapidly emerging evidence on the introduction of DBT in breast screening. The third part pinpoints the evidence needed if and when breast tomosynthesis is adopted routinely into service screening for breast cancer.

TECHNICAL BACKGROUND

MAMMOGRAPHY

Screen-film mammography

Mammography is an X-ray examination of the breast used for decades in diagnosis of breast disease and as a screening modality. In analog mammography, also called SFM, the X-ray beams are captured on a film cassette. The films are then developed and reviewed on a light-box by the physician. Breast cancer is not one single disease entity; it rather comprises a wide range of types, growth rates, and growth patterns which is also mirrored in the X-ray image of the breast. Hence, the radiographic appearance

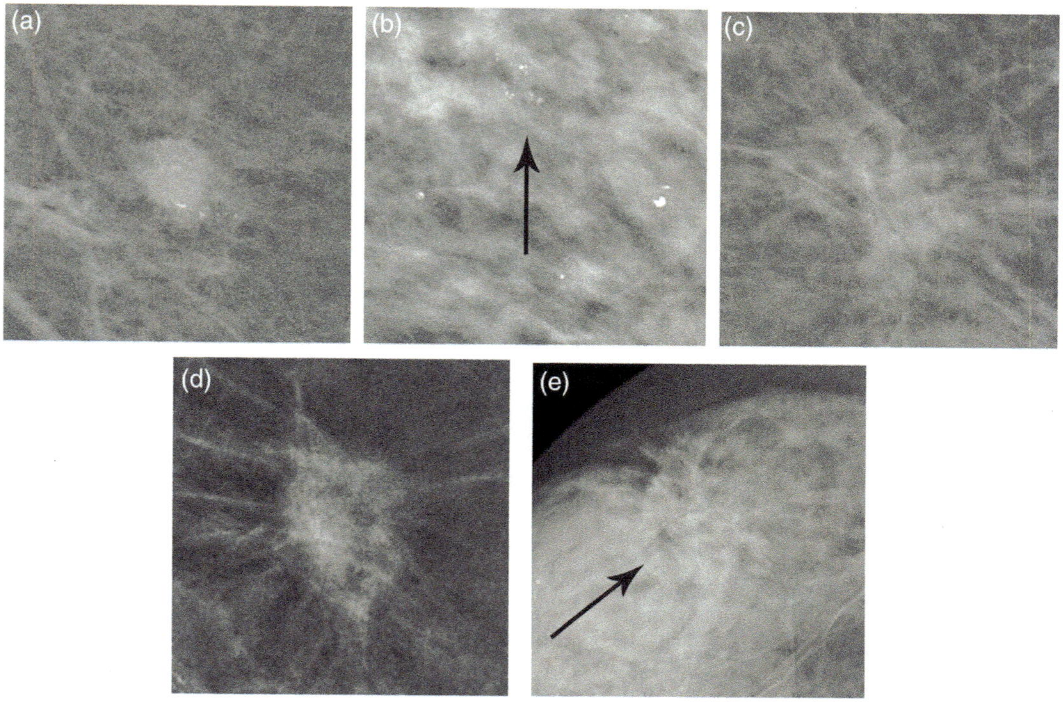

FIGURE 13.1

Examples of tumor appearances on mammography images illustrating the wide range of growth patterns for breast cancers where some are more easily detectable than others. (a) A well-defined mass in a fatty breast; (b) microcalcifications; (c) an ill-defined mass with slight retraction; (d) a spiculated tumor; and (e) an architectural distortion in a dense breast.

Reproduced from Ref. 60 with permission from SAGE publications.

of breast cancer ranges from barely detectable, minimal signs to apparent cancer growth and hence a clearly visible abnormality. Some radiographic patterns of breast cancer are readily detected when relatively small (at an early stage), such as spiculated lesions and tumors presenting with calcifications, whereas other lesions are challenging to detect such as tumors causing only a nonspecific density or areas with subtle architectural distortion (Fig. 13.1).

Therefore, mammography is one of the most technically challenging areas in radiography since it requires a high spatial resolution, for fine details like microcalcifications, and outstanding soft-tissue contrast to enable visualization of soft-tissue lesions such as tumors. Moreover, a low radiation dose is crucial since the breast is a radiosensitive organ. SFM was hence refined to get high-resolution images of both soft-tissue lesions and calcifications. The randomized trials in mammography screening were all performed with SFM systems and hard copy (film) reading. Still, far from all screening centers have transitioned to DM, due to costs inherent in changing workflow from analog to digital and due to image storage issues.

Full-field digital mammography

Along the development of digital imaging, flat panel detectors were developed enabling so-called FFDM, which has been broadly used in diagnostic and screening practice since 2006. In FFDM a specially designed digital detector captures the X-rays (replacing the film) and converts the information to a digital image, which is displayed on a high-resolution computer monitor, and transmitted and stored just like computer files. Before the introduction of DM into practice, it was questioned whether the image quality and especially the spatial resolution of DM was sufficient for detection of minimal calcifications. It was concluded, however, that even if the spatial resolution of DM commonly was inferior to SFM due to technical reasons, the resolution is good enough for breast cancer diagnostics.[1,2] The digital technique provided a number of other advantages compared to SFM, such as elimination of film-related inefficiencies, contrast resolution, quick transfer/teleradiology, and simplified storage of images in picture archiving and communication systems and image processing.[3] It also reduces the need for technical repeats, because the radiographer can immediately see whether the image fulfills the quality standards or not and the woman does not need to come back for a new visit due to technical failure. Furthermore, digital images allows for potential application of computer-aided detection and other advanced applications.

DIGITAL BREAST TOMOSYNTHESIS

The development of tomosynthesis

Tomosynthesis is a relatively new tomographic X-ray technique with the capability to significantly reduce the confounding effect of overlapping normal anatomy. The story of tomosynthesis development began in the beginning of the 20th century. It was not until the early 1970s that the idea was realized by a group at Johns Hopkins University, Baltimore, United States[4] and further developed by the same group by inventing a simple reconstruction method.[5] Since the applications considered for tomosynthesis were thereafter taken over by the introduction of spiral computered tomography in the late 1980s, the development of tomosynthesis came to a halt. Along with the digitalization of radiography, more powerful computers, and the development of high-quality flat panel detectors, tomosynthesis reemerged again for breast, lung, and skeletal applications.[6] In breast imaging, the study of Niklason et al. started the new era for breast tomosynthesis by describing and evaluating a breast tomosynthesis imaging method based on a FFDM system.[7]

Tomosynthesis technique

In tomosynthesis,[7–10] low-dose images are acquired of the compressed breast from different angles (usually 11–25 by number), as the X-ray tube moves along a limited arc, typically between 15 and 50 degrees (see Fig. 13.2).[6]

The low-dose images (so-called projection images) are mathematically reconstructed to a stack of usually 1 mm thin slices, parallel to the detector plane. The slices can be viewed as a cine-loop or through scrolling/viewing single slices. Each slice contains much less of the overlapping tissue compared to a standard mammography image, and hence much of the superimposition effect of dense glandular tissue and parenchymal structures (potentially masking tumors) is reduced. The total examination time is about the same as for a mammography examination. The time that the breast needs to be compressed during image acquisition varies depending mainly on how wide the acquisition angle that

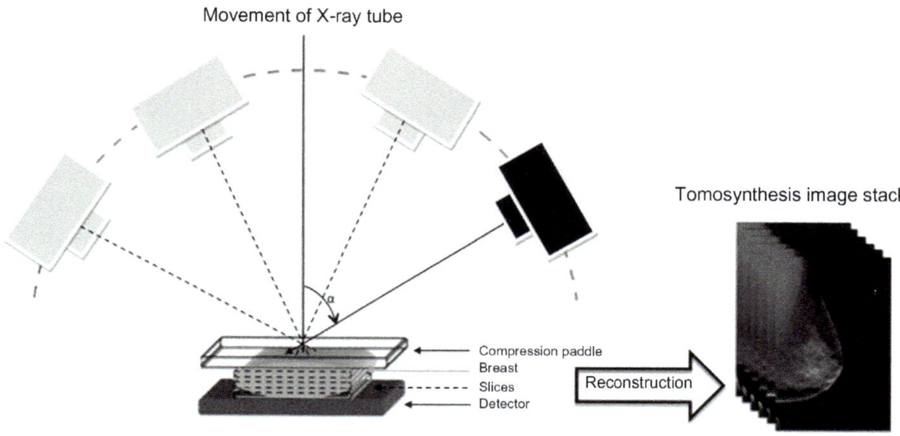

FIGURE 13.2

A schematic presentation of the tomosynthesis principle. The X-ray tube moves in an arch (typically 15–50 degrees varying between systems, α = the acquisition angle) over the compressed breast and acquires multiple low-dose projection images from different angles. The projection images are mathematically reconstructed parallel to the detector plane into usually 1 mm thin slices of the breast, which can be viewed either as a cine-loop or as individual images when scrolling through the image volume. A standard breast usually results in around 50 slices. Tomosynthesis reduces the overlapping effect of breast parenchyma that on a conventional 2D image may hide or simulate a tumor.

is used. Scan times for one projection have been reported to range between 8 and 25 s.[11] Any of the traditional mammography views can be used, such as craniocaudal, mediolateral-oblique, and lateral views, etc.

The projection images first sampled need to be reconstructed and processed to get good images for review and interpretation. Much research efforts have been put into optimization of image reconstruction. Initially, filtered back-projection was the most common reconstruction method[12] and the same as used in CT, although in later years iterative reconstruction has been introduced.[13] Iterative reconstruction may be less insensitive to noise and incomplete sampling data but usually takes longer time compared to filtered back-projection. No conclusion has been reached on which method is more superior.

Synthetic views

Without any additional radiation exposure, it is possible to derive a so-called *synthetic mammogram* from the tomosynthesis volume. Some tomosynthesis systems are approved by the US Food and Drug Administration only for the clinical use of the combination of tomosynthesis and mammography, which entails almost double the radiation dose if obtained as dual acquisition.[14] Furthermore, there was initially a belief that microcalcification detection would be inferior in tomosynthesis compared to mammography. There are conflicting results regarding the sensitivity of tomosynthesis for microcalcification, whereas some publications suggest tomosynthesis is inferior in calcification detection compared to mammography,[15–17] other studies suggest similar capability for the two modalities,[18–22] and one study suggesting that tomosynthesis may be more specific but slightly less sensitive than DM in characterizing microcalcification.[23] Such differences between study findings on microcalcification may be partially due to the fact that many are observer studies and not actually embedded in routine screening reporting, therefore more realistic estimates for detection of microcalcification are available from the prospective trials (see paragraph on prospective trials of DBT). A synthetic mammogram may be of help or could save time judging whether there actually is a microcalcification cluster present, since individual calcifications from a cluster may appear in different adjacent tomosynthesis slices. In addition, a synthetic mammogram could provide an overview of potential lesions within the 3D volume and help when comparing tomosynthesis to prior mammograms. The combination of two-view tomosynthesis and synthetic (C-view) mammogram has been investigated in the Oslo Tomosynthesis Screening Trial (OTST) with promising initial results.[24] In that study, using synthesized two-dimensional (2D) images plus DBT data during the interpretation of screening mammograms, the radiologists' overall performance levels were comparable to when using standard FFDM plus DBT, with cancer detection rates of 7.8 and 7.7 per 1000 screens for FFDM plus DBT and for current synthesized 2D images plus DBT, respectively (false-positive scores, 4.6% and 4.5%, respectively). The radiation dose to the breast was reduced by 45% with the combination of synthesized 2D images and DBT. Availability of synthetic mammograms, if tomosynthesis is to be used in screening, will probably be pivotal to minimize the radiation dose for screening populations, by avoiding dual acquisition of DBT and DM. Evidence from additional studies addressing the issue of synthetic 2D in population screening would be valuable, and at least one prospective population-based trial (STORM 2: screening with tomosynthesis or mammography 2) is anticipated to report its findings in the near future.

EVIDENCE ON SCREENING FROM DIFFERENT TECHNICAL ERAS

FFMD VERSUS SFM

The implementation of mammography screening is based on the results from the former RCTs where SFM was used,[14] see also chapter "Estimates of Screening Benefit: The Randomized Trials of Breast Cancer Screening", Nelson et al., in this book which outlines the evidence from the mammography screening trials. These trials had long-term follow-up and breast cancer–specific mortality as endpoint. The majority of the studies comparing the screening performance of FFDM versus SFM are observational, comparative studies.[25–36] The only RCT is the Oslo II[37] trial. The main results of these studies and the Oslo trial are described in Table 13.1. It is worth noting that despite higher cancer detection at FFDM in the Oslo trial, there was no significant reduction in interval cancer rates.[37]

There are large variations in the results from the nonrandomized studies, which may have several explanations. The study designs vary and include prospective, paired testing using both techniques, or retrospective comparisons of cohorts screened with either FFDM or SFM and used different screen-reading and recall strategies.[38] Regarding cancer detection, FFDM seems to perform equally or better than SFM, and in the RCT higher cancer detection was shown for FFDM.[37] Considering the recall rates for FFDM and SFM, these show large variability across studies and in several of these studies recall was actually slightly increased by FFDM.[26,27,30,35] It has been suggested that the higher recall rate at FFDM in most of the studies may be explained by the higher contrast resolution and increased cancer conspicuity for subtle "minimal sign" lesions and microcalcifications at FFDM, although there are no studies that have explicitly investigated this.[27] Furthermore, differences in reading strategies and

Table 13.1 Studies Comparing Screen-Film Mammography and Full-Field Digital Mammography: Estimates of Breast Screening Performance[a]

Study (First Author)	Age Group (Years)	Number of Screening Examinations		Recall Rate (%)		Cancer Detection Rate (%) (Invasive and DCIS)		Positive Predictive Value for Recall (%)	
		SFM	FFDM	SFM	FFDM	SFM	FFDM	SFM	FFDM
Colorado–Massachusetts (Lewin et al., 2001[25])	>40	6736	6736	14.9	11.8[b]	0.49	0.40	3.3	3.4
Oslo I (Skaane et al., 2005[26])	50–59	3683	3683	3.5	4.6[b]	0.71	0.54	20.2	11.8
Oslo II (Skaane et al., 2007[37])	45–69	16,985	6944	2.5	4.2[b]	0.38	0.59[b]	15.1	13.9
DMIST (Pisano et al., 2005[28])	47–62	42,555	42,555	8.6	8.6	0.41	0.44	4.7	5.1
Helsingborg (Heddson et al., 2007[29])	46–74	25,901	9841	1.4	1.0[b]	0.31	0.49[b]	21.8	47.1[b]
Florence (Del Turco et al., 2007[30])	50–69	14,395	14,385	3.5	4.3[b]	0.58	0.72	14.7	15.9
Vestfold County (Vigeland et al., 2008[31])	50–69	324,763	18,239	4.2	4.1	0.65	0.77	15.1	18.5[b]
East London (Vinnicombe et al., 2009[32])	≥50	31,720	8478	3.4	3.2	0.72	0.68	14.6	14.2
Barcelona (Sala et al., 2009[33])	50–69	12,958	6074	5.5	4.2[b]	0.40	0.40	7.5	9.7
Utrecht (Karssemeijer et al., 2009[34])	50–75	311,082	56,518[c]	1.3	2.1	0.51	0.56	39.5	25.5[b]
INBSP[d] (Hambly et al., 2009[35])	50–64	153,619	35,204	3.1	4.0[b]	0.52	0.63[b]	16.7	15.7
Flanders (Van Ongeval et al., 2010[36])	50–69	23,325	11,355	2.4	2.6	0.64	0.59	24.8	24.0

Reproduced from Ref. 38, with permission from Elsevier.
SFM, screen-film mammography; FFDM, full-field digital mammography; DMIST, Digital Mammographic Imaging Screening Trial.
[a] *Adapted, in part, from a review by Skaane (2009)*[27].
[b] *Indicates statistically significant difference ($p < 0.05$) for comparison between SFM and FFDM.*
[c] *Full-field digital mammography with computer-aided detection.*
[d] *Irish National Breast Screening Programme.*

whether single- or double-reading was performed may explain the large variations in results regarding recall rates.

A systematic review with a metaanalysis of eight studies concludes that FFDM results in a slightly higher detection rate (11 additional cancers per 10,000 screening mammograms (95%CI 4 to 18)) for FFDM, particularly at age 60 years and younger, but no clear modality difference in recall rates or positive predictive values.[32]

Some interesting findings were shown in subgroup analyses in some of the above-reported studies. The Digital Mammography Imaging Screening Trial (DMIST), showed overall equal accuracy for FFDM and SFM, although in women 50 years and younger as well as in women with heterogeneously or extremely dense breasts the accuracy was higher for FFDM.[28] In the Florence study, which was performed within a population-based screening program, similar results were found in younger women.[30]

DIGITAL BREAST TOMOSYNTHESIS

Observer studies

When DBT units became available either as prototype systems or commercially available systems, there was a great interest in evaluating the technique in clinical settings as well as extensive technical engagement for improving the systems.[39] The majority of the initial studies on DBT were performed on enriched populations (ie, with a high proportion of cancers in relation to normal cases and mostly done using retrospective mammogram sets) as outlined in a review that captured the literature until 2012.[40] In the overview from Houssami and Skaane,[40] the following summary findings were highlighted (here updated with literature until 2015):

- One-view DBT has at least equal or better accuracy than standard (two-view) DM.
- Two-view DBT has at least equal or better accuracy than standard (two-view) DM based on comparative accuracy for these modalities.
- The *addition* of DBT to standard two-view mammography (DBT with DM or film-screen mammography for diagnosis or triage of screen-recalled abnormalities) *significantly* improves accuracy—partly or predominantly through reduced false-positive interpretations.
- Comparisons of DBT and DM using enriched reader studies yielded variable estimates for accuracy and/or sensitivity and specificity pairs, which may be due to reader differences or differences in the research methods used in these studies. Overall, improved accuracy from DBT (relative to, or added to, mammography), appears to be due to increased cancer detection or due to a reduction of false-positive recalls or both.
- Many observer or reader studies did not find significant differences in interpretive accuracy between DBT and DM: this may be a true reflection of lack of a difference, or more likely a limitation of the "selection" of cases (from DM-defined detection) and also due to underpowered analyses since some studies had modest subject numbers.
- Subjective interpretation of cancer conspicuity or lesion visibility (evaluated qualitatively in feature analysis or quantitatively scored) consistently showed that cancers were equally conspicuous or more conspicuous on DBT relative to FFDM.

Using the framework of the literature review from Houssami and Skaane,[40] we updated the evidence summary on studies of DBT (other than the screening trials described in the paragraph "prospective screening trials with DBT") comprising cancer-enriched studies: the updated findings were generally similar to those discussed in the published overview[40] with more consistent evidence in observer studies that adding DBT improves interpretive accuracy. Furthermore, one-view DBT was shown to have higher diagnostic accuracy compared to two-view DM in an extended study by Svahn et al.[41] We present our updated study-specific summary in Table 13.2.

Table 13.2 Evidence on the Accuracy of Digital Breast Tomosynthesis (DBT) Compared to Standard Mammography

Study	Study Design	Subjects Age (Timeframe of Cases Collected)	Summary of Findings on Accuracy
Gilbert et al., (TOMMY) (2015)[a]	Multicentre retrospective reader study of enriched mammogram set collected prospectively from women recalled for assessment of *DM screen-detected* finding in the UK national program *or* women having screen because of family history (7060 screens: 1160 BC) read by 26 radiologists	Mean 56 (range 29–85) (2011–13)	[b]AUC from ROC analysis: • DM 0.84 vs DM + DBT 0.89 ($p < 0.001$) • DM 0.84 vs $DM_{synthetic}$+DBT 0.88 ($p < 0.001$) [b]AUC from ROC analysis (data restricted to screens with breast density ≥50%): • DM 0.83 vs DM + DBT 0.89 ($p < 0.001$) • DM 0.83 vs $DM_{synthetic}$+DBT 0.87 ($p < 0.001$)
Alakhras et al. (2015)[c]	Retrospective reader study of enriched mammogram set (50 cases: 27 BC) read by 26 radiologists	NR	[b]AUC from ROC analysis (all readers combined): • DM 0.681 vs DM + DBT 0.788 ($p < 0.001$) [d]Jacknife FROC analysis: • DM 0.621 vs DM + DBT 0.745 ($p < 0.001$)
Morel et al. (2014)[e]	Retrospective reader study of enriched mammogram set from women recalled to assessment of *DM screen-detected* finding *or* symptomatic women having work-up imaging (341 cases, 354 lesions: 103 BC), 7 readers	Mean NR (range 35–73) years (2010–11)	[b]AUC from ROC analysis: • DM + coned compression magnification views 0.87 vs DM + one-view DBT 0.93 ($p = 0.001$)
Thibault et al. (2013)[f]	Retrospective reader study of enriched mammogram set from women with image-detected (DM or ultrasound) findings *or* symptoms (130 cases, 55 BC), 7 readers	Mean NR (≥40) years (NR)	[b]AUC from ROC analysis showed *no statistical difference* for various modalities (ordered from highest to lowest AUC): DBT + DM(CC-only): 0.7795 DBT (MLO-only): 0.7783 DM (two-view) + ultrasound: 0.7697 DM + ultrasound + DBT (MLO): 0.7628 DM (two-view): 0.7556

(*Continued*)

Table 13.2 Evidence on the Accuracy of Digital Breast Tomosynthesis (DBT) Compared to Standard Mammography (Continued)

Study	Study Design	Subjects Age (Timeframe of Cases Collected)	Summary of Findings on Accuracy
Rafferty et al. (2013)[g] (Rafferty, 2014)[h]	Retrospective reader studies of enriched mammogram sets collected prospectively from women having screening *or* diagnostic (pre-biopsy) mammography: • Study 1 (312 mammograms: 48 BC) read by 12 radiologists • Study 2 (310 mammograms: 51 BC) read by 15 radiologists • (2014 study, similar design based on same mammogram set from 2013 study; 310 exams: 51 BC, read by 15 radiologists)	NR (2006–07)	[b]AUC from (pooled) ROC analysis: • Study 1: DM 82.1% vs DM + DBT 89.4% ($p < 0.001$) →7.2% increase in AUC • Study 2: DM 82.8% vs DM + DBT 89.5% ($p < 0.001$) →6.8% increase in AUC • (2014: DM 82.8% vs DM + one view DBT 86.4% ($p = 0.009$); DM 82.8% vs DM+ two view DBT 89.5% ($p < 0.001$))
Wallis et al. (2012)[i]	Test set (130 subjects: 40 BC, 24 benign lesions, 66 normal) observer study; read by two groups of 10 experienced readers *Prototype DBT system	Mean 56.3 (range 40–80) with BIRADS density 2–4 (2008–09)	[b]AUC from ROC analysis: • 2D mammography 0.772 vs two-view tomosynthesis 0.851 ($p = 0.021$) • 2D mammography 0.774 vs one-view (MLO) tomosynthesis 0.775 ($p = 0.79$)
Michell et al (2012)[j]	Prospective study of women recalled (738 consecutive recalls, both FFDM and DBT were performed: 204 BC) to assessment based on positive *film-screen* mammography at assessment, and double-read by experienced breast radiologists	NR (2009–10)	[b]AUC from ROC analysis: • 2D film-screen mammography alone 0.788 vs combined film-screen and FFDM 0.895 vs DBT *added* to combined film-screen and FFDM 0.967 ($p = 0.0001$) Addition of DBT resulted in more normal/benign cases correctly classified (for 74% of normal/benign screens)
Skaane et al. (2012)[k]	Clinical series of 129 subjects (27 BC) with symptoms or recalled for screen-detected abnormality or having surveillance; read by experienced breast radiologists (1 with limited experience). DBT reported 2–4 weeks after (and blinded to) standard assessment	Mean 57 (range 30–87) years (NR)	FFDM (with standard work-up) vs DBT (blinded to result of assessment): DBT concordant with assessment (identified all 25 BC): DBT-only recalled 4 other cases (2 of these had BC)→8% incremental detection with DBT
Svahn et al. (2012)[l]	Clinical series of 185 subjects, 89 with BC, observer study; read by 5 experienced breast radiologists; constrained cases selected with subtle screen-detected abnormalities or diagnostic (symptomatic) cases. (Extension of the study by Svahn 2010)	Mean 60 (range 42–79) years (2006–08)	Jacknife alternative FROC[d] analysis (mean figure of merit) • DBT (one-view) 0.809 vs two-view DM 0.706 ($p = 0.0031$) • Sensitivity 90% vs 79% • Similar false-positive fraction between methods

(*Continued*)

Table 13.2 Evidence on the Accuracy of Digital Breast Tomosynthesis (DBT) Compared to Standard Mammography (Continued)

Study	Study Design	Subjects Age (Timeframe of Cases Collected)	Summary of Findings on Accuracy
Gur et al. (2012)[m]	Test set (228 breasts/114 mammograms: 48 BC, 6 high-risk and 30 benign lesions, 144 normal) observer study; read by 10 tomosynthesis-trained radiologists. (Tested version of synthetically reconstructed 2D-images (2Dsynthetic))	Mean 51 (range 36–77) years (2008–09)	Average *sensitivity* • FFDM + DBT 82.6% vs 2Dsynthetic + DBT 77.2% (difference 5.4%; $p = 0.017$ or $p = 0.053$ for fixed or random reader effects) Average *false-positive* (FP) recall • FFDM + DBT 29.8% vs 2Dsynthetic + DBT 29.7% (no difference)
Bernardi et al. (2012)[n]	Prospective (simulation) study integrating DBT to triage screening recalls (158 consecutively recalled screens: 21 BC); 7 radiologists provided opinion on DBT prior to assessment	Mean 51.8 (range 35–77) years (2011)	Screens recalled on FFDM vs whether would recall with *added* DBT • DBT would have recalled all 21 screens found to have BC • DBT would *not* have recalled 74% of screens (102/137) that had negative work-up
Noroozian et al. (2012)[o]	Test set (67 subjects with breast masses: 30 BC, 37 benign lesions) observer study; read by 4 radiologists experienced in breast imaging; reads separated in time and by random allocation	Mean NR (range 34–88) years (cases collected 2006–08)	[b]AUC from ROC analysis comparing digital spot compression vs DBT of breast containing lesion: • Spot compression (range) 0.88–0.93 vs DBT (range) 0.89–0.93 (no difference in overall accuracy)
Svane et al. (2011)[p]	Clinical series ($n = 144$: 76 BC) selected with suspicious lesions on mammogram; read by 2 breast radiologists with limited tomosynthesis training *Prototype DBT system	Mean 56.8 (range 40–85) years; (2007–09)	[b]AUC from ROC: • 2D mammography 0.942 vs one-view (MLO) tomosynthesis 0.935 (no significant difference) Sensitivity: 2D mammography 93.4% vs one-view tomosynthesis 89.5% (no significant difference) Specificity: 2D mammography 80.9% vs one-view tomosynthesis 86.0% (no significant difference)
Tagliafico et al. (2011)[q]	Prospective study of abnormalities recalled from screening for mammographic work-up (52 consecutive recalls: 9 BC); 2 experienced breast radiologists independently provided opinion on spot compression views and DBT	Mean 51 years (2010)	AUC comparing digital spot compression vs DBT of the breast containing FFDM-recalled abnormality: • Spot compression 0.963 vs DBT 1.00 (no difference in overall accuracy)

(*Continued*)

Table 13.2 Evidence on the Accuracy of Digital Breast Tomosynthesis (DBT) Compared to Standard Mammography (Continued)

Study	Study Design	Subjects Age (Timeframe of Cases Collected)	Summary of Findings on Accuracy
Gennaro et al. (2010)[r]	Clinical/diagnostic series (200 subjects: 63 BC) selected with equivocal or suspicious lesions on mammogram and/or ultrasound; interpreted by 6 breast radiologists with experience in conventional mammography *Prototype DBT system	Age (NR) (2007–08)	[b]AUC from ROC analysis • 2D-FFDM 0.836 vs one-view DBT 0.851 ($p = 0.64$) *Mean* sensitivity and specificity for FFDM vs one-view DBT did *not* significantly differ: • Sensitivity 74.3% vs 69.8% • Specificity 84.8% vs 88.9%
Svahn et al. (2010)[s]	Test set (50 subjects) observer study; read by 5 experienced breast radiologists; constrained cases selected with subtle screen-detected abnormalities or diagnostic (symptomatic) cases *Prototype DBT system	NR (NR)	Jacknife alternative FROC[d] analysis (mean figure of merit) • DM + DBT (one view of each) 0.818 vs two-view DM 0.771 vs one-view (MLO) DBT 0.705 Combined DM + DBT higher summary accuracy vs two-view DM ($p < 0.05$); no difference found for other comparisons
Teertstra (2010)[t]	Clinical series of 513 subjects referred for work-up of abnormal screen or with symptoms, and followed-up for 2 years for incident cancer (112 incident BC); blinded reading of DBT and FFDM by one radiologist *Prototype DBT system	Mean 52 (range 29–92) years (2006–07)	FFDM vs DBT: 8 of 112 BC missed by each method; sensitivity 93% for each of FFDM and DBT Similar specificity: FFDM 86.1% vs DBT 84.4%
Gur et al. (2009)[u] (Gur et al., 2011)[v]	Test set (125 subjects: 35 BC, 90 no cancer) observer study, comparing *4 reading modalities*; read by 8 experienced radiologists. (Gur et al., 2011) was based on the same study-set but used different analytic methods)	NR (NR)	Overall (all readers) sensitivity and specificity pairs: • 2D-FFDM: 88%, 60% • Frames (11 projections)[d]: 89%, 60% • Reconstructed DBT: 93%, 64% • FFDM + DBT: 93%, 72% (Same study-set with FROC[d] analysis reported in 2011: combined FFDM + DBT improved accuracy index by an average 16% (95% CI: 7–26%; $p < 0.01$) over FFDM alone)

(*Continued*)

Table 13.2 Evidence on the Accuracy of Digital Breast Tomosynthesis (DBT) Compared to Standard Mammography (Continued)

The table updates and modifies a published overview from Houssami and Skaane [40].
The table summarizes the evidence on studies[a,c,e–v] that have used breast cancer-enriched sets of mammographic examinations to evaluate digital breast tomosynthesis (DBT) accuracy: these are mostly retrospective observer (reader) studies[a,c,f–i,m,o,s,u,v], or clinical series that included a mix of symptomatic and screen-recalled cases with known abnormalities[e,k,l,p,r,t] or investigated DBT in subjects recalled for work-up[j,n,q] on the basis of DM-positive[n,q] or film-screen mammography positive screens[j].BC, breast cancer; DBT, digital breast tomosynthesis; FFDM, full-field digital mammography; DM, digital mammography; MLO, mediolateral oblique; AUC, area under curve; ROC, receiver operating characteristic; 2D, 2-dimensional.
[a]*Gilbert FJ, Tucker L; Gillan MG; Willsher P; Cooke J; et al. Accuracy of Digital Breast Tomosynthesis for Depicting Breast Cancer Subgroups in a UK Retrospective Reading Study (TOMMY Trial). Radiology 2015; 277:697–706.*
[b]*Estimated area under curve (AUC) for multiple-reader multiple-case receiver operating characteristic (ROC) analysis (from data of all readers, averaged or pooled estimate of AUC—statistical methods varied between studies).*
[c]*Alakhras MM, Brennan PC, Rickard M, Bourne R, Mello-Thoms C. Effect of radiologists' experience on breast cancer detection and localization using digital breast tomosynthesis. Eur Radiol 2015;***25***: 402–9.*
[d]*The free-response receiver operating characteristic (FROC) method involves analysis of detection and location-specific data, and also the rating of each suspected abnormality, to give a summary (composite) accuracy index. The jackknife alternative free-response receiver operating characteristic (JAFROC) method uses a similar approach to calculate the mean figure of merit (FOM) which is also a summary measure of reader accuracy (further details of the exact FROC analytic methods applied are reported by Gur et al[v] and Svahn et al[s]).*
[e]*Morel JC, Iqbal A, Wasan RK, Peacock C, Evans DR, Rahim R, et al. The accuracy of digital breast tomosynthesis compared with coned compression magnification mammography in the assessment of abnormalities found on mammography. Clin Radiol 2014;***69***: 1112–6.*
[f]*Thibault F, Dromain C, Breucq C, Balleyguier CS, Malhaire C, Steyaert L, et al. Digital breast tomosynthesis versus mammography and breast ultrasound: a multireader performance study. Eur Radiol 2013;***23***: 2441–9.*
[g]*Rafferty EA, Park JM, Philpotts LE, Poplack SP, Sumkin JH, Halpern EF, et al. Assessing radiologist performance using combined digital mammography and breast tomosynthesis compared with digital mammography alone: results of a multicenter, multireader trial. Radiology 2013;***266***: 104–13.*
[h]*Rafferty EA, Park JM, Philpotts LE, Poplack SP, Sumkin JH, Halpern EF, et al. Diagnostic accuracy and recall rates for digital mammography and digital mammography combined with one-view and two-view tomosynthesis: results of an enriched reader study. AJR Am J Roentgenol 2014;***202***: 273–81.*
[i]*Wallis et al.[21]*
[j]*Michell MJ, Iqbal A, Wasan RK, Evans DR, Peacock C, Lawinski CP, et al. A comparison of the accuracy of film-screen mammography, full-field digital mammography, and digital breast tomosynthesis. Clin Radiol 2012;***67***: 976–81.*
[k]*Skaane P, Gullien R, Bjorndal H, Eben EB, Ekseth U, Haakenaasen U, et al. Digital breast tomosynthesis (DBT): initial experience in a clinical setting. Acta Radiol2012;***53***: 524–9.*
[l]*Svahn et al.[41]*
[m]*Gur D, Zuley ML, Anello MI, Rathfon GY, Chough DM, Ganott MA, Hakim CM, et al. Dose reduction in digital breast tomosynthesis (DBT) screening using synthetically reconstructed projection images: an observer performance study. Acad Radiol 2012;***19***: 166–71.*
[n]*Bernardi D, Ciatto S, Pellegrini M, Tuttobene P, Fanto C, Valentini M, et al. Prospective study of breast tomosynthesis as a triage to assessment in screening. Breast Cancer Res Treat 2012;***133***: 267–71.*
[o]*Noroozian M, Hadjiiski L, Rahnama-Moghadam S, Klein KA, Jeffries DO, Pinsky RW, et al. Digital breast tomosynthesis is comparable to mammographic spot views for mass characterization. Radiology 2012;***262***: 61–8.*
[p]*Svane et al.[20]*
[q]*Tagliafico A, Astengo D, Cavagnetto F, Rosasco R, Rescinito G, Monetti F, et al. One-to-one comparison between digital spot compression view and digital breast tomosynthesis. Eur Radiol 2012;***22***: 539–44.*
[r]*Gennaro G, Toledano A, di Maggio MC, Baldan E, Bezzon E, La Grassa M, et al. Digital breast tomosynthesis versus digital mammography: a clinical performance study. Eur Radiol 2010;***20***: 1545–53.*
[s]*Svahn T, Andersson I, Chakraborty D, Svensson S, Ikeda D, Fornvik D, et al. The diagnostic accuracy of dual-view digital mammography, single-view breast tomosynthesis and a dual-view combination of breast tomosynthesis and digital mammography in a free-response observer performance study. Radiat Prot Dosimetry 2010;***139***: 113–7.*
[t]*Teertstra et al.[18]*
[u]*Gur D, Abrams GS, Chough DM, Ganott MA, Hakim CM, Perrin RL, et al. Digital breast tomosynthesis: observer performance study. AJR Am J Roentgenol 2009;***193***: 586–91.*
[v]*Gur D, Bandos AI, Rockette HE, Zuley ML, Sumkin JH, Chough DM, et al. Localized detection and classification of abnormalities on FFDM and tomosynthesis examinations rated under an FROC paradigm. AJR Am J Roentgenol 2011;***196***: 737–41.*

Prospective screening trials with DBT

Three pivotal prospective trials embedded within organized population screening programs have provided key evidence on screen-detection measures for DBT. They are briefly described next and their main findings summarized in Table 13.3.

The STORM trial

The STORM (Screening with Tomosynthesis or Standard Mammography) trial, from Ciatto and colleagues,[42] was the first population-based prospective trial of DBT to report its final results and was the smallest of the three prospective trials (7292 screens). STORM investigated screen-reading in two *sequential* phases (DM-only and then integrated DM + DBT), and recruited asymptomatic women aged ≥48 years who had screening through two Italian services (Trento and Verona) in 2011–12. Double-reading was used to decide recall based on positive mammography at either screen-reading phase.[42]

The STORM study showed that standard DM alone and also DM + DBT detected 39 (of the 59) cancers identified at screening, but 20 additional cancers were detected only with DM + DBT compared with *none* detected at DM screen-reading ($p < 0.0001$). The estimated *incremental* cancer detection rate attributed to screening with DM + DBT was 2.7/1000 screens (95% CI: 1.7–4.2) which represented around one-third of the detected breast cancers in the trial's population. An extended analysis of the STORM trial factoring 12 months follow-up estimated an interval cancer rate of 0.82/1000 screens (95% CI: 0.30–1.79/1000) but the investigators acknowledged the uncertainty around this estimate and the limited follow-up.[43]

Data on FPR form STORM are summarized in Table 13.3 and show that the overall recall rate was 5.5% (95% CI: 5.0–6.0), of which more FPR were due to DM-alone screen-reading than those caused by adding DBT. The trial estimated that *conditional* recall (see Table 13.3) could have *reduced* FPR rates by approximately 17% however it should be noted that approximately 1% of false-positive screens were caused by adding DBT to screening.[42]

The Oslo trial (OTST)

The OTST from Skaane and colleagues,[44] aimed to enroll 25,000 women aged 50–69 years from a population-based screening program in Oslo, Norway. The study had four arms using different screen-reading strategies: conventional two-view DM (2D); conventional DM plus computer-aided detection (2D + CAD); conventional DM plus two-view tomosynthesis (2D + 3D); and synthesized 2D plus tomosynthesis resulting in 2Dsynthetic + 3D. Several publications based on interim results of the OTST report different comparisons in this four-arm study. The interim results of the OTST that reported data on 2Dsynthetic + 3D are discussed earlier in this chapter.[24]

In the published interim analysis comparing single-reading of 2D with single-reading of 2D + 3D, which included 12,631 women, cancer detection rates, including invasive and in situ cancers, were 6.1 per 1000 examinations for DM and 8.0 per 1000 examinations for DM + DBT (data are summarized in Table 13.3). This corresponds to an incremental increase in cancer detection of 1.9/1000 women screened or 27% increase (adjusted for reader; $p = 0.001$). There was a 15% decrease in FPR *before* arbitration with 61.1 per 1000 examinations with mammography alone and 53.1 per 1000 examinations with mammography plus tomosynthesis (adjusted for reader; $p < 0.001$).[44] Because the study had multiple arms (which could "add up" to increased overall recall across all arms) the investigators focused their FPR results on prearbitration estimates.

Table 13.3 Studies Evaluating 3D-Mammography (Digital Breast Tomosynthesis) for Population Breast Screening

	Study Characteristics		Breast Cancer Detection		Recall Measures	
First Author, Year Published	**Study Design (Number of Screens)**	**Screen-Reading Practice & Context**	**Cancer Detection Rates (CDR)/1000 Screens**	**Absolute Effect of 3D[a] on CDR Compared to 2D-alone**	**Recall Rates (Overall Recall, False-Positive (FP) Data Where Specified)**	**Absolute Effect of 3D[a] on FPR Compared to 2D-Alone**
Prospective Trials Embedded in Population Breast Screening Programs						
Ciatto et al. (2013) (STORM trial) *Lancet Oncol*[b]	Prospective trial (7292) in Italian screening program, comparing 2D and integrated 2D/3D screening (sequential read of each screen)	Sequential read of 2D then 2D/3D; independent double-reading, recall by either reader at either read; population-based program	2D: 5.3 2D/3D: 8.1 $p < 0.001$	↑2.7/1000	Recall for 2D-alone *or* 2D/3D: 5.5% Recall *conditional* to 2D/3D-positive: 3.5%	(Estimated not actual) ↓2.0%[c]
Houssami et al. (2014) (STORM 12-month follow-up) *Eur J Cancer*[d]	Extended analysis of STORM trial (7292) comparing several screening strategies (single or double-reading) with follow-up for year-1 *interval cancers*		2D double-read 5.3 vs 2D/3D single-read 7.5; $p < 0.001$ (reports other comparisons)	↑2.2/1000	(Modeling of recall data from STORM trial, various comparisons reported)	(Estimated not actual) ↓1.2%[c]
Skaane et al. (2013)$_A$ (*Interim* report Oslo trial) *Radiology*[e]	Prospective trial (12,631) in Norwegian screening program, comparing 2D and 2D/3D screening (study has four arms to compare different strategies)	Four reading arms (2 readers per arm): independent double-reading with arbitration; population-based program	2D: 6.1 2D/3D: 8.0 (reader-adjusted) $p = 0.001$	↑1.9/1000	2D: 6.1% 2D/3D: 5.3% (15% decrease of FR, adjusted for reader; $p < 0.001$)	↓0.8%
Skaane et al. (2013)$_B$ *Eur Radiol*[f]	Interim analysis from the Oslo trial based on double-reading		Double-reading 2D: 7.1 2D/3D: 9.4 $p < 0.001$	↑2.3/1000	FP scores (prearbitration) 2D: 10.3% 2D/3D: 8.5% $p < 0.001$ Overall recall rate (after arbitration): 2D: 2.9% 3D: 3.7% $p < 0.05$	↓1.8% of FP scores but increased *overall* recall rate by 0.8%
Lång et al. (2016) (*Interim* report MBTST)[g] *Eur Radiol*[h]	Prospective trial (7500 in interim analysis) random sample invited in Swedish screening program: 2D (two views) vs stand-alone one-view 3D-mammography (DBT)[g]	Independent double-reads; population-based program	2D (two-view): 6.3 3D (one-view): 8.9[g] $p < 0.0001$	↑2.6/1000	Overall recall rate (after arbitration): 2D: 2.6% 3D: 3.8% $p < 0.0001$	↑0.9%

(*Continued*)

Table 13.3 Studies Evaluating 3D-Mammography (Digital Breast Tomosynthesis) for Population Breast Screening (Continued)

	Study Characteristics		Breast Cancer Detection		Recall Measures	
First Author, Year Published	**Study Design (Number of Screens)**	**Screen-Reading Practice & Context**	**Cancer Detection Rates (CDR)/1000 Screens**	**Absolute Effect of 3D[a] on CDR Compared to 2D-alone**	**Recall Rates (Overall Recall, False-Positive (FP) Data Where Specified)**	**Absolute Effect of 3D[a] on FPR Compared to 2D-Alone**
Retrospective Evaluations in Hospital-Based Imaging or Breast Services and/or Community-Based Radiology Services						
Rose et al. (2013) *AJR*[i]	Retrospective: before vs after (13,856 vs 9499) introduction of 3D as adjunct to 2D screening	Single-reading; readers from several radiology services, United States	2D: 4.0 2D/3D: 5.4; $p = 0.18$ *For Invasive cancer* 2D: 2.8 2D/3D: 4.3; $p = 0.07$	↑1.4/1000 (NS)	Overall recall 2D: 8.7% 2D/3D: 5.5% $p < 0.001$	↓3.2%
Haas et al. (2013) *Radioogy*[j]	Retrospective: services using 2D vs services using 2D/3D (7058 vs 6100) in same year.	Single-reading; readers from breast or radiology services, United States	2D: 5.2 2D/3D: 5.7; $p = 0.70$	↑0.5/1000 (NS)	Overall recall 2D: 12.0% 2D/3D: 8.4%; $p < 0.01$	↓3.6%
Friedewald et al. (2014) *JAMA*[k]	Retrospective: before vs after (281,187 vs 173,663) introduction of 3D as adjunct to 2D mammography screening	Single-reading; readers from 13 radiology services, Unites States	2D: 4.2 2D/3D: 5.4; $p < 0.001$ *For Invasive ca* 2D: 2.9 2D/3D: 4.1; $p < 0.001$	↑1.2/1000 ↑1.2/1000	Overall recall 2D: 10.7% 2D/3D: 9.1%; $p < 0.001$	↓1.6%
Greenberg et al. (2014) *AJR*[l]	Retrospective: women opting for 3D vs 2D (23,149 vs 54,684) mammography screening, concurrent groups	Single-reading; readers from several radiology or imaging services, United States	2D: 4.9 2D/3D: 6.3; $p = 0.035$	↑1.3/1000 (adjusted)	Overall recall 2D: 16.2% 2D/3D: 13.6%; $p < 0.001$	↓2.6%
McCarthy et al. (2014) *JNCI*[m]	Retrospective: before vs after (15,571 vs 10,728) introduction of 3D as adjunct to 2D mammography screening	Single-reading; several readers from one imaging service, United States	2D: 4.6 2D/3D: 5.5; $p = 0.32$	↑0.9/1000 (NS)	Overall recall 2D: 10.4% 2D/3D: 8.8%; $p < 0.001$	↓1.6%

Durand et al. (2015) *Radiology* (overlaps with Haas 2013)[n]	Retrospective: women who received 2D/3D vs those who received 2D[o] (8591 vs 9364) based on 3D availability across services or patients' preference	Single-reading; readers from several radiology or imaging services, United States	2D: 5.7 2D/3D: 5.9; $p = 0.88$	↑0.2/1000 (NS)	Overall recall 2D: 12.3 2D/3D: 7.8; $p < 0.001$	↓4.5%
Lourenco et al. (2015) *Radiology*[p]	Retrospective: before vs after (12,577 vs 12,921) introduction of 3D as adjunct to 2D mammography screening	Single-reading; several readers at one imaging service, United States	2D: 5.4 2D/3D: 4.6; $p = 0.44$	↓0.8/1000 (NS)	Overall recall 2D: 9.3 2D/3D: 6.4; $p < 0.001$	↓2.9%

Key: ↑*refers to increase;* ↓ *refers to decrease; 2D refers to digital mammography acquisition of two-view mammographic images, 3D refers to digital breast tomosynthesis acquisitions for two-views except where otherwise specified (see Lång et al., 2016).NS, not statistically different; STORM, Screening with Tomosynthesis or Mammography trial; MBTST, Malmo Breast Tomosynthesis Screening Trial.*

[a] *3D refers to 3D as adjunct to 2D except for the study from Lång et al. (2016) which reported data for 3D-alone.*

[b] *Ciatto et al.*[42]

[c] *Decrease in FPR achieved only if recall conditional to 3D-positivity (analytic estimate, not actual rate achieved in trial).*

[d] *Houssami et al.*[43]

[e] *Skaane et al.*[44]

[f] *Skaane et al.*[45]

[g] *Study from Lång et al. (2016) (MBTST) is the only study reporting screen-detection metrics for 3D-alone versus 2D (all other studies in evidence table compare 2D + 3D vs 2D).*

[h] *Lang et al.*[46]

[i] *Rose et al.*[51]

[j] *Haas et al.*[49]

[k] *Friedewald et al.*[47]

[l] *Greenberg et al.*[48]

[m] *McCarthy et al.*[53]

[n] *Durand et al.*[52]

[o] *Durand (2015): Age, breast density, and risk factor (including personal history of BC) distribution differed between the group who had 2D/3D and the grp who had 2D-only.*

[p] *Lourenco et al.*[50]

In a further report of the OTST interim analysis (Table 13.3), comparing double-reading strategies as commonly practiced in European programs, the incremental cancer detection attributed to adding 3D to 2D was 2.3 per 1000 screening examinations. As also given in Table 13.3, the absolute increase in overall recall rate *after* arbitration was 0.8%. The recall rates *after* arbitration increased in the OTST with double-reading (2.9% for mammography compared to 3.7%, $p < 0.05$ for the combination mode), comprising a relative increase of both true- and false-positive cases.[45]

The Malmö trial (MBTST)

The Malmö Breast Tomosynthesis Screening Trial (MBTST) enrolled 15,000 women aged 40–74 years, 2010–15. In contrast to STORM and OTST, the investigators of the MBTST explored the possibility of using one-view tomosynthesis (MLO) alone in screening, with the aim of enhancing translation of 3D-screening by reducing the burden of both reading time and radiation exposure. A paired study design was used, with 15,000 women randomly selected from the population-based screening program in the city of Malmö, Sweden. At one screening occasion, the women had both a single-view DBT and a two-view screening DM. The trial had two independent reading arms with double-reading for DM and DBT, respectively.[46]

The interim analysis of the first 7500 women screened in the MBTST showed that 67 women were detected with breast cancer in Reading arm DBT and 47 in Reading arm DM, respectively.[46] Of these, 46 cancer cases were detected in both reading arms. Hence, 21 cancer cases were detected by DBT alone and one cancer by DM alone. The detection rate for DBT versus DM was 8.9 per 1000 screens (95% CI: 6.9–11.3) versus 6.3 per 1000 screens (4.6–8.3), respectively. This corresponds to an *incremental* increase in cancer detection of 2.6 per 1000 women screened with one-view DBT compared to DM or a 43% relative increase (95% CI: 21–68; $p < 0.0001$), see also Table 13.3. All cancers found with DBT were detected in the first reading step, that is, by DBT alone.

Table 13.3 also summarizes the FPR of the MBSTS. The recall rate after arbitration for DBT and DM was 3.8% (95% CI: 3.3–4.2) and 2.6% (2.3–3.0), respectively. The positive predictive value after arbitration was 24% (67/282) for DBT as well as for DM (47/197). The final results from the MBTST are expected in 2016/17 including data on interval cancer rates.

Nonprospective screening studies

Several retrospective studies have taken place in the United States, studying the effect of adding two-view tomosynthesis to mammography. The retrospective studies have limitations in that they compare different cohorts or timeframes and therefore there may be differences in the groups of women compared that account for the different findings on screen-detection using DBT. A summary of the studies and their findings are listed in Table 13.3. In contrast to the prospective trials, the majority of the retrospective studies did not show a statistically significant increase in cancer detection rate,[47–53] although cancer detection rates were generally improved using DBT in all but one study.[50] Two of the retrospective studies, Friedewald et al.[47] and Greenberg et al.,[48] reported a significant increase in cancer detection rates attributed to DBT. It is worth noting that McCarthy et al. found that DBT significantly increased cancer detection in women aged younger than 50 years (2.2 for DM vs 5.7 for DM + DBT; $p = 0.02$).[53]

The retrospective studies all showed decreased recall rates, although it is important to consider that the recall rates in the United States are higher than the recommended standards for European programs (where the prospective trials were performed), and that all were based on single-reading. In Europe, the recall rate is recommended to be below 7% at prevalence screening and below 5% in incidence screening (women with prior screening examinations).[54] In the United States, the recall rate is typically higher than in Europe, and is recommended not to exceed 12%.[55] Therefore, it seems likely that the effect of DBT on false recall rates will vary according to the magnitude of FPR at "baseline" 2D-mammography and according to the reading strategy.

WHAT EVIDENCE IS NEEDED BEFORE WE CHANGE A SCREENING MODALITY?

The evolution of breast cancer screening from analog to DM was gradual but inevitable in the digital era, once it had been proven that the performance of SFM and FFDM was at least equal. Also, of importance, health economic evaluation supports that mammography screening can be cost-effective among women 50–69 years of age in countries with a high incidence of breast cancer.[14]

With DBT now emerging as a new (third) player in breast cancer population screening, history seems to be repeating itself: the same issues previously raised regarding SFM versus FFDM (eg, the ability to detect microcalcifications, or conflicting data on recall rates), come up again. In the initial phase of evaluating a new screening technique, it is always difficult to judge what the true effect would be in real life (service screening) in contrast to what was shown in trials. Because in initial trials a new technique has an inherent disadvantage due to the fact that radiologists have a learning curve and long experience with the "conventional" technique, and the further limitation of "no prior DBT" screens to compare with, this could underestimate the effect of the new technique. On the other hand, pioneering trials often include the expertise of early adopters, and frequently represent prevalent screening, both of which could overestimate the effect of the new technique. There is no doubt that DBT significantly increases breast cancer detection, at least in the first screening round, that is, the prevalence screen. So far, there are no reported data on repeated screens with DBT and hence no information on cancer detection at incidence screens with DBT, but we should expect the detection rate to be somewhat lower.[56] The most important question, however, is whether the increased breast cancer detection with DBT actually translates into reduced breast cancer mortality or is merely contributing to overdetection of indolent cancers. None of the current prospective trials were powered or designed for assessment of breast cancer mortality, since they are detection studies. For this purpose, very large RCTs would be needed and with long follow-up, since the expected difference in breast cancer mortality for women screened with FFDM compared to DBT would be modest. Such RCTs are unlikely to ever be performed, and recommendations around DBT screening are unlikely to wait for another decade or longer, hence, alternate approaches are needed.

A way to indirectly get information on the potential of DBT screening to have an effect on mortality is through assessing its impact on meaningful surrogate (intermediate) screening outcomes, such as interval cancer rates.[57] If DBT increases breast cancer detection rates, and subsequently *reduces* interval cancer rates in those who had DBT screening (compared to a contemporary DM screened population) then it could be reasonably inferred that DBT is detecting relevant cancers and is likely to extend screening benefit.

The recently published summary paper "Breast-Cancer Screening—Viewpoint of the IARC Working Group" concludes that there is no evidence around mortality effect or reduction on interval cancers from DBT screening published so far.[14] However, new data are awaited and expected in the near future, such as the full reports from the OTST and MBTST, including estimates for interval cancer rates. Furthermore, it seems likely that the OTST and the STORM trials will have subpopulations that continue screening with second rounds of DBT which may provide data for repeat DBT screening.

Last, but not least, health economic evaluations of population screening with DBT are of great importance and will be essential to inform future recommendations on DBT screening. A simulation modeling study, using input parameters from several sources including the Breast Cancer Surveillance Consortium and the Oslo trial, reported that adding DBT to FFDM approaches the cost-effectiveness threshold for US women aged 50–74 with dense breasts.[58] This study estimated that in this population of women, adding DBT would avert 0.5 breast cancer deaths after 12 screening rounds.[58] Health-economic analyses conducted as part of screening trials would provide more robust evidence, and are anticipated from the MBTST which has integrated cost-effectiveness evaluation as part of the study.

ADVANCED IMAGING MODALITIES

New imaging modalities are under investigation for breast cancer detection (see also chapter: Screening for Breast Cancer in Women with Dense Breasts): ultrasound, 3D automated ultrasound, contrast enhanced mammography, spectral mammography, scintimammography, breast computered tomography, optical imaging, and dedicated breast positron emission tomography to mention some. There is also great interest in magnetic resonance imaging (MRI). Several of the techniques not only provide structural (anatomical) information, but also functional and molecular information[59] giving information on the expression and activity of specific molecules which may help visualize tumor heterogeneities regarding, for example, aggressiveness and prognosis and also in treatment surveillance. Since a screening test needs to be not just accurate but also fast and not too expensive, several of these techniques have drawbacks, for example, requiring use of intravenous contrast agents and having long examination times. As the IARC group indicated, there is at present no evidence supporting use of breast imaging technologies for population breast screening other than mammography.[14]

CONCLUSION

The technical evolution of mammographic imaging has taken great leaps since the introduction of mammography screening. The shift from SFM to FFDM is now definitive and relies on the fact that the diagnostic accuracy is at least similar and brings the efficiencies of the digital era. Regarding the use of DBT for population screening, either stand-alone or in combination with DM or synthetic 2D reconstructed from the DBT acquisition, the evidence is promising and is emerging quickly. Nonetheless, despite the evidence that DBT improves screen-detection metrics, the data from published studies are heterogeneous and the evidence on screening benefit is limited. Extended data from trials with DBT screening are expected in the near future and could provide key evidence on screening outcomes at follow-up of women screened with DBT.

LIST OF ACRONYMS AND ABBREVIATIONS

2D Two-dimensional
3D Three-dimensional
CC Craniocaudal

DBT	Digital breast tomosynthesis
DCIS	Ductal cancer in situ
DM	Digital mammography
DMIST	Digital Mammography Imaging Screening Trial
FFDM	Full-field digital mammography
FPR	False-positive rate
IARC	International Agency for Research on Cancer
JAFROC	Jacknife Alternative Free-Response Receiver Operating Characteristics
MBTST	Malmö Breast Tomosynthesis Screening Trial
MLO	Mediolateral oblique
MRI	Magnetic resonance imaging
OTST	Oslo Tomosynthesis Screening Trial
RCT	Randomized controlled trial
STORM	Screening with Tomosynthesis OR standard Mammography Trial
US	United States

REFERENCES

1. Pisano ED, Yaffe M. Digital mammography. *Breast Dis* 1998;**10**(3–4):127–35.
2. Fischer U, Hermann KP, Baum F. Digital mammography: current state and future aspects. *Eur Radiol* 2006;**16**(1):38–44.
3. Pisano ED, Yaffe MJ. Digital mammography. *Radiology* 2005;**234**(2):353–62.
4. Garrison JB, Grant DG, Guier WH, Johns RJ. Three dimensional roentgenography. *Am J Roentgenol Radium Ther Nucl Med* 1969;**105**(4):903–8.
5. Grant DG. Tomosynthesis: a three-dimensional radiographic imaging technique. *IEEE Trans Biomed Eng* 1972;**19**(1):20–8.
6. Dobbins III JT. Tomosynthesis imaging: at a translational crossroads. *Med Phys* 2009;**36**(6):1956–67.
7. Niklason LT, Christian BT, Niklason LE, Kopans DB, Castleberry DE, Opsahl-Ong BH, et al. Digital tomosynthesis in breast imaging. *Radiology* 1997;**205**(2):399–406.
8. Tingberg A. X-ray tomosynthesis: a review of its use for breast and chest imaging. *Radiat Prot Dosimetry* 2010;**139**(1-3):100–7.
9. Helvie MA. Digital mammography imaging: breast tomosynthesis and advanced applications. *Radiol Clin North Am* 2010;**48**(5):917–29.
10. Baldwin P. Digital breast tomosynthesis. *Radiol Technol* 2009;**81**(1):57M–74M.
11. Sechopoulos I. A review of breast tomosynthesis. Part I. The image acquisition process. *Med Phys* 2013;**40**(1):014301.
12. Dobbins III JT, Godfrey DJ. Digital X-ray tomosynthesis: current state of the art and clinical potential. *Phys Med Biol* 2003;**48**(19) R65-106.
13. Sechopoulos I. A review of breast tomosynthesis. Part II. Image reconstruction, processing and analysis, and advanced applications. *Med Phys* 2013;**40**(1):014302.
14. Lauby-Secretan B, Scoccianti C, Loomis D, Benbrahim-Tallaa L, Bouvard V, Bianchini F, et al. Breast-Cancer Screening—Viewpoint of the IARC Working Group. *N Engl J Med* 2015.
15. Rafferty EA. Digital mammography: novel applications. *Radiol Clin North Am* 2007;**45**(5):831–43. vii.
16. Poplack SP, Tosteson TD, Kogel CA, Nagy HM. Digital breast tomosynthesis: initial experience in 98 women with abnormal digital screening mammography. *AJR Am J Roentgenol* 2007;**189**(3):616–23.

17. Spangler ML, Zuley ML, Sumkin JH, Abrams G, Ganott MA, Hakim C, et al. Detection and classification of calcifications on digital breast tomosynthesis and 2D digital mammography: a comparison. *AJR Am J Roentgenol* 2011;**196**(2):320–4.
18. Teertstra HJ, Loo CE, van den Bosch MA, van Tinteren H, Rutgers EJ, Muller SH, et al. Breast tomosynthesis in clinical practice: initial results. *Eur Radiol* 2010;**20**(1):16–24.
19. Kopans D, Gavenonis S, Halpern E, Moore R. Calcifications in the breast and digital breast tomosynthesis. *Breast J* 2011;**17**(6):638–44.
20. Svane G, Azavedo E, Lindman K, Urech M, Nilsson J, Weber N, et al. Clinical experience of photon counting breast tomosynthesis: comparison with traditional mammography. *Acta Radiol* 2011;**52**(2):134–42.
21. Wallis MG, Moa E, Zanca F, Leifland K, Danielsson M. Two-view and single-view tomosynthesis versus full-field digital mammography: high-resolution X-ray imaging observer study. *Radiology* 2012;**262**(3):788–96.
22. Andersson I, Ikeda DM, Zackrisson S, eRuschin M, Svahn T, Timberg P, et al. Breast tomosynthesis and digital mammography: a comparison of breast cancer visibility and BIRADS classification in a population of cancers with subtle mammographic findings. *Eur Radiol* 2008;**18**(12):2817–25.
23. Tagliafico A, Mariscotti G, Durando M, Stevanin C, Tagliafico G, Martino L, et al. Characterisation of microcalcification clusters on 2D digital mammography (FFDM) and digital breast tomosynthesis (DBT): does DBT underestimate microcalcification clusters? Results of a multicentre study. *Eur Radiol* 2015;**25**(1): 9–14.
24. Skaane P, Bandos AI, Eben EB, Jebsen IN, Krager M, Haakenaasen U, et al. Two-view digital breast tomosynthesis screening with synthetically reconstructed projection images: comparison with digital breast tomosynthesis with full-field digital mammographic images. *Radiology* 2014;**271**(3):655–63.
25. Lewin JM, Hendrick RE, D'Orsi CJ, Isaacs PK, Moss LJ, Karellas A, et al. Comparison of full-field digital mammography with screen-film mammography for cancer detection: results of 4,945 paired examinations. *Radiology* 2001;**218**(3):873–80.
26. Skaane P, Skjennald A, Young K, Egge E, Jebsen I, Sager EM, et al. Follow-up and final results of the Oslo I Study comparing screen-film mammography and full-field digital mammography with soft-copy reading. *Acta Radiol* 2005;**46**(7):679–89.
27. Skaane P. Studies comparing screen-film mammography and full-field digital mammography in breast cancer screening: updated review. *Acta Radiol* 2009;**50**(1):3–14.
28. Pisano ED, Gatsonis C, Hendrick E, Yaffe M, Baum JK, Acharyya S, et al. Diagnostic performance of digital versus film mammography for breast-cancer screening. *N Engl J Med* 2005;**353**(17):1773–83.
29. Heddson B, Ronnow K, Olsson M, Miller D. Digital versus screen-film mammography: a retrospective comparison in a population-based screening program. *Eur J Radiol* 2007;**64**(3):419–25.
30. Del Turco MR, Mantellini P, Ciatto S, Bonardi R, Martinelli F, Lazzari B, et al. Full-field digital versus screen-film mammography: comparative accuracy in concurrent screening cohorts. *AJR Am J Roentgenol* 2007;**189**(4):860–6.
31. Vigeland E, Klaasen H, Klingen TA, Hofvind S, Skaane P. Full-field digital mammography compared to screen film mammography in the prevalent round of a population-based screening programme: the Vestfold County Study. *Eur Radiol* 2008;**18**(1):183–91.
32. Vinnicombe S, Pinto Pereira SM, McCormack VA, Shiel S, Perry N, Dos Santos Silva IM. Full-field digital versus screen-film mammography: comparison within the UK breast screening program and systematic review of published data. *Radiology* 2009;**251**(2):347–58.
33. Sala M, Comas M, Macia F, Martinez J, Casamitjana M, Castells X. Implementation of digital mammography in a population-based breast cancer screening program: effect of screening round on recall rate and cancer detection. *Radiology* 2009;**252**(1):31–9.
34. Karssemeijer N, Bluekens AM, Beijerinck D, Deurenberg JJ, Beekman M, Visser R, et al. Breast cancer screening results 5 years after introduction of digital mammography in a population-based screening program. *Radiology* 2009;**253**(2):353–8.

35. Hambly NM, McNicholas MM, Phelan N, Hargaden GC, O'Doherty A, Flanagan FL. Comparison of digital mammography and screen-film mammography in breast cancer screening: a review in the Irish breast screening program. *AJR Am J Roentgenol* 2009;**193**(4):1010–8.
36. Van Ongeval C, Van Steen A, Vande Putte G, Zanca F, Bosmans H, Marchal G, et al. Does digital mammography in a decentralized breast cancer screening program lead to screening performance parameters comparable with film-screen mammography? *Eur Radiol* 2010;**20**(10):2307–14.
37. Skaane P, Hofvind S, Skjennald A. Randomized trial of screen-film versus full-field digital mammography with soft-copy reading in population-based screening program: follow-up and final results of Oslo II study. *Radiology* 2007;**244**(3):708–17.
38. Houssami N, Ciatto S. The evolving role of new imaging methods in breast screening. *Prev Med* 2011;**53**(3):123–6.
39. Tingberg A, Zackrisson S. Digital mammography and tomosynthesis for breast cancer diagnosis. *Expert Opin Med Diagn* 2011;**5**(6):517–26.
40. Houssami N, Skaane P. Overview of the evidence on digital breast tomosynthesis in breast cancer detection. *Breast* 2013;**22**(2):101–8.
41. Svahn TM, Chakraborty DP, Ikeda D, Zackrisson S, Do Y, Mattsson S, et al. Breast tomosynthesis and digital mammography: a comparison of diagnostic accuracy. *Br J Radiol* 2012;**85**(1019):e1074–82.
42. Ciatto S, Houssami N, Bernardi D, Caumo F, Pellegrini M, Brunelli S, et al. Integration of 3D digital mammography with tomosynthesis for population breast-cancer screening (STORM): a prospective comparison study. *Lancet Oncol* 2013;**14**(7):583–9.
43. Houssami N, Macaskill P, Bernardi D, Caumo F, Pellegrini M, Brunelli S, et al. Breast screening using 2D-mammography or integrating digital breast tomosynthesis (3D-mammography) for single-reading or double-reading—evidence to guide future screening strategies. *Eur J Cancer* 2014;**50**(10):1799–807.
44. Skaane P, Bandos AI, Gullien R, Eben EB, Haakenaasen U, Izadi M, et al. Comparison of digital mammography alone and digital mammography plus tomosynthesis in a population-based screening program. *Radiology* 2013;**267**(1):47–56.
45. Skaane P, Bandos AI, Gullien R, Eben EB, Ekseth U, Haakenaasen U, et al. Prospective trial comparing full-field digital mammography (FFDM) versus combined FFDM and tomosynthesis in a population-based screening programme using independent double reading with arbitration. *Eur Radiol* 2013;**23**(8):2061–71.
46. Lång K, Andersson I, Rosso A, Tingberg A, Timberg P, Zackrisson S. Performance of one-view breast tomosynthesis as a stand-alone breast cancer screening modality: results from the Malmo Breast Tomosynthesis Screening Trial, a population-based study. *Eur Radiol* 2016;**26**(1):184–190.
47. Friedewald SM, Rafferty EA, Rose SL, Durand MA, Plecha DM, Greenberg JS, et al. Breast cancer screening using tomosynthesis in combination with digital mammography. *JAMA* 2014;**311**(24):2499–507.
48. Greenberg JS, Javitt MC, Katzen J, Michael S, Holland AE. Clinical performance metrics of 3D digital breast tomosynthesis compared with 2D digital mammography for breast cancer screening in community practice. *AJR Am J Roentgenol* 2014;**203**(3):687–93.
49. Haas BM, Kalra V, Geisel J, Raghu M, Durand M, Philpotts LE. Comparison of tomosynthesis plus digital mammography and digital mammography alone for breast cancer screening. *Radiology* 2013;**269**(3):694–700.
50. Lourenco AP, Barry-Brooks M, Baird GL, Tuttle A, Mainiero MB. Changes in recall type and patient treatment following implementation of screening digital breast tomosynthesis. *Radiology* 2015;**274**(2):337–42.
51. Rose SL, Tidwell AL, Bujnoch LJ, Kushwaha AC, Nordmann AS, Sexton Jr. R. Implementation of breast tomosynthesis in a routine screening practice: an observational study. *AJR Am J Roentgenol* 2013;**200**(6):1401–8.
52. Durand MA, Haas BM, Yao X, Geisel JL, Raghu M, Hooley RJ, et al. Early clinical experience with digital breast tomosynthesis for screening mammography. *Radiology* 2015;**274**(1):85–92.
53. McCarthy AM, Kontos D, Synnestvedt M, Tan KS, Heitjan DF, Schnall M, et al. Screening outcomes following implementation of digital breast tomosynthesis in a general-population screening program. *J Natl Cancer Inst* 2014;**106**(11). Available from: http://dx.doi.org/10.1093/jnci/dju316.

54. Perry N, Broeders M, de Wolf C, Törnberg S, Holland R, von Karsa L. European guidelines for quality assurance in breast cancer screening and diagnosis. Fourth edition—summary document. *Ann Oncol* 2008;**19**(4):614–22.
55. Seidenwurm D, Rosenberg R. Breast cancer screening with tomosynthesis and digital mammography. *JAMA* 2014;**312**(16):1695.
56. Houssami N. Digital breast tomosynthesis (3D-mammography) screening: data and implications for population screening. *Expert Rev Med Devices* 2015;**12**(4):377–9.
57. Barratt A. Overdiagnosis in mammography screening: a 45 year journey from shadowy idea to acknowledged reality. *BMJ* 2015;**350**:h867.
58. Lee CI, Cevik M, Alagoz O, Sprague BL, Tosteson AN, Miglioretti DL, et al. Comparative effectiveness of combined digital mammography and tomosynthesis screening for women with dense breasts. *Radiology* 2015;**274**(3):772–80.
59. Alcantara D, Leal MP, Garcia-Bocanegra I, Garcia-Martin ML. Molecular imaging of breast cancer: present and future directions. *Front Chem* 2014;**2**:112.
60. Sartor H, Borgquist S, Hartman L, Olsson A, Jawdat F, Zackrisson S. Do mammographic tumor features in breast cancer relate to breast density and invasiveness, tumor size, and axillary lymph node involvement? *Acta Radiol* 2015;**56**(5):536–44.

CHAPTER

ETHICAL AND SOCIETAL CONSIDERATIONS IN BREAST CANCER SCREENING

14

Lisa M. Parker and Stacy M. Carter

Centre for Values, Ethics and the Law in Medicine (VELiM), The University of Sydney, Sydney, NSW, Australia

CHAPTER OUTLINE

PLAIN LANGUAGE SUMMARY

Breast screening is a large public health program with a significant reach. It is shaped by existing patterns of acting and reasoning, and challenges us to think differently about society and ethics.

Social attitudes about the breast affect attitudes toward breast cancer. The symbolism of the breast (motherhood, sexuality) means breast cancer is a highly emotive issue and breast screening is a popular

Breast Cancer Screening. DOI: http://dx.doi.org/10.1016/B978-0-12-802209-2.00014-0

media story. This may contribute to the popularity of breast screening. Screening may, in turn, affect social attitudes about breast cancer via its contribution toward increasing public familiarity with this disease. Breast screening has arisen within the context of (and may have contributed toward) increasing tendencies in society to place responsibility for health upon individuals, and to be aware of and averse to risks. Similarly, breast screening has arisen within and may have contributed toward a biomedical culture that exhibits strong support for early detection of cancer, technological innovation, and evidence-based medicine. Breast screening is a powerful public health institution. Part of its success may be due to key stakeholders having multiple reasons to support and promote its continuation, strong breast cancer advocacy, and political popularity.

There are several ethical principles relevant to breast screening. There are debates over the extent to which breast screening respects these principles, and over how to prioritize principles in order to deliver the most ethically justifiable program.

Breast screening should deliver benefits, avoid delivering harms where possible, and should deliver more benefits than harms. It seems likely that breast screening reduces population breast cancer mortality in women aged 50–69 years and delivers a range of harms, but there are debates about the extent and significance of each of these consequences. Benefits and harms appear to be closely balanced. Involving consumers at various levels may help with comparing benefits and harms, and negotiating between principles. Breast screening should deliver the most benefits possible within the resources available. The cost-effectiveness of breast screening compared to other healthcare expenditure is controversial, and cost-effectiveness arguments relating to participation rates may be problematic. Breast screening should respect and support individual autonomy: facilitating informed choice is an important part of this. There is disagreement over the impact of informed choice policies on costs and participation rates, and over how much this matters. Breast screening communications with consumers should be honest, and decision-making procedures should be transparent and just. Breast screening policies may be biased if decision-makers have vested interests, including professional interests. Honest communications may be facilitated by removing participation targets or using independent experts. Vested interests could be declared, or managed by excluding conflicted parties from decision-making. Breast screening should operate justly, providing fair screening opportunities, and achieving fair breast cancer and general health outcomes. Implications of the principles of reciprocity and solidarity for breast screening remain complex and caution is warranted. Like any public health program, breast screening inevitably has social and ethical implications: we suggest these will become increasingly central in future policy and practice.

INTRODUCTION

In this chapter we consider the social and ethical dimensions of breast screening. Breast screening is grounded in science, but it is also part of society. Like any large-scale public health program, breast screening exists in a two-way relationship with the society in which it is located, being subject to the values and conventions of that society,[1,2] but also influencing future social attitudes, values, and practices.[3] We will look at the many ways in which social structures and conventions, and moral and ethical thinking, interact with breast screening policies and practices. Our discussion is in two main sections. First we consider social aspects of breast screening: societal attitudes and ideas that influence or are influenced by breast screening. Second we examine ethical aspects: considerations about right and wrong with regard to breast screening.

SOCIAL ASPECTS OF BREAST SCREENING

Social norms and structures interact with breast screening in many ways. They may act as facilitators or barriers to the implementation of and public participation in breast screening, and may themselves be influenced by breast screening policies and practices. Below we discuss key aspects of the interactions between society and breast screening, focusing on those that have been most studied and discussed in academic and lay literature.

SOCIAL ATTITUDES TOWARD BREASTS AND BREAST CANCER

Breast screening is influenced by more general social norms and values regarding the breast itself. Because the breast is associated with sexuality and motherhood,[4] disease and treatment of this organ is highly emotive and associated with particular fear and anxiety.[5] Women may feel embarrassed about breast disease, and hesitate to seek medical attention for breast symptoms. Breasts, particularly youthful looking breasts, are a popular topic for the media, raising the profile of breast cancer higher than might be expected from its medical impact alone and higher than for any other cancer.[6,7] This media coverage is an important source of information for many women[8] but is also skewed toward reporting breast cancer in young and attractive women,[9] despite breast cancer incidence being much higher in older women.[8,10]

Many authors have suggested that both breast screening itself, and public communication encouraging women to participate in screening, have changed the way that breast cancer is understood in society, and may also have changed the profile of the disease itself. Most authors agree that the introduction of screening has coincided with a sharp and sustained increase in breast cancer incidence and prevalence. The rise in incidence may be at least partly due to overdiagnosis.[10,11] Similarly the rise in prevalence may be inflated by a combination of increased lead time and improved survival as a result of screening, along with contemporaneous improvements in treatment.[12–14] The impact of this increase on the number of breast cancer patients and survivors has been discussed by many writers, some of whom hold potentially conflicting views. It is suggested that breast screening may have:

1. reduced embarrassment and nihilism about symptomatic disease, thus facilitating earlier presentation;[15]
2. artificially inflated fear of breast cancer death;[16,17]
3. artificially inflated belief in breast screening benefits;[16,18] and
4. made women vulnerable to overmedicalization, leading them to demand screening and precautionary treatment even when it is unlikely to be beneficial.[19]

Some authors are particularly critical of the use of fear in breast cancer or breast screening communication. They point to the media presentation of breast cancer as a mysterious, increasing, frightening "epidemic," predominantly striking premenopausal white women in their prime years. These authors point to the inaccuracy of this depiction, and some suggest it has been deliberately engineered as a tool to encourage participation in screening.[9,10,20,21]

Summary: social attitudes toward breasts and breast cancer

- The symbolism of the breast (motherhood and sexuality) means breast cancer is highly emotive and breast screening is a popular media story, potentially contributing toward attitudes toward breast screening.
- Screening may affect social attitudes about breast cancer via its contribution toward increasing public familiarity with the disease.

SOCIOLOGY OF HEALTH AND ILLNESS

Breast screening resonated with general cultural and social trends in the second half of the twentieth century relating to health risks and responsibilities. Many authors note an increasing expectation, beginning in the 1970s and 1980s, that individuals could and indeed, should, make "lifestyle choices" to improve their health.[6,9,21] These authors suggest the introduction of breast screening has contributed to a "personal responsibility" model of breast cancer, by providing an opportunity for women to take individual responsibility for breast health.[6,22] There are two concerns with this model: firstly, the opportunity to participate in breast screening may have become a social obligation, with normative repercussions and judgment against those who do not screen, especially if they get breast cancer.[6,22,23] Secondly, there is concern that preoccupation with screening may have deflected attention from studying other methods of breast cancer control such as primary prevention.[6,9,24,25]

Other writers have noted an increasing tendency to subject ourselves to medical attention,[26] including widespread general enthusiasm for testing and screening.[27] Relatedly, sociologists have extensively documented the increasing risk awareness and risk aversiveness that characterizes contemporary society. This seems especially pertinent here, as women have been shown to be particularly aware of themselves as being at-risk for breast cancer as opposed to other conditions,[28] and to overestimate both their risk of dying from breast cancer and the protective benefit of mammography.[16,18]

Summary: sociology of health and illness

- Breast screening fits with the increasing tendencies of society to place responsibility for health upon individuals, and to be aware of and averse to risks.

BIOMEDICAL CULTURE

Breast screening has arisen in the context of prevailing biomedical paradigms regarding cancer growth and control, the use of technology and evidence in medicine. Breast screening, as an important practice in preventive health and medicine, has arguably contributed to these paradigms. We discuss each of them below.

The first example of the relationship between breast screening and biomedical paradigms relates to the conceptualization of breast cancer as a disease. For decades breast cancer has been (dominantly) understood as having a linear growth pattern progressing from a localized focus of dysplasia or in situ disease, to invasive and potentially metastatic cancer.[5,29] This helps to explain the inherent acceptability of breast screening as a policy. The most successful methods of control for women without specific genetic abnormalities have been assumed to be early detection and intervention and this has contributed greatly to the widespread support for breast cancer screening among the medical profession. Although this paradigm is still dominant, some writers are challenging its hegemony, suggesting that some breast cancers may regress[30] or adhere to nonlinear growth patterns.[31] It remains to be seen whether these or other theories become more widely accepted and influence the future of breast screening.

Breast screening is seen by some writers as an example of the technological imperative in action: that is, some propose that screening was adopted in part because both women and experts believed in the technology itself.[32] The implication here is that belief in the technology may have been at least as significant a factor in the popularity of breast screening as evidence of benefit.[33] This is particularly discussed in relation to the encouragement of women under 50 to participate in breast screening, despite lack of evidence about benefit for this age group in early randomized controlled trials (RCTs).[9,29,34] More recent developments in breast screening suggest that the technological imperative may be losing force as we learn from past experience: newer screening modalities that appear to offer increased test sensitivity are being approached with some caution and concern regarding overdiagnosis.[35]

The rise of evidence-based medicine (EBM) has paralleled the production of evidence about breast screening. Breast screening proved to be highly conducive to epidemiological study, and the large amount of RCT and other evidence generated around this topic was an important reason for its broad acceptance by the biomedical community. In turn, it may be that the perceived success of (evidence-based) mammographic screening programs gave a boost to the EBM approach.

Summary: biomedical culture

- Breast screening has arisen within the context of, and has contributed toward, the culture of biomedicine.
- Breast screening has supported and been supported by approaches to the early detection of cancer, technological innovation, and EBM.

COMMERCIAL AND INSTITUTIONAL ASPECTS OF BREAST SCREENING

Breast screening has become heavily institutionalized in Western society and culture. Many writers express concern about commercial interests in this process. They point to a range of actors including pharmaceutical companies, equipment manufacturers, professional medical organizations, and corporate donors who are doubtless motivated strongly by the desire to prevent women from dying of breast cancer, but have additional commercial interests.[9,24,36]

Breast cancer advocacy is one notable institution related to breast screening. Breast cancer advocacy groups are large, powerful, and highly visible social institutions with recognizable symbols (pink ribbons) and traditions, such as the Komen Foundation Race for the Cure.[15] Although not the first major disease-specific advocacy group (this belongs to HIV) breast cancer advocacy has, arguably, led the way in ensuring that consumer voices are taken seriously as a legitimate form of public opinion and power. Many breast cancer advocacy groups believe strongly in early detection by screening[37] and campaign for screening resources and services.[6] Some authors suggest that the symbolic significance of the breast previously discussed makes it easier to raise funds for breast cancer causes (including breast screening) than for some other conditions,[9,24] helping to explain the relatively strong funding base and profile for breast cancer advocacy.

Summary: commercial and institutional aspects

- Key stakeholders may have commercial interests that influence their participation in breast screening.
- Breast cancer advocacy is powerful and bolsters support for breast screening.

THE POLITICAL NATURE OF BREAST SCREENING

Many authors have ascribed the political popularity of breast screening partly to its easily quantifiable outcomes, which can be readily presented as success stories, but more importantly to its role as a "women's issue" that will attract votes.[25,38,39] Breast screening is seen as a "safe and noncontroversial" women's issue, unlike, for example, abortion or domestic violence. This is illustrated by the willingness of women in political life to be candid about their breast cancer experiences (think here of Betty Ford or Happy Rockefeller).[32] By contrast when Janette Howard, wife of the then Prime Minister of Australia, was diagnosed with cervical cancer her disease was not made public.[40]

The lively advocacy environment surrounding breast screening also illustrates its political nature[7,9,19,32,38] and contributes to the frequent politicization of breast screening. For example, when the 1997 Consensus Conference by the US National Institutes of Health (NIH) removed its endorsement of routine screening for women aged 40–49 years, suggesting instead that it be a personal decision, many advocates organized against the change. Their political influence was strong enough to encourage the US Senate to pass a resolution urging the NIH to reconsider, and ultimately the NIH re-endorsed routine, annual mammography for this age group.[25] Twelve years later, breast screening again returned to the center of political attention. In 2009 the United States Preventive Services Task Force (USPSTF) also recommended that screening for younger women (aged 40–49) be an individual choice rather than standard practice, provoking immediate and intense condemnation by advocacy and clinical leaders. The US Department of Health and Human Services quickly issued a statement to distance itself from the recommendations, stating that federal breast screening policy would remain unchanged and assuming that private health insurers would follow their lead. The US federal health insurance program *Medicare* continues to provide coverage for annual breast screening from age 40.[41,42]

Summary: politics

- Breast screening tends to be both politically popular and politically contested, which influences the design of policy and practice.

ETHICAL ISSUES IN BREAST SCREENING

Readers will be familiar with the idea of planning and evaluating screening programs against public health, economic, and perhaps legal criteria.[43,44] Although many of these evaluative criteria include implicit ethical principles (such as maximizing benefits, minimizing harms, and more recently, respect for autonomy voiced as requirement for informed consent) a formal ethical approach can provide additional value. First, it can provide depth of analysis, making arguments for why principles are important and should be upheld. Second, it draws our attention to additional considerations that have not traditionally appeared in screening ethics frameworks. For example, ethicists focused on screening have not only written about why it might be important to obtain informed consent for screening[45–47] but also about the tensions between promoting individual health, promoting community health and respecting autonomy.[48] They have also considered the ethical implications of professional, institutional and consumer tendencies to start and, once started, to continue preventive screening programs and to under-recognize the potential for this screening to do more harm than good.[47,49]

The ethics of screening are made more complicated by its location on the boundary between clinical and public health practice. Although some of the ethical issues faced by clinical medicine versus public health are similar, others are quite different. Many readers will be familiar with the Beauchamp–Childress principles for clinical ethics (respect autonomy, do good, avoid harm, seek justice): in recent years authors have proposed alternative sets of principles for public health ethics.[50–54] We will consider both clinical and public health principles, beginning with those that are more frequently discussed and debated within breast screening. Note that some of these principles are more contentious, and so require more space to discuss. This is not meant to imply any greater importance, but might suggest these issues are deserving of greater societal debate.

The public health ethics and screening ethics literatures[45,51–54] suggest the importance of these ethical issues when evaluating breast screening[46–50]:

- Maximize health benefits
- Minimize harms
- Deliver more benefits than harms
- Deliver the most benefit possible within the resources available
- Respect autonomy
- Maintain transparency, including communicating honestly
- Distribute benefits and burdens justly
- Uphold reciprocal obligations
- Act in solidarity with others

We will consider each of these in turn.

MAXIMIZING HEALTH BENEFITS THROUGH BREAST SCREENING

The goal of improving the health of populations is central to public health practice. There has been considerable debate over the degree to which public health policies should deliberately contribute to individual and societal well-being beyond physical health, an issue we will consider later in this chapter. In this section we concentrate specifically on health benefits. In general, a program that delivers greater health benefit can be considered more justifiable, primarily because—in many ethical traditions—good consequences have moral value in themselves. In addition, delivering these benefits keeps the promises implicitly or explicitly made about the program.

Public health is generally characterized as being concerned with health benefits in *populations* rather than primarily focusing on *individuals*.[55] In population breast screening, for example, a public health perspective would predominantly focus on the degree to which screening increases the longevity and quality of life of women on average across a population, rather than being concerned with benefit delivered to individual women. It is useful to consider the distinction between benefits to populations and benefits to individuals since it is less clear than it may seem, especially for an activity like screening. This is in part because benefits to populations are of more than one type. They include all of the benefits experienced by individuals added up (*aggregative benefits*) but many public health programs also provide an additional benefit, sometimes called a *corporate benefit*, that occurs at the population level only.[56] For example, vaccination programs deliver aggregated benefits (all of the instances of personal protection via immunization, added up) but also corporate benefits (the herd immunity that arises only after a certain proportion of the population is vaccinated, and which protects even those who are not vaccinated). The various aggregate and corporate benefits of breast screening are discussed below.

Breast cancer mortality benefits

Breast cancer screening delivers breast cancer (disease specific) mortality benefit for some age groups.[57] The introduction of breast cancer screening into a population has been shown to result in a reduced population breast cancer mortality rate. This is mainly because some women who are screened derive benefit from their participation (the sum of which provides an aggregative benefit) although the existence of breast screening may also provide corporate benefits to women in general (discussed below).

For some public health programs, aggregative population benefit is widely and equally distributed among most people. For example, in vaccination programs where most children participate, the benefit is approximately the same for each child. Not so for the breast cancer mortality benefit of screening: most women who attend breast screening receive no breast cancer mortality benefit at all, and attending screening will not make any difference to whether or not they die of breast cancer. This is because most women, screened and unscreened, will not develop breast cancer. Of those women, screened and unscreened, who do develop breast cancer, many will not die from it if they undergo current treatment regimes. Still others, sadly, will die from it regardless of whether or not they attended screening. It has been calculated that less than one in seven women who are screen-diagnosed and treated for breast cancer receive mortality benefit from their screening.[58] Thus the aggregative disease-specific benefits of screening clearly exist, but are unequally distributed in the population, being derived from a small number of women.

This aggregative benefit from a small number of women remains the dominant driving force behind mammography screening. Recent attempts to quantify breast cancer mortality benefit suggest that screening is less beneficial than was calculated in most of the early RCTs, partly because of revised calculations from the original studies,[57,59] and partly because of recent improvements in treatment, which reduces the margin for benefit from interventions such as screening.[14] Writers also express concern that breast cancer screening has very little impact on *all-cause* mortality.[60]

The likelihood of deriving breast cancer mortality benefit from screening may vary between women and between populations of women. Individual women at increased risk of dying from breast cancer will be more likely to derive benefit from screening, and conversely those at decreased risk will be less likely to derive benefit. The latter group includes young women (since they are much less likely to get breast cancer than older women) and women who are more likely to die from other causes (eg, due to age or significant comorbidities). Similarly, populations of women with a higher incidence of breast cancer will derive more absolute mortality benefit from screening, and populations with a lower incidence (eg, communities in many parts of Asia[61]) will derive less benefit. This raises questions regarding screening policy, and the extent to which programs should consider themselves obliged to focus screening on those subpopulations of women which are most likely to experience an (aggregative) mortality benefit. Thus far, within a given population, outside of age and (uncommon) genetic markers, most risk factors for breast cancer are modest and thus of limited use in stratifying screening.[62] Recent research on risk factors such as family history of breast cancer in first-degree relatives, and personal breast density may alter this. Women in their 40s at high risk of breast cancer may have similar benefits and harms from breast screening as average risk women aged 50–74, and thus might consider screening at an earlier age.[63–65]

Breast cancer morbidity benefits

Breast cancers identified through screening programs tend to be smaller and more amenable to breast conserving treatment than cancers that present symptomatically. This is often mentioned as a benefit of breast screening programs but is controversial. If the breast cancer detected was destined to progress and become more difficult to treat, then the woman concerned has certainly experienced a morbidity benefit. However some researchers are concerned that many small, asymptomatic cancers identified through breast screening are indolent—cancers that would never otherwise have come to the attention of the woman.[11,66] If this is so, breast-conserving treatment cannot be counted as a benefit, since no treatment was necessary. This problem of unnecessary diagnosis and management of nonprogressive cancers produces the overdiagnosis in breast screening programs; there is little consensus on how common it is. Overdiagnosis is discussed in more detail later in this chapter. In addition, several writers have expressed concern that screening has led to an increase, rather than a decrease, in mastectomy rates, due to the screen-detection of multifocal noninvasive disease that confers an increased risk of developing invasive breast cancer and is unsuitable for localized treatments.[11,67] This remains controversial.[68]

Psychological benefits

Since the majority of women are not destined to develop breast cancer, most women will receive a negative screen. While some argue that the reassurance of a negative screen can justifiably be counted as a benefit of screening, others disagree. Those who object give several reasons, including that in some cases the screening result will be wrong (a false-negative), so screening may sometimes deliver false reassurance.[11] More generally, though, since it has been consistently shown that both the fear of breast cancer death and the expectation of mortality benefit from screening are inflated relative to what the evidence would support,[16,69] it is argued that a woman's *subjectively experienced* reassurance from a negative screen may be considerably inflated relative to our best estimates of her *objective risk* of developing breast cancer. This distorted perception of risk may have at least in part arisen from the communication campaigns of public health communication about breast screening.[11] If this is true, without denying women's subjective experience of reassurance, we should question the justifiability of including it as a benefit of screening. In addition, a wrong may be done to women if they are implicitly or explicitly misled them about the degree to which they are at risk and the degree to which participating in screening may prevent their death.

Does breast screening offer corporate benefits?

Many people consider that a population's benefits for cancer screening are accrued only as aggregative benefits: the sum of benefits experienced by (a few) individuals as a result of participating in screening. Others describe several corporate benefits, added benefits that accrue to an entire community as a result of breast screening policies and practices. First, screening promotion campaigns have arguably improved public awareness and knowledge about breast cancer and, as noted earlier, this familiarity with disease may facilitate earlier presentation among women with symptomatic breast disease.[70] Second, operating a breast screening program within a population may generate a sense that society cares about women, and is willing to support them and provide them with services. (This is considered in more detail below.) Finally, although it is impossible to assert a causal link, the introduction of breast screening is widely considered to have catalyzed better breast cancer management, facilitating an improvement in the coordination and operation of breast cancer treatment through better experience, training and monitoring of medical specialists, and the introduction of multidisciplinary team care.[71] This has meant better outcomes and experiences for all women with breast cancer. Note, however, that these latter benefits have, to a large extent, already been delivered and are likely to continue, whatever happens to screening. Thus they seem relevant for an evaluation of past screening programs, but arguably are not relevant to our assessment of how screening should occur in future. This is in contrast, for example, to herd immunity, the corporate benefit of vaccination programs, which depends entirely on their continuing operation.

Summary: benefits

- Breast screening delivers breast cancer–specific mortality benefits and may deliver all-cause mortality benefits.
- Breast screening may deliver morbidity benefits (less aggressive treatments but possibly some unnecessary treatments).
- Consumer reassurance may or may not be a legitimate benefit for many women who participate in screening.
- Introduction of breast screening has stimulated additional, population-wide benefits (eg, improved management) but this may not be a pertinent justification for future screening programs.

Avoiding or Minimizing Harms

Evaluations of public health programs often focus on delivery of benefits. However any intervention on an individual or population can also do harm. In clinical medicine, this concept is covered by the principle of nonmaleficence: avoiding doing harm associated with patient investigation or treatment. While nonmaleficence is an ancient and widely recognized principle of clinical medicine, the idea that public health policies such as screening can do harm is less-well recognized.[47] It may not be possible to completely avoid harms in public health programs, but in general a more ethically justifiable program is thought to be one that minimizes harms for participants and populations.

There are several types of harms common to any screening program. The discussion below relates specifically to breast screening. Some of these are examined in more detail elsewhere in this book.

Inconveniences and financial costs of participation

It is well recognized that participation in breast screening incurs inconveniences and difficulties such as taking time away from work or child care to attend appointments, psychological anxiety, and pain.[72] Although these are generally perceived as being relatively inconsequential, they are persistently cited by consumers as notable aspects of the breast screening experience and policymakers should continue to work toward addressing such concerns. In many countries, a screening mammogram and any associated investigations also incurs financial costs.[73]

Harms related to the test

Radiation harms associated with modern mammographic screening are widely recognized to be acceptably low for women 40 and older.[74] The radiation dose is higher for women who have dense breasts and for women with very large breasts, thus radiation exposure may be more problematic for premenopausal women and large-breasted women, particularly if having frequent (eg, annual) mammographic screening.[75] Greater radiation exposure associated with adding newer tomography screening modalities is currently of concern, and work is continuing to address this.[76]

Harms related to test results

Harms associated with test results include technical faults and false-positive results requiring recall and repeat testing, and false-negative results. Recall for technical faults or false-positive screens deliver physical harms of additional mammograms and possibly fine needle or core biopsies. In addition to physical harm, these also carry risks of psychological harm and, in many countries, extra financial costs.[73] It has been estimated that the psychological distress associated with false-positive mammography can last for over 3 years.[77] The likelihood of a woman receiving a false-positive diagnosis during a lifetime of screening varies greatly with the location and parameters of the screening program. It also accumulates such that a regularly screened woman's risk of having a false-positive in her lifetime is much higher than her risk of having a false-positive as a result of a single test.[78–81] False-negative results are much less common but may also cause harm through false reassurance and delayed presentation of symptomatic disease.[82]

Harms arising from the limitations of screening

Some of the cancers diagnosed through breast screening may never progress and, without screening, would not have come to the attention of the individual in her lifetime. This includes both invasive breast cancers and noninvasive breast cancers—ductal carcinoma in situ (DCIS) and lobular carcinoma in situ (LCIS). This phenomenon is called overdiagnosis or overdetection and is discussed in detail in chapters "Weighing the Benefits and Harms: Screening Mammography in the Balance"; "Challenges in Understanding and Quantifying Overdiagnosis and Overtreatment"; and "Treatment of Screen-Detected Breast Cancer: Can We Avoid or Minimize Overtreatment?". At present indolent cancers cannot be distinguished from progressive, potentially lethal cancers, so all cancers are treated. Treatment is generally unpleasant and may be financially burdensome for the individual (eg, in the United States, even those with health insurance suffer considerable "financial toxicity" after a cancer diagnosis due to the rising costs of patient copayments for cancer treatment[83]). Very occasionally treatment will result in patient death. Thus at a population level, breast screening may be associated with unnecessary morbidity and mortality due to overdiagnosis. Although it is not possible to determine whether overdiagnosis has occurred in any one individual woman, we know that it is one of the harms associated with breast screening because it can be identified at a population level (see chapter: Challenges in Understanding and Quantifying Overdiagnosis and Overtreatment). Despite intensive research, there is currently no firm consensus on rates of overdiagnosis within breast screening.[66,84,85]

Breast screening does not always deliver certainty about breast health: sometimes screening uncovers changes in the breast (such as LCIS and atypical hyperplasia) that are not cancerous, but are associated with increased susceptibility to breast cancer in that individual. That is, unlike DCIS, which is regarded as a nonobligate precursor to invasive cancer, certain "high-risk" lesions (including LCIS and atypical hyperplasias) are widely regarded as indicative of generalized increase in the likelihood of breast cancer. This type of result might be seen as a harm because it produces heightened anxiety about breast cancer, but does not deliver an expected level of certainty about risk to the individual and may require substantial removal of noncancerous breast tissue (eg, single or double mastectomy) to reduce the woman's risk and anxiety levels to those of an age-matched cohort without identified breast disease.[86]

Are harms justifiable?

There are several important points to consider when evaluating whether or not the harms associated with breast screening are justifiable. These include the size of the harm and how this should be measured, the extent to which harms can be predicted, whether it is possible to minimize harms and if so what other consequences may follow, and finally whether action should be taken to minimize harms. We consider each of these points below.

How much harm?

It has proven difficult to gain consensus on the amount of harm associated with breast screening. As noted above, despite many years of operation and many studies and metaanalyses, there remains substantial variation in calculations of cumulative false-positive and overdiagnosis rates. At least some of the variation may be real: it may be that different screening protocols and different populations produce different amounts of population harm. Some of the variation may be methodological: differences in overdiagnosis calculations may contribute to the considerable disparity between estimates.[84,85,87] Writers have urged breast screening experts to reach consensus about how to measure overdiagnosis in order to make progress on this controversial topic.[88]

Anticipating harms

Some harms, particularly false-positives and false-negatives, are well anticipated prior to the implementation of organized screening, and programs only go ahead if and when it is possible to minimize these harms. Other harms are less well anticipated. For example, the possible harms associated with ionizing radiation were unknown when mammographic screening was initially introduced sporadically in the 1950s and then widely implemented through several states in the United States in the 1960s and 1970s in the Breast Cancer Detection and Demonstration Projects.[32] (Since that time, mammography units have much improved and radiation doses considerably reduced.) Similarly, while overdiagnosis was discussed prior to widespread breast screening,[89,90] it was generally assumed this would not be a significant problem. In particular, overdiagnosis of DCIS was not seriously considered since DCIS is usually impalpable (asymptomatic) and was a rare diagnosis prior to the onset of screening. Recently, there have been calls for researchers to make a more deliberate effort to anticipate, investigate, and report on possible harms associated with proposed (and existing) screening programs[91] particularly in relation to the diagnosis of inconsequential disease.[44]

Minimizing harms

When harms are anticipated (or should reasonably be able to be anticipated), ethical obligations to avoid harming imply that programs should be designed to not only maximize benefits, but also to minimize harms. In the context of breast screening this includes close attention to quality control, and requires careful and ongoing monitoring of screening program procedures, parameters, and outcomes in order to identify and correct technical and procedural problems.[92] Program policies should incorporate activities before and after the testing stage, with identifiable standards and quality checks for all steps including, for example, recruitment and communication, repeat testing, and follow-up. There is some concern that private opportunistic screening providers may not engage with the same quality control standards and parameters that public, nationally organized providers adhere to.[80,93] Notwithstanding these needs for quality control, the nature of screening means that harms cannot be avoided: minimizing harms from false-positive tests is likely to increase harms from false-negative tests and vice versa. Program operators must decide how to balance their programs such that the various harms are best minimized.

Summary: harms

- Breast screening delivers harms to the participating population.
- There is no consensus on how much harm is delivered by breast screening.
- Close attention to quality control is required to minimize harms.

DELIVERING MORE BENEFITS THAN HARMS

We have shown above that there are potentially both positive and negative consequences of breast screening: benefits and harms. For most people, having benefits outweigh harms is a necessary criterion for an ethically justified public health program. (We would add: necessary *but not sufficient*. That is, other morally relevant factors such as autonomy, transparency, and distributive justice should also be considered, and we discuss these and other principles below.) The process of weighing up benefits against harms is multilayered. It includes, in no particular order: quantitative measurements of benefits and harms (which is controversial in breast screening, as discussed above); comparisons between qualitatively different benefits and harms; and the relative weightings ascribed to maximizing benefits and minimizing harms.

Comparing qualitatively different benefits and harms

Benefits and harms may be disparate in nature, making meaningful comparisons difficult. How, for example, should we compare population breast cancer mortality reductions against (possible) population breast cancer morbidity increases? The logic underpinning endorsed public health activities is that they should result in population health benefits that are clearly more substantial than the harms, and this has generally been the case with breast screening. For example, when organized breast cancer screening was introduced in Australia, the benefits from reducing breast cancer deaths was widely accepted to considerably outweigh the harms associated with occasional false-positive or false-negative tests. Since that time, as discussed above, estimates of screening benefit have decreased and anticipated harms have increased and it is now frequently suggested that the benefits and harms accruing from breast screening are closely balanced.[70,94] In such a scenario, qualitative differences between screening outcomes make comparisons particularly troublesome. Translating screening outcomes into comparable units may have some similarities with the somewhat controversial use of QALYs (quality-adjusted life years) for comparing disease outcomes. It is not clear who might be best placed to make such translations.

Should we prioritize maximizing benefits or minimizing harms?

The relative importance ascribed to maximizing benefits and minimizing harms may vary according to context and individual preferences.[95] In some circumstances, or for some people, avoiding harm may be considered a prioritized principle, that can rarely be traded off against benefit or any other principle. Again, where the differences between benefits and harms are clearly great, personal preferences about the importance of each principle may not significantly affect the outcome of balancing benefits against harms in population-level policymaking. For breast screening, where benefits and harms appear more closely balanced, individual differences in prioritizing each principle may become more important.

Who should decide whether benefits outweigh harms?

Many writers think it important to involve consumers in such calculations. Consumers can be involved at policy level and at a personal participation level. Firstly, deliberative democracy methods, such as citizens juries, can be used to determine public perspectives on comparing qualitatively different benefits and harms, and on the weightings that should be ascribed to maximizing benefits and minimizing harms.[96] The rationale here is that lay people may value and trade off the various possible benefits and harms differently to experts. Secondly, many people suggest that individuals who are considering participating in breast screening can and should be more involved in deciding whether or not benefits outweigh harms in their particular case, because they are best placed to know their own attitudes toward these benefits and harms.[97] Consumer decision-making is valued here for its usefulness as being the best way of deciding between somewhat similar or incomparable outcomes, independent of the intrinsic value of being able to make decisions for oneself (see more on this in the next section on respect for autonomy). This reasoning contributes to new breast screening communications with consumers, that seek to present both benefits and harms and encourage informed choices about screening participation.[98]

Note however, that obtaining informed consent does not remove responsibility from providers to minimize harms,[46] and breast screening policymakers arguably have a duty to deliver screening policies that the majority of the target population will accept. Many consider that benefits of screening remain substantial enough to outweigh harms and so breast screening should continue unchanged. Others disagree, and, notwithstanding the use of deliberative democratic methods to help ascertain public opinion, many writers are suggesting that breast screening programs should be more tailored to individual risk profiles in order to facilitate a better benefit to harm ratio. For example, that those at higher risk of dying from breast cancer, for whom benefits of screening are likely to be greater, should have more screening than those who are at lower risk of dying from breast cancer and are therefore less likely to benefit from screening. Tailored screening programs are discussed in greater detail in chapters "Challenges and Opportunities in the Implementation of Risk-Based Screening for Breast Cancer"; "Breast Cancer Screening in the Older Woman"; "Screening Women in Their Forties"; "Screening for Breast Cancer in Women with Dense Breasts"; "Screening Women with Known or Suspected Cancer Gene Mutations"; and "Imaging Surveillance of Women with a Personal History of Breast Cancer."

Summary: delivering more benefits than harms

- The benefit to harm ratio in breast screening is more closely balanced than previously thought.
- Given the qualitative differences between benefits and harms, and variations in how much to prioritize the principles of maximizing benefits and minimizing harms, it is hard to know where, exactly, the balance between breast screening benefits and harms lies.
- Involving consumers at the levels of policymaking and individual decision-making may assist with making this calculation.

DELIVERING THE MOST BENEFIT POSSIBLE WITHIN THE RESOURCES AVAILABLE

Given that resources for healthcare are always finite, resource allocation and the amount of benefit received for a given investment is worthy of ethical consideration. In the context of breast screening it is relevant to not only explore how much benefit can be delivered while minimizing harms, but also how to maximize the benefits that matter *within a healthcare budget.*

Population breast screening is an expensive program, even when taking into account healthcare savings associated with earlier diagnosis and treatment, and containment of costs that might otherwise accrue from unregulated, opportunistic screening.[99,100] The high cost of breast screening programs does not mean they should not be funded, but it does mean there are opportunity costs to other potential areas of expenditure, and we should consider how breast screening costs compare with other healthcare expenses. There is controversy over this,[101–103] partly due to lack of consensus over mortality benefit and overdiagnosis figures. We should also consider ways to keep breast screening as cost-efficient as possible. Attaining and maintaining a high level of public participation is often suggested as being important for cost-efficiency[93] but this is contestable. For many screening programs, the main expenses are the variable (participant related) costs associated with actually performing the screens and follow up tests, rather than the fixed (setup and infra-structure) costs, and as such, screening can be cost-effective even with low rates of participation.[104,105] Given this, the common link made from cost-effectiveness to participation rates may be less certain than is sometimes suggested.

Summary: the most benefits within resources

- Cost-effectiveness of breast screening compared to other healthcare expenditure is controversial.
- For cancer screening generally, it is not clear that high participation rates are required to achieve cost effectiveness.

RESPECTING AND SUPPORTING AUTONOMY

Respecting, or supporting, the autonomy of individual patients, consumers, or citizens is a fundamental principle in healthcare ethics. For the purposes of this discussion, we regard an autonomous person as one who: sees herself as in being charge of her own life; believes this to be appropriate; and has the freedom, opportunity, skills and capacities required to make choices, take action, and live in a manner that is consistent with her sense of who she is.[106] Being autonomous thus relies not just on the person herself, but also the people, systems, and society that surround her. These relationships and systems can either support or diminish her autonomy.

Informed decision-making in breast screening

The facilitation of informed decision-making in breast screening is an important part of supporting and respecting autonomy. Many writers have expressed concern that breast screening communication with consumers should: (1) include evidence-based information about risks and benefits; and (2) be designed to inform women in a balanced way rather than persuade them to participate.[107,108] Many countries have recently released or will shortly release new information pamphlets.[93,98] We mentioned above that facilitating informed decision-making about breast screening may be more likely to produce beneficial outcomes. This may be for several reasons: for example, the experience of having one's autonomy supported may increase one's sense of wellbeing; also, if we believe that we are all best able to know our own interests, the choices we make for ourselves may be more likely to be beneficial to us. In this section, however, we present autonomy as something to be valued in its own right irrespective of the resulting consequences, and suggest that facilitating informed choice has independent value from whether or not it improves the benefit to harm ratio.[109]

How else should we support and respect women's autonomy in breast screening?

Providing opportunities for informed decision-making is only one part of supporting and respecting autonomy. Other aspects of respecting and supporting autonomy in the breast screening context include, for example:

- Communication that indicates women have the authority to decide whether or not participation is right for them (rather than suggesting that they should not question participation, or are in no position to decide);
- Ensuring that women understand the implications of participating or not participating in screening; and
- Ensuring that women have an opportunity to consider screening in the context of their own values and sense of self.[110]

How important is supporting and respecting autonomy?

Respecting autonomy is considered a very important concept in healthcare ethics. In the Four Principles approach within clinical ethics discussed earlier, respect for autonomy has been referred to as the "first among equals."[111] Writers on public health ethics have recently tended to criticize excessive importing of clinical ethics concerns, particularly respect for autonomy, into public health contexts, arguing that this potentially overrides community-orientated principles such as justice, solidarity, and reciprocity which are fundamental to public health practice. Certainly the extensive evidence that individual health is heavily influenced by social, as well as personal, factors suggests that it may be misguided to conceptualize respect for autonomy as independence of choice, or to prioritize this as a good.[112]

The principle of respecting autonomy may conflict with other principles discussed here. For example, it may be very hard to engage large numbers of women in informed shared decision-making for a complex topic like breast screening, especially if they are not well-informed to begin with.[16] Some writers argue that enabling all consumers to make their own, fully informed, choices about screening would be so resource-intensive and challenging that it would seriously undermine the cost-effectiveness of screening.[48] Others disagree, arguing that informing women about breast screening is not especially difficult [97] or that respecting autonomy should be such a high priority that we may be obliged to offer such information and support if breast screening is to continue, regardless of cost. Respecting autonomy may also influence the level of benefit delivered by screening. There has been concern that embarking upon an informed consent process for breast screening may worry consumers, and reduce public participation in breast screening programs.[113,114] Despite this, varied stakeholders support the principle of respecting autonomy strongly enough that there is reasonably widespread international support for shared decision-making and informed choice in cancer screening.[113–115]

Summary: respecting or supporting autonomy

- Facilitating informed choice is an important aspect of respecting autonomy in breast screening.
- There is disagreement over whether or not facilitating informed choice might be excessively expensive or decrease public participation rates, and over how to balance support and respect for autonomy against other ethical principles.

HONESTY, TRANSPARENCY, AND PROCEDURAL JUSTICE

Ethically justified and legitimate public health decisions and actions will generally have the qualities of honesty, integrity, and openness. This is relevant to the substance of communication, and the process of decision-making and implementation.

Ethically justified programs will pursue full and honest disclosure of information that might be considered relevant for consumer decision-making. Communicating honestly is, in part, a way to show respect for individuals and their autonomy as discussed above, but many would also regard it as being important in its own right. That is, many think that governments should, as a general rule, be open and up-front when communicating about their policies and programs. Transparency is the full and honest disclosure of how, and by whom, decisions and policies are made. This includes the disclosure of possible vested interests among policymakers and advisors in order to facilitate accountability and take account of possible bias. Procedural justice is about fairness in decision-making: for example, ensuring that all relevant stakeholders are included, that decisions are made for good reasons, that decisions are open to revision if new evidence or arguments emerge, and that the influence of biases and vested interests are minimized in order to ensure decisions are made in the best interests of the public.[53]

Vested interests in breast screening

Communication with breast screening consumers is often produced by breast screening providers who are required to meet participation targets. Truthful communication about breast screening may be facilitated by changing the key performance indicators for breast screening services from rates of consumer participation in screening to rates of consumer understanding and participation in shared decision-making.[97,116] It may also be preferable for information to be written by independent experts.[117]

Breast screening policy decisions are often heavily influenced by government or independent experts who review existing evidence and issue comments or guidelines. As in any public health program, experts may have commercial, political, or professional interests in a particular outcome that may bias the policymaking process. Debates about vested professional interests are a particularly common topic in breast screening. The breast screening evidence is complex and contradictory and there have been many reviews of the multiple breast screening trials and studies that have presented variable conclusions regarding the benefits and harms associated with breast screening. There has been widespread and public accusation about vested interests of key expert clinicians and researchers with a long history of practice or publication related to breast screening who promote or criticize screening. The declaration of *commercial* interests is a widely accepted tradition, but some writers suggest the principle of transparency also demands that all *professional* interests should be declared (eg, the reputational interests of experts in continuing to defend a long-held position).[118] Others advocate that procedural justice requires accepting only independent experts as advisors or decision-makers, excluding practicing clinicians and academics who have previously published on the topic,[57,118] or to ensure that all legitimate stakeholders are involved in decision-making in order to reduce the chance of any one vested interest dominating the process.[53]

Summary: honesty, transparency, and procedural justice

- Breast screening communication and decision-making may be biased due to vested interests, including professional vested interests, in a particular outcome.
- Honest communications about breast screening may be facilitated by strategies such as removing participation targets or using independent experts.
- Those with professional vested interests could be asked to declare their interests, or be excluded from decision-making.

DISTRIBUTIVE JUSTICE

Distributive justice is about fairness: fairness of opportunity (eg, the opportunity for all individuals to pursue good health) and fairness of outcome (eg, everyone in a society achieving at least a basic or threshold level of good health). Achieving justice does not necessarily mean that everyone is treated equally: more effort may need to be expended on some individuals than others in order to attain the same opportunity for, or achievement of, good health. Thus, justice may demand that those with the more limited health opportunities or the poorest predicted health outcomes receive priority.

Justice in opportunity

The opportunity for women to attend breast screening remains an important issue. Several barriers to breast screening opportunities have been identified, including geographic, sociocultural, and financial.[80,119] Many programs have sought to remove or ameliorate these barriers through actions such as: mobile breast screening services, culture- and language-specific consumer communication strategies, and reduced cost or free screening. These policies may be expensive, and may bring the principle of justice into conflict with other principles, such as delivering the most benefits within available resources.[80]

Justice in health outcomes

Is breast screening a fair strategy in terms of population health outcomes? Certainly breast screening only benefits a minority of the population, but given that people with breast cancer are more likely to have poorer health outcomes, it would seem to be consistent with the principle of justice to expend effort on trying to improve this outcome. Some writers disagree: while breast cancer may affect any woman, it is more common among those with higher socioeconomic status—that is, women from the group who are, on average, more likely to have good health and opportunities to achieve it. It has been suggested that the breast cancer focus is discriminatory,[37] and a fairer public health system would be one that targets the needs of people who have poorer health outcomes—for example, those with significant social disadvantages or physical disabilities. In this view a more just approach might be one that focuses less on early detection of breast cancer, and more on providing basic social and health infrastructure for all (eg, public transport, a healthy food supply, and affordable treatment services) as well as targeted programs to address the needs of those groups with the worst health outcomes. Notice, though, that this takes for granted that it is reasonable to trade these health-related goods off against one another within a limited health budget. It is likely that many high-income countries could afford both breast screening and interventions to reduce structural disadvantage if they reduced spending in other, arguably less important, policy areas.

Summary: distributive justice

- Many breast screening programs have policies that aim to give all women fair opportunities to attend screening.
- Some writers suggest breast screening makes a relatively small contribution toward the fairness of distribution of health outcomes.

RECIPROCITY

The principle of reciprocity is generally used to refer to concepts such as returning a favor that is done to us, sharing in carrying public burdens, and supporting and compensating those who carry the heaviest burdens.[120,121]

Reciprocity, individuals, and breast screening

The principle of reciprocity would suggest that individuals who live in and therefore gain health benefits from a society that offers breast screening should be cognizant and supportive of these benefits. In particular, they should not act so as to reduce the opportunity for others to receive similar benefits. This may suggest certain limited obligations for women: for example, to actively attend, cancel, or reschedule appointments so as not to prevent or delay another woman from accessing the service. Whether there is any more substantial reciprocal obligation for women is arguable. We discussed possible corporate benefits of breast screening programs in a previous section (eg, improved breast cancer treatment). We argued that such benefits, which have already been achieved, are not clearly contingent on women's continued participation. This suggests that individual women should not consider themselves obliged to participate in exchange for these existing corporate benefits. Some might suggest that the existence of a publically funded healthcare service is a benefit to all, and that in return, citizens should take reasonable care of their health, which includes attending screening services when advised to do so.[33] It is now common in public health generally to emphasize the importance of individual behaviors,[21,122] often framed in terms of individual responsibility and duty. This moral language can suggest some kind of reciprocal obligation on individuals. However many would reject this, arguing, for example, that breast screening is not a *necessary* way for a society to demonstrate its commitment to women's health, so women do not have any reciprocal responsibility to participate (or not participate) in breast screening in particular.

Reciprocity is also relevant to breast screening as a driving force in screening advocacy. Individuals who have been diagnosed with illness through screening may feel they have benefited from that program and wish to return the good. Thus the concept of reciprocity may be invoked by screening consumers who seek to "give back" to society through involvement in activities related to screening promotion and advocacy. This is a sensitive issue, particularly if the positions of those advocates, often resolutely proscreening,[37] seem to ignore more recent evidence about the uncertain balance between benefits and harms of screening.[97] Despite this potential to distort the accuracy of communication, it seems important to recognize the moral value of these advocates' desire to reciprocate, as this provides a stronger basis from which to engage respectfully.

Reciprocity, the state, healthcare systems, and breast screening

The principle of reciprocity requires that breast screening programs should seek to minimize disproportionate burdening of any one individual or group of individuals and should support and compensate those who carry burdens, particularly the heaviest burdens. For example when countries offer organized, publicly funded breast screening, the absence of a financial barrier could be seen as a reciprocal exchange to these women for their status as taxpayers and for their willingness to participate in a service that is unlikely to benefit them personally. Screening programs that include free follow-up testing to the point of diagnosis ensure that women who receive false-positive tests and thus already carry a disproportionately heavy burden of screening (associated with inevitably imperfect quality control) are not further burdened by financial costs. Privately operated breast screening, by contrast, may simply charge per item. This not only means that women must pay to participate, but also that women who receive false-positive screening tests due to limitations of mammography pay more for their screening event than other women. Part of the discomfort that we may feel about this arrangement is likely to be recognition that it contravenes the principle of reciprocity.

Summary: reciprocity

- In a society that offers breast screening, women may be bound by the principle of reciprocity to at least consider screening, and to accept or cancel screening appointments.
- Privately funded screening programs may contravene reciprocity by failing to ameliorate the disproportionate burdens of screening carried by those who receive false-positive tests.

SOLIDARITY

Commitment to solidarity has been implicit in public health since its earliest origins, although explicit discussions of solidarity in public health ethics have emerged more recently.[123] Solidarity is "pulling together" toward a common (collective) cause on the understanding that there is mutual respect and obligation between members of a community,[124] and a sharing of burdens and threats.[123] Readers might note some overlap between reciprocity and solidarity: both are grounded in ideas about mutual obligation and collective interests.

Solidarity expressed by individuals

Individuals may participate in breast screening for reasons of solidarity—that is, partly to contribute toward benefits for others. Karen Willis,[33] for example, has shown empirically that women in rural Australia are motivated to visit mobile breast screening vans partly to show support for services that may be needed by others in the future. It is possible to recognize the moral value of this expression of solidarity, but question the reasoning that underpins it. In many cases, for example, lack of attendance should not necessarily threaten the viability or continuation of breast screening. Fine-tuning screening according to risk profile may over time decrease the perception that participation by low-risk women is a valuable expression of solidarity with high-risk women.

Uses of solidarity by the state (or by organized screening programs)

Solidarity may be used by the state to justify promotional activities aiming for high breast screening participation rates. That is, while it is recognized that screening will not benefit most people, and will be (mildly, moderately, or severely) inconvenient or harmful to many people, it may be acceptable that screening is promoted in order to maintain a politically and economically viable program that delivers large benefits to some.

While the concept of solidarity remains a strong driver for public policy, it is not clear how much burden many members of a society should be expected to shoulder in order to deliver benefit to a few. Some argue that the amount of societal burden attached to breast screening is large and the amount of benefit is small, and it is therefore unreasonable for the state to decide that the public should shoulder that burden. Others argue that the benefits are large and the burdens small, and therefore operating a breast screening program is entirely justifiable. It may be useful to explore community ideas about the importance of solidarity in the context of breast screening; this could be done, for example, by using a citizens' jury to answer the question of whether or not the state is justified in asking people to shoulder the expected burdens of breast screening in order to deliver the predicted level of population benefit.

This way of looking at solidarity and breast screening views breast screening as a topic in isolation. An alternative way of looking at solidarity is to look more generally at population health or even population well-being. At this more holistic level, we might ask the question of how we, as a society, should pull together in order to facilitate well-being in others, and consider the impact of a particular policy, such as breast screening, on the flourishing of the community. This would require a holistic assessment of the extent and distribution of the benefits and burdens of breast screening in the context of other possible health-supporting programs, and deciding how best to recognize the importance of community interests and act for the well-being of each other.

Summary: solidarity

- Individuals may attend, and states may promote, breast screening for reasons of solidarity: while solidarity in itself may have moral value, its use to promote breast screening deserves close scrutiny.
- Prioritizing solidarity may require that we consider breast screening in the context of the broadest range of possible health-supporting programs and community interests.

CONCLUSION

Breast screening is a large public health program with a significant reach. It is not a static entity, but one that varies with time and place. Our discussion of contemporary social issues and ethical principles, and how they are relevant in the context of current and future breast screening, adds to and complements biomedical perspectives on this important program. Armed with this knowledge and understanding, consumers, providers, researchers, and policymakers will be well placed to make an ethical analysis of breast screening: to consider the different ways that principles are being traded off against each other and to contemplate the extent to which these trade-offs are ethically justifiable. They may identify aspects that could be altered in order to make breast screening a more ethically sound program. Just as the evidence base for healthcare is constantly being updated, social values and institutions change over time. Given the range of social and ethical issues that we have shown to be relevant to breast screening, it seems important to explicitly reconsider these dimensions of breast screening programs when evaluating their success and future. As breast screening continues to evolve in the twenty-first century, we expect that social and ethical considerations will be increasingly recognized as critical in policymaking and screening practice.

GLOSSARY

Aggregative benefits In public health, aggregative benefits of a program or policy consist of all of the benefits experienced by individuals added up; for example, in breast screening, aggregative benefits are the sum of benefits experienced by (a few) individuals as a result of participating in screening. (See also: corporate benefits).

Autonomy An autonomous person is one who sees herself as in being charge of her own life; believes this to be appropriate; and has the freedom, opportunity, skills and capacities required to make choices, take action, and live in a manner that is consistent with her sense of who she is.

Citizens' jury (also known as community jury) A deliberative democratic method whereby a group of 12–24 individuals are recruited to meet for a period ranging from 1–7 days and produce a set of recommendations, or a decision on one or more defined questions. The jury receives information and evidence, cross-examines witnesses, and then deliberates on the issue at hand. (See also: deliberative democracy methods).

Corporate benefits In public health, the corporate benefits of a program or policy are those benefits that occur at the population level only; for example, in breast screening, corporate benefits are the added benefits (beyond aggregative benefits) that accrue to an entire community as a result of breast screening policies and practices. A clear example of a corporate benefit in public health is the herd immunity that results from achieving a certain vaccination rate in a population. (See also: aggregative benefits).

Deliberative democratic methods Ways of engaging citizens in formal iterative dialogue on important and complex problems. The main goal is to use the considered opinions and values of informed members of the public in a policy process; deliberative methods tend to provide participants with information, involve a range of people with diverse perspectives, and provide opportunities for reflection, critique and discussion. The two-way process of information exchange distinguishes deliberative democratic methods from other methods of communication with the public, which are dominated by one or other party informing the other (eg, consumer information pamphlets, public polling). Policies that incorporate public opinions obtained through deliberative democracy methods can be more legitimate, justifiable and feasible than those that don't. Different deliberative democratic methods include citizens' juries, consensus conferences, study circles, and citizens' assemblies. (See also: citizens' jury).

Distributive justice This concept is about fairness, including fairness of opportunity (eg, the opportunity for all individuals to pursue good health), and fairness of outcome (eg, everyone in a society achieving at least a basic or threshold level of good health.

Informed decision-making In healthcare, informed decision-making implies that patients or consumers have information and understanding about their health conditions and the nature and purpose of available interventions including benefits, harms and risks of choosing to participate, or not participate. It generally requires meaningful dialogue with healthcare workers, and the opportunity for people to make choices that are in their own best interests.

Nonmaleficence The principle of nonmaleficence imposes an obligation not to inflict harm on others. In healthcare, nonmaleficence demands that healthcare workers avoid inflicting harm on patients or consumers.

Overdetection A health-related finding in a person, probably through using testing technology, which does not produce a net benefit for that person. (See also: overdiagnosis).

Overdiagnosis Diagnosis of a condition in a person, where that diagnosis would be considered correct, but it does not produce a net benefit for that person, for example, diagnosis through screening of an indolent breast cancer that would never progress, or progress so slowly that, without screening, it would not have come to the attention of the individual in her lifetime. (See also: overdetection).

Overmedicalization Altering the meaning or understanding of experiences, so that health-related findings are reinterpreted as medical problems requiring medical treatment, without net benefit to patients or citizens.

Procedural justice Fairness in decision-making; for example, in breast screening procedural justice might require ensuring that all relevant stakeholders are included, that decisions are made for good reasons, that decisions are open to revision if new evidence or arguments emerge, and that biases and vested interests are minimized in order to ensure decisions are made in the best interests of the public. (See also: distributive justice).

Reciprocity Returning a favor that is done to you, sharing with others in the carrying of public burdens, and supporting and compensating those who carry the heaviest burdens.

Solidarity "Pulling together" toward a common (collective) cause on the understanding that there is mutual respect and obligation between members of a community and a sharing of burdens and threats.

Technological imperative A rule or belief that if a new technology exists, we need it. That is, we tend to believe that because we have the technology available, we must use it, sometimes before it has been proven safe or effective.

Transparency The full and honest disclosure of how, and by whom, decisions and policies are made. This includes the disclosure of possible vested interests among policymakers and advisors.

LIST OF ACRONYMS AND ABBREVIATIONS

DCIS Ductal carcinoma in situ
EBM Evidence-based medicine

HIV	Human immunodeficiency virus
LCIS	Lobular carcinoma in situ
NIH	(United States) National Institutes of Health
QALYs	Quality-adjusted life years
RCT	Randomized controlled trial
USPSTF	United States Preventive Services Task Force

REFERENCES

1. Sismondo S. *An introduction to science and technology studies*, 2nd ed. Chichester, England: Wiley-Blackwell; 2010.
2. Liverani M, Hawkins B, Parkhurst JO. Political and institutional influences on the use of evidence in public health policy. A systematic review. *PLoS One* 2013;**8**(10):e77404.
3. Bashford A, Strange C. Thinking historically about public health. *Med Humanit* 2007;**33**(2):87–92.
4. Yalom M. *A history of the breast*. New York, NY: Knopf; 1997.
5. Lerner BH. Fighting the war on breast cancer: debates over early detection, 1945 to the present. *Ann Intern Med* 1998;**129**(1):74–8.
6. Griffiths F, Bendelow G, Green E, Palmer J. Screening for breast cancer: medicalization, visualization and the embodied experience. *Health (London)* 2010;**14**(6):653–68.
7. Gardner KE. *Early detection: women, cancer, and awareness campaigns in the twentieth-century United States*. Chapel Hill, NC: University of North Carolina Press; 2006.18.53
8. Jones, SC, Rossiter, JRBreast cancer detection messages in Australian print media advertising—are they promoting correct information? In: *Proceedings of the 31st European marketing academy conference (EMAC), Braga, Portugal*; May 28–31, 2002.
9. Kaufert PA. Women and the debate over mammography: an economic, political and moral history. In: Sargent CF, Brettell CB, editors. *Gender and health: an international perspective*. New Jersey: Simon & Schuster; 1996. p. 167–86.
10. Lanz PM, Booth KM. The social construction of the breast cancer epidemic. *Soc Sci Med* 1998;**46**(7):907–18.
11. Welch HG. Overdiagnosed: making people sick in the pursuit of health. Boston, MA: Beacon Press; 2011.73.89
12. Bray F, Ren JS, Masuyer E, Ferlay J. Global estimates of cancer prevalence for 27 sites in the adult population in 2008. *Int J Cancer* 2013;**132**(5):1133–45.
13. Coleman MP, Quaresma M, Berrino F, Lutz JM, De Angelis R, Capocaccia R, et al. Cancer survival in five continents: a worldwide population-based study (CONCORD). *Lancet Oncol* 2008;**9**(8):730–56.
14. Early Breast Cancer Trialists' Collaborative Group (EBCTCG) Effects of chemotherapy and hormonal therapy for early breast cancer on recurrence and 15-year survival: an overview of the randomised trials. *Lancet* 2005;**365**(9472):1687–717.
15. Ferguson S, Kasper A. Living with breast cancer. In: Kasper A, Ferguson S, editors. *Breast cancer: society shapes an epidemic*. New York, NY: St Martin's Press; 2000. p. 1–24.
16. Black WC, Nease Jr. RF, Tosteson AN. Perceptions of breast cancer risk and screening effectiveness in women younger than 50 years of age. *J Natl Cancer Inst* 1995;**87**(10):720–31.
17. Chamot E, Perneger TV. Misconceptions about efficacy of mammography screening: a public health dilemma. *J Epidemiol Community Health* 2001;**55**:799–803.
18. Gigerenzer G, Mata J, Frank R. Public knowledge of benefits of breast and prostate cancer screening in Europe. *J Natl Cancer Inst* 2009;**101**(17):1216–20.
19. Reynolds H. The big squeeze: a social and political history of the controversial mammogram *The House that mammography built*. New York, NY: Cornell University Press; 2012.72.83 [Chapter 7].

20. Hann A. 'Controversy'. Propaganda versus evidence based health promotion: the case of breast screening. *Int J Health Plann Manage* 1999;**14**(4):329–34.
21. Lupton D. Femininity, responsibility, and the technological imperative: discourses on breast cancer in the Australian press. *Int J Health Serv* 1994;**24**(1):73–89.
22. Kaufert PA. Screening the body: the pap smear and the mammogram. In: Lock M, Young A, Cambrosio A, editors. *Living and working with the new medical technologies*. Cambridge, MA: Cambridge University Press; 2000. p. 165–83.
23. Lupton D. Risk as moral danger: the social and political functions of risk discourse in public health. *Int J Health Serv* 1993;**23**(3):425–35.
24. King S. *Pink ribbons, Inc. Breast cancer and the politics of philanthropy*. Minneapolis, MN: University of Minnesota Press; 2006.
25. Wells J. Mammography and the politics of randomised controlled trials. *BMJ* 1998;**317**(7167):1224–9.
26. Moynihan R, Smith R. Too much medicine? *BMJ* 2002;**324**(7342):859–60.
27. Schleifer D, Rothman DJ. The ultimate decision is yours": exploring patients' attitudes about the overuse of medical interventions. *PLoS One* 2012;**7**(12):e52552.
28. Robertson A. Embodying risk, embodying political rationality: women's accounts of risks for breast cancer. *Health Risk Soc* 2010;**2**(2):219–35.
29. Aronowitz RA. Do not delay: breast cancer and time, 1900–1970. *Milbank Q* 2001;**79**(3):355–86.
30. Zahl PH, Maehlen J, Welch HG. The natural history of invasive breast cancers detected by screening mammography. *Arch Intern Med* 2008;**168**(21):2311–6.
31. Baum M. Modern concepts of the natural history of breast cancer: a guide to the design and publication of trials of the treatment of breast cancer. *Eur J Cancer* 2013;**49**(1):60–4.
32. Aronowitz RA. Unnatural history: breast cancer and American society *Crisis in Prevention*. Cambridge, UK: Cambridge University Press; 2007.235.55 [Chapter 10].
33. Willis K. Choice, trust and risk: the policy context and mammography screening. In: Uchiyama N, Zanchetta Do Nascimento M, editors. *Mammography: recent advances*. Croatia, Shanghai: InTech Publishers; 2012. p. 3–24.
34. Gold RH, Yagmai AA, Bassett LW. The history of breast imaging. In: Bassett LW, Jackson VP, Jahan R, Fu YS, Gold RH, editors. *Diagnosis of diseases of the breast*. Philadelphia, PA: WB Saunders Company; 1997. p. 3–26.
35. Houssami N, Macaskill P, Bernardi D, Caumo F, Pellegrini M, Brunelli S, et al. Breast screening using 2D-mammography or integrating digital breast tomosynthesis (3D-mammography) for single-reading or double-reading—evidence to guide future screening strategies. *Eur J Cancer* 2014;**50**(10):1799–807.
36. Baines CJ. The Canadian national breast screening study: science meets controversy. In: Temple N, Thompson A, editors. *Excessive medical $pending*. Abingdon, UK: Radcliffe Publishing; 2007. p. 121–4.
37. Moffett J. Moving beyond the ribbon: an examination of breast cancer advocacy and activisim in the US and Canada. *Cultur Dyn* 2003;**15**(3):287–306.
38. Hann A. The decision to screen. In: Mills M, editor. *Prevention, health and british politics*. Aldershot: Avebury; 1993. p. 40–51.
39. Lupton D. The establishment of mass mammographic screening programs: in whose interests? *Aust J Soc Issues* 1992;**27**(2):112–24.
40. Wray N, Markovic M, Manderson L. Discourses of normality and difference: responses to diagnosis and treatment of gynaecological cancer of Australian women. *Soc Sci Med* 2007;**64**(11):2260–71.
41. Woolf SH. The 2009 breast cancer screening recommendations of the US preventive services task force. *JAMA* 2010;**303**(2):162–3.
42. Reynolds H. The big squeeze: a social and political history of the controversial mammogram *Pulling the plug on granny*. New York, NY: Cornell University Press; 2012.62.71 [Chapter 6].

43. Wilson J, Junger G. *Principles and practices of screening for disease*. Geneva: WHO; 1968. [Public Health Papers No. 34].
44. Barratt A, Mannes P, Irwig L, Trevena L, Craig J, Rychetnik L. Cancer screening. *J Epidemiol Community Health* 2002;**56**(12):899–902.
45. Skrabanek P. Why is preventive medicine exempted from ethical constraints? *J Med Ethics* 1990;**16**(4):187–90.
46. Shickle D, Chadwick R. The ethics of screening: is 'screeningitis' an incurable disease? *J Med Ethics* 1994;**20**(1):12–18.
47. Marshall KG. Prevention. How much harm? How much benefit? 4. The ethics of informed consent for preventive screening programs. *CMAJ* 1996;**155**(4):377–83.
48. Juth N, Munthe C. *The Ethics of screening in health care and medicine: Serving society or serving the patient*. Dordrecht: Springer; 2012.
49. Mant D, Fowler G. Mass screening: theory and ethics. *BMJ* 1990;**300**(6729):916–8.
50. Beauchamp T, Childress J. *Principles of biomedical ethics*, 7th ed. New York, NY, USA: Oxford University Press; 2012.
51. Kass NE. An ethics framework for public health. *Am J Public Health* 2001;**91**(11):1776–82.
52. Childress JF, Faden RR, Gaare RD, Gostin LO, Kahn J, Bonnie RJ, et al. Public health ethics: mapping the terrain. *J Law Med Ethics* 2002;**30**(2):170–8.
53. Upshur REG. Principles for the justification of public health intervention. *Can J Public Health* 2002;**93**(2):101–3.
54. ten Have M, de Beaufort ID, Mackenbach JP, van der Heide A. An overview of ethical frameworks in public health: can they be supportive in the evaluation of programs to prevent overweight? *BMC Public Health* 2010;**10**:638.
55. Dawson A. Resetting the parameters: public health as the foundation for public health ethics. In: Dawson A, editor. *Public health ethics: key concepts and issues in policy and practice*. Cambridge, MA: Cambridge University Press; 2011. p. 1–19.
56. Widdows H, Cordell S. Why communities and their goods matter: illustrated with the example of biobanks. *Public Health Ethics* 2011;**4**(1):14–25.
57. Independent UK Panel on Breast Cancer Screening The benefits and harms of breast cancer screening: an independent review. *Lancet* 2012;**380**(9855):1778–86.
58. Welch HG, Frankel BA. Likelihood that a woman with screen-detected breast cancer has had her "life saved" by that screening. *Arch Intern Med* 2011;**171**(22):2043–6.
59. Gotzsche PC, Nielsen M. Screening for breast cancer with mammography. *Cochrane Database Syst Rev* 2011;**1**.
60. Baum M. Harms from breast cancer screening outweigh benefits if death caused by treatment is included. *BMJ* 2013;**346**:f385.
61. Key TJ, Verkasalo PK, Banks E. Epidemiology of breast cancer. *Lancet Oncol* 2001;**2**(3):133–40.
62. Fletcher SW. Breast cancer screening: a 35-year perspective. *Epidemiol Rev* 2011;**33**(1):165–75.
63. van Ravesteyn NT, Miglioretti DL, Stout NK, Lee SJ, Schechter CB, Buist DS, et al. Tipping the balance of benefits and harms to favor screening mammography starting at age 40 years: a comparative modeling study of risk. *Ann Intern Med* 2012;**156**(9):609–17.
64. Mandelblatt J, Cronin K, de Koning H, Miglioretti DL, Schechter C, Stout NK. *Collaborative modeling of U.S. Breast cancer screening strategies*. Rockville, MD: Agency for Healthcare Research and Quality; 2015.
65. US Preventive Services Task Force. Draft recommendation statement: breast cancer: screening. Available from: <http://www.uspreventiveservicestaskforce.org/Page/Document/RecommendationStatementDraft/breast-cancer-screening1/>; May 2015 [cited 26.06.15].
66. Jorgensen KJ, Gotzsche PC. Overdiagnosis in publicly organised mammography screening programmes: systematic review of incidence trends. *BMJ* 2009;**339**:b2587.

67. Dixon JM. Breast screening has increased the number of mastectomies. *Breast Cancer Res* 2009;**11**(Suppl. 3):S19.
68. Paci E, Duffy SW, Giorgi D, Zappa M, Crocetti E, Vezzosi V, et al. Are breast cancer screening programmes increasing rates of mastectomy? Observational study. *BMJ* 2002;**325**(7361):418.
69. Domenighetti G, D'Avanzo B, Egger M, Berrino F, Perneger T, Mosconi P, et al. Women's perception of the benefits of mammography screening: population-based survey in four countries. *Int J Epidemiol* 2003;**32**(5):816–21.
70. Welch HG. Screening mammography—a long run for a short slide? *N Engl J Med* 2010;**363**(13):1276–8.
71. Forrest AP, Anderson ED. Breast cancer screening and management. *Med J Aust* 1999;**171**(9):479–84.
72. Brotherton J, Taylor R, Ivanov O, Tewson R, Page A. It's much easier than going to the dentist": high levels of satisfaction in a mammography screening program. *Aust N Z J Public Health* 2007;**31**(4):353–9.
73. Alcusky M, Philpotts L, Bonafede M, Clarke J, Skoufalos A. The patient burden of screening mammography recall. *J Womens Health (Larchmt)* 2014;**23**(Suppl. 1):S11–9.
74. Yaffe MJ, Mainprize JG. Risk of radiation-induced breast cancer from mammographic screening. *Radiology* 2011;**258**(1):98–105.
75. Miglioretti DL, Lange J, van Revesteyn NT, van den Broek J, Lee CI, Melnikow J. *Radiation-induced breast cancer and breast cancer death from mammography screening [abstract]*. Rockville, MD: Agency for Healthcare Research and Quality; 2015.
76. Houssami N, Skaane P. Overview of the evidence on digital breast tomosynthesis in breast cancer detection. *Breast* 2013;**22**(2):101–8.
77. Bond M, Pavey T, Welch K, Cooper C, Garside R, Dean S, et al. Systematic review of the psychological consequences of false-positive screening mammograms. *Health Technol Assess* 2013;**17**(13):1–170. v-vi.
78. Pace LE, Keating NL. A systematic assessment of benefits and risks to guide breast cancer screening decisions. *JAMA* 2014;**311**(13):1327–35.
79. Hofvind S, Ponti A, Patnick J, Ascunce N, Njor S, Broeders M, et al. False-positive results in mammographic screening for breast cancer in Europe: a literature review and survey of service screening programmes. *J Med Screen* 2012;**19**(Suppl. 1):57–66.
80. Miles A, Cockburn J, Smith RA, Wardle J. A perspective from countries using organized screening programs. *Cancer* 2004;**101**(5 Suppl):1201–13.
81. Hubbard RA, Kerlikowske K, Flowers CI, Yankaskas BC, Zhu W, Miglioretti DL. Cumulative probability of false-positive recall or biopsy recommendation after 10 years of screening mammography: a cohort study. *Ann Intern Med* 2011;**155**(8):481–92.
82. Petticrew MP, Sowden AJ, Lister-Sharp D, Wright K. False-negative results in screening programmes: systematic review of impact and implications. *Health Technol Assess* 2000;**4**(5):1–120.
83. Zafar SY, Peppercorn JM, Schrag D, Taylor DH, Goetzinger AM, Zhong X, et al. The financial toxicity of cancer treatment: a pilot study assessing out-of-pocket expenses and the insured cancer patient's experience. *Oncologist* 2013;**18**(4):381–90.
84. Biesheuvel C, Barratt A, Howard K, Houssami N, Irwig L. Effects of study methods and biases on estimates of invasive breast cancer overdetection with mammography screening: a systematic review. *Lancet Oncol* 2007;**8**(12):1129–38.
85. Carter JL, Coletti RJ, Harris RP. Quantifying and monitoring overdiagnosis in cancer screening: a systematic review of methods. *BMJ* 2015;**350**:g7773.
86. Morrow M, Schnitt SJ, Norton L. Current management of lesions associated with an increased risk of breast cancer. *Nat Rev Clin Oncol* 2015;**12**(4):227–38.
87. Carter SM, Williams J, Parker L, Pickles K, Jacklyn G, Rychetnik L, et al. Screening for cervical, prostate, and breast cancer: interpreting the evidence. *Am J Prev Med* 2015;**49**(2):274–85.
88. Barratt A. Overdiagnosis in mammography screening: a 45 year journey from shadowy idea to acknowledged reality. *BMJ* 2015;**350**:h867.

89. Skrabanek P. Mass mammography: the time for reappraisal. *Int J Technol Assess Health Care* 1989;**5**(03):423–30.
90. Schmidt JG. The epidemiology of mass breast cancer screening—a plea for a valid measure of benefit. *J Clin Epidemiol* 1990;**43**(3):215–25.
91. Heleno B, Thomsen MF, Rodrigues DS, Jorgensen KJ, Brodersen J. Quantification of harms in cancer screening trials: literature review. *BMJ* 2013;**347**:f5334.
92. Raffle AE, Muir Gray JA. *Screening: Evidence and practice*. Oxford: Oxford University Press; 2007.
93. Moutel G, Duchange N, Darquy S, de Montgolfier S, Papin-Lefebvre F, Jullian O, et al. Women's participation in breast cancer screening in France—an ethical approach. *BMC Med Ethics* 2014;**15**:64.
94. Jorgensen KJ, Keen JD, Gotzsche PC. Is mammographic screening justifiable considering its substantial overdiagnosis rate and minor effect on mortality? *Radiology* 2011;**260**(3):621–7.
95. Autier P, Esserman L, Flowers C, Houssami N. Breast cancer screening: the questions answered. *Nat Rev Clin Oncol* 2012;**9**(10):599–605.
96. Rychetnik L, Carter SM, Abelson J, Thornton H, Barratt A, Entwistle VA, et al. Enhancing citizen engagement in cancer screening through deliberative democracy. *J Natl Cancer Inst* 2013;**105**(6):380–6.
97. Stefanek ME. Uninformed compliance or informed choice? A needed shift in our approach to cancer screening. *J Natl Cancer Inst* 2011;**103**(24):1821–6.
98. Informed choice about cancer screening. NHS breast screening: helping you decide. Available from: <http://www.informedchoiceaboutcancerscreening.org/wp-content/uploads/2013/05/Breast-screening-leaflet_8August2013_Final_ready-for-print-version.pdf/>; 2013 [cited 30.04.15].
99. de Gelder R, Bulliard JL, de Wolf C, Fracheboud J, Draisma G, Schopper D, et al. Cost-effectiveness of opportunistic versus organised mammography screening in Switzerland. *Eur J Cancer* 2009;**45**(1):127–38.
100. Duckett S. Commonwealth/state relations in health. In: Hancock L, editor. *Health policy in the market state*. St. Leonards: Allen & Unwin; 1999. p. 71–86.
101. Carter R, Glasziou P, van Oortmarssen G, de Koning H, Stevenson C, Salkeld G, et al. Cost-effectiveness of mammographic screening in Australia. *Aust J Public Health* 1993;**17**(1):42–50.
102. Wright CJ, Mueller CB. Screening mammography and public health policy: the need for perspective. *Lancet* 1995;**346**(8966):29–32.
103. Pharoah PD, Sewell B, Fitzsimmons D, Bennett HS, Pashayan N. Cost effectiveness of the NHS breast screening programme: life table model. *BMJ* 2013;**346**:f2618.
104. Torgerson DJ, Donaldson C. An economic view of high compliance as a screening objective. *BMJ* 1994;**308**(6921):117–9.
105. Howard K, Salkeld G, Irwig L, Adelstein BA. High participation rates are not necessary for cost-effective colorectal cancer screening. *J Med Screen* 2005;**12**(2):96–102.
106. Mackenzie C. Autonomy. In: Arras J, Fenton E, Kukla R, editors. *Routledge companion to bioethics*. New York, NY: Routledge; 2014.
107. Slaytor EK, Ward JE. How risks of breast cancer and benefits of screening are communicated to women: analysis of 58 pamphlets. *BMJ* 1998;**317**(7153):263–4.
108. Gummersbach E, Piccoliori G, Zerbe CO, Altiner A, Othman C, Rose C, et al. Are women getting relevant information about mammography screening for an informed consent: a critical appraisal of information brochures used for screening invitation in Germany, Italy, Spain and France. *Eur J Public Health* 2010;**20**(4):409–14.
109. Hoffmann TC, Del Mar CB. Shared decision making: what do clinicians need to know and why should they bother? *Med J Aust* 2014;**201**(9):513–4.
110. Rimer BK, Briss PA, Zeller PK, Chan ECY, Woolf SH. Informed decision making: what is its role in cancer screening? *Cancer* 2004;**101**(S5):1214–28.
111. Gillon R. Ethics needs principles—four can encompass the rest—and respect for autonomy should be "first among equals." *J Med Ethics* 2003;**29**(5):307–12.

112. Dawson A. The future of bioethics: three dogmas and a cup of hemlock. *Bioethics* 2010;**24**(5):218–25.
113. Austoker J. Gaining informed consent for screening. Is difficult—but many misconceptions need to be undone. *BMJ* 1999;**319**(7212):722–3.
114. Raffle AE. Information about screening—is it to achieve high uptake or to ensure informed choice? *Health Expect* 2001;**4**(2):92–8.
115. Hoffman RM, Elmore JG, Fairfield KM, Gerstein BS, Levin CA, Pignone MP. Lack of shared decision making in cancer screening discussions: results from a national survey. *Am J Prev Med* 2014;**47**(3):251–9.
116. Strech D. Participation rate or informed choice? Rethinking the European key performance indicators for mammography screening. *Health Policy* 2014;**115**(1):100–3.
117. Jorgensen KJ, Gotzsche PC. Content of invitations for publicly funded screening mammography. *BMJ* 2006;**332**(7540):538–41.
118. Guyatt G, Akl EA, Hirsh J, Kearon C, Crowther M, Gutterman D, et al. The vexing problem of guidelines and conflict of interest: a potential solution. *Ann Intern Med* 2010;**152**(11):738–41.
119. Rimer BK, Meissner H, Breen N, Legler J, Coyne CA. Social and behavioural interventions to increase breast cancer screening. In: Schneiderman N, Speers MA, Silva JM, Tomes H, Gentry JH, editors. *Integrating behavioural and social sciences with public health.* Washington, DC: American Psychological Association; 2001. p. 177–202.
120. Gouldner AW. The norm of reciprocity: a preliminary statement. *Am Sociol Rev* 1960;**25**(2):161–78.
121. Viens AM, Bensimon CM, Upshur REG. Your liberty or your life: reciprocity in the use of restrictive measures in contexts of contagion. *Bioeth Inq* 2009;**6**:207–17.
122. Nettleton S. Governing the risky self: how to become healthy, wealthy and wise. In: Peterson A, Bunton R, editors. *Foucault, health and medicine*. London: Routlege; 1997. p. 207–22.
123. Dawson A, Verweij M. Solidarity: a moral concept in need of clarification. *Public Health Ethics* 2012;**5**(1):1–5.
124. ter Meulen R, Wright K. Family solidarity and informal care: the case of care for people with dementia. *Bioethics* 2012;**26**(7):361–8.

CHAPTER

TREATMENT OF SCREEN-DETECTED BREAST CANCER: CAN WE AVOID OR MINIMIZE OVERTREATMENT?

15

J. Michael Dixon[1] and David Cameron[2]

[1]*Edinburgh Breast Unit, Western General Hospital, Edinburgh, United Kingdom,*
[2]*Edinburgh Cancer Research Centre, Western General Hospital, Edinburgh, United Kingdom*

CHAPTER OUTLINE

PLAIN LANGUAGE SUMMARY

Women with screen-detected breast cancers have better survival than those with symptomatic breast cancers. Many screen-detected cancers are low risk because they are unlikely to recur or to cause death, with between 11% and 19% of screen-detected cancers considered as being overdiagnosed, that means that these women have been diagnosed and treated for breast cancer but if they had not been screened then they would not have known they had breast cancer (nor required treatment for it) in

Breast Cancer Screening. DOI: http://dx.doi.org/10.1016/B978-0-12-802209-2.00015-2

their lifetime. As well as overdiagnosis, some screen-detected breast cancers are probably overtreated, meaning women receive more aggressive treatment than necessary to control their cancer. There is a need to better match treatment not only to the patient's characteristics and the tumor stage but also to the tumor biology. Some patients with noninvasive cancers–known as ductal carcinoma in situ (DCIS)-are overtreated and ongoing studies are looking at whether low grade DCIS needs any treatment at all. Although the numbers of patients having breast conserving surgery has increased over time, many patients are unnecessarily treated with mastectomy. Whole breast radiotherapy after breast conserving surgery is the standard for women with invasive cancer but not all women with screen-detected invasive breast cancer need it. Likewise not all women with screen-detected invasive cancer need axillary surgery. Similarly systemic therapies after a diagnosis of screen-detected breast cancer may be over used in some women. The increased use of molecular profiling should limit the use of chemotherapy but the threshold for using adjuvant endocrine treatment is such that few women are not prescribed this. Chemotherapy and hormone therapy are not without morbidity. It is essential that overdiagnosis and overtreatment of screen-detected breast cancer are addressed in future studies.

INTRODUCTION

The method of detection of breast cancer appears in a number of studies to be an independent prognostic variable. When controlled for age, nodal status, and tumor size, a study of 1983 Finnish women with invasive breast cancer reported that screen-detected cancers had a lower risk of relapse compared with symptomatic cancers and had an improved overall survival after adjusting for other prognostic factors.[1] Women whose cancers were detected outside screening had an increased death rate (HR) 1.90 (95% confidence interval (CI), 1.15–3.11) compared to women with screen-detected breast cancer, even though symptomatic women were more likely to receive adjuvant systemic therapy.[1] In another study of three randomized screening trials (Health Insurance Plan, National Breast Screening Study NBSS-1, and NBSS-2) in the analysis adjusted for known prognostic parameters, patients whose cancer was found via screening had a more favorable prognosis than women with symptomatic cancers.[2] The relative risks for death were 1.53 (95% CI, 1.17–2.00) for interval and incident cancers, compared with screen-detected cancers and 1.36 (95% CI, 1.10–1.68) for cancers in the symptomatic group, compared with screen-detected cancers.[2] A study of 5604 English women with breast cancer diagnosed between 1998 and 2003 also found that women with screen-detected cancers fared better than their symptomatic counterparts (Fig. 15.1).[3] The HR for survival of screen-detected versus symptomatic women was 0.79 (95% CI, 0.63–0.99).[3] These various observations are consistent with the view that many screen-detected breast cancers are low risk and that some of these cancers require less or even no treatment because they would not have caused problems in the patient's lifetime. It is well recognized that a proportion of screen-detected breast cancers do indeed represent overdiagnosis and that this is of the order of 11% from a population perspective, or approximately 19% from the perspective of a woman invited to screening.[4] Chapter "Challenges in Understanding and Quantifying Overdiagnosis and Overtreatment" of this book provides additional information on estimates of overdiagnosis from breast screening.

There is also clearly overtreatment of screen-detected breast cancer. Overtreatment can be considered to occur in two ways, although these are related. First, in overdiagnosed cases, since by definition these cancers did not need to be found (as they would not have become clinically apparent in the

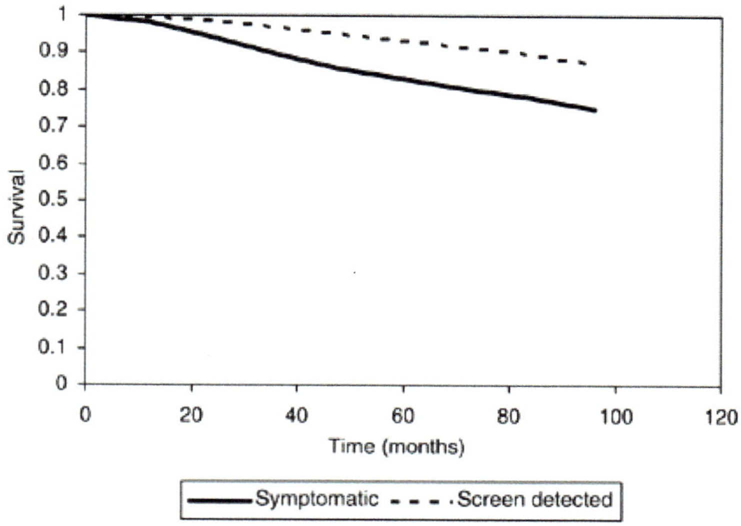

FIGURE 15.1

Survival by detection mode.

Reprinted by permission from Macmillan Publishers Ltd on behalf of Cancer Research UK: British Journal of Cancer (Ref. 3).

absence of screening), any treatment is unnecessary in these women and so represents overtreatment. Diagnosing less low risk cancers or renaming some of these cancers are potential methods of limiting overtreatment. There has been renaming of cancers at other sites, such as the bladder and the cervix, and this has produced less overdiagnosis and has reduced overtreatment[5]. It has also reduced anxiety and improved the quality of life in these women.

The second aspect of overtreatment is the administration of therapies that are unnecessary to treat the early stage cancers detected through breast screening.[6,7] The one-size-fits-all philosophy of treating in situ or invasive breast cancer based on tumor size and node status is inappropriate and takes no account of the range of biology of cancers seen within the screen-detected population. There is a real need to tailor treatment not only to the patient and tumor stage but also to the biology of the cancer, both for screen-detected as well as nonscreen-detected cancers.

There is some evidence that tailoring treatment to the cancer is occurring in terms of surgical treatment.[8] The absolute numbers of breast conserving surgery episodes has increased over time and the absolute numbers of mastectomies has fallen. Nonetheless, there remains enormous variation in the rates of breast conserving surgery for cancers with a total size less than 15 mm throughout the UK and North America, and the message of reducing the extent of surgery has not reached all surgeons[9] (Fig. 15.2). Some of this variation may be patient driven but thus there is a need to ensure patients are educated that more extensive surgery is not beneficial. The rate of mastectomy in the UK is actually higher for noninvasive breast cancers (27% in 2011/12) compared with invasive breast cancer (23%).[10] As a result of breast screening the actual numbers of women having mastectomy for noninvasive cancer has increased every year in the UK for the past 15 years.[10] The incidence of DCIS increased from 5.8 per 100,000 women in the 1970s to 32.5 per 100,000 women in the US in 2004 and then reached a

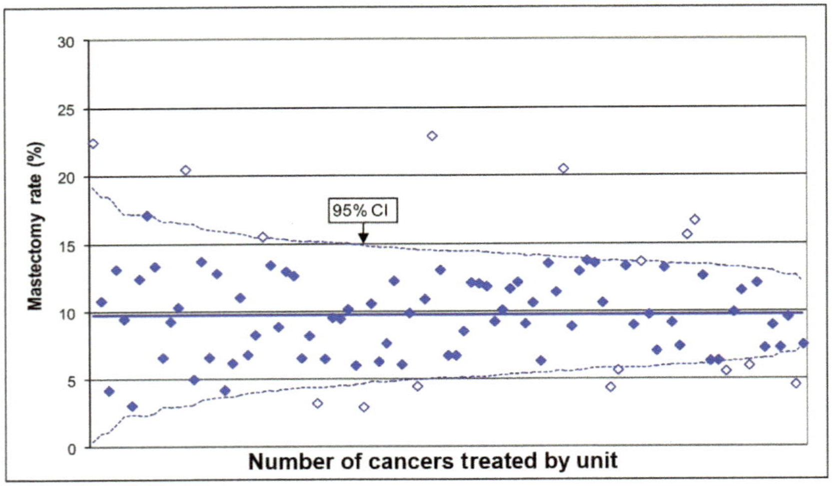

FIGURE 15.2

Percentage of patients with screen-detected breast cancers whole size ≤ 15 mm treated by mastectomy in the UK in 2009/10–2011/12. Each symbol represents an individual Breast Unit and the number of cases of breast cancer treated by that Unit is platted on the X axis. Six units lie above the 95% confidence intervals of the mean.

From Ref. 10.

plateau. Over 60,000 women will be diagnosed with DCIS in the USA in 2015.[11–14] This needs to be addressed by the surgical community. Most women detected with breast cancer through screening are node-negative and there has been a move to reduce the number of women having axillary clearance even in patients with 1 or 2 positive sentinel nodes. Sentinel node is a step in the right direction but do women with small low risk cancers require any axillary surgery?

Whole breast radiotherapy after breast conserving surgery is now standard but do all screen-detected women require whole breast radiotherapy? Is there any role for partial breast radiotherapy and can some women avoid radiotherapy altogether? Ongoing studies are providing evidence that one can identify women at low risk in whom radiotherapy can be omitted. Whole breast radiotherapy is used following breast conserving surgery for DCIS but again not all women need it. This means that many women receive treatment they may not need and experience the associated side effects, yet have little potential gain. Current evidence shows that the breast cancer specific mortality at 20 years is only 3.3% and was not influenced by the use of radiotherapy. Using genomic tests to identify women with low risk DCIS is one avenue of research that is showing promise. There is also an onus on the oncological community to ensure that systemic adjuvant therapies are administered on the basis of tumor characteristics rather than just stage at diagnosis. Systemic therapies can produce significant and long-term adverse effects on quality of life so it is essential that these treatments are tailored to the patient and their cancer.

REDUCING CANCER DIAGNOSES

Many core biopsies are performed for calcifications detected on mammography that have a low risk of being invasive cancer or DCIS, but a high likelihood of being benign. Should these really be a target for screening? If lesions that had a greater than 50% risk of representing DCIS or greater than 10% risk of being invasive cancer were targeted, would it be possible to reduce overdiagnosis and also the numbers of interventions? A study by Flowers and Esserman[5] using these criteria found that the biopsy rate fell by almost half from 100% to 52%. The cancer to biopsy yield rose from 28% to 47% and only a single invasive cancer would have been missed: a 3 mm Grade 1 invasive cancer.[5] Redefining what lesions are biopsied is one potential method of reducing overdiagnosis and thus reducing over treatment.

Lobular carcinoma in situ (LCIS) is a rare form of mammary cancer first described in 1941 by Foote and Stewart.[15] LCIS was initially considered a form of breast cancer and was treated by mastectomy but later it became reclassified as a marker of generalized breast cancer risk with a relative risk of breast cancer of between 8 to 10 times that of the women of the same age without LCIS.[16,17] The rate of invasive breast cancer in women with LCIS is approximately 1% per year.[18,19] Atypical lobular hyperplasia (ALH) is diagnosed when there is a lesser degree of lobular expansion with the same cells as seen in LCIS and has an increased risk of invasive breast cancer, between 4–5 times that of the general population. Because of the difficulties of separating LCIS and ALH, the term lobular intraepithelial neoplasia (LIN) has been introduced to include both lesions. LCIS is diagnosed by screening in somewhere between 0.5% and 2% of all core biopsies. The current North American NCCN guidelines and the UK guidelines are that patients with LCIS or ALH on core biopsy should have surgical excision.[20,21] This is based on studies that have shown upgrade rates to invasive cancer or to DCIS as high as 50%. The logic of excision is that there is likely to be a worse lesion in the breast. There are however problems with the studies investigating women with LCIS on core biopsy because they have contained small numbers of women and have reported a huge variation in upgrade rates varying from 0% to 50%. More recently there has been an attempt to correlate radiology with pathology and two groups can be identified: a concordant group where the histologic findings in the core biopsy adequately explain the findings on imaging and a discordant group where the histological findings on the core biopsy do not adequately explain the findings on imaging studies. The upgrade rate of core biopsy diagnosed LCIS and ALH in patients with concordant imaging findings is small.[22–24] A recent prospective multi-institutional study by Nakhlis enrolled 79 patients.[25] In 74 women who had LIN as the worst lesion on core biopsy with concordant imaging, 73 had no upgrade on surgical excision with only one upgrade to DCIS.[25] From a total of 335 cases from five different publications in the literature where there was concordance between histology and imaging there have been just six upgrades (1.8%). Five of these were to DCIS (1.5%) and one was a 2 mm grade I invasive cancer. There is now growing evidence that excision biopsy can be avoided in patients diagnosed with LIN on core biopsy where there is concordance with imaging. If however there is atypical ductal hyperplasia (ADH) or pleomorphic LCIS is diagnosed on core biopsy then excision is still required. The upgrade rate for pleomorphic LCIS is much higher than for nonpleomorphic LCIS and varies from 17% to 46% in three small series.[22–24]

Similar arguments can be made for avoiding excision of radial scars and papillary lesions that have been adequately sampled with a large core vacuum assisted device. Radial scars are found in association with low or intermediate grade DCIS or low grade invasive breast cancers in between 3% and 40% of patients.[26] If these lesions are adequately sampled however the upgrade rate following surgical excision is small enough to believe that excision is unnecessary unless there are concerns of malignancy on large bore biopsy.[27] The same is true for papillary lesions and formal excision is required only where a large bore core biopsy shows atypia. Radial scars and papillary lesions diagnosed on 14 gage core biopsy should be further sampled by a large gage vacuum assisted device and only where there is concern histologically should excision be advised. This would avoid a significant number of the excision biopsy procedures currently performed in women with radial scars and papillary lesions.

CHANGING TERMINOLOGY

DCIS was uncommon before mammographic breast screening was introduced but since the introduction of breast screening there has been a 500% increase in the number of DCIS cases diagnosed (Fig. 15.3). Between 20–30% of all cancers diagnosed through screening are now DCIS. What happened to these women with DCIS before breast screening? A study by Welsh et al. looked at seven series of women who died without breast cancer and had their breasts examined at autopsy.[28] The prevalence of invasive cancer in this population was 1.3% with a range of 0% to 18%. The prevalence of DCIS was 8.9% with a range of 0% to 14%. In women aged 40–70 who had more than 50 slides examined the prevalence of DCIS was 14.5%. Currently, as a result of breast screening many of these women with

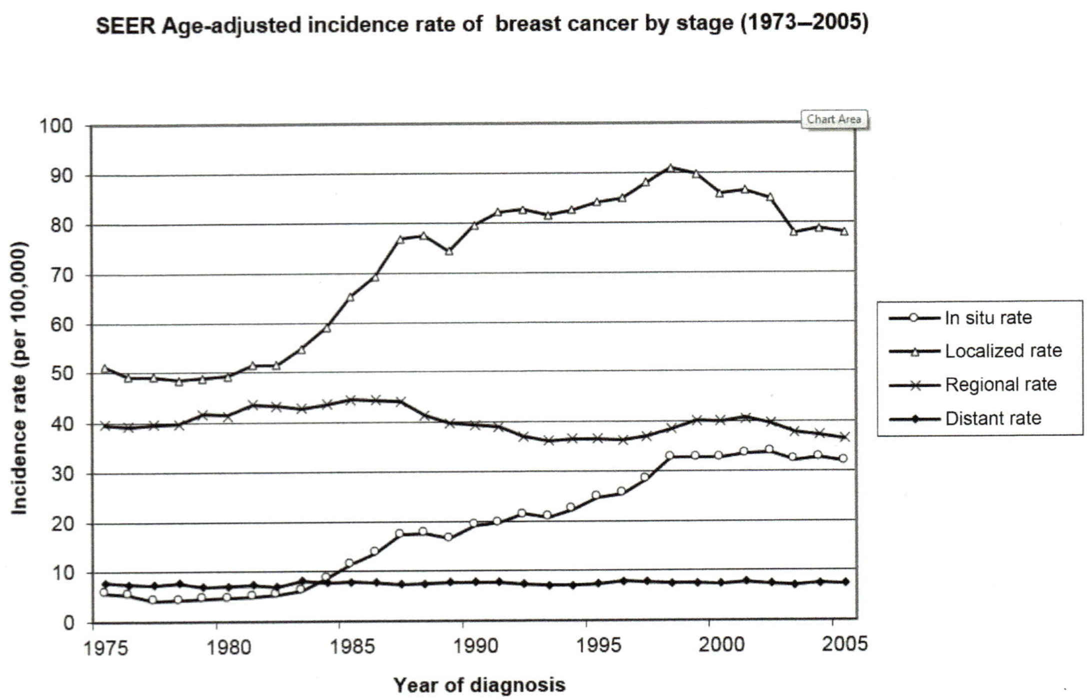

FIGURE 15.3

Rates of Breast Cancer in the USA looking specifically at the numbers of women with in situ, localized, and distant disease.

DCIS are identified even though many would have died of other causes and the DCIS would never have become symptomatic. The reason for detecting DCIS is that this should in theory reduce the rate of subsequent breast cancer development. There is, however, limited evidence that there has been a major reduction in the subsequent rates of invasive cancer or any a reduction in the numbers of women with advanced disease has not been as large as one might have hoped.[29]

The current dilemma relates to whether all patients with DCIS require treatment and should all DCIS be considered cancer? A cancer or a neoplasm is defined as an abnormal mass of tissue whose growth is in excess of, or uncoordinated with that of surrounding normal tissue and whose growth continues in the same excessive manner after the removal of the stimulus which evoked the change. Not all DCIS progresses and not all DCIS lesions continue to grow in an excessive manner after development. The question is can we identify those DCIS cases that are true neoplasms and those that continue to grow and progress to cancer?

DCIS is diagnosed if histologically there are two complete spaces filled or there is greater than 2 mm of an intraductal proliferation with significant atypia.[30] If there are less than 2 complete spaces in the terminal duct lobular unit or less than 2 mm of disease even if significant atypia is present, then this is classified as ADH. There is no real scientific basis for this definition of DCIS based on number of spaces or size of the lesion. Not all pathologists adhere to this definition and this has led to significant variation in how small areas of epithelial proliferation within the terminal duct lobular unit are classified. Studies show up to a third of pathologists will diagnose DCIS if a single 1.5 mm ductal space is filled with low grade atypical epithelium with no necrosis and a classical cribriform architecture, yet based on the currently agreed criteria this should be diagnosed as ADH.[31] The problem is that there is a lack of diagnostic concordance between pathologists in interpreting these difficult lesions. A recent study showed excellent concordance in the diagnosis of invasive cancer (96%) but a lower concordance in DCIS (84%) and a lower still concordance in atypia (48%).[32] Variation in diagnosis potentially leads to variation in treatment for women with histologically identical lesions.

There have been huge advances in molecular pathology and when the genomics of ADH is compared with DCIS, ADH has most of the features of DCIS.[33] ADH is not reversible, is often clonal and it can progress to invasive cancer, although this is rare. Genomic studies have shown that ADH and low grade DCIS are more closely related to LCIS than to high grade DCIS.[34] This has led some to argue that low grade DCIS and ADH should be reclassified together as a single entity-ductal intraepithelial neoplasia or DIN as they are clearly different abnormalities compared to high grade DCIS. Distinguishing ADH from low grade DCIS does appear somewhat illogical. The term LIN was introduced to combine LCIS an ALH because the two are so obviously related and there was a lack of consistency between pathologists. Classifying low grade DCIS as neoplasia rather than cancer does seem sensible based on what we know. This reclassification would follow the lead from other organs. Areas of atypia and carcinoma in situ (CIS) in the cervix are now incorporated into the condition of cervical intraepithelial neoplasia or CIN. Is it time for a similar approach to low grade and some intermediate grade DCIS?

The 5-year risk of developing ipsilateral invasive breast cancer among women diagnosed with LIN but having no treatment is about 3–5% and the 10 year risk between 5–10%.[35] For ADH and low risk DCIS without treatment the rate is pretty similar at 3–5% at 5 years and 5–10% at 10 years. The risk associated with intermediate risk DCIS is a little higher at about 4–5% at 5 years and 7–12% at 10 years. The risk is much higher for high risk DCIS and without treatment is about 7–5% at 5 years and 15–20% at 10 years. It is thus evident that different grades and risk categories of DCIS have differences in their natural history and yet they are all classified together as DCIS.[35]

There is also concern that some lesions classified currently as DCIS may be invasive cancers.[32,36] Tabár and colleagues have reported that patients who have extensive DCIS and have casting-type calcification have a high rate of developing invasive recurrence after mastectomy.[36] How does this happen? Pathologists argue that they examine only a fraction of the disease and that invasion can be present in the breast but that this is missed because only a small proportion of disease is sampled. In some patients tumor cells are seen in lymphatics and even in lymph nodes yet there is no histological evidence of invasion identified in the breast. Is this just a sampling issue or is it that histological assessment cannot differentiate in situ from invasive cancer? Patients that have invasive cancer that is missed are at risk of being undertreated. There is an urgent need to develop better ways of assessing the presence of invasion and the likely biological behavior of DCIS, so that both overtreatment and undertreatment are avoided.

LESS SURGERY FOR IN SITU BREAST CANCER

One of the consequences of the increase in the number of women with DCIS detected through breast screening is that over the period 2001–2015 the number of women in the UK having mastectomy for DCIS has more than doubled.[37] There is also evidence from the USA that mastectomy rates have increased. The explanation is that although a higher percentage of women with DCIS are now having breast conserving surgery, the number of women diagnosed with DCIS over this period of time has more than doubled. In 2011–12 the mastectomy rate for invasive cancer was 23% but for non or micro invasive cancer it was 27%.[10] There were relatively few cases of low grade DCIS so it is difficult to estimate the numbers having mastectomy for low grade DCIS. The counterargument is that patients who have extensive DCIS in association with invasive cancer are treated by mastectomy, so if all women with DCIS eventually develop invasive disease mastectomy might not be overtreatment. Post-mortem studies suggest however that not all DCIS becomes symptomatic. There needs to be greater effort in DCIS to minimize treatment and this is the basis of the upcoming trials of low grade DCIS discussed later. The whole ethos behind screening is to detect disease early so as to improve outlook and to reduce the treatment required. There is an urgent need to reduce the number of women with DCIS having more extensive surgery and to reduce the overall burden of treatment for this condition that in some women would never have caused problems in their lifetime.

Within the UK screening program the Sloane project collected prospectively, surgery, pathology, and radiotherapy data on patients with in situ cancers diagnosed and treated between 2003 and 2012.[38] Approximately 50% of all DCIS cases have been captured in this data set. Patients who had successful breast conserving surgery at one operation had a mean pathology size of 12 mm and the size increased to 17 mm for patients who had successful breast conserving surgery at two operations. For those who had breast conserving surgery and then subsequently went on to mastectomy, their average pathology size was 40 mm. There were 1969 women who had a mastectomy for DCIS over 20 mm and 510 women who had mastectomy for DCIS that measured less than 20 mm. In patients who had a mastectomy for DCIS under 20 mm, radiology often overestimated tumor size. The average overestimate in these patients was 19.86 mm. The Sloane data set shows clearly that many women who currently have mastectomies for DCIS could be treated by breast conserving surgery. It would appear that up to a half of women in the UK who have a mastectomy for screen-detected DCIS, based on size alone, do not require it. There is also a huge variation in the percentage of women having unnecessary mastectomies between hospitals. Women with DCIS diagnosed through screening should have biopsies at both ends

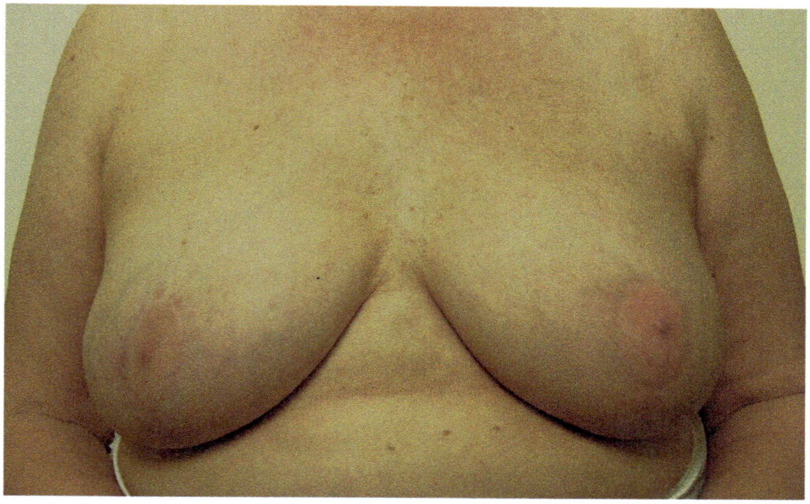

FIGURE 15.4

Excellent result from therapeutic mammaplasty.

M Dixon, Edinburgh Breast Unit, Edinburgh, UK.

of the mammographic lesion and have a careful evaluation of the extent of disease before any decision is made on surgery. Performing a mastectomy routinely on the basis of the calcification measuring 4 cm or more, with a single biopsy demonstrating DCIS, is inappropriate. National guidelines on an acceptable rate of mastectomy for small areas of DCIS are required and centers that have rates that fall well outside these guidelines need to provide an adequate explanation.

Although the international standard care for patients with DCIS measuring 4 cm in size or over has been mastectomy, wide excision and radiotherapy offers equivalent outcomes providing all the DCIS is adequately excised. A number of units scattered throughout the UK have developed methods for excising large areas of DCIS and conserving the breast in women with DCIS >40 mm in extent. This involves multiple wire localizations to mark all visible disease and combining the excision with a therapeutic mammaplasty. Such procedures produce excellent cosmetic results (Fig. 15.4), have a high rate of complete excision and to date a low rate of subsequent recurrence. In Edinburgh these are performed as bilateral procedures by a team of a breast and plastic surgeons operating simultaneously. Complications are infrequent and complete excision rates over 90%. Follow-up is limited but there have been no recurrences in the Edinburgh series so far.[39–41] This approach is becoming more widespread in Europe, in North and South America, and in Australasia. The issue for many of these women is that even if they are treated by mastectomy and breast reconstruction to get symmetry, a contralateral procedure is required. Bilateral therapeutic mammaplasty can be performed without drains as a day patient or a short stay procedure and recovery is quicker, complications are fewer, and overall costs reduced compared with mastectomy and whole breast reconstruction.

The role of MRI in DCIS has recently been reviewed.[42] The results of MRI in DCIS are similar to those of MRI in invasive cancer. MRI has a high false-positive rate and so cannot be relied upon with any certainty to delineate the extent of disease. DCIS is frequently over treated surgically as a consequence of MRI false-positives and overestimation of disease extent.[42] Recurrence rates after breast conserving surgery are falling and for all women diagnosed with DCIS, a multidisciplinary approach is required with mastectomy being indicated only where breast conservation is not feasible or the patient herself choses this option.[37,39,40]

REDUCED TREATMENT FOR DCIS

There are now a number of national and international trials looking at reducing treatment for women with low risk DCIS. Data from the UK Sloane Project which includes over 10,000 cases showed that 66% of DCIS is high grade, 25% intermediate, and 9% low grade.[38] Grading of DCIS by pathologists is inconsistent and many classify anything other than high grade as low risk DCIS. The UK trial of low risk DCIS study (LORIS) requires that all pathology is reviewed centrally and those deemed to have low grade, or DCIS at the boundary between low and intermediate grade, are eligible for entry into the study.[43] Eligible patients with low risk DCIS are offered randomization to surgery, endocrine therapy, or observation alone.[43] A recent US study has shown that the benefit of any surgery in low grade DCIS is very limited.[44] Of 57,222 cases of DCIS, for low grade DCIS the 10-year breast cancer specific survival of the nonsurgery group was 98.8% and for the surgery group was 98.6% ($p = 0.95$). Further prospective studies, such as the one ongoing in the UK, will provide better insight into the natural history of low risk DCIS diagnosed through breast screening treated by endocrine therapy or managed by observation alone. It should provide a better evidence base for identifying those women with DCIS who need excision with or without radiotherapy. Other similar trials of low grade DCIS are underway in Europe and in the USA.

LIMITING RADIOTHERAPY IN PATIENTS WITH DCIS

Numerous randomized trials have shown the benefits of whole breast radiotherapy in patients with DCIS following breast conserving surgery. The first trial was performed by the NSABP, but large trials have also been performed in Europe.[45] The largest European study enrolled over 1000 patients with DCIS less than 5 cm in size, 50% of whom received radiotherapy after surgical excision. The 15-year cumulative incidence of DCIS recurrence in the surgery group was 14.9% compared to 7.5% in those patients who had both surgery and radiotherapy.[46] The rates of development of invasive disease in the treated breast was 15.5% in the surgery-only group and 9.8% when surgery was combined with radiotherapy[45]. The rate of DCIS or invasive cancer in the treated breast in this trial was thus over 1% per year even after wide excision and radiotherapy. It is perhaps surprising therefore that no survival advantage for radiotherapy was found, because it reduced the rate of invasive cancer development and the women who developed invasive cancer had a significantly worse survival compared with women who had DCIS recurrence or no recurrence at all. The majority of DCIS recurrences occurred within the first 5 years after treatment and the greatest effect of radiotherapy on reducing invasive recurrence was also in the first 5 years. The risks of developing any recurrence was however more or less continuous over 15 years of follow-up and this may explain the lack of any impact of radiotherapy on long-term outcome. The lack of a survival benefit for radiotherapy is clear even when all the randomized studies are combined. Since these initial trials, the rates of local recurrence in invasive cancer have fallen over time and there is now evidence that the rates of local recurrence following breast conservation for

DCIS is also falling.[47,48] Thus a 1% per year rate of recurrence in the European trial with surgery and radiotherapy is no longer seen and the rate is closer to 0.5% per year. The relevance of these older trials to current practice is thus not entirely clear.

Tamoxifen has been shown in randomized trials to reduce the rates of DCIS recurrence and invasive breast cancer development in patients with ER positive DCIS. Similarly aromatase inhibitors reduce recurrence rates.[49] These agents are used widely in the US in ER positive DCIS but their use, at least in the UK, is not routine. Given the low rate of mortality from DCIS at 20 years and the morbidity of these treatments it is easy to understand why endocrine therapy use in DCIS is not in routine use in many centers.

An initial analysis of factors related to recurrence after DCIS treatment was undertaken in the European Organisation of Research and Treatment of Cancer (EORTC) study and showed that there was a higher rate of local recurrence in patients who presented symptomatically compared with being screen-detected. Those with close or positive versus clear margins, who had cribriform, solid, or comedo DCIS versus other types, had intermediate or high grade DCIS versus low grade DCIS, or were younger than 40 versus over 40 all had higher rates of recurrence.[46] It is now common in Europe and North America for lower risk groups of patients with screen-detected DCIS to be treated by wide local excision alone and to add radiotherapy only for higher risk women. There have been some studies of wide excision alone that have shown reasonable rates of local control. The ECCOG-5194 study enrolled 670 women with grade 1 or 2 DCIS of noncomedo type of less than 2.5 cm or grade III and comedo DCIS <1 cm in size treated by excision alone without any radiotherapy. Women had to have a negative margin width of greater than 3 mm and tamoxifen treatment after surgery was optional. This study was published and reported a 5-year recurrence rate of 6.1% in those stratified as low or intermediate risk.[50] The median tumor size of the low and intermediate grade DCIS was 6 mm and for the high grade DCIS it was 5 mm. In the high grade DCIS group even though they were relatively small lesions the recurrence rate was 15.3% at a median follow-up period of 6.7 years.

Following the success of tumor profiling of invasive cancers and the development of a 21 gene recurrence score for predicting in-breast tumor recurrence and breast cancer survival,[51] a 12 gene DCIS score has been developed and been evaluated in two separate studies.[35,50] These 12 genes, a subset of the 21 genes, include five proliferation genes, the progesterone receptor gene, and GSTM1 or glutathione S transferase, as well as five reference genes. Three groups of patients can be defined at low, intermediate, and high risk of recurrence. In the ECOG 5194 study the low risk group comprised 146 patients who had a 10-year risk of recurrence of 12%. In the 45 women in the intermediate group the 10-year risk was 24.5% and in the 36 patients in the high risk group the 10-year rate of recurrence was 27.3% (Fig. 15.5a and 15.5b).[35] The invasive breast cancer rate was 5.1% in the low risk group, 8.9% in the intermediate group, and 19.1% in the high risk group. In a multivariate analysis the 12 gene recurrence score, tumor size, and postmenopausal status were significant predictors of recurrence in ECOG 5194. A validation study presented at San Antonio 2014 from Canada confirmed the utility of the DCIS recurrence score. Although traditionally pathologic features have been used to predict patients likely to get recurrence, this genomic based assay has the ability to identify a group of women who have a low risk of recurrence and may therefore avoid radiation after wide local excision.[52]

Other methods of predicting DCIS recurrence are already used in clinical practice. The Van Nuys classification includes patient age, width of margin of excision, DCIS extent, and pathology.[53] Each of these 4 factors is scored 1, 2, or 3 and an overall score out of 12 is calculated with higher scores having greater rates of recurrence. This index has clinical utility but it is starting to be replaced by the 12 gene recurrence score. One reason is that even in patients with low Van Nuys scores, there is

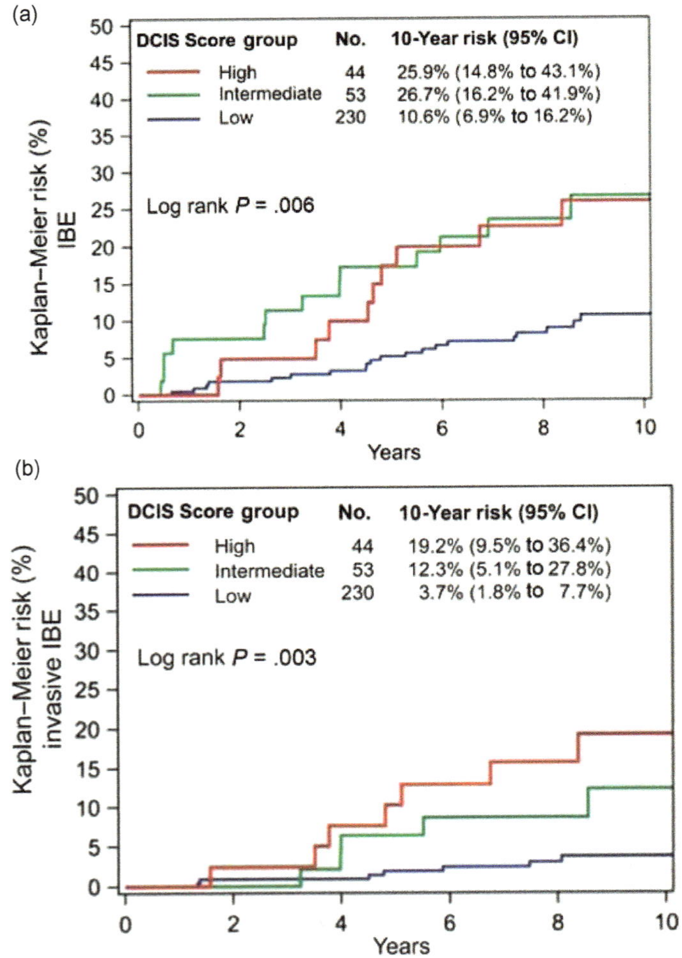

FIGURE 15.5

Ten-year Ipsilateral Breast Events (IBE) by Risk Group subdivided by DCIS score using the 12 gene assay in the ECOG 5194 study. (a) Probability of developing an IBE based on the DCIS Score according to the three prespecified risk groups. (b) Probability of developing an invasive IBE based on the DCIS Score according to the three prespecified risk groups.

From Ref. 35, reproduced by permission of Oxford University Press.

evidence that radiotherapy reduces significantly the rate of recurrence following surgery. There is also now less emphasis on wide margins, given their impact on cosmetic outcome and the uncertainty that wider margins do reduce rates of local recurrence. There is undoubtedly a group of women who do not require radiotherapy after wide excision. It is imperative that further research is performed to identify these women. The 12 gene recurrence score is being used more widely in the United States to identify those women with low risk DCIS who can safely avoid radiotherapy but as yet this score has not been incorporated into clinical practice in Europe.[54–57]

NEOADJUVANT ENDOCRINE THERAPY FOR DCIS

One potential way to reduce extensive surgery for DCIS is to reduce the size of the DCIS prior to surgery. More than half of DCIS is ER rich. A number of studies have evaluated the role of endocrine agents in DCIS. Tamoxifen in ER positive women produces a 60% reduction in the rate of local recurrence at 9 years.[58] Studies have shown that short periods of preoperative therapy with aromatase inhibitors in patients with DCIS can produce dramatic reductions in proliferation.[59,60] Hwang and Esserman in 2004 demonstrated that it is possible to show a reduction in extent of DCIS on imaging with neoadjuvant endocrine therapy.[61] We have treated 20 women with neoadjuvant endocrine therapy prior to surgery in our own practice in Edinburgh. In many of these cases, the surgery performed was therapeutic mammoplasty to excise large areas of DCIS.[40] Using a combination of neoadjuvant endocrine therapy and therapeutic mammoplasty we have a very low rate of margin involvement of less than 5%, which is surprisingly low given the high rates of margin involvement normally reported for breast conserving surgery in DCIS.[39] Some individual patients have had either no residual disease or ADH only following neoadjuvant endocrine therapy. Others have had reduction in the extent on disease visible on imaging.[61] Further evaluations of the role of endocrine therapy before surgery in women with ER positive DCIS to avoid mastectomy are required urgently.

ANTI-HER2 THERAPY

Many DCIS lesions are HER2 positive. Neoadjuvant trastuzumab in HER2 positive cancers in addition to chemotherapy dramatically improves the rates of complete pathology response with no invasive or in situ cancer remaining. It is evident that in many patients with extensive DCIS in association with invasive breast cancer chemotherapy and trastuzumab eliminates the DCIS.[62] Ongoing studies giving trastuzumab during radiotherapy after surgery for DCIS will determine whether anti-HER2 therapies when combined with radiotherapy improve outcomes.[63] Whether anti-HER2 therapy in DCIS is another example of overtreatment only time will tell.

REDUCING MASTECTOMY FOR INVASIVE CANCER

One meta-analysis of nine trials that compared breast conserving surgery and mastectomy in women with invasive breast cancer found no significant difference in the risk of death at 10 years: the relative risk reduction for breast-conserving surgery compared with mastectomy was 0.02 (95% CI, −0.05 to +0.09).[64] There was also no difference in the rates of local recurrence in six randomized controlled trials involving 3006 women where data were available: the relative risk reduction for mastectomy versus breast-conserving surgery was 0.04 (95% CI, −0.04 to +0.12).[65] There is no group of women with invasive breast cancer who are suitable for breast conserving surgery and whole breast radiotherapy where mastectomy alone does improve outcome. Some studies have even suggested better outcomes for breast conserving surgery with no excess of local recurrences (Fig. 15.6).[66] Despite this there is a trend for increasing rates of mastectomy and for increasing rates of bilateral mastectomy. This has been driven in part by the women themselves and in part reflects our inability to educate patients as to the benefits of

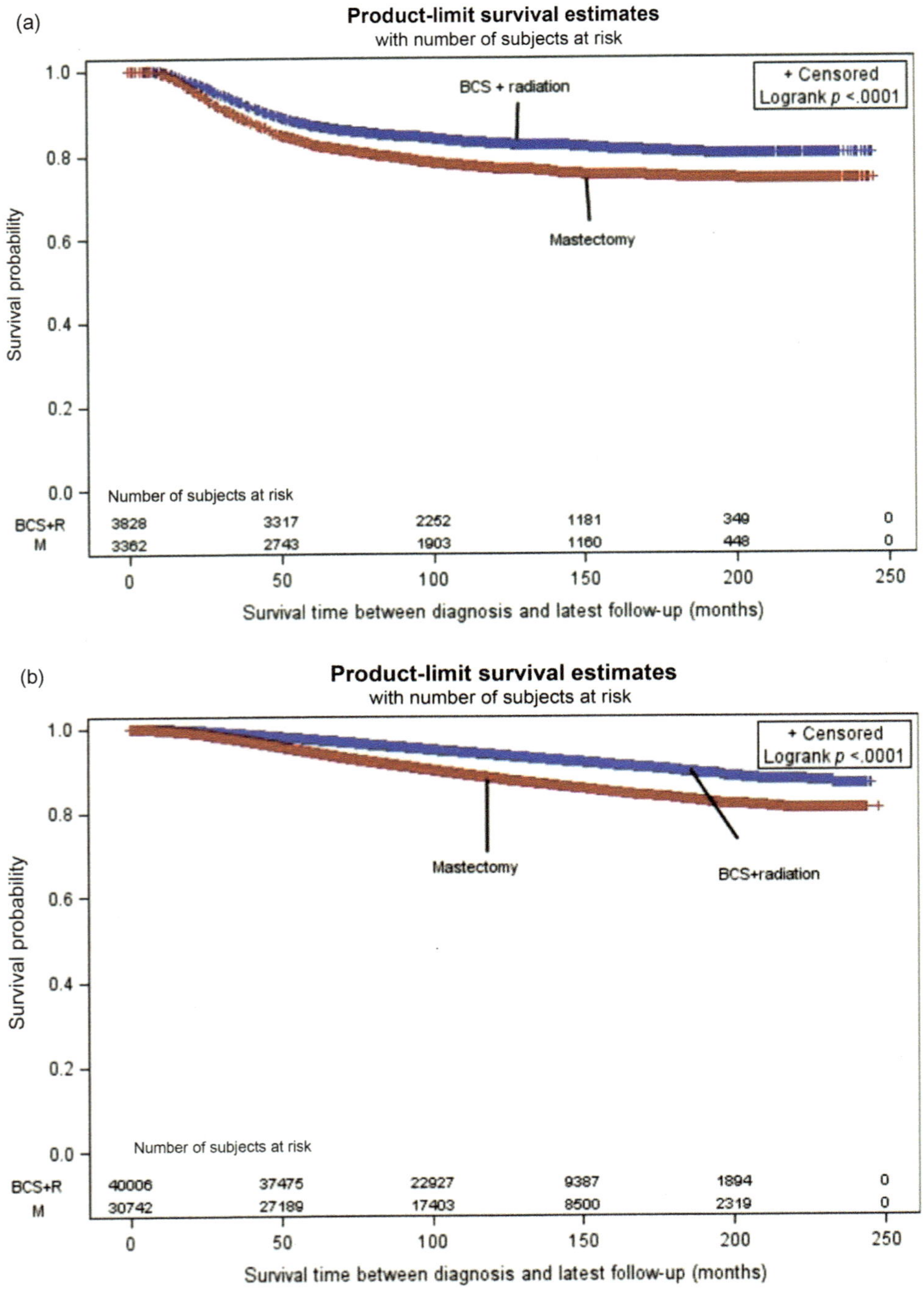

FIGURE 15.6

Kaplan-Meier overall survival estimates are shown for hormone receptor (HR)-negative patients, age <50 years at diagnosis (a) and age >50 years at diagnosis (b): comparison of breast-conserving therapy (breast-conserving therapy (BCS) with radiation (R)) and mastectomy (M) groups.

From Ref. 66, reproduced by permission of Wiley Materials.

breast conservation. Fear of recurrence has driven the increase in mastectomy although local recurrence rates after breast conserving surgery are falling and are no longer greater than seen after mastectomy. Mastectomy rates vary widely within countries (Fig. 15.2) and within the same unit depending on which surgeon a patient sees. The use of preoperative MRI also increases the rate of mastectomy.[67–70] Surgeons and multidisciplinary teams have a huge role to play in presenting the patient with the best current evidence. Mastectomy is overtreatment for most screen-detected breast cancers and local recurrence rates now for breast conservation are less than 5% at 10 years. There is also increasing evidence that breast conserving surgery results in better survival rates compared with mastectomy.[66] In a recent study from the Netherlands breast conserving surgery had a hazard ratio for survival of 0.87 versus mastectomy in a multivariable analysis in a population of 173,797 female patients.[71] It is no longer acceptable to assume that a high mastectomy rate in any hospital compared with another in the same country represents patient choice. Other factors including the surgeon's advice and the availability of all treatments locally have a huge impact (Fig. 15.2). The evidence that choice is influenced by the surgeon and the attitude of the multidisciplinary team is very clear from the literature. Most women with screen-detected breast cancer can have breast conserving surgery as a day patient combined with a sentinel node biopsy. Most women should get an excellent or good cosmetic outcome and excellent long-term control of disease and survival after breast conserving treatment, and therefore mastectomy offers these women no advantage.

REDUCING THE NUMBER OF PATIENTS WHO GET RADIOTHERAPY AFTER BREAST CONSERVING SURGERY FOR INVASIVE BREAST CANCER

The current standard of care for patients treated by breast conserving surgery for invasive breast cancer irrespective of age or other risk factors is to give whole breast radiotherapy plus or minus a boost to the tumor bed.[72] The data on the impact of age on local recurrence following breast conserving surgery suggests that in-breast tumor recurrences falls with increasing age.[73] Adjuvant tamoxifen with or without adjuvant radiotherapy reduces the risk of recurrence and so the question that has been addressed by a number of trials is whether low risk older women with ER positive invasive cancer require both adjuvant endocrine therapy and whole breast radiation to maintain satisfactory rates of local control. The PRIME II trial randomized women aged 65 or older with ER positive invasive breast cancer whose cancers measured under 3 cm in size, were completely excised and were node-negative to endocrine therapy alone or endocrine therapy and radiotherapy.[74] At a median of 5 years follow-up radiotherapy provided a 2.8% (95% CI, 1.9–4%) absolute reduction in breast tumor recurrence. The majority of patients in the PRIME trial had grade I–II, T1-2 cancer with clear margins and were low risk. The cancer and leukemia group (CALGB) 9343 trial tested the omission of adjuvant whole breast radiotherapy in an even lower risk group of older women, namely those with T1 tumors up to 2 cm in women greater than 70 years of age receiving adjuvant tamoxifen after breast conserving surgery.[75] As in the PRIME trial, there was a 3% improvement in locoregional control from the addition of radiotherapy at 5 years and a 7% gain at 10 years. The BASO II trial included patients with invasive breast cancers less than 2 cm in size that were Grade I or special type cancers and randomized these women to four arms: no treatment, radiotherapy, radiotherapy + tamoxifen, or tamoxifen alone.[76] The mean age of women in this trial was 57 years. At a median follow-up of 167 months the annual rate of recurrence was 0.8% for the tamoxifen alone arm and 0% when tamoxifen was combined with whole breast radiotherapy. The German Breast Cancer Study

Group reported in a similar low risk group of women aged 45 years or older, an in-breast tumor recurrence rate of 6% with adjuvant endocrine therapy alone and 2% when adjuvant therapy was combined with radiotherapy.[77] In an Italian trial patients aged between 55 and 70 years with cancers measuring 2–5 cm or less without an extensive in situ component who received systemic therapy were randomized to radiotherapy or no radiotherapy and the in-breast tumor recurrence rates were 3.1% with radiotherapy and 4.4% in the surgery alone group.[78] In summary, various trials have shown that in low risk women, and this includes many of those with screen-detected breast cancers, radiotherapy can be omitted safely. In the PRIME trial, a hypothesis generating observation was that in the subgroup of patients with ER rich tumors treated with endocrine therapy the benefit of radiotherapy was even lower. In this subgroup the 5-year local recurrence rate was 3.3% at 5 years. This rate of local control is better than seen in younger women treated by wide excision, systemic therapy, and radiotherapy. The CALGB 9434 trial had little apparent impact on the use of radiotherapy in the USA. The US National Cancer Institute (NCI) guidelines now allow the omission of radiotherapy in older suitable patients after breast conserving surgery.[79] The majority of women with screen-detected invasive breast cancer will not die from breast cancer. By far and away the majority die from other causes. Many of the patients who develop recurrence after wide excision and adjuvant endocrine therapy have the option of a further excision and radiotherapy. This contrasts to patients who develop recurrence after whole breast radiotherapy who usually require mastectomy. It is time to apply the results of the many clinical trials and reduce the use of whole breast radiotherapy in lower risk women with screen-detected invasive breast cancers.

Another option is to use partial breast radiotherapy. A number of studies have evaluated partial breast radiotherapy after breast conserving surgery. The TARGIT trial looked at intraoperative radiotherapy.[80] The risks of local recurrence in the TARGIT arm were in reality similar to the rates of local recurrence seen in the PRIME II trial without radiotherapy. In another partial breast radiotherapy trial 1305 patients were randomized (654 to external radiotherapy and 651 to intraoperative radiotherapy) between November 2000 and December 2007. After a medium follow-up of 5.8 years (IQR 4.1–7·7), 35 patients in the intraoperative radiotherapy group and four patients in the external radiotherapy group had had an IBTR ($p < 0.0001$). The 5-year event rate for IBRT was 4.4% (95% CI, 2.7–6.1) in the intraoperative radiotherapy group and 0.4% (0.0–1.0) in the external radiotherapy group (hazard ratio 9.3 (95% CI, 3.3–26.3))[81] (Fig. 15.7). Follow-up in most partial breast radiotherapy trials, and in particular in TARGIT, are short and those with longer follow-up have shown increasing local recurrence rates over time. Most of the patients included in TARGIT study were low risk. There are clear advantages of intraoperative radiotherapy or limiting the length of treatment of radiotherapy compared to more prolonged treatments. Ongoing studies are evaluating shorter courses of whole breast radiotherapy and their efficacy and comparing these with the more prolonged treatment courses that have been traditionally used. The current view is that there is insufficient longterm data from large randomized trials of partial breast radiotherapy to recommend its use, even in a screen-detected low risk population. The current choice is therefore whole breast radiotherapy or no radiotherapy.

REDUCING SURGERY IN THE AXILLA IN WOMEN WITH SCREEN-DETECTED INVASIVE BREAST CANCER

The surgical approach to the axilla in invasive breast cancer has changed dramatically over the last decade. Although the status of the axillary lymph nodes continues to be a significant prognostic marker

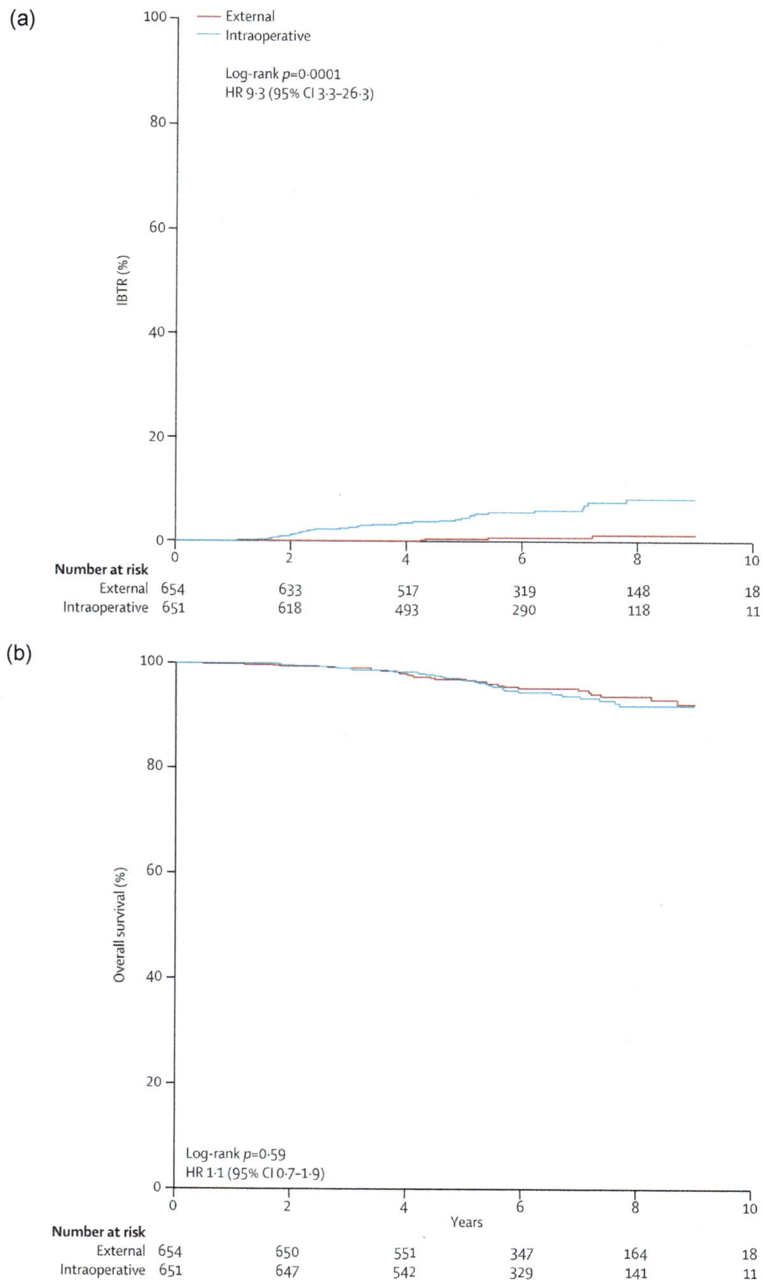

FIGURE 15.7

Cumulative incidence of (a) ipsilateral breast tumor recurrence and (b) overall survival (intention-to-treat population) in a trial of intraoperative or external beam radiotherapy conducted by Veronesi et al.

From Ref. 81, reprinted from The Lancet with permission of Elsevier.

in the management of breast cancer patients, removal of lymph nodes carries no survival benefit. As such, the purpose of axillary surgery is primarily for staging and local control. Historically, a complete axillary node dissection with removal of level I and II lymph nodes or even levels I–III was standard and while this operation provided excellent prognostic data and local control, it was associated with significant morbidity in terms of lymphoedema and decreased range of movement of the shoulder. Through the pioneering efforts of Cabanas,[82] who first coined the term "sentinel node" based on cadaveric studies of penile cancer, and the work of Donald Morton in melanoma,[83] sentinel node biopsy has revolutionized breast cancer treatment. The concept of sentinel node biopsy is that one can map the lymphatic drainage of a tumor to the first draining lymph nodes and these nodes will be representative of other nodes in the lymphatic basin. Large validation studies have confirmed that sentinel node biopsy is a safe, reliable, minimally invasive procedure that accurately stages the axilla.[84] The National Surgical Adjuvant Breast and Bowel Project B-32 trial found overall survival, disease-free survival, and locoregional recurrence were equivalent between patients who were randomized to sentinel node biopsy followed by routine axillary dissection compared with sentinel node biopsy (SNLB) alone in sentinel node-negative patients.[85] Given these data and those from numerous other studies, sentinel node biopsy is now the standard of care in the management of patients with clinically node-negative breast cancer. As most patients with such screen-detected breast cancer do not have involved nodes, sentinel lymph node biopsy is now in routine use for such women.

IS AXILLARY NODE DISSECTION NECESSARY IN ALL NODE-POSITIVE PATIENTS?

The American College of Surgeons Oncology Group (ACOSOG) Z-0011 trial randomized 891 sentinel node-positive patients to complete axillary node dissection versus no axillary node dissection.[86] All patients received whole breast tangential irradiation, which in some cases covered the lower axilla. The median total number of nodes removed was 17 in the axillary lymph node dissection (ALND) group and 2 in the women having sentinel lymph node biopsy group alone. A total of 27.3% of patients having a subsequent axillary dissection had further node metastases. At a median follow-up of 6.3 years, there was no significant difference in axillary recurrence between patients who had a complete axillary node dissection (0.5%) and those who did not (0.9%). Disease-free survival did not differ significantly between the two treatment arms; the 5-year disease-free survival was 83.9% (95% CI, 80.2–87.9%) for the sentinel lymph node biopsy alone group and 82.2% (95% CI, 78.3–86.3%) for the ALND group. At a median follow-up of 6.3 years, there was also no evidence that sentinel lymph node biopsy alone compared with ALND resulted in a statistically significant inferior survival. The unadjusted hazard ratio between the two groups was in favor of sentinel lymph node biopsy with a hazard ratio of 0.79 (90% CI, 0.56–1.11). The hazard ratio for overall survival adjusting for adjuvant therapy and age was 0.87 (90% CI, 0.62–1.23). The rates of wound infections, axillary seromas, and paresthesia were significantly higher for the ALND group (70% vs 25%, $P < 0.001$). Lymphoedema was also significantly more common in the ALND group ($P < 0.001$).

For many surgeons, this trial has been practice changing and questions the need for routine axillary dissection in the setting of a positive sentinel node. It should be noted, however, that this study had several important limitations affecting its generalizability, and its findings apply only to those defined under the trial's eligibility criteria. Patients who had locally advanced disease or who underwent neoadjuvant chemotherapy were not candidates for the trial. Further, only patients with fewer than three positive nodes were eligible. Patients all had breast conserving surgery with whole breast irradiation (accelerated partial breast irradiation or brachytherapy was an exclusion factor), and most had systemic adjuvant therapy. Some would consider the follow-up, especially for luminal breast cancers, to be short relative to the natural history of those cancers, and although the statistical end-point of this study was achieved, due to low local recurrence rates to date, it was underpowered to show a small effect on outcome. There are, however, large amounts of other supporting data from patients who have involved nodes treated by sentinel node biopsy alone, so the results of the Z-0011 data do not stand alone in indicating that it should no longer be routine practice to advise complete axillary dissection for all patients with a positive sentinel node. ASCO guidelines now state that patients with 1 or 2 positive sentinel nodes having breast conserving surgery and whole breast radiotherapy who fulfill Z-0011 entry criteria do not require routine axillary clearance.[87]

The International Breast Cancer Study Group (IBCSG) 23-01 reported a trial where patients with sentinel nodes containing micrometastases were randomized to either complete axillary node dissection or no complete axillary node dissection.[88] Unlike the ACOSOG Z-0011 trial, only 75% of patients had breast-conserving surgery; 89% of patients in the group randomized to axillary node dissection received adjuvant breast or chest wall radiation therapy, and 92% of patients randomized to no complete axillary dissection received radiation. Five-year disease-free survival was 87.3% for the 464 patients who underwent axillary node dissection and 88.4% for the 467 patients who did not undergo this procedure, with low rates of axillary recurrence in both groups. Locoregional recurrences were seen in five patients (1.1%) having no axillary dissection: two in the axilla alone, one in the axilla together with internal mammary nodes, one in the breast and axilla, and one in the internal mammary nodes alone. There was only one patient in the axillary dissection group (0.2%) who developed locoregional recurrence and this was an isolated axillary recurrence. Overall survival was 98% at 5 years in both groups. These and other data show that patients with micrometastases in a sentinel node biopsy do not require axillary dissection and this includes screen-detected patients.

The EORTC 10981 "After Mapping of the Axilla, Radiotherapy or Surgery?" (AMAROS) trial assessed whether surgery or axillary radiation ART produced similar outcomes in sentinel node-positive patients.[89] AMAROS enrolled 4806 patients who had clinically node-negative disease. Those who subsequently had a positive SNLB were randomized to ALND or ART. At 5-year follow-up, the rates of lymphoedema were 28% after ALND and 14% after ART ($p < 0.0001$). Axillary recurrence rates at the same time point were 0.54% (47/744) after ALND versus 1.03% (7/681) after ART. Unfortunately, the intended noninferiority test did not have sufficient statistical power due to the unexpectedly low number of recurrences. There was no significant difference in either disease-free ($p = 0.18$) or overall survival ($p = 0.34$) rates. The results suggest that both ALND and ART can provide excellent regional control but with a more significant cost in terms of morbidity after ALND. Patients with screen-detected breast cancer treated with breast conserving surgery and radiotherapy who also have involved lymph nodes who are considered after a multidisciplinary discussion to require further axillary treatment should now be offered the option of either axillary dissection or axillary radiation.

DO PATIENTS REQUIRE ANY AXILLARY SURGERY?

Fisher[90,91] and Baum and Coyle[92] were the first to show that a "wait and see" policy regarding axillary nodes is an option in breast cancer without loss of local control of disease, and that it is safe in terms of overall survival. Other studies of different therapeutic strategies, ranging from no intervention[93,94] to radiation therapy to the lower[95] or the entire axilla,[96] have generally confirmed good local disease control and overall survival. The rate of axillary relapse from such approaches has been small,[94–96] and even in those who did recur salvage surgery has produced satisfactory control rates.[93] The risk of relapse in the axilla is mainly related to the size of the primary tumor (2% for T1a cancer to 18% for T2). However, it is now well established that lymph node metastases are "indicators but not governors" of survival[97] and thus in women who have no axillary treatment, the appearance of an axillary metastasis does not necessarily indicate a poor prognosis or a potential source of metastatic spread. Any axillary surgery is likely overtreatment for most women with T1 breast cancer and particularly in T1a and T1b tumors, because the rate of axillary node involvement and thus axillary relapse is actually very low in both. Even in the T2 group, a high rate of successful salvage surgery for axillary relapse indicates that up-front axillary surgery not be always required. While at present the standard in clinically node-negative women is to do a sentinel node biopsy, further trials of no axillary surgery are required. One can see in the future that women with small screen-detected breast cancers will have an axillary ultrasound plus or minus FNA and in those without evidence of axillary metastases on imaging, either no further axillary procedure will be performed, or at least a choice of avoiding axillary intervention will be part of standard care. For higher risk node-negative women a sentinel lymph node biopsy seems appropriate. Even in those women with proven node-positive disease it is clear that for many women axillary dissection is overtreatment. A more rational evidence-based approach to the axilla is required. There is huge variation between the USA and Europe in the implementation of the Z-0011 results. Waiting another decade for the results of new trials is inappropriate. There is an urgent need for international guidelines based on best evidence rather than on consensus to be published and adhered to. The latter allows individual opinion to influence the final statement which should be based entirely on the clinical evidence.

SYSTEMIC THERAPY IN OVERDIAGNOSED CANCERS

In addition to local therapy, patients with a screen-detected malignancy will, via the normal multidisciplinary team meeting discussions, be considered for adjuvant systemic therapy. For those with overdiagnosed cancers, adjuvant systemic therapy will constitute a further example of overtreatment, with the consequent toxicities and risks. However, this dilemma is not *intrinsically* different from that facing any woman with a potentially curable symptomatic breast cancer. It is not currently possible to identify the subset of patients for whom adjuvant systemic therapy will control or eradicate micrometastatic disease that would otherwise lead to their demise. While meta-analyses have demonstrated significant survival benefits for women receiving systemic therapies, the absolute percentage gain in survival is modest, and since the benefits are relative reductions in recurrence and death, the absolute benefits are small for those with a lower risk of relapse.

Given that it is likely that most disease that is overdiagnosed by screening is either DCIS or low-grade cancer,[4] the main consideration in these women is the role of endocrine therapy, as only a minority are likely to be considered for chemotherapy. Currently most patients with hormone receptor positive breast cancer are offered at least 5 years' endocrine therapy, which is not without toxicity. Patients with DCIS in the UK are not usually offered endocrine therapy as the risk of dying of breast cancer is low—so any mortality benefits from therapy are too small to justify the toxicity. In contrast endocrine therapy is used widely in the USA. Some patients and/or clinicians use systemic endocrine therapy to reduce the risk of developing a second cancer as much as to treat the primary cancer. There are no data to suggest that the risks of a second cancer after a screen-detected cancer are profoundly different from that in nonscreen-detected disease. But the risks of dying from a second breast cancer in a treated or contralateral breast are small. If the rationale for using endocrine therapy is prevention of subsequent cancers, then it would not really be "overtreatment," if a patient with a screen-detected malignant lesion is treated with endocrine treatment as she is at some increased risk of a contralateral cancer relative to a nonaffected woman. One can argue the potential benefits of tamoxifen as a preventative agent are unproven in terms of a reduction in mortality but in terms of reduction in breast cancer incidence the evidence clearly favors tamoxifen use.[98]

So how much harm is done by the use of adjuvant endocrine therapy in an invasive breast cancer that was screen-detected? The simple answer is that we don't know, as we don't know how many or which screen-detected lesions can be left untreated. Risk of relapse relates to the biology of the cancer, and while multigene parameters such as Oncotype Dx and MammaPrint provide a measure of risk of relapse, none were designed to address who should get adjuvant endocrine therapy. Indeed Oncotype was developed on the background of trials where every patient received endocrine therapy. Thus in order to determine when the use of adjuvant endocrine therapy may offer little benefit, clinicians still use traditional prognostics, such as tumor size, grade, ER, HER2 and node status, alone or as part of online tools such as Adjuvant! Online or Predict! and the challenge is intrinsically no different for a screen-detected cancer than a symptomatic one. One advantage of using Predict! Is that it includes in its calculations whether the cancer is symptomatic or screen-detected. Screen-detected lesions tend to be smaller and of lower grade, but in many hospitals there is no universally accepted threshold of risk below which adjuvant hormonal therapy is not used. There is therefore a risk that screen-detected lesions will be subject, along with many symptomatic cancers, to "overtreatment" with adjuvant endocrine therapy. Perhaps given the low rate of relapse in smaller grade 1 and 2 cancers seen in the BASO trial[76] there is a case for avoiding endocrine therapy in some women, although even in this low risk trial the endocrine therapy significantly reduced subsequent breast cancer events. What is not clear in women with low risk breast cancer is whether the benefits of tamoxifen exceed the risk of increased DVT and PE, and endometrial cancer? This is a decision that needs to be taken after discussion of the pros and cons with the patient.

Chemotherapy is given to about 25% of UK screen-detected cancers, but only those at higher risk (eg, those with positive nodes hence with evidence of disease progression). While it cannot be proven, it is likely that few if any of the "overdiagnosed" cancers are given chemotherapy since one anticipates that the "overdiagnosed" cancers will be noninvasive or small more indolent lesions (tumor characteristics not suggestive of high risk) where chemotherapy is not usually indicated. There is a lack of data outside of the UK on the proportion of women with screen-detected breast cancer who receive chemotherapy. Thus while one cannot exclude the possibility of some overdiagnosed cancers being given chemotherapy, in reality this is unlikely to be a significant number of cases. Some of the online tools do provide information on screen-detected versus symptomatic breast cancers separately. Thus it is possible using Predict! to assess the benefits of chemotherapy for patients with either screen-detected or symptomatic cancers, and take into account of the better overall prognosis of such detected cancers.

There are also the newer molecular profiles that assist in determining the likely benefit of chemotherapy. The most widely used are Oncotype and MammaPrint. The problem is that their use identifies some patients who as a group benefit, but the Oncotype score does not tell with any certainty whether an individual patient needs chemotherapy or will benefit from it.

There is also the group with intermediate recurrence scores where it is not at all clear chemotherapy is of benefit. Although ongoing studies are investigating the efficacy of chemotherapy in these intermediate risk patients, it is unlikely results will be separated into symptomatic and screen-detected patients. Thresholds for chemotherapy do vary between countries and even within countries.

The magnitude of any overtreatment of screen-detected breast cancers with chemotherapy is likely to be small.[99] In contrast many women get hormone therapy who may not need it and get no benefit, but this situation is little different to women with symptomatic breast cancers. Although these have been attempts to identify those who will benefit none are accurate enough to incorporate into routine use. Given the numbers of women involved and the toxicity of the treatments, more studies in women with screen-detected breast cancers are indicated.

REFERENCES

1. Joensuu H, Lehtimäki T, Holli K, Elomaa L, Turpeenniemi-Hujanen T, Kataja V, et al. Risk for distant recurrence of breast cancer detected by mammography screening or other methods. *J Am Med Assoc* 2004;**292**(9):1064–73.
2. Shen Y, Yang Y, Inoue LY, Munsell MF, Miller AB, Berry DA. Role of detection method in predicting breast cancer survival: analysis of randomized screening trials. *J Natl Cancer Inst* 2005;**97**(16):1195–203.
3. Wishart GC, Greenberg DC, Britton PD, Chou P, Brown CH, Purushotham AD, et al. Screen-detected vs symptomatic breast cancer: is improved survival due to stage migration alone? *Br J Cancer* 2008;**98**(11):1741–4.
4. Marmot MG, Altman DG, Cameron DA, Dewar JA, Thompson SG, Wilcox M. The benefits and harms of breast cancer screening: an independent review. *Br J Cancer* 2013;**108**(11):2205–40.
5. Flowers CI, O'Donoghue C, Moore D, Goss A, Kim D, Kim HJ, et al. Reducing false-positive biopsies: a pilot study to reduce benign biopsy rates for BI-RADS 4A/B assessments through testing risk stratification and new thresholds for intervention. *Breast Cancer Res Treat* 2013;**139**(3):769–77.
6. Barth RJ, Gibson GR, Carney PA, Mott LA, Becher RD, Poplack SP. Detection of breast cancer on screening mammography allows patients to be treated with less-toxic therapy. *Am J Roentgenol* 2005;**184**(1):324–9.
7. Duffy SW, Tabar L. Screening for breast cancer. *Lancet* 1995;**346**(8978):852.
8. Paci E, Duffy SW, Giorgi D, Zappa M, Crocetti E, Vezzosi V, et al. Are breast cancer screening programmes increasing rates of mastectomy? Observational study. *Br Med J* 2002;**325**(7361):418.
9. The Canadian Institute for Health Information. *Breast Cancer surgery in Canada 2007–2008 and 2009–2010*. Ottawa, ON: CIHI. Online: <https://secure.cihi.ca/free_products/BreastCancer_7-8_9-10_EN.pdf>; 2012 [accessed 10.19.15].
10. National Health Service Breast Screening Programme and Association of Breast Surgery. *An audit of screen-detected breast cancers for the year of screening April 2011 to March 2012*. NHSBSP & ABS. Online: <http://www.cancerscreening.nhs.uk/breastscreen/publications/baso2011-2012.pdf>; 2013, [accessed 01.09.15].
11. Allegra CJ, Aberle DR, Ganschow P, Hahn SM, Lee CN, Millon-Underwood S, et al. National Institutes of Health State-of-the-science conference statement: diagnosis and management of ductal carcinoma in situ September 22–24, 2009. *J Natl Cancer Inst* 2010;**102**(3):161–9.
12. Brinton LA, Sherman ME, Carreon JD, Anderson WF. Recent trends in breast cancer among younger women in the United States. *J Natl Cancer Inst* 2008;**100**:1643.

13. Virnig BA, Tuttle TM, Shamliyan T, Kane RL. Ductal carcinoma in situ of the breast: a systematic review of incidence, treatment, and outcomes. *J Natl Cancer Inst* 2010;**102**:170.
14. American Cancer Society. Cancer Facts & Figures 2012. *Atlanta: American Cancer Society*. Online: http://www.cancer.org/acs/groups/content/@epidemiologysurveilance/documents/document/acspc-031941.pdf; 2012, [accessed 10.19.15].
15. Foote FW, Stewart FW. Lobular Carcinoma in situ: a rare form of mammary cancer. *Am J Pathology* 1941;**17**(4):491–6.
16. Salvadori B, Bartoli C, Zurrida S, Delledonne V, Squicciarini P, Rovini D, et al. Risk of invasive cancer in women with lobular carcinoma in situ of the breast. *Eur J Cancer* 1991;**27**(1):35–7.
17. Ottesen GL, Graversen HP, Blichert-Toft M, Zedeler K, Andersen JA. Lobular carcinoma in situ of the female breast. Short-term results of a prospective nationwide study. The Danish Breast Cancer Cooperative Group. *Am J Surg Pathol* 1993;**17**(1):14–21.
18. Fisher ER, Land SR, Fisher B, Mamounas E, Gilarski L, Wolmark N. Pathologic findings from the National Surgical Adjuvant Breast and Bowel project: twelve-year observations concerning lobular carcinoma in situ. *Cancer* 2004;**100**(2):238–44.
19. Chuba PJ, Hamre MR, Yap J, Severson RK, Lucas D, Shamsa F, et al. Bilateral risk for subsequent breast cancer after lobular carcinoma-in-situ: analysis of surveillance, epidemiology, and end results data. *J Clin Oncol* 2005;**23**(24):5534–41.
20. Association of Breast Surgery at BASO 2009 Surgical Guidelines for the management of breast cancer. *Eur J Surg Oncol* 2009;**35**(Suppl. 1):1–22.
21. National Comprehensive Cancer Network Clinical Practice Guidelines in Oncology (NCCN Guidelines®). *Breast Cancer version 3*. Online: http://www.nccn.org/professionals/physician_gls/pdf/breast.pdf; 2015, [accessed 01.09.15].
22. Hwang H, Barke LD, Mendelson EB, Susnik B. Atypical lobular hyperplasia and classic lobular carcinoma in situ in core biopsy specimens: routine excision is not necessary. *Mod Pathol* 2008;**21**(10):1208–16.
23. O'Neil M, Madan R, Tawfik OW, Thomas PA, Fan F. Lobular carcinoma in situ/atypical lobular hyperplasia on breast needle biopsies: does it warrant surgical excisional biopsy? A study of 27 cases. *Ann Diagn Pathol* 2010;**14**(4):251–5.
24. Atkins KA, Cohen MA, Nicholson B, Rao S. Atypical lobular hyperplasia and lobular carcinoma in situ at core breast biopsy: use of careful radiologic-pathologic correlation to recommend excision or observation. *Radiology* 2013;**269**(2):340–7.
25. Nakhlis F, Gilmore L, Gelman R, Bedrosian I, Ludwig K, Hwang E, et al. The Incidence of adjacent synchronous invasive carcinoma and/or DCIS in patients with lobular neoplasia on core biopsy: results from a prospective multi-institutional registry (TBCRC 020). *Ann Surg Oncol* 2015;**22**(Suppl. 1):S17.
26. Morgan C, Shah ZA, Hamilton R, Wang J, Spiegel J, DeLeon W, et al. The radial scar of the breast diagnosed at core needle biopsy. *Proceedings (Baylor University Medical Center)* 2012;**25**(1):3–5.
27. Wilson R, Kavia S. Comparison of large-core vacuum-assisted breast biopsy and excision systems. *Recent Results Cancer Res* 2009;**173**:23–41.
28. Welsh HG, Black WC. Using autopsy series to estimate the disease 'reservoir' for ductal carcinoma in situ of the breast: how much more breast cancer can we find? *Ann Intern Med* 1997;**127**(11):1023–8.
29. Bleyer A, Welch HG. Effect of three decades of screening mammography on breast-cancer incidence. *N Engl J Med* 2012;**367**(21):1998–2005.
30. Page DL, Jensen RA. Evaluation and management of high risk and premalignant lesions of the breast. *World J Surg* 1994;**18**(1):32–8.
31. Ghofrani M, Tapia B, Tavassoli FA. Discrepancies in the diagnosis of intraductal proliferative lesions of the breast and its management implications: results of a multinational survey. *Virchows Arch* 2006;**466**(6):609–16.
32. Elmore JG, Longton GM, Carney PA, Geller BM, Onega T, Tosteson AN, et al. Diagnostic concordance among pathologists interpreting breast biology specimens. *J Am Med Assoc* 2015;**313**(11):1122–32.

33. Tavassoli FA. Breast pathology: rationale for adopting the ductal intraepithelial neoplasia (DIN) classification. *Nat Clin Pract Oncol* 2005;**2**(3):116–7.
34. Pinder SE, Ellis IO. The diagnosis and management of pre-invasive breast disease: ductal carcinoma in situ (DCIS) and atypical ductal hyperplasia (ADH) – current definitions and classification. *Breast Cancer Res* 2003;**5**(5):254–7.
35. Solin LJ, Gray R, Baehner FL, Butler SM, Hughes LL, Yoshizawa C, et al. A multigene expression assay to predict local recurrence risk for ductal carcinoma in situ of the breast. *J Natl Cancer Inst* 2013;**105**(10):701–10.
36. Holmberg L, Wong YN, Tabár L, Ringberg A, Karlsson P, Arnesson LG, et al. Mammography casting-type calcification and risk of local recurrence in DCIS: analyses from a randomised study. *Br J Cancer* 2013;**108**(4):812–9.
37. Dixon JM. Breast screening has increased the number of mastectomies. *Breast Cancer Res* 2009;**11**(Suppl. 3): S19.
38. Thomas J, Evans A, Macartney J, Pinder SE, Hanby A, Ellis I, et al. Radiological and pathological size estimations of pure ductal carcinoma in situ of the breast, specimen handling and the influence on the success of breast conservation surgery: a review of 2564 cases from the Sloane project. *Br J Cancer* 2010;**102**(2): 285–93.
39. Schaverien MV, Raine C, Majdak-Paredes E, Dixon JM. Therapeutic mammaplasty – extending indications and achieving low incomplete excision rates. *Eur J Surg Oncol* 2013;**39**(4):329–33.
40. Majdak-Paredes E, Schavarien M, Zychta P, Raine C, Dixon JM. Intraoperative digital specimen radiology reduces re-operation rates in therapeutic mammoplasty for breast cancer. *Breast* 2015;**24**(5)556–9.
41. Kunkler IH, Kerr GR, Thomas JS, Jack WJ, Bartlett JM, Pedersen HC, et al. Impact of screening and risk factors for local recurrence and survival after conservative surgery and radiotherapy for early breast cancer: results from a large series with long-term follow-up. *Int J Radiat Oncol Biol Phys* 2012;**83**(3):829–38.
42. Fancellu A, Turner RM, Dixon JM, Pinna A, Cottu P, Houssami N. Meta-analysis of the effect of preoperative breast MRI on the surgical management of ductal carcinoma in situ. *Br J Surg* 2015;**102**(8):883–93.
43. Francis A, Bartlett JMS, Billingham LJ, Bowden SJ, Brookes CL, Dodwell DJ, et al. The LORIS trial: a multicentre, randomized phase III trial of standard surgery versus active monitoring in women with newly diagnosed low risk ductal carcinoma in situ. *Cancer Res* 2013;**73** (sup): OT2-3-01.
44. Sagara Y, Mallory MA, Wong S, Aydogan F, DeSantis S, Barry WT, et al. Survival benefit of breast surgery for low-grade ductal carcinoma in situ: a population-based cohort study. *JAMA Surg* 2015;**150**(8):739–45.
45. Wapnir IL, Dignam JJ, Fisher B, Mamounas EP, Anderson SJ, Julian TB, et al. Long-term outcomes of invasive ipsilateral breast tumor recurrences after lumpectomy in NSABP B-17 and B-24 randomized clinical trials for DCIS. *J Natl Cancer Inst* 2011;**103**(6):478–88.
46. EORTC Breast Cancer Cooperative Group, EORTC Radiotherapy Group, Bijker N Breast-conserving treatment with or without radiotherapy in ductal carcinoma-in-situ: ten year results of European Organisation for Research and treatment of cancer randomized phase III trial 10853 – a study by EORTC Breast Cancer Cooperative Group and EORTC Radiotherapy Group. *J Clin Oncol* 2006;**24**(21):3381–7.
47. Dixon JM. Breast conserving surgery: the balance between good cosmesis and local control vol. ed. In: Dixon JM, editor. *A Companion to specialist surgical practice: Breast surgery* 5th ed. Edinburgh: Elsevier; 2014. p. 51–70.
48. Houssami N, Macaskill P, Marinovich ML, Dixon JM, Irwig L, Brennan ME, et al. Meta-analysis of the impact of surgical margins on local recurrence in women with early-stage invasive breast cancer treated with breast-conserving therapy. *Eur J Cancer* 2010;**46**(18):3219–32.
49. Goss PE, Ingle JN, Alés-Martínez JE, Cheung AM, Chlebowski RT, Wactawski-Wende J, et al. Exemestane for breast-cancer prevention in postmenopausal women. *N Engl J Med.* 2011;**364**(25):2381–91.
50. Hughes LL, Wang M, Page DL, Gray R, Solin LJ, Davidson NE, et al. Local excision alone without irradiation for ductal carcinoma in situ of the breast: a trial of the Eastern Cooperative Oncology Group. *J Clin Oncol* 2009;**27**(32):5319–24.

51. Thaker NG, Hoffman KE, Strauder MC, Shaitelman SF, Strom EA, Tereffe W, et al. The 21-gene recurrence score complements IBTR! Estimates in early-stage, hormone receptor-positive, HER2-normal, lymph node-negative breast cancer. *Springerplus* 2015;**4**:36.
52. Rakovitch E, Nofech-Mozes S, Hanna W, Baehner FL, Saskin R, Butler SM, et al. A large prospectively designed study of the DCIS score: predicting recurrence risk after local excision for ductal carcinoma in situ patients with and without irradiation. 2014 San Antonio Breast Cancer Symposium. Abstract S5–04.
53. Silverstein MJ, Lagios MD, Craig PH, Waisman JR, Lewinsky BS, Colburn WJ, et al. A prognostic index for ductal carcinoma in situ of the breast. *Cancer* 1996;**77**(11):2267–74.
54. Silverstein MJ, Lagios MD, Groshen S, Waisman JR, Lewinsky BS, Martino S, et al. The influence of margin width on local control of ductal carcinoma in situ of the breast. *N Engl J Med* 1999;**340**(19):1455–61.
55. Goodwin A, Parker S, Ghersi D, Wilcken N. Post-operative radiotherapy for ductal carcinoma in situ of the breast – a systematic review of the randomised trials. *Breast* 2009;**18**(3):143–9.
56. Fisher B, Dignam J, Wolmark N, Wickerham DL, Fisher ER, Mamounas E, et al. Tamoxifen in treatment of intraductal breast cancer: National Surgical Adjuvant Breast and Bowel Project B-24 randomised controlled trial. *Lancet* 1999;**353**(9169):1993–2000.
57. Houghton J, George WD, Cuzick J, Duggan C, Fentiman IS, Spittle M, et al. Radiotherapy and tamoxifen in women with completely excised ductal carcinoma in situ of the breast in the UK, Australia, and New Zealand: randomised controlled trial. *Lancet* 2003;**362**(9378):95–102.
58. Allred DC, Anderson SJ, Paik S, Wickerham DL, Nagtegaal ID, Swain SM, et al. Adjuvant tamoxifen reduces subsequent breast cancer in women with estrogen receptor-positive ductal carcinoma in situ: a study based on NSABP protocol B-24. *J Clin Oncol* 2012;**30**(12):1268–73.
59. Ozanne EM, Shieh Y, Barnes J, Bouzan C, Hwang ES, Esserman LJ. Characterising the impact of 25 years of DCIS treatment. *Breast Cancer Res Treat* 2011;**129**(1):165–73.
60. Meyerson AF, Lessing JN, Itakura K, Hylton NM, Wolverton DE, Joe BN, et al. Outcome of long term active surveillance for estrogen receptor-positive ductal carcinoma in suit. *Breast* 2011;**20**(6):529–33.
61. Hwang ES, Esserman L. Neoadjuvant hormonal therapy for ductal carcinoma in situ: trial design and preliminary results. *Ann Surg Oncol* 2004;**11**(Suppl. 1):37S–43S.
62. Gunia SR, Patel MS, Mamounas EP. Pathologic complete response of HER-2 Neu-Positive invasive ductal carcinoma and ductal carcinoma in situ following Neoadjuvant Chemotherapy plus Trastuzumab: a case report and review of literature. *Case Rep Surg* 2012;454273.
63. Kuerer HM, Buzdar AU, Mittendorf EA, Esteva FJ, Lucci A, Vence LM, et al. Biologic and immunologic effects of preoperative trastuzumab for ductal carcinoma in situ of the breast. *Cancer* 2011;**117**(1):39–47.
64. Morris AD, Morris RD, Wilson JF, White J, Steinberg S, Okunieff P, et al. Breast conserving therapy versus mastectomy in early stage breast cancer: a meta-analysis of 10 year survival. *Cancer J Sci Am* 1997;**3**(1):6–12.
65. Early Breast Cancer Trialists' Collaborative Group Effects of radiotherapy and surgery in early breast cancer: an overview of the randomised trials. *N Engl J Med* 1995;**333**(22):1444–55.
66. Hwang ES, Lichtensztajn DY, Gomez SL, Fowble B, Clarke CA. Survival after lumpectomy and mastectomy for early stage invasive breast cancer: the effect of age and hormone receptor status. *Cancer* 2013;**119**(7):1402–11.
67. Katipamula R, Degnim AC, Hoskin Boughey JC, Loprinzi C, Grant CS, et al. Trends in mastectomy rates at the Mayo Clinic Rochester: effect of surgical year and preoperative magnetic resonance imaging. *J Clin Oncol* 2009;**27**(25):4082–8.
68. Bleicher RJ, Ciocca RM, Egleston BL, Sesa L, Evers K, Sigurdson ER, et al. Association of routine pretreatment magnetic resonance imaging with time to surgery, mastectomy rate and margin status. *J Am Coll Surg* 2009;**209**(5):679.
69. Sorbero ME, Dick AW, Beckjord EB, Ahrendt G. Diagnostic breast magnetic resonance imaging and contralateral prophylactic mastectomy. *Ann Surg Oncol* 2009;**16**(6):1597–605.

70. Weber JJ, Bellin LS, Milbourn DE, Verbanac KM, Wong JH. Selective preoperative magnetic resonance imaging in women with breast cancer: no reduction in the reoperation rate. *Arch Surg* 2012;**147**(9):834–9.
71. Saadatmand S, Bretveld R, Siesling S, Tilanus-Linthorst MMA. Influence of tumor stage at breast cancer detection on survival in modern times: population based study in 173 797 patients. *B Med J* 2015;**351**. Available from: http://dx.doi.org/10.1136/bmj.h4901
72. National Institute for Health and Care Excellence. *Breast cancer quality standard: NICE quality standards (QS12)*. <https://www.nice.org.uk/guidance/qs12>; 2011.
73. Veronesi U, Luini A, Del Vecchio M, Greco M, Galimberti V, Merson M, et al. Radiotherapy after breast-preserving surgery in women with localized cancer of the breast. *N Engl J Med* 1993;**328**(22):1587–91.
74. Kunkler IH, Williams LJ, Jack WJ, Cameron DA, Dixon JM. Breast-conserving surgery with or without irradiation in women aged 65 years or older with early breast cancer (PRIME II): a randomised controlled trial. *Lancet Oncol* 2015;**16**(3):266–73.
75. Hughes KS, Schnaper LA, Bellon JR, Cirrincione CT, Berry DA, McCormick B, et al. Lumpectomy plus tamoxifen with or without irradiation in women age 70 years or older with early breast cancer: long-term follow-up of CALGB 9343. *J Clin Oncol* 2013;**31**(19):2382–7.
76. Blamey RW, Bates T, Chetty U, Duffy SW, Ellis IO, George D, et al. Radiotherapy or tamoxifen after conserving surgery for breast cancer of excellent prognosis: British Association of Surgical Oncology (BASO) II trial. *Eur J Cancer* 2013;**49**(10):2294–302.
77. Winzer KJ, Sauerbrei W, Braun M, Liersch T, Dunst J, Guiski H, et al. Radiation therapy and tamoxifen after breast-conserving surgery: updated results of a 2× 2 randomised clinical trial in patients with low risk of recurrence. *Eur J Cancer* 2010;**46**(1):95–101.
78. Tinterri C, Gatzemeier W, Zanini V, Regolo L, Pedrazzoli C, Rondini E, et al. Conservative surgery with and without radiotherapy in elderly patients with early-stage breast cancer: a prospective randomised multicentre trial. *Breast* 2009;**18**(6):373–7.
79. Carlson RW, Moench S, Hurria A, Balducci L, Burstein HJ, Goldstein LJ, et al. NCCN Task Force Report: breast cancer in the older woman. *J Natl Compr Canc Netw* 2008;**6**(Suppl. 4):S1–25.
80. Vaidya JS, Wenz F, Bulsara M, Tobias JS, Joseph DJ, Keshtgar M, et al. Risk-adapted targeted intraoperative radiotherapy versus whole breast radiotherapy for breast cancer: 5 year results for local control and overall survival from the TARGIT-A randomised trial. *Lancet* 2014;**383**(9917):603–13.
81. Veronesi U, Orecchia R, Maisonneuve P, Viale G, Rotmensz N, Sangalli C, et al. Intraoperative radiotherapy versus external radiotherapy for early breast cancer (ELIOT): a randomised controlled equivalence trial. *Lancet Oncol* 2013;**14**(13):1269–77.
82. Cabanas RM. An approach for the treatment of penile carcinoma. *Cancer* 1977;**39**(2):456–66.
83. Morton DL, Thompson JF, Essner R, Elashoff R, Stern SL, Nieweg OE, et al. Validation of the accuracy of intraoperative lymphatic mapping and sentinel lymphadenectomy for early-stage melanoma: a multicenter trial. Multicenter Selective Lymphadenectomy trial group. *Ann Surg* 1999;**230**(4):453–63.
84. Kim T, Giuliano AE, Lyman GH. Lymphatic mapping and sentinel lymph node biopsy in early-stage breast carcinoma: a meta-analysis. *Cancer* 2006;**106**(1):4–16.
85. Krag DN, Anderson SJ, Julian TB, Brown AM, Harlow SP, Costantino JP, et al. Sentinel-lymph-node resection compared with conventional axillary-lymph-node dissection in clinically node-negative patients with breast cancer: overall survival findings from the NSABP B-32 randomised phase 3 trial. *Lancet Oncol* 2010;**11**(10):927–33.
86. Giuliano AE, Hunt KK, Ballman KV, Beitsch PD, Whitworth PW, Blumencranz PW, et al. Axillary dissection vs no axillary dissection in women with invasive breast cancer and sentinel node metastasis: a randomized clinical trial. *J Am Med Assoc* 2011;**305**(6):569–75.
87. Lyman GH, Temin S, Edge SB, Newman LA, Turner RR, Weaver DL, et al. Sentinel lymph node biopsy for patients with early-stage breast cancer: American Society of Clinical Oncology clinical practice guideline update. *J Clin Oncol* 2014;**32**(13):1365–83.

88. Galimberti V, Cole BF, Zurrida S, Viale G, Luini A, Veronesi P, et al. Axillary dissection versus no axillary dissection in patients with sentinel-node micrometastases (IBCSG 23-01): a phase 3 randomised controlled trial. *Lancet Oncol* 2013;**14**(4):297–305.
89. Rutgers EJ, Donker M, Straver ME, Meijnen P, van de Velde CHJ, Mansel RE, et al. Radiotherapy or surgery of the axilla after a positive sentinel node in breast cancer patients: Final analysis of the EORTC AMAROS trial. *J Clin Oncol* 2013;**31** (suppl; abstr LBA1001).
90. Fisher B, Montague E, Redmond C, Barton B, Bortland D, Fisher ER, et al. Comparison of radical mastectomy with alternative treatments for primary breast cancer: a first report of results from prospective randomized clinical trial. *Cancer* 1977;**39**(Suppl. 6):2827–39.
91. Fisher B, Redmond C, Fisher E, Bauer M, Wolmark N, Wickerham DL, et al. Ten-year results of randomized trial comparing radical mastectomy and total mastectomy with or without radiation. *N Engl J Med* 1985;**312**(11):674–81.
92. Baum M, Coyle PJ. Simple mastectomy for early breast cancer and the behaviour of the untreated axillary nodes. *Bull Cancer* 1977;**64**(4):603–10.
93. Baxter N, McCready D, Chapman JA, Fish E, Kahn H, Hanna W, et al. Clinical behavior of untreated axillary nodes after local treatment for primary breast cancer. *Ann Surg Oncol* 1996;**3**(3):235–40.
94. Halverson KJ, Taylor ME, Perez CA, Garcia DM, Myerson R, Philpott G, et al. Regional nodal management and patterns of failure following conservative surgery and radiation therapy for stage I and II breast cancer. *Int J Radiat Oncol Biol Phys* 1993;**26**(4):593–9.
95. Kuznetsova M, Graybill JC, Zusag TW, Hartsell WF, Griem KL. Omission of axillary lymph node dissection in early-stage breast cancer: effect on treatment outcome. *Radiology* 1995;**197**(2):507–10.
96. Hafty BG, McKhann C, Beinfield M, Fischer D, Fischer JJ. Breast conservation therapy without axillary dissection. *Arch Surg* 1993;**128**(12):1315–9.
97. Cady B. Case against axillary lymphadenectomy for most patients with infiltrating breast cancer. *J Surg Oncol* 1997;**66**(1):7–10.
98. Cuzick J, Sestak I, Cawthorn S, Hamed H, Holli K, Howell A, et al. Tamoxifen for prevention of breast cancer: extended long-term follow-up of the IBIS-I breast cancer prevention trial. *Lancet* 2015;**16**(1):67–75.
99. Coldman AJ, Phillips N, Speers C. A retrospective study of the effect of participation in screening mammography on the use of chemotherapy and breast conserving surgery. *Int J Cancer* 2007;**120**(10):2185–90.

CHAPTER

INFORMED AND SHARED DECISION MAKING IN BREAST SCREENING

16

Jolyn Hersch, Jesse Jansen and Kirsten McCaffery

Screening and Test Evaluation Program (STEP) and Centre for Medical Psychology and Evidence-based Decision-making (CeMPED), Sydney School of Public Health, The University of Sydney, Sydney, NSW, Australia

CHAPTER OUTLINE

PLAIN LANGUAGE SUMMARY

Breast cancer screening has been going on for many years now, and research suggests that most women in the community feel positive about screening as a way to reassure them that they are well or to find early signs of cancer that can then be treated. Women have been told a lot about the potential benefits of screening, such as helping some women to avoid dying from breast cancer. But more recently, experts have gained a better understanding of the potential downsides of screening. In particular, some of the women who go for breast screening will be diagnosed and treated for a cancer that would never have caused them any trouble if it were not found through screening. This is called overdiagnosis (or overdetection).

Putting together the research about the chances of benefit and harm from screening, experts have moved toward the view that women in the community should be given the opportunity to consider the

Breast Cancer Screening. DOI: http://dx.doi.org/10.1016/B978-0-12-802209-2.00016-4

important information about screening for themselves and make up their own minds about whether it seems worthwhile. The final decision is likely to vary from woman to woman, as it depends on how she personally weighs up the pros and cons. This idea—that people should have a say in what is the best healthcare for them—fits with a broad approach called shared decision making, which is about encouraging people to be involved in health decisions together with their doctor. In many countries, women are offered breast screening directly through an organized program so they do not necessarily discuss it with a doctor. Therefore, we often use the terms informed decision making and informed choice, rather than shared decision making, in this context. Regardless of the term or setting, a key feature of these approaches is making sure women are aware of important things that could happen if they choose to screen or not screen.

Decision aids are tools designed to support people in getting the best information and deciding what is the best thing to do in a particular situation—for example, deciding whether to screen. In this chapter, we discuss research on decision aids and other ways of informing women about screening and finding out their thoughts and feelings toward it. We also discuss the challenges involved in moving to an informed choice approach. More work is needed to figure out the best ways of achieving good-quality, informed decision making for women who are considering breast screening.

INTRODUCTION

Cancer screening leads to a complex array of potential consequences for participants. Quantitative estimates of the outcomes of breast screening are outlined elsewhere in this book, so in this chapter we focus on informed and shared decision making. Policy makers face a difficult task in weighing the value of different screening outcomes and judging whether the benefits outweigh the harms.[1] It has been argued that the balance between benefits and harms in breast cancer screening may be considered a close call on which reasonable individuals may vary in their choices.[2] These judgements are at least partly driven by the values of the people making the decisions. The fact that the values of policy makers may not accord with those of individuals who are subsequently offered screening underscores the need for balanced, evidence-based information to be presented to members of the public to enable them to participate in screening decisions.[1] A woman's choice to attend screening or not should be determined by how she values the small possibility of a large clinical benefit (ie, extension of life) compared with the higher probability of undesirable events such as unnecessary investigations and overtreatment.[3] After all, the woman who undergoes screening must live with the decision and its repercussions.[4]

PUBLIC PERCEPTIONS OF SCREENING

Achievement of informed decision making in mammography screening faces several challenges,[5,6] not least for women themselves. There are widely held positive attitudes and often uncritical support for mammography and screening generally. A landmark 2002 survey that documented widespread public enthusiasm for cancer screening in the United States, with 87% of respondents considering routine cancer screening "almost always a good idea,"[7] was partially repeated in a large British sample in 2012 with very similar results.[8] Also, a 2013 systematic review of patient or public expectations of the benefits and harms of medical interventions found that participants tended to overestimate benefits and underestimate harms of a broad range of treatments and tests including breast cancer screening.[9]

Studies employing qualitative methods such as interviews and focus groups have been useful in eliciting women's reasoning about different aspects of screening and their own participation. Table 16.1 provides examples of women's attitudes to mammography using selected quotations from research participants. Though there may be cultural influences on screening attitudes, many beliefs recur across socioeconomic and cultural boundaries.[10]

Table 16.1 Women's Perspectives on Breast Cancer Screening: Selected Quotations From Qualitative Research Literature

Theme	Example Statement About Breast Screening	Reference
Enthusiasm for testing	I feel that it is very important whether you are 30 or... 80 [that] you have any tests that you can.	Schonberg[11]
	I do know that an intelligent person needs the tests routinely, just to make sure everything is cool.	Denberg[10]
Faith in sensitive technology	Once you have the mammography you think "well, they've checked it now, that's that done"... so you know there's nothing there.	Griffiths[12]
	Machines that are cleverer than you are looking at you every three years which is a reassurance really.	Griffiths[12]
Value of reassurance	I feel happy having a mammogram, seeing some kind of in depth look at you, to see if you're all right	Griffiths[12]
	[The] greatest benefit is learning you don't have cancer.	Denberg[10]
	I feel good when I receive that letter and all is well. Then I feel safe.	Solbjor[13]
Attitudes to risk	If someone objected to having it done, why they're taking their own life in their hands I guess.	Silverman[14]
	Even if statistical risk (of getting breast cancer) is low I still want screening, there is still a chance.	Davey[15]
Trust vs skepticism	I just have a trust that the NHS wouldn't haul us all out if statistically there wasn't some evidence that, by and large, some people get saved, you know, and that not many people get disadvantaged.	Waller[16]
	If my doctor told me not to have a mammogram, I would think something is wrong with her.	Allen[17]
Accepting without question	I just think, something that you've got to have done. They send the letter through the door, up to you to just go. I don't necessarily think about it.	Griffiths[12]
	Yes I've always been and it doesn't worry me. At a certain age, you get a letter from the doctor to attend that sort of thing. I don't really read about it all.	Griffiths[12]
Anxiety about results	But of course, when you receive that letter you're a bit tense anyway about what it'll tell... Before you open the envelope, you feel a sting, like.	Solbjor[13]
	Is it or isn't it, do I have this? ... The recalls are traumatic... I try not to worry about it, but I still do.	Greco[18]
Critical views on testing	Personally I am of the opinion that you shouldn't cross your bridges until you come to them.	Osterlie[6]
	If it's the case that you don't feel anything from it, then you should let sleeping dogs lie.	Lagerlund[19]

As Table 16.1 shows, taking the opportunity for early detection through breast screening is perceived as a way of minimizing potential regret, whereas failure to be screened puts one at risk of a preventable death.[14] Women acknowledge some anxiety about going for screening mammograms, awaiting their results, and having the follow-up tests that false-positive results entail. Some are concerned about the possibility of false-negative results, but many women express strong confidence in the sensitivity of mammography and emphasize the sense of reassurance gained from receiving the "all clear" (Table 16.1). The reassurance of being cancer-free that a normal mammogram result provides may be a key motivator for women to undergo screening,[20] but this reassurance is sometimes false.[21] Moreover, publicity about screening may be partly responsible for raising breast cancer anxiety in the first place, making it questionable whether anxiety reduction can legitimately be considered a benefit of screening.[22]

THE CONVENTIONAL APPROACH TO INFORMATION PROVISION

The public perception of mammography as undeniably valuable is partly due to the persuasive impact of decades of screening promotion campaigns by the health sector.[7,11,23] Public health campaigns and messages about cancer screening over many decades have largely reflected a positive view of screening widely held among public health organizations, professional associations, patient advocacy groups, academics, and clinicians.[24] The main approach has been to deploy powerfully persuasive communication tools to convince individuals to screen, with the overall goal of maximizing screening uptake in the population. A standard "recipe" for such communication has been described as follows: induce feelings of fear and vulnerability, then offer hope by framing screening as a simple way to protect oneself.[24] Also consistent with this screening communication approach is presenting "a lopsided view" with an emphasis on (often exaggerated) benefits and minimization of harms.[24,25] Such communications have created strongly positive views of screening in the community, which in turn feed normative expectations that screening is the "right" thing to do.[12,26]

This simplistic positive messaging has increasingly come under criticism in recent years. Several international reviews have pointed out that information materials produced and distributed by breast screening services and other relevant groups have overestimated benefits and underplayed harms.[27–29] The direct communications women receive about breast screening, as described above, occur within a broader context of media stories about medical testing that frequently overlook harms.[30] The heated debates that occur among researchers and health professionals do not necessarily filter through into the public sphere.[13,31] It is therefore unsurprising that women in screened societies find the idea of scientific uncertainty about breast screening difficult to accept, and are skeptical about attempts to raise awareness of controversies.[17–19] Nevertheless, research suggests that many women do desire better information.[15,32] In a Swiss survey, 89% of respondents wanted information on limits of mammography screening and 82% wanted to know reasons why some people oppose screening.[32]

THE NEED FOR SHARED/INFORMED DECISION MAKING IN SCREENING

There is now growing consensus that harm and benefit information must be communicated clearly and transparently to women offered mammography screening, so that they can make informed decisions.[33–35] Screening can trigger a cascade of serious and stressful interventions with lasting implications; therefore, cancer screening decisions are a good example of where helping people to be engaged and involved in decision making is valuable.[36] Experts familiar with the evidence on breast screening recognize that women may weigh things up differently depending on their context and personality—some might appropriately decline screening while others consider the risks acceptable and choose to do it.[25,37,38] The importance of this is even greater due to the fact that screening involves offering an intervention to apparently healthy people, as opposed to providing symptomatic patients with medical help they are seeking out.[39]

As outlined above, the task of informing the public in a transparent way has largely been performed inadequately thus far.[25,37] This necessitates a shift in the approach to screening communications such that efforts are focused on educating people and respecting their informed decisions, rather than persuading them to a particular course of action as if there were an a priori best choice for each individual.[24,25]

WHAT IT MEANS TO MAKE AN INFORMED DECISION ABOUT SCREENING

Shared decision making is a highly influential model of how patient involvement in medical decision making can be conceived. It has been defined as follows[40]: "Shared decision making enables a clinician and patient to participate jointly in making a health decision, having discussed the options and their benefits and harms, and having considered the patient's values, preferences and circumstances. It is not a single step to be added into a consultation, but a process that can be used to guide decisions about screening, investigations and treatments." While shared decision making is applicable to many (if not most) clinical decision situations, it is especially important where a preference-sensitive decision is involved.[40] As discussed above, choosing whether to undergo breast cancer screening may be considered such a decision.

Both shared decision making and the related term, informed decision making, can be used to encompass the broader concept of people's involvement in decision making about their health and healthcare. Shared decision making, as defined above, is conceptualized in terms of patient–clinician consultations in which both parties have input. But many health decisions are made outside of the clinical encounter and without any direct input from a healthcare provider. Deciding whether to accept or decline a screening offer made within a population-based screening program is an example. In this case, informed decision making might be considered the more appropriate term.

Statements endorsing informed decision making are strengthening across the medical literature and health policy landscape.[41–44] Across a range of clinical contexts, incorporating patient preferences in decision making is recommended as a core aspect of fulfilling the fundamental principles of ethical medical practice.[45] Yet despite a growing consensus that people should be provided with information to enable informed choice, there remains little agreement on precisely what this means in practice.[46]

One way in which informed decision making has been operationalized in research is through the construct of informed choice, which relates to whether people's decisions in a specific health context are consistent with their informed values or attitudes.[47,48] Informed choice may be assessed by combining measures of a person's knowledge, attitudes, and actual choice.[49] For example, an informed choice about whether to undergo screening may be defined as one in which knowledge is adequate, with screening attitudes and intentions being consistent (ie, positive attitudes with positive intentions, or negative attitudes with negative intentions). This conceptualization of informed choice, in terms of knowledge, attitudes, and choice made (in this case measured as intentions), is presented in Table 16.2.

Table 16.2 Framework for Determining Informed Choice in a Screening Decision Aid Trial [50]

	Adequate Knowledge	Positive Attitude	Intending to Screen
Informed Choice-Adequate Knowledge and Consistent Attitudes+ Intentions			
Accept screening	✓	✓	✓
Decline screening	✓	×	×
Partly Uninformed Choice			
Accept	✓	×	✓
Decline	✓	✓	×
Accept	×	✓	✓
Decline	×	×	×
Completely Uninformed Choice			
Accept	×	×	✓
Decline	×	✓	×

An essential aspect of defining an informed choice is the decision maker's knowledge of the potential for benefit and harm from the whole screening process. But even if experts agree broadly that some such understanding is necessary, exactly what level of knowledge is sufficient for making an informed decision is subject to varying opinions and hard to pin down.[46] Critics of "the quantitative imperative" have claimed that giving numerical risk information (ie, probabilities of specific benefits and harms) is appropriate for some situations and patients, but not others, because many people may have trouble understanding it.[51] Yet prominent experts assert the centrality of quantitative information within the scope of necessary knowledge about possible outcomes of options in preference-sensitive decisions, arguing that knowing the approximate chances, if not exact probabilities, is crucial.[35,45,52]

SUPPORTING SHARED/INFORMED DECISION MAKING WITH DECISION AIDS

Methods are available with the potential to achieve better shared and/or informed decision making in breast screening. Decision aids can address the need for better communication of important possible outcomes of breast screening.[25,53] These are interventions designed to support people in making decisions about treatment or screening when there is more than one reasonable option available, with benefits and harms that people may value differently—in other words, decisions where personal preferences are relevant.[54,55] Decision aids make the decision explicit (eg, to be screened or not), describe why choice exists, provide information about the options and their associated outcomes, and are intended to help people consider and deliberate about the options from their own personal perspective.[55,56] Some decision aids include explicit methods for helping users to clarify their values in relation to the decision (values clarification exercises), but the evidence supporting these is uncertain as studies have found mixed results regarding whether they improve decision making.[57,58]

When presenting quantitative information about decision outcomes, such as the frequencies of important benefits and harms, risk communication experts recommend using either simple percentage (eg, $x\%$) or simple frequency formats (eg, x in 100, where x is a whole number) that explicitly specify the reference class over time.[59,60] Icon arrays (or "pictographs") are a type of visual graphic display representing the numerator and denominator together via differently colored filled circles arranged in a matrix, thus depicting the part-whole relationship. Visual displays such as icon arrays are supported by a solid body of research evidence and considered best practice.[45] Presenting numerical information in pictographs has been shown to improve comprehension, including among people with low literacy and numeracy.[59,61]

Extensive randomized controlled trial evidence in a variety of settings has shown that decision aids improve knowledge and accuracy of risk perceptions, stimulate people to take a more active decision making role, and can improve congruence between the chosen option and the person's values.[55] Studies have also demonstrated that decision aids can improve the rate of informed decision making about participation in screening programs, including those for cancer.[62] For example, two Australian randomized trials of mammography screening decision aids for women aged 40 and 70 (ie, outside the national screening program's target age range) showed that the interventions increased knowledge and reduced the proportion of women who remained undecided.[63,64] Amongst participants who made a decision, older women's screening intentions and behavior were not altered; for younger women, fewer of those viewing the decision aid intended to start screening now compared to controls, but most were still in favor of screening.

Although current guidance directs clinicians to involve patients in decisions,[43] some are concerned that taking a more active role in screening choices is too daunting or burdensome for lay people.[65] Breast screening program staff thought the information in a mammography decision aid might be too detailed and cause worry, but users considered it clear and understandable, with 97% of participants completing the trial.[63] A trial to evaluate a bowel cancer screening decision aid for adults with low education and literacy[66] achieved an 85% consent rate in a socioeconomically disadvantaged population, with 93% of those randomized actually completing the trial. The decision aid increased by 22% the proportion of people making an informed choice,[66] providing further evidence that informed decision making about screening can be accessible to the wider community.

ALTERNATIVES TO INDIVIDUAL INFORMED CHOICE

Research suggests that a structured, balanced presentation of health information can empower people to assume a more active decision-making role than they initially intend.[67] Nevertheless, some women may not wish to individually evaluate detailed information on the outcomes of mammography screening, including quantified risk data, when they are deciding whether to take part. Determining the extent to which there is a need for promoting individual-level deliberation about this particular health decision could be based on examining the distribution of preferences amongst fully informed women.[2] In turn, these preferences could be elicited in various ways. One strategy known as "community sampling" requires fully informing a random sample of eligible women and asking each person whether she would choose screening.[2] A somewhat different method involves engaging a representative "citizens jury" to deliberate together in considering benefits and harms.[68] Citizens juries are a method of deliberative democracy which can be used to engage citizens in formal iterative dialog on important and complex problems. These methods provide balanced factual information to people with diverse perspectives and potentially conflicting views, and create opportunities to discuss issues freely and test competing claims.[26] A deliberative citizens jury approach has been demonstrated to be a feasible way of eliciting a well-informed, considered community view in the context of mammography screening policy[69] as well as in prostate cancer screening.[70]

Diversity of screening preferences amongst fully informed women would support the need for detailed individual consent,[2] whereas a community consensus in favor of screening would suggest that alternative approaches may be appropriate. For example, providers could assist people to "consider an offer" of screening.[71] This involves helping people evaluate the trustworthiness and personal relevance of the screening offer, while acknowledging that it might reasonably be declined. Personal preferences determine whether the individual requires further information such as data on outcomes or community views.[71] The "consider an offer" concept provides the basis for the novel approach adopted in England since 2013 regarding information for people invited for cancer screening.[72] Each eligible person receives a letter of invitation (which may be seen as a recommendation in itself). Alongside the letter, people receive a leaflet developed at arm's length from the screening program, with balanced information about benefits and harms. The leaflet aims to encourage the reader to assess the offer of screening, rather than simply encouraging screening, and to make it clear that declining the offer may be reasonable.[72]

COMMUNICATING ABOUT OVERDIAGNOSIS

One highly contentious issue in breast screening is overdiagnosis (or overdetection). The medical community has long recognized that diagnosing and treating inconsequential disease is an important potential harm of screening.[22] However, public awareness about nonprogressive cancer is extremely limited. A 1997 postal survey among US women showed that only 6% knew that some breast cancers grow so slowly as to not affect health.[73] In 2010 an online survey of Americans aged 50–69 who had been invited to cancer screening by their doctor found that only 8% of women had been informed about the risk of overdiagnosis and overtreatment.[74] Similarly, in an Australian telephone survey conducted in 2014, just 10% of women who reported having had a mammogram said they were told about the risk of overdiagnosis.[75]

Questions of how information about overdiagnosis in breast screening could be communicated to women, and how such information may affect decisions about whether to undergo screening, have been identified in the screening and shared decision making literature as important targets for empirical investigation. The first research to address these questions in depth was an Australian qualitative study involving a series of focus groups held in 2011.[76] During the focus groups, the investigators explained the concept of overdiagnosis and explored women's responses to different estimates of its rate—1–10%, 30%, and 50%—reflecting the varied estimates published at that time. Participants were women in the age range eligible for mammography screening. These women had virtually no awareness of overdiagnosis in breast screening and reacted with surprise, raising many questions about the new information. Most women reached a basic understanding of overdiagnosis by the end of these sessions, and they expressed diverse attitudes towards. Participants suggested a range of ways in which their approaches to screening might be affected, from no change whatsoever to potentially declining screening altogether. Their screening intentions overall were quite sensitive to the magnitude of overdiagnosis, with higher estimates more likely to prompt careful consideration. It was interesting that a number of women interpreted the information as more pertinent to how screen-detected cancers should be managed, rather than whether to undergo screening in the first place. Overall, most participants felt that information on overdiagnosis was important and should be available to women to enable informed decision making.[76] Focus groups conducted in 2012 in England[16] echoed the findings that women were unaware of overdiagnosis but could understand the concept, recognized the information as important, and believed women should be informed about it. There was, however, a broad consensus that the risk of overdiagnosis with screening was preferable to the risk of delayed diagnosis without it.[16]

The above evidence from qualitative studies of women's understanding of overdiagnosis highlighted the urgent need to investigate whether a meaningful explanation of overdiagnosis could be condensed into a concise written format, and to evaluate its effects quantitatively. A randomized controlled trial in Australia assessed the potential consequences of informing women about overdiagnosis using a decision aid.[50] This paper-based resource presented the probabilities, cumulated over 20 years of screening, of avoiding death from breast cancer, experiencing overdiagnosis, and having a false-positive—three outcomes that are considered important to decisions about mammography screening.[3,25,27,28,35,53] Fig. 16.1 shows extracts from the decision aid illustrating how it explained the concept and risk of overdiagnosis. By comparing this with a control decision aid omitting the overdiagnosis component, the trial addressed the question of whether including the overdiagnosis content specifically improved the rate of informed choice.[50]

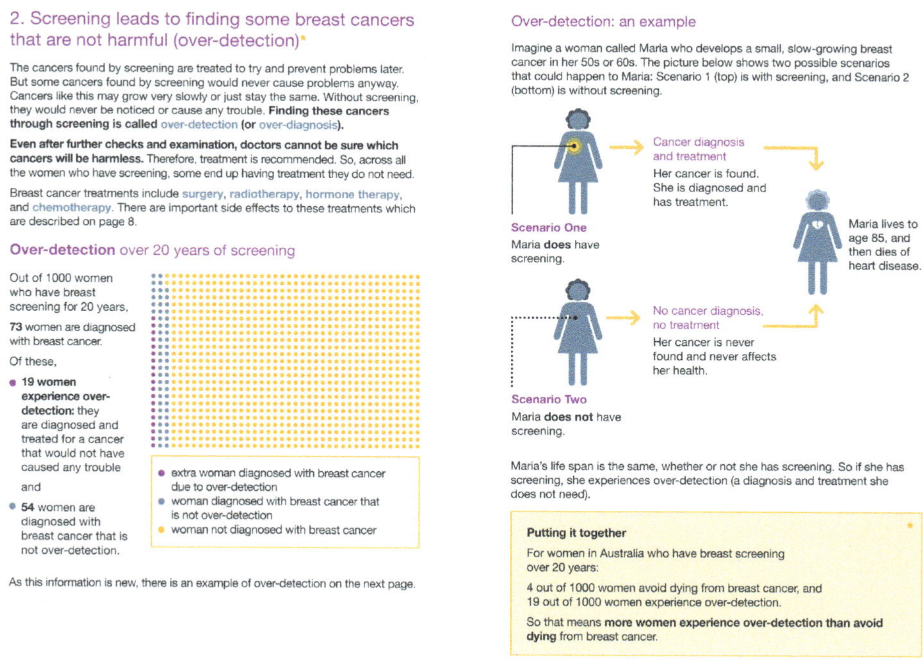

FIGURE 16.1

Extracts from a breast screening decision aid[50] illustrating how it explained the concept and risk of overdiagnosis (using the term overdetection).

The key finding from the randomized controlled trial[50] was that a decision aid which explained the risk of overdiagnosis in breast screening increased knowledge and enabled more women to make an informed choice, compared with a control decision aid which omitted the overdiagnosis information (Table 16.3). This showed that women could understand information about overdiagnosis and incorporate it into their reasoning about screening. The information did not adversely affect women by raising anxiety or decisional conflict, in fact it slightly reduced levels of worry about developing breast cancer. Another finding of interest was that being better informed about potential consequences made women feel a little less positive about undergoing breast screening, and somewhat reduced intentions to be screened in the next few years (Table 16.3). This suggests that some women, when better informed about the balance of harm and benefit, might make different decisions about whether to have breast screening[50]—a finding consistent with a 2013 UK survey[77] and a small pilot study of a mammography decision aid for US women over 75.[78]

INFORMED CHOICE IN BREAST SCREENING: MAKING IT WORK

It is important to recognize that the principles of shared decision making do not imply that individuals have to take sole responsibility for complex medical choices, without recourse to expert guidance.[79] Rather, the critical first step is helping people see that there are multiple options and that their preferences are relevant—notions which may be contrary to their expectations. Only once this understanding is established and the basic essential information outlined, should the person's informed preferences for degree of involvement and responsibility in decision making come into play.[80] These informed preferences might still include seeking and even deferring to the views of others.[79]

People's literacy and numeracy may influence how effectively they can use decision support tools, and involving vulnerable populations in medical decisions may be seen as a particular challenge for shared decision making.[80–82] For example, some people with lower education might be inclined to dismiss quantitative risk information if they lack confidence in their numeracy ability.[83] Important concerns have therefore been raised about the risk of inadvertently widening health inequalities if such approaches preferentially benefit those who already have better health associated with higher social status.[84,85] A review of patient decision aid trials to 2010 noted that health literacy had been insufficiently considered in the existing literature, but highlighted some encouraging results suggesting that efforts to better address the needs of lower literacy users can be effective.[81] Another review of the literature to 2012 indicated that shared decision making interventions (including decision aids) have been shown to significantly improve various key outcomes for people from disadvantaged groups (eg, low education or literacy).[82]

Additional research is necessary to ensure that decision support is genuinely accessible across all sectors of the community so as not to contribute to social inequity.[86] This is likely to require testing alternative approaches that might involve simpler resources but possibly more assistance from care providers.[83] There may, however, be unavoidable trade-offs between the completeness of the information presented—in particular the quantitative data—and the degree to which it will be understood by people with limited numeracy.[51] On the other hand, well-presented risk information may be valuable even when not fully understood—it can be a powerful tool for communicating vital basic messages: that multiple options exist, these involve considerable trade-offs, and there are no guarantees either way.[87]

Ultimately, people will vary in their desire, and perhaps ability, to engage with evidence and make an individual decision when it comes to screening.[71] In a sense, information can be thought of like a

Table 16.3 Analysis of Informed Choice and Components for Intervention and Control Groups in a Randomized Trial[50]

	Intervention Group $n = 419$		Control Group $n = 419$		Difference (95% CI)		p value
Knowledge (Conceptual & Numeric Combined)							
Breast cancer mortality benefit	272	(65%)	256	(61%)	3.8	(−2.7 to 10.4)	0.25
False-positives	244	(58%)	278	(66%)	−8.1	(−14.7 to −1.6)	0.02
Overdetection	230	(55%)	112	(27%)	28.2	(21.8 to 34.5)	<0.001
Adequate knowledge across all 3 subscales	122	(29%)	71	(17%)	12.2	(6.5 to 17.8)	<0.001
Attitudes Toward Having Breast Screening[a]							
Mean (SD) total attitudes score	24.5	(4.4)	26.1	(4.1)	−1.5	(−2.1 to −0.9)	<0.001
Positive attitudes to screening (scores ≥ 24)	282	(69%)	340	(83%)	−14.4	(−20.1 to −8.6)	<0.001
Most positive (scores 29–30)	100	(24%)	156	(38%)	−13.8		
Scores 24–28	182	(44%)	184	(45%)	−0.6		
Scores 18–23	93	(23%)	55	(13%)	9.3		
Least positive (scores 6–17)	34	(8%)	13	(3%)	5·1		
Intentions About Having Breast Screening							
Intending to be screened (definitely *or* likely)	308	(74%)	363	(87%)	−13.1	(−18.5 to −7.8)	<0.001
Definitely will	197	(47%)	268	(64%)	−16.9		
Likely to	111	(26%)	95	(23%)	3.8		
Unsure	69	(16%)	30	(7%)	9.3		
Not likely to *or* definitely will not	42	(10%)	26	(6%)	3.8		
Informed Choice[b]							
Made an informed choice	99	(24%)	63	(15%)	8.8	(3.3 to 14.2)	0.002

Data are number of participants (%) unless otherwise stated.

[a]*Six attitude items were each rated strongly disagree 1 to strongly agree 5. Total scores could range from 6 to 30: higher scores indicate more positive attitudes. Data were missing for 21 women.*

[b]*Informed choice was defined as adequate knowledge and intentions consistent with attitudes (positive or negative). Participants with missing data for attitudes were excluded from the analysis of informed choice.*

drug—it must be given in the right dose.[88] Responding to these varied information needs and preferences poses a challenge for information providers. In the future, methods for delivery of information may need to become more flexible and incorporate tailoring according to personal characteristics.[72] Furthermore, most of the formative work in the shared decision making field has taken place in the western world. The field has not extensively engaged with the diversity of cultural beliefs and value systems which may be relevant.[89,90] Future research could test the effectiveness of "cultural targeting and tailoring" as next steps toward improving informed decision making in multicultural societies.[90]

There is clearly a potential contradiction—real or perceived—between government-endorsed screening programs traditionally focused on maximizing uptake, and future communication methods that encourage informed choice and might thereby reduce participation. It is likely that in practice many women will view the receipt of an offer of screening as an implicit indication that health authorities consider participation worthwhile.[91] Continuing to monitor this aspect of how people process new information will be important as the communication landscape evolves. Further research is also needed to determine how screening programs could be evaluated on the basis of their success in providing informed choice to the public. Conducting informed choice studies that are embedded within screening programs would help to progress the field toward achieving this important goal.

COMMUNICATION IN CONTEXT

Crucially, evidence-based information such as that presented in a decision aid is just one of many factors that shape health choices.[83,87] Decisions are influenced by preferences and emotions as well as, if not more than, provision of information derived from scientific evidence.[91,92] People's sense of their own risk is often more about feelings than facts, which might limit the impact of new factual information.[93] Feelings can also influence people's ability to understand and reason about numeric facts and figures.[94] Although many medical decisions involve considerable uncertainty and complex trade-offs, mammography screening could be singled out as an exemplar of the tension between the powerful role of emotions and the objective assessment of harm and benefit.[95] This tension contributes fundamentally to the challenge of successfully communicating to women the potential harms of breast screening. If the problem of overdiagnosis does not resonate emotionally, this risk may continue to be effectively "invisible" despite improved education efforts.[95]

One of the influential factors likely to feed into decision making about screening is the source and setting of information provision. This can shape how women interpret new information they receive. For example, effects of information observed in a research study might be attenuated by skepticism about the motives and trustworthiness of academic scientists. In comparison, government-supported screening services might be perceived as more credible information sources. Clinicians may also be more respected sources of advice, possibly seen as more in touch with the individual's personal reality.

If future invitations encourage women to be involved in a more careful decision making process, clinicians might be called on to help women understand the evidence and guide them in clarifying their informed preferences. This highlights the need for clinicians to be better informed themselves about overdiagnosis. Currently it seems many clinicians have limited understanding of overdiagnosis[96] and perform suboptimally in terms of explaining screening downsides to patients.[74,97] Primary care doctors may not yet have the capacity and training to contribute usefully to shared decision making about screening, and messages conveyed by doctors now may be inconsistent with recently developed screening information.[72] An important goal of future research should therefore be to better understand clinicians' perspectives and develop ways to support them to communicate more effectively with patients about overdiagnosis and other challenging topics. This may involve producing communication tools and resources to better equip clinicians for such discussions.

Working toward better and more nuanced understanding of harms and benefits of screening among journalists and policy makers is also important, to improve the quality of public discourse on the topic.[91] Women's knowledge, attitudes, and expectations are partly a function of their cultural context and the prevailing positive messages about screening. Contextual factors shape the underlying schema or conceptual framework through which people interpret and engage with new information. The fact that women are accustomed to receiving only positive information on screening might lead them to perceive more balanced materials as against screening.[50,64] As long as women continue to expect breast screening information to strongly endorse participation, finding ways to give balanced information that is perceived as such will remain a challenge.

CONCLUSION

The traditional approach to informing women about mammography screening, aimed at promoting uptake by emphasizing benefits and downplaying harms, was once considered quite appropriate. But the growing realization that benefit and harm may be finely balanced—and particularly evidence that screening leads to overdiagnosis and overtreatment—has led to a profound questioning of the ethics of offering breast screening without providing adequate information on benefit and harm. Arguments have been made for why women should be able to make their own informed decisions about whether to undergo breast screening, and why they need high-quality and accessible information on screening outcomes, including overdiagnosis. Evidence is now starting to emerge regarding women's perspectives on this complex and unfamiliar issue—how it could be effectively communicated to them, and whether becoming informed about overdiagnosis will matter to their views and decisions about screening.

Research has shown that, notwithstanding some challenges, it is possible for rigorously developed and piloted information resources to help women become better informed about breast screening, including its benefit and its potentially harmful consequences. Of critical importance is the finding that women vary in the degree to which they view their new knowledge about overdiagnosis as necessitating a shift in their (largely positive) screening attitudes and intentions. Speculative assumptions and assertions that women would not care at all about overdiagnosis thus are incorrect. Likewise, concerns that women might suddenly decide en masse to abandon screening altogether do not seem to have been borne out. Instead, based on the evidence to date,[50] it appears that the majority of women who have been informed about overdiagnosis would still prefer to be screened, after evaluating balanced information and incorporating it into their decisions. If patients or people are really to be at the heart of the healthcare system, then engaging and supporting individuals to construct and enact their own informed preferences in making decisions about their health is vital.[36,45] The diversity of breast screening preferences when women are better informed suggests that this is indeed a preference-sensitive decision, which underscores the need for individual choice to be available.[2]

If cancer screening programs are to be judged, in future, by their achievement of informed choice rather than by their participation rates,[2,23,98] the challenge remains to determine how to implement such a change in practice. Researchers in the US have advocated for discussions about screening trade-offs to be measured in healthcare systems to help monitor preference-based screening, in a move toward more useful and meaningful metrics than crude participation rates.[25,92] Yet breast screening services in many other countries are set up to interact with women directly, without the need for any clinician contact. Many challenges are entailed, and considerable resources required, in seeking to provide adequate information to each individual being offered screening in such programs and ensuring equity of access to the information.[2] Nonetheless, a new approach has already been introduced in the UK, based on the "consider an offer" concept, aiming to offer and support informed choice about breast screening. The authorities involved have argued that their new approach is justified on ethical grounds, while calling for its effects on women's decision quality to be evaluated.[72] These types of changes to cancer screening programs are now being considered around the world.

GLOSSARY

Citizens jury a deliberative democracy method which brings together a diverse group of citizens to deliberate on a particular issue. Jurors are exposed to balanced factual information about the issue, discuss among themselves, and then produce a decision or recommendations.

Decision aid a tool to support people in making a treatment or screening decision when there is more than one reasonable option, with benefits and harms that people may value differently. Decision aids give information to help people consider the options from their own perspective.

Decision support a more generic term for any method that attempts to support individuals facing decisions. The intervention may be a service, a system, or items such as decision aids, used either in dialog with an agent (eg, a health care professional) or independently of such dialogs.

Health literacy the capacity to obtain, process, and understand basic health information and services needed to make appropriate health decisions.

Icon array a type of visual graphic display used for presenting numerical information, for example in decision aids. An icon array represents the numerator and denominator together via differently colored filled circles arranged in a matrix, thus depicting the part-whole relationship.

Informed choice a decision (eg, whether to have screening) based on: (1) adequate relevant knowledge and (2) agreement between the person's values and their behavior or intentions.

Informed decision making a situation where the decision maker understands the advantages and disadvantages of the options and where their decision reflects their informed preference.

Numeracy how competent people are with basic probability and mathematical concepts.

Overdetection detection of a hidden illness through screening that would otherwise never cause any symptoms or health problems in the person's life.

Overdiagnosis diagnosis of a person with a medical condition that would otherwise never cause symptoms or death. This can occur through screening asymptomatic populations, increasingly sensitive tests, incidental findings, widened disease definitions, or medicalization of normal life.

Overtreatment treatment occurring as a consequence of overdiagnosis.

Preference-sensitive (a decision) likely to be influenced by individual preferences and values.

Reference class the relevant denominator pertaining to a specific number (eg, in a decision aid).

Shared decision making an approach to clinical consultations in which clinician and patient participate jointly in making health decisions. The process involves discussing the options and their benefits and harms, and considering the patient's values, preferences and circumstances.

REFERENCES

1. Barratt A, Trevena L, Davey HM, McCaffery K. Use of decision aids to support informed choices about screening. *Br Med J* 2004;**329**:507–10.
2. Irwig L, Glasziou P. Informed consent for screening by community sampling. *Eff Clin Pract* 2000;**3**:47–50.

3. Kinsinger LS, Harris R. Breast cancer screening discussions for women in their forties. *Breast Dis* 2001;**13**:21–31.
4. Thornton H. Pairing accountability with responsibility: the consequences of screening 'promotion'. *Med Sci Monit* 2001;**7**:531–3.
5. Rimer BK, Briss PA, Zeller PK, Chan ECY, Woolf SH. Informed decision making: what is its role in cancer screening? *Cancer* 2004;**101**:1214–28.
6. Osterlie W, Solbjor M, Skolbekken JA, Hofvind S, Saetnan AR, Forsmo S. Challenges of informed choice in organised screening. *J Med Ethics* 2008;**34**:e5.
7. Schwartz LM, Woloshin S, Fowler Jr. FJ, Welch HG. Enthusiasm for cancer screening in the United States. *J Am Med Assoc* 2004;**291**:71–8.
8. Waller J, Osborne K, Wardle J. Enthusiasm for cancer screening in Great Britain: a general population survey. *Br J Cancer* 2015;**112**:562–6.
9. Hoffmann TC, Del Mar C. Patients' expectations of the benefits and harms of treatments, screening, and tests: a systematic review. *JAMA Intern Med* 2015;**175**:274–86.
10. Denberg TD, Wong S, Beattie A. Women's misconceptions about cancer screening: implications for informed decision-making. *Patient Educ Couns* 2005;**57**:280–5.
11. Schonberg MA, Ramanan RA, McCarthy EP, Marcantonio ER. Decision making and counseling around mammography screening for women aged 80 or older. *J Gen Intern Med* 2006;**21**:979–85.
12. Griffiths F, Bendelow G, Green E, Palmer J. Screening for breast cancer: medicalization, visualization and the embodied experience. *Health* 2010;**14**:653–68.
13. Solbjor M, Skolbekken JA, Osterlie W, Forsmo S. Women's experiences with mammography screening through 6 years of participation – a longitudinal qualitative study. *Health Care Women Int* 2015;**36**:558–77.
14. Silverman E, Woloshin S, Schwartz LM, Byram SJ, Welch HG, Fischhoff B. Women's views on breast cancer risk and screening mammography: a qualitative interview study. *Med Decis Making* 2001;**21**:231–40.
15. Davey C, White V, Gattellari M, Ward JE. Reconciling population benefits and women's individual autonomy in mammographic screening: in-depth interviews to explore women's views about 'informed choice'. *Aust NZ J Public Health* 2005;**29**:69–77.
16. Waller J, Douglas E, Whitaker KL, Wardle J. Women's responses to information about overdiagnosis in the UK breast cancer screening programme: a qualitative study. *BMJ Open* 2013;**3**:e002703.
17. Allen JD, Bluethmann SM, Sheets M, Opdyke KM, Gates-Ferris K, Hurlbert M, et al. Women's responses to changes in U.S. Preventive Task Force's mammography screening guidelines: results of focus groups with ethnically diverse women. *BMC Public Health* 2013;**13**:1169.
18. Greco KE, Nail LM, Kendall J, Cartwright J, Messecar DC. Mammography decision making in older women with a breast cancer family history. *J Nurs Scholarsh* 2010;**42**:348–56.
19. Lagerlund M, Widmark C, Lambe M, Tishelman C. Rationales for attending or not attending mammography screening – a focus group study among women in Sweden. *Eur J Cancer Prev* 2001;**10**:429–42.
20. Miller AB. Conundrums in screening for cancer. *Int J Cancer* 2010;**126**:1039–46.
21. Welch HG, Schwartz LM, Woloshin S. *Over-diagnosed: making people sick in the pursuit of health*. Boston, MA: Beacon Press; 2011.
22. Barratt A, Irwig L, Glasziou P, Cumming RG, Raffle A, Hicks N, et al. Users' guides to the medical literature: XVII. How to use guidelines and recommendations about screening. *J Am Med Assoc* 1999;**281**:2029–34.
23. Welch HG. Screening mammography – a long run for a short slide? *N Engl J Med* 2010;**363**:1276–8.
24. Woloshin S, Schwartz LM, Black WC, Kramer BS. Cancer screening campaigns – getting past uninformative persuasion. *N Engl J Med* 2012;**367**:1677–9.
25. Stefanek ME. Uninformed compliance or informed choice? A needed shift in our approach to cancer screening. *J Natl Cancer Inst* 2011;**103**:1821–6.
26. Rychetnik L, Carter SM, Abelson J, Thornton H, Barratt A, Entwistle VA, et al. Enhancing citizen engagement in cancer screening through deliberative democracy. *J Natl Cancer Inst* 2013;**105**:380–6.

27. Zapka JG, Geller BM, Bulliard J-L, Fracheboud J, Sancho-Garnier H, Ballard-Barbash R, et al. Print information to inform decisions about mammography screening participation in 16 countries with population-based programs. *Patient Educ Couns* 2006;**63**:126–37.
28. Jorgensen KJ, Gotzsche PC. Content of invitations for publicly funded screening mammography. *Br Med J* 2006;**332**:538–41.
29. Gummersbach E, Piccoliori G, Zerbe CO, Altiner A, Othman C, Rose C, et al. Are women getting relevant information about mammography screening for an informed consent: a critical appraisal of information brochures used for screening invitation in Germany, Italy, Spain and France. *Eur J Public Health* 2010;**20**:409–14.
30. Wilson AJ, Robertson J, Ewald BD, Henry D. What the public learns about screening and diagnostic tests through the media. *Med J Aust* 2012;**197**:324–6.
31. Chen JY, Eborall H, Armstrong N. Stakeholders' positions in the breast screening debate, and media coverage of the debate: a qualitative study. *Critical Public Health* 2014;**24**:62–72.
32. Chamot E, Charvet AI, Perneger TV. Variability in women's desire for information about mammography screening: implications for informed consent. *Eur J Cancer Prev* 2005;**14**:413–8.
33. Gotzsche PC, Jorgensen KJ. Screening for breast cancer with mammography. *Cochrane Database Syst Rev* 2013;**6** CD001877.
34. Independent UK Panel on Breast Cancer Screening. The benefits and harms of breast cancer screening: an independent review. *Lancet* 2012;**380**:1778–86.
35. Welch HG, Passow HJ. Quantifying the benefits and harms of screening mammography. *JAMA Intern Med* 2014;**174**:448–54.
36. Barry MJ, Edgman-Levitan S. Shared decision making – pinnacle of patient-centered care. *N Engl J Med* 2012;**366**:780–1.
37. Heath I. It is not wrong to say no. *Br Med J* 2009;**338** b2529.
38. Kirwan CC. Breast cancer screening: what does the future hold? *Br Med J* 2013;**346**:f87.
39. Skrabanek P. Mass mammography. The time for reappraisal. *Int J Technol Assess Health Care* 1989;**5**:423–30.
40. Hoffmann TC, Legare F, Simmons MB, McNamara K, McCaffery K, Trevena LJ, et al. Shared decision making: what do clinicians need to know and why should they bother? *Med J Aust* 2014;**201**:35–9.
41. 111th United States Congress. Patient protection and affordable care act. *Public Law* 2010:111–48.
42. Australian Commission on Safety and Quality in Health Care. *Australian safety and quality framework for health care*; 2010.
43. General Medical Council. *Consent: patients and doctors making decisions together*. London; 2008.
44. UK Department of Health. *Equity and excellence: liberating the NHS*. London; 2010.
45. Stiggelbout AM, Van der Weijden T, De Wit MP, Frosch D, Legare F, Montiori VM, et al. Shared decision making: really putting patients at the centre of healthcare. *Br Med J* 2012;**344**:e256.
46. Biesecker BB, Schwartz MD, Marteau TM. Enhancing informed choice to undergo health screening: a systematic review. *Am J Health Behav* 2013;**37**:351–9.
47. Elwyn G, O'Connor A, Stacey D, Volk R, Edwards A, Coulter A, et al. Developing a quality criteria framework for patient decision aids: online international Delphi consensus process. *Br Med J* 2006;**333**:417.
48. Sepucha KR, Borkhoff CM, Lally J, Levin CA, Matlock DD, Ng CJ, et al. Establishing the effectiveness of patient decision aids: key constructs and measurement instruments. *BMC Med Inform Decis Mak* 2013;**13**:S12.
49. Marteau TM, Dormandy E, Michie S. A measure of informed choice. *Health Expect* 2001;**4**:99–108.
50. Hersch J, Barratt A, Jansen J, Irwig L, McGeechan K, Jacklyn G, et al. Use of a decision aid including information on overdetection to support informed choice about breast cancer screening: a randomised controlled trial. *Lancet* 2015;**385**:1642–52.
51. Schwartz PH. Questioning the quantitative imperative: decision aids, prevention, and the ethics of disclosure. *Hastings Cent Rep* 2011;**41**:30–9.
52. Barry MJ. Too much information? *Hastings Cent Rep* 2012;**42**:4.
53. Pace LE, Keating NL. A systematic assessment of benefits and risks to guide breast cancer screening decisions. *J Am Med Assoc* 2014;**311**:1327–35.

54. Joseph-Williams N, Newcombe R, Politi M, Durand MA, Sivell S, Stacey D, et al. Toward minimum standards for certifying patient decision aids: a modified Delphi consensus process. *Med Decis Making* 2014;**34**:699–710.
55. Stacey D, Legare F, Col NF, Eden KB, Holmes-Rovner M, Llewellyn-Thomas H, et al. Decision aids for people facing health treatment or screening decisions. *Cochrane Database Syst Rev* 2014;**1** CD001431.
56. Elwyn G, Frosch D, Volandes AE, Edwards A, Montori VM. Investing in deliberation: a definition and classification of decision support interventions for people facing difficult health decisions. *Med Decis Making* 2010;**30**:701–11.
57. Fagerlin A, Pignone M, Abhyankar P, Col N, Feldman-Stewart D, Gavaruzzi T, et al. Clarifying values: an updated review. *BMC Med Inf Decis Mak* 2013;**13**:S8.
58. Garvelink MM, ter Kuile MM, Stiggelbout AM, de Vries M. Values clarification in a decision aid about fertility preservation: does it add to information provision? *BMC Med Inf Decis Mak* 2014;**14**:68.
59. Trevena LJ, Zikmund-Fisher BJ, Edwards A, Gaissmaier W, Galesic M, Han PK, et al. Presenting quantitative information about decision outcomes: a risk communication primer for patient decision aid developers. *BMC Med Inform Decis Mak* 2013;**13**:S7.
60. Zipkin DA, Umscheid CA, Keating NL, Allen E, Aung K, Beyth R, et al. Evidence-based risk communication: a systematic review. *Ann Intern Med* 2014;**161**:270–80.
61. Tait AR, Voepel-Lewis T, Zikmund-Fisher BJ, Fagerlin A. Presenting research risks and benefits to parents: does format matter? *Anesth Analg* 2010;**111**:718–23.
62. van Agt HM, Korfage IJ, Essink-Bot ML. Interventions to enhance informed choices among invitees of screening programmes – a systematic review. *Eur J Public Health* 2014;**24**:789–801.
63. Mathieu E, Barratt A, Davey HM, McGeechan K, Howard K, Houssami N. Informed choice in mammography screening: a randomized trial of a decision aid for 70-year-old women. *Arch Intern Med* 2007;**167**:2039–46.
64. Mathieu E, Barratt AL, McGeechan K, Davey HM, Howard K, Houssami N. Helping women make choices about mammography screening: an online randomized trial of a decision aid for 40-year-old women. *Patient Educ Couns* 2010;**81**:63–72.
65. Suss R. The problem with choice: what my mechanic taught me about PSA screening. *Can Fam Physician* 2008;**54**:1287–8.
66. Smith SK, Trevena L, Simpson JM, Barratt A, Nutbeam D, McCaffery KJ. A decision aid to support informed choices about bowel cancer screening among adults with low education: randomised controlled trial. *Br Med J* 2010;**341**:c5370.
67. van Tol-Geerdink JJ, Stalmeier PF, van Lin EN, Schimmel EC, Huizenga H, van Daal WA, et al. Do prostate cancer patients want to choose their own radiation treatment? *Int J Radiat Oncol Biol Phys* 2006;**66**:1105–11.
68. Smith G, Wales C. The theory and practice of citizens' juries. *Policy Politics* 1999;**27**:295–308.
69. Paul C, Nicholls R, Priest P, McGee R. Making policy decisions about population screening for breast cancer: the role of citizens' deliberation. *Health Policy* 2008;**85**:314–20.
70. Rychetnik L, Doust J, Thomas R, Gardiner R, Mackenzie G, Glasziou P. A Community Jury on PSA screening: what do well-informed men want the government to do about prostate cancer screening–a qualitative analysis. *BMJ Open* 2014;**4**:e004682.
71. Entwistle VA, Carter SM, Trevena L, Flitcroft K, Irwig L, McCaffery K, et al. Communicating about screening. *Br Med J* 2008;**337**:a1591.
72. Forbes LJ, Ramirez AJ, Expert group on Information about Breast Screening. Offering informed choice about breast screening. *J Med Screen* 2014;**21**:194–200.
73. Schwartz LM, Woloshin S, Sox HC, Fischhoff B, Welch HG. US women's attitudes to false-positive mammography results and detection of ductal carcinoma in situ: cross sectional survey. *Br Med J* 2000;**320**:1635–40.
74. Wegwarth O, Gigerenzer G. Overdiagnosis and overtreatment: evaluation of what physicians tell their patients about screening harms. *JAMA Intern Med* 2013;**173**:2086–7.
75. Moynihan R, Nickel B, Hersch J, Beller E, Doust J, Compton S, et al. Public opinions about overdiagnosis: a national community survey. *PLoS One* 2015;**10**:e0125165.

76. Hersch J, Jansen J, Barratt A, Irwig L, Houssami N, Howard K, et al. Women's views on overdiagnosis in breast cancer screening: a qualitative study. *Br Med J* 2013;**346**:f158.
77. Waller J, Whitaker KL, Winstanley K, Power E, Wardle J. A survey study of women's responses to information about overdiagnosis in breast cancer screening in Britain. *Br J Cancer* 2014;**111**:1831–5.
78. Schonberg MA, Hamel MB, Davis RB, Griggs MC, Wee CC, Fagerlin A, et al. Development and evaluation of a decision aid on mammography screening for women 75 years and older. *JAMA Intern Med* 2014;**174**:417–24.
79. Politi MC, Dizon DS, Frosch DL, Kuzemchak MD, Stiggelbout AM. Importance of clarifying patients' desired role in shared decision making to match their level of engagement with their preferences. *Br Med J* 2013;**347**:f7066.
80. Barry MJ. Shared decision making: informing and involving patients to do the right thing in health care. *J Ambulatory Care Manage* 2012;**35**:90–8.
81. McCaffery KJ, Holmes-Rovner M, Smith SK, Rovner D, Nutbeam D, Clayman ML, et al. Addressing health literacy in patient decision aids. *BMC Med Inf Decis Mak* 2013;**13**:S10.
82. Durand MA, Carpenter L, Dolan H, Bravo P, Mann M, Bunn F, et al. Do interventions designed to support shared decision-making reduce health inequalities? A systematic review and meta-analysis. *PLoS One* 2014;**9**:e94670.
83. Smith SK, Kearney P, Trevena L, Barratt A, Nutbeam D, McCaffery KJ. Informed choice in bowel cancer screening: a qualitative study to explore how adults with lower education use decision aids. *Health Expect* 2014;**17**:511–22.
84. Coulter A, Ellins J. Effectiveness of strategies for informing, educating, and involving patients. *Br Med J* 2007;**335**:24–7.
85. Thomson R, Murtagh M, Khaw FM. Tensions in public health policy: patient engagement, evidence-based public health and health inequalities. *Qual Saf Health Care* 2005;**14**:398–400.
86. Irwig L, McCaffery K, Salkeld G, Bossuyt P. Informed choice for screening: implications for evaluation. *Br Med J* 2006;**332**:1148–50.
87. Gruman J. Too much information? *Hastings Cent Rep* 2012;**42**:4–5.
88. Epstein RM, Peters E. Beyond information: exploring patients' preferences. *J Am Med Assoc* 2009;**302**:195–7.
89. Mullen PD, Allen JD, Glanz K, Fernandez ME, Bowen DJ, Pruitt SL, et al. Measures used in studies of informed decision making about cancer screening: a systematic review. *Ann Behav Med* 2006;**32**:188–201.
90. Alden DL, Friend J, Schapira M, Stiggelbout A. Cultural targeting and tailoring of shared decision making technology: a theoretical framework for improving the effectiveness of patient decision aids in culturally diverse groups. *Soc Sci Med* 2014;**105**:1–8.
91. Johansson M, Brodersen J. Informed choice in screening needs more than information. *Lancet* 2015;**385**:1597–9.
92. Onega T, Beaber EF, Sprague BL, Barlow WE, Haas JS, Tosteson AN, et al. Breast cancer screening in an era of personalized regimens: a conceptual model and National Cancer Institute initiative for risk-based and preference-based approaches at a population level. *Cancer* 2014;**120**:2955–64.
93. Rosenbaum L. "Misfearing" – culture, identity, and our perceptions of health risks. *N Engl J Med* 2014;**370**:595–7.
94. Nelson W. Too much information? *Hastings Cent Rep* 2012;**42**:5–6.
95. Rosenbaum L. Invisible risks, emotional choices – mammography and medical decision making. *N Engl J Med* 2014;**371**:1549–52.
96. Wegwarth O, Schwartz LM, Woloshin S, Gaissmaier W, Gigerenzer G. Do physicians understand cancer screening statistics? A national survey of primary care physicians in the United States. *Ann Intern Med* 2012;**156**:340–9.
97. Hoffman RM, Elmore JG, Fairfield KM, Gerstein BS, Levin CA, Pignone MP. Lack of shared decision making in cancer screening discussions: results from a national survey. *Am J Prev Med* 2014;**47**:251–9.
98. Canadian Partnership Against Cancer. *Quality determinants of breast cancer screening with mammography in Canada*. Toronto: Canadian Partnership Against Cancer; 2013.

Index

Note: Page numbers followed by "*f*" and "*t*" refer to figures and tables, respectively.

P

Q

R